Critical decisions
in emergency

Volume 37 Number 1 January 2023

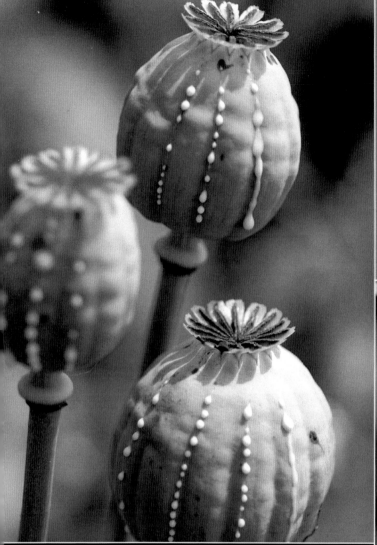

Safety First

Opioids have been used and prescribed in emergency departments for decades to treat a variety of ailments, but there are misconceptions about and nuances to their use. Emergency physicians must have a thorough understanding of dosing, formulation, alternatives, and side effects to improve pain relief and patient safety.

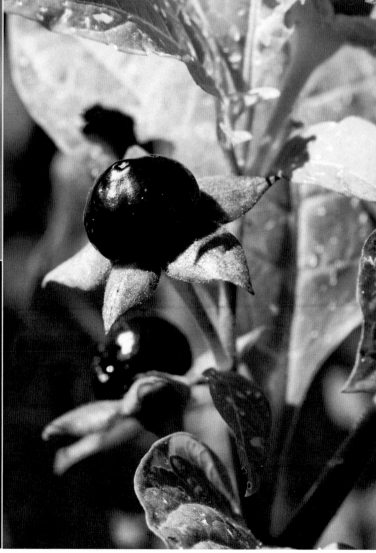

Poison Control

Ingestion of toxic substances and unintentional overdoses cause a variety of signs and symptoms and can be life-threatening, even when symptoms are slow to appear. Emergency physicians must be aware of the many presentations of toxic substance ingestions in children to accurately diagnose and manage these conditions.

THE OFFICIAL CME PUBLICATION OF THE AMERICAN COLLEGE OF EMERGENCY PHYSICIANS

Individuals in Control of Content

1. Matthew Augusta – Faculty
2. Jeremy Berberian, MD – Faculty
3. William J. Brady, MD, FACEP – Faculty
4. Lindsey Chaudoin, MD – Faculty
5. Jonathan Glauser, MD, MBA, FACEP – Faculty
6. Dominic Nicacio, MD – Faculty
7. Aria C. Shi, MD – Faculty
8. Joseph Tagliaferro III, DO, FACEP – Faculty
9. Micaela Simon, FNP-C, AAHIVS – Faculty
10. Malcolm Velasco, MD – Faculty
11. Tareq Al-Salamah, MBBS, MPH, FACEP – Faculty/Planner
12. Joshua S. Broder, MD, FACEP – Faculty/Planner
13. Andrew J. Eyre, MD, MS-HPEd – Faculty/Planner
14. John Kiel, DO, MPH, FACEP, CAQSM – Faculty/Planner
15. Frank LoVecchio, DO, MPH, FACEP – Faculty/Planner
16. Sharon E. Mace, MD, FACEP – Faculty/Planner
17. Amal Mattu, MD, FACEP – Faculty/Planner
18. Christian A. Tomaszewski, MD, MS, MBA, FACEP – Faculty/Planner
19. Steven J. Warrington, MD, MEd, MS – Faculty/Planner
20. Michael S. Beeson, MD, MBA, FACEP – Planner
21. Wan-Tsu Chang, MD – Planner
22. Ann M. Dietrich, MD, FAAP, FACEP – Planner
23. Kelsey Drake, MD, MPH, FACEP – Planner
24. Walter L. Green, MD, FACEP – Planner
25. John C. Greenwood, MD – Planner
26. Danya Khoujah, MBBS, MEHP, FACEP – Planner
27. Nathaniel Mann, MD – Planner
28. George Sternbach, MD, FACEP – Planner
29. Joy Carrico, JD – Planner/Reviewer

Contributor Disclosures. In accordance with the ACCME Standards for Integrity and Independence in Accredited Continuing Education, all relevant financial relationships, and the absence of relevant financial relationships, must be disclosed to learners for all individuals in control of content 1) before learners engage with the accredited education, and 2) in a format that can be verified at the time of accreditation. The following individuals have reported relationships with ineligible companies, as defined by the ACCME. These relationships, in the context of their involvement in the CME activity, could be perceived by some as a real or apparent conflict of interest. All relevant financial relationships have been mitigated to ensure that no commercial bias has been inserted into the educational content. Joshua S. Broder, MD, FACEP, is a founder and president of OmniSono Inc, an ultrasound technology company, and a consultant on the Bayer USA Cardiac Imaging Advisory Board. Sharon E. Mace, MD, FACEP, performs contracted research funded by Biofire Corporation, Genetesis, Quidel, and IBSA Pharma. Frank LoVecchio, DO, MPH, FACEP, receives speaking fees from ABBVIE for antibiotics. All remaining individuals with control over content have no relevant financial relationships to disclose.

This educational activity consists of two lessons, eight feature articles, a post-test, and evaluation questions; as designed, the activity should take approximately 5 hours to complete. The participant should, in order, review the learning objectives for the lesson or article, read the lesson or article as published in the print or online version until all have been reviewed, and then complete the online post-test (a minimum score of 75% is required) and evaluation questions. Release date: January 1, 2023. Expiration date: December 31, 2025.

Accreditation Statement. The American College of Emergency Physicians is accredited by the Accreditation Council for Continuing Medical Education to provide continuing medical education for physicians.

The American College of Emergency Physicians designates this enduring material for a maximum of 5 *AMA PRA Category 1 Credits™.* Physicians should claim only the credit commensurate with the extent of their participation in the activity.

Each issue of *Critical Decisions in Emergency Medicine* is approved by ACEP for 5 ACEP Category I credits. Approved by the AOA for 5 Category 2-B credits.

Commercial Support. There was no commercial support for this CME activity.

Target Audience. This educational activity has been developed for emergency physicians.

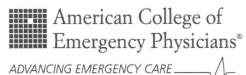

American College of Emergency Physicians®

ADVANCING EMERGENCY CARE

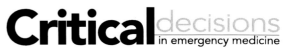

Critical decisions *in emergency medicine*

Critical Decisions in Emergency Medicine is the official CME publication of the American College of Emergency Physicians. Additional volumes are available.

EDITOR-IN-CHIEF

Michael S. Beeson, MD, MBA, FACEP
Northeastern Ohio Universities, Rootstown, OH

SECTION EDITORS

Joshua S. Broder, MD, FACEP
Duke University, Durham, NC

Andrew J. Eyre, MD, MS-HPEd
Brigham and Women's Hospital/
Harvard Medical School, Boston, MA

John Kiel, DO, MPH, FACEP, CAQSM
University of Florida College of Medicine,
Jacksonville, FL

Frank LoVecchio, DO, MPH, FACEP
Valleywise, Arizona State University, University of Arizona,
and Creighton Colleges of Medicine, Phoenix, AZ

Sharon E. Mace, MD, FACEP
Cleveland Clinic Lerner College of Medicine/
Case Western Reserve University, Cleveland, OH

Amal Mattu, MD, FACEP
University of Maryland, Baltimore, MD

Christian A. Tomaszewski, MD, MS, MBA, FACEP
University of California Health Sciences,
San Diego, CA

Steven J. Warrington, MD, MEd, MS
MercyOne Siouxland, Sioux City, IA

ASSOCIATE EDITORS

Tareq Al-Salamah, MBBS, MPH, FACEP
King Saud University, Riyadh, Saudi Arabia/
University of Maryland, Baltimore, MD

Wan-Tsu Chang, MD
University of Maryland, Baltimore, MD

Ann M. Dietrich, MD, FAAP, FACEP
University of South Carolina College of Medicine,
Greenville, SC

Kelsey Drake, MD, MPH, FACEP
St. Anthony Hospital, Lakewood, CO

Walter L. Green, MD, FACEP
UT Southwestern Medical Center, Dallas, TX

John C. Greenwood, MD
University of Pennsylvania, Philadelphia, PA

Danya Khoujah, MBBS, MEHP, FACEP
University of Maryland, Baltimore, MD

Nathaniel Mann, MD
Greenville Health System, Greenville, SC

George Sternbach, MD, FACEP
Stanford University Medical Center, Stanford, CA

EDITORIAL STAFF

Suzannah Alexander, Editorial Director
salexander@acep.org

Joy Carrico, JD
Managing Editor

Alex Bass
Assistant Editor

Kyle Powell
Graphic Artist

ISSN2325-0186 (Print)   ISSN2325-8365 (Online)

Contents

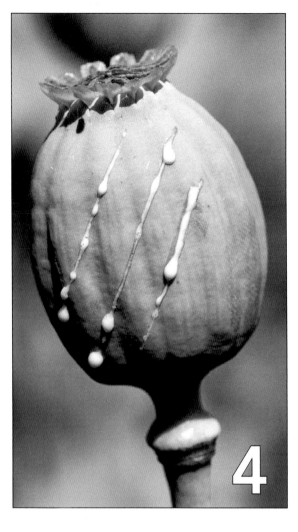

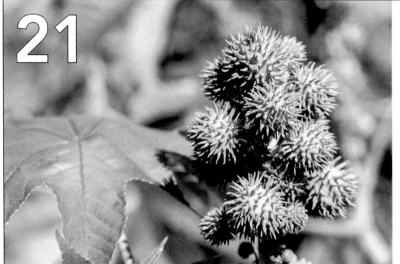

FEATURES

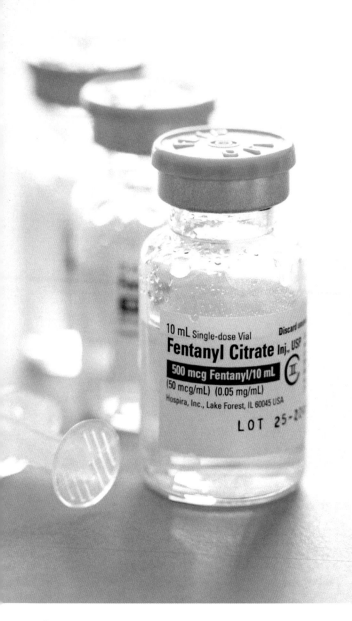

Safety First

Best Practices for Opioid Administration

LESSON 1

By Malcolm Velasco, MD; and
John Kiel, DO, MPH, FACEP, CAQSM
Dr. Velasco is an emergency medicine resident and Dr. Kiel is an assistant professor in the Department of Emergency Medicine and the Department of Orthopedics and Sports Medicine at the University of Florida College of Medicine – Jacksonville.

Reviewed by Tareq Al-Salamah, MBBS, MPH, FACEP

Objectives

On completion of this lesson, you should be able to:

1. Describe which clinical presentations require opioids in the emergency department.
2. Choose the correct opioid for the correct patient.
3. Discuss how to correctly titrate various opioids to pain.
4. Select the correct opioid to discharge a patient on.
5. Modify opioid selection and doses for patients who are older, have kidney or liver disease, or are opioid dependent.

From the EM Model

17.0 Toxicologic Disorders
    17.1 Drug and Chemical Classes
        17.1.2 Analgesics
            17.1.2.3 Opioids

▬ CRITICAL DECISIONS ▬

- Which patients should receive opioids in the emergency department?

- Which parenteral opioids are most effective?

- What is the correct opioid dose for adequate analgesia?

- Which opioids should a patient be discharged on?

- How do comorbidities and special circumstances affect which opioids are administered?

Research estimates that nearly 30% of patients addicted to opioids get their first prescription from the emergency department. Opioids have been used and prescribed in emergency departments for decades to treat a variety of ailments, but there are misconceptions about and nuances to their use. Improved understanding of dosing, formulation, alternatives, and side effects can improve pain relief and patient safety.

CASE ONE

A 35-year-old man without a significant medical history presents for abdominal pain that has persisted for the past 2 days. He appears to be in considerable distress. His vital signs are stable except for a fever of 38.9°C (102°F). He weighs 180 lbs (81.6 kg). The physical examination is significant for severe pain in the right lower quadrant. Appendicitis is suspected, and 4 mg of morphine is ordered.

CASE TWO

An 88-year-old woman with a history of stage 3 chronic kidney disease, hypertension, atrial fibrillation, and congestive heart failure presents with an obvious hip deformity after a fall. During examination, she is lying in bed in obvious discomfort. Her left hip is shortened and externally rotated. The workup includes an opioid as a first-line analgesic.

CASE THREE

A 67-year-old man with a history of nonalcoholic fatty liver disease–related cirrhosis arrives complaining of fever, shortness of breath, and chronic back pain. He has a productive cough with yellow sputum. He appears in mild distress. His vital signs are BP 150/90, P 108, R 20, and T 38.3°C (100.9°F); SpO_2 is 90% on room air. Chest x-ray reveals a lobar pneumonia, so the patient is given the appropriate antibiotics. When he learns that he needs to be admitted to the hospital, he requests medication for his chronic back pain. The physician orders 8 mg of morphine.

Introduction

In 2016, 53% of patients who presented to the emergency department received an opioid during their visit, and 35% of patients were also discharged with an opioid prescription.[1] Opioid prescriptions, however, come from a broad range of physicians — emergency physicians prescribe only a small fraction. Treating patients with opioids for an acute or chronic condition is not without consequence. Across the larger health care landscape, more than 500,000 deaths from opioid overdose have occurred since 2009.[2] Accordingly, medical systems have sought alternative options to control pain, including regional anesthesia (often termed nerve blocks), nonopioid analgesics, and other nonpharmacologic interventions. However, some patients, especially those with acute pathology or trauma, often require opioids to adequately manage their pain. With the wide variety of opioids available, some of which have lesser-known side effects and pharmacokinetics, choosing the correct opioid at the correct dose for the correct patient can be difficult.

CRITICAL DECISION

Which patients should receive opioids in the emergency department?

The American College of Emergency Physicians (ACEP) updated its stance on acute pain treatment in the emergency department in 2017. It recommends nonopioid pain medications — including analgesic ceiling doses of NSAIDs, acetaminophen, nerve blocks (regional anesthesia), subdissociative-dose ketamine, and intravenous and topical lidocaine — as alternatives to opioids.[3] In many patients with acute pain, nonopioid medications are effective. Several studies have shown that when ibuprofen is administered at its analgesic ceiling dose of 400 mg alongside acetaminophen at its analgesic ceiling dose of 1,000 mg, they are noninferior to opioids.[4,5] Nerve blocks are especially effective at controlling pain that is isolated to a specific nerve distribution, as in cases of fractures, dislocations, and dental emergencies. Lidocaine patches and other topical agents are effective for muscular pain or postherpetic neuralgia. ACEP recommends using opioids only for severe acute pain or for pain refractory to other modalities. Opioids can be prescribed as the initial analgesic for long-bone fractures or severe acute abdominal pain. Despite concerns that opioid administration in patients with acute abdominal pain could reduce the diagnostic accuracy of the physical examination, it has not been shown to do so and, thus, is a good option for patients with moderate to severe abdominal pain.[6]

ACEP also recommends that physicians encourage patients to be proactive in making decisions about their medical treatment.[3] To do so, patients should be counseled on the risks of opioids, including respiratory depression, tolerance, hyperalgesia, and opioid use disorder. Discussions with patients should also be patient centered. Studies have shown that emergency physicians often lack a patient-centered approach and dominate the conversation.[7] Physicians who take extra time to discuss the risks of various medications, treatment options, and expectations can help reduce opioid use and improve patient outcomes.

Drug	Pharmacokinetics	Side Effects
Morphine IV	Onset: 1-2 minutes Peak effect: 3-5 minutes Duration: 1-2 hours	Hypotension, nausea, and vomiting from histamine release
Fentanyl IV	Onset: <1 minute Peak effect: 2-5 minutes Duration: 30-60 minutes	Chest wall rigidity with high doses
Hydromorphone IV	Onset: 5-15 minutes Peak effect: 10-20 minutes Duration: 2-4 hours	Euphoria
Morphine PO	Onset: 30 minutes Peak effect: 1 hour Duration: 3-5 hours	Hypotension, nausea, and vomiting from histamine release
Hydrocodone/ acetaminophen PO	Onset: 30-60 minutes Duration: 4-6 hours	Nausea, increased risk of acetaminophen overdose when combined with OTC acetaminophen
Oxycodone PO	Onset: 10-15 minutes Duration: 3-6 hours	Nausea, increased risk of acetaminophen overdose when combined with OTC acetaminophen
Codeine PO	Onset: 30-60 minutes Duration: 4-6 hours	GI side effects, increased risk of acetaminophen overdose when combined with OTC acetaminophen
Tramadol PO	Onset: 1 hour Duration: 4-6 hours	CNS side effects

TABLE 1. Opioid pharmacokinetics and side effects[8]

CRITICAL DECISION

Which parenteral opioids are most effective?

The three primary parenteral opioids available in the emergency department are morphine, fentanyl, and hydromorphone. Each medication has its benefits and drawbacks. The primary considerations when choosing an opioid are time of onset, time to peak effect, duration of action, and side effects (*Table 1*).

Morphine

Morphine is one of the most frequently used parenteral opioids. When given intravenously, its onset is within 1 to 2 minutes, its time to peak is around 3 to 5 minutes, and its duration is between 1 to 2 hours. Morphine's primary side effects, induced by histamine release, are hypotension, nausea, and vomiting.[8] About 10% of patients who receive morphine experience these symptoms. An alternative to morphine should be used in patients who present with nausea and vomiting because morphine can worsen these existing symptoms.

Fentanyl

Fentanyl is known for being significantly more potent than morphine. It is frequently chosen for trauma patients because of its nearly immediate time to onset — less than 1 minute. Its effect peaks between 2 to 5 minutes. However, fentanyl does have a shorter duration of action, between 30 and 60 minutes, and, therefore, must be dosed more frequently. Fentanyl also depresses the cardiovascular system less than morphine but, at high doses, is associated with chest wall rigidity.[8]

Hydromorphone

Hydromorphone also has a short onset of action (5-15 minutes) and peak effect time (10-20 minutes) but has a longer duration of action than morphine and fentanyl, at 2 to 4 hours. Hydromorphone is often chosen for pain that is refractory to other opioids.[9] However, hydromorphone is associated with more euphoria than other opioids, making it more likely to be requested by patients and making it the most valuable opioid on the black market.[8]

Common misconceptions surround opioids. One of the most common is that hydromorphone is a substantially better analgesic than morphine. A metanalysis by Felden et al found that hydromorphone has only a slight analgesic difference from morphine, and Chang et al found no difference between the drugs when used in older adults.[10,11] The analgesic difference between morphine and fentanyl has also been called into question. In a study of trauma patients, no analgesic differences between morphine and fentanyl were found.[12] In all likelihood, the difference in pain relief experienced by patients receiving different intravenous opioids has more to do with the dosage than the choice of opioid (*Table 2*).

In summary, fentanyl is the most appropriate intravenous opioid for acute traumatic injuries. Between hydromorphone and morphine, morphine is the better choice because it has the same analgesic effect as hydromorphone without its euphoric effects, which increase the potential for abuse (*Figure 1*). Morphine, however, should be avoided in patients with active nausea and vomiting; antiemetics can be given alongside morphine in other patients to reduce the likelihood of these symptoms.

CRITICAL DECISION

What is the correct opioid dose for adequate analgesia?

Many factors must be considered when selecting the correct opioid dose for a patient. Health conditions such as kidney and liver disease and age-related changes in drug metabolism affect dosing. Also, many patients who chronically take opioids do not achieve adequate analgesia from standard dosing. Standard dosing suggestions discussed are based on nongeriatric patients in moderate to severe pain who do not normally take opioids.

Morphine

The most cited morphine dose in textbooks is 0.1 mg/kg, but for most patients, this dose does not significantly relieve pain.[13] There is no one optimal morphine dose for adequate pain relief, so titration to effect is important. An initial dose of 0.1 mg/kg of morphine followed by 0.05-mg/kg boluses every 30 minutes may be a better approach for titrating morphine to pain relief.[14]

Fentanyl

Surprisingly few studies have evaluated the effectiveness of different doses of fentanyl at managing pain in the emergency department. Miner et al found that 1.5 μg/kg is an effective dose in children.[15] Reasonably, 0.5 to 1 μg/kg of fentanyl can be used to titrate to effect.

Hydromorphone

The optimal starting dose for hydromorphone is also controversial. Patients given a 0.0075-mg/kg dose often do not have adequate pain control, and 2-mg doses are associated with hypoxia.[11,16] A better alternative is a 1-mg bolus followed by smaller doses titrated to pain relief.

CRITICAL DECISION

Which opioids should a patient be discharged on?

When discharging patients on opioids, physicians must consider and discuss the risks of opioid dependence and abuse. Physicians must also remember that oral opioids are valuable when sold

Drug	Equipotent IV Dose	Equipotent PO Dose	Oral Morphine Milligram Equivalent Conversion Factor
Morphine IV	10 mg	60 mg (acute) and 30 mg (chronic)	1
Fentanyl IV	100 μg	200 μg (transmucosal)	2.4 (transdermal in μg/hr)
Hydromorphone IV	1.5 mg	7.5 mg	4
Hydrocodone	N/A	30 mg	1
Oxycodone	N/A	20 mg	1.5
Codeine	120 mg	200 mg	0.15
Tramadol	N/A	300 mg	0.1

TABLE 2. Opioid equivalency table[8]

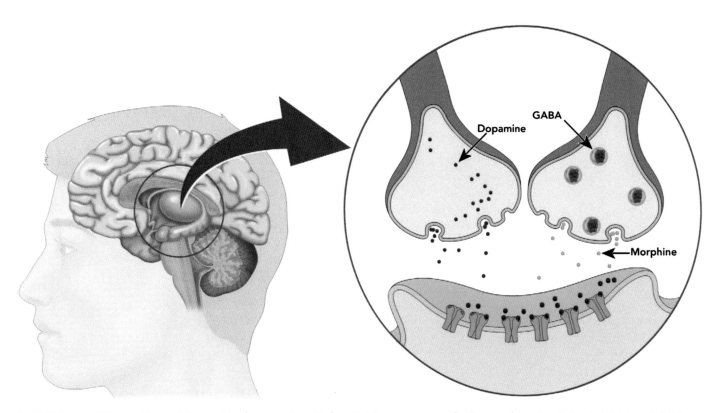

FIGURE 1. Effect of opioids. Aside from pain relief, opioids can create feelings of euphoria by inhibiting GABA, which in turn increases dopamine activity. *Credit:* ACEP.

illegally and that some patients may intend to sell them. In one small study, 29% of patients who later became addicted to opioids got their first prescription from the emergency department.[17]

The primary oral opioids commonly available and prescribed in US pharmacies are hydrocodone, oxycodone, and morphine sulfate. In the United States, hydrocodone is available only in combination with acetaminophen. Combination formulations are designed to include other analgesics to reduce the dosage of opioids. In the emergency department, prescriptions for opioids should be written as immediate-release formulations only, and patients should be counseled on any additional medications in combination formulations to avoid unintentional overdose. Patients should generally be started on the lowest effective dose for their pain, usually 5 mg for hydrocodone, 5 mg for oxycodone, and 7.5 mg for morphine.

Contrary to commonly held beliefs among emergency physicians, oxycodone, hydrocodone, and morphine all appear to have the same analgesic effect.[18-20] Oxycodone is one of the most addictive and, behind hydromorphone, most valuable opioids on the black market; it is more likely than the other oral opioids to potentiate euphoria, which can be accounted for by its higher lipophilicity and ability to cross the blood-brain barrier.[19,21] Morphine, by contrast, appears to have weaker reinforcing effects and less potential for abuse.[21] Perhaps this is why morphine has less demand than oxycodone and hydrocodone when sold illegally.[22] Morphine may also have a lower incidence of inducing nausea and vomiting than previously believed.[23] Overall, morphine sulfate, in its immediate-release preparation, may be the best opioid to prescribe in the emergency department for a short course of pain relief.

Codeine and tramadol have more recently fallen out of favor in emergency departments. Codeine is heavily dependent on metabolism, a highly variable factor, for its analgesic effect. A significant percentage of the population cannot metabolize codeine at all and, therefore, receive no analgesia from it. Codeine also has failed to prove any more

effective at analgesia than acetaminophen combined with ibuprofen.[24] Similar to codeine, tramadol is dependent on metabolism for its analgesic effects. Tramadol inhibits the reuptake of norepinephrine and serotonin to cause central analgesia that is associated with significant side effects, including dizziness, nausea, constipation, and headache.[8] In patients on other serotonergic medications who take tramadol, serotonin syndrome is another concern. Tramadol can also lower the threshold for seizures and has been linked to a higher 1-year mortality compared to NSAIDs when used to treat osteoarthritis.[25] Neither codeine nor tramadol is recommended for use in the emergency department or at discharge.

CRITICAL DECISION

How do comorbidities and special circumstances affect which opioids are administered?

Liver Disease

The liver is the primary site where opioids are metabolized. In patients with liver disease, opioids and other sedatives commonly

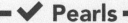

Pearls

- Opioids should only be used after other forms of analgesia have failed or when acute pain is severe, like in cases of traumatic injuries.

- Opioids should be titrated to effect. For instance, morphine is most effective when used at a 0.1-mg/kg initial dose and titrated by 0.05-mg/kg doses until pain relief is achieved.

- Fentanyl is the best opioid choice for patients with liver and kidney failure.

induce hepatic encephalopathy. More specifically, opioid metabolism primarily occurs through the various CYP450 enzymes and glucuronidation, both of which are affected by liver disease — although glucuronidation is generally thought to be affected less.[26] Dosing and drug selection are a priority primarily in patients with cirrhosis. Morphine has significantly increased bioavailability and decreased clearance in these patients, so it should generally be avoided.[27] Fentanyl may be a better option because its pharmacokinetics do not appear to be significantly altered in patients with cirrhosis.[27] Oral opioids such as hydrocodone and oxycodone that undergo first-pass metabolism may also be more bioavailable. Some sources recommend reducing these opioids' doses by 50% and increasing dosing frequency in patients with liver disease.[28]

Kidney Disease

The kidneys play an equally important role in opioid metabolism. In theory, opioid doses could be adjusted based on a patient's glomerular filtration rate (GFR), but in the emergency department, an accurate GFR is rarely known on initial evaluation. Factors other than GFR such as pH also influence how a drug is filtered by the kidneys. Morphine has three main metabolites that are excreted by the kidneys. In patients with renal failure, the accumulation of one of these metabolites, morphine-6-glucuronide, can cause respiratory depression.[29] Like in patients with liver failure, fentanyl is generally safer than morphine in patients with renal failure because it is metabolized into inactive agents by the liver. However, in patients with severe uremia, a dose reduction in fentanyl should be considered because some incidences of respiratory depression have been reported in these patients.[30] Like parenteral opioids, oral opioids are also cleared by the kidneys. For this reason, Pham et al recommend hydrocodone at a 50% dose reduction for patients with stage 4 or 5 chronic kidney disease.[31]

Older Patients

Acute pain in the geriatric population is a common problem in the emergency department. Pain is a complaint for 25% to 50% of older persons living in the community and up to 70% of those living in nursing homes.[32] Opioid pharmacokinetics can be altered with normal senescence: GI transit time is increased, adipose tissue is increased, and total body water is decreased.[32] These factors combined with polypharmacy and multiple comorbidities make choosing and dosing opioids difficult. Other analgesics like NSAIDs often carry a higher risk of side effects if used chronically in geriatric patients, which can leave opioids as one of the few options for pain control. In older patients, opioids should be started at 25% to 50% of the normal dose. The doses can then be titrated up by 50% to 100% for adequate analgesia. Opioids like tramadol that have psychoactive components should be avoided entirely in older patients.

Opioid-Dependent Patients

Managing acute pain in opioid-dependent patients can be especially difficult. Physiologic adaptations occur on multiple levels, including changes in opioid receptors, cellular messaging, neurologic networks, and synaptic plasticity.[33] If opioid-dependent patients present with new acute pain, their home opioid dose (when known) can be resumed, and their new pain can be treated with a multimodal approach that may include new, short-acting opioids. In patients who use opioids recreationally, the baseline opioid

requirements are more difficult to estimate. As these patients' acute pain resolves, short-acting opioids used in treatment can be titrated down. In patients who use opioids chronically, an opioid converter should be used to estimate daily morphine equivalent doses for appropriate dosing. These conversions greatly reduce the likelihood of underdosing patients and increase the likelihood of adequately addressing pain.

Occasionally in an episode of acute pain, patients tolerate some opioids better than the opioid they take at home. An opioid equivalency table gives estimates of equivalent doses between different opioids (see *Table 2*). The new opioid is usually started at roughly two-thirds the dose of the previous opioid because the degree of cross-tolerance between two opioids is relatively unpredictable.[33]

Opioid-induced hyperalgesia is another common problem in the emergency department. Although the underlying mechanism is incompletely understood, the NMDA receptor is believed to be involved. For this reason, subdissociative-dose ketamine may be a good option for patients with this type of hyperalgesia. Previous studies have shown that ketamine decreases total morphine equivalents in patients experiencing postoperative hyperalgesia.[34]

Summary

Although the use of opioids in the emergency department has been well established for many years, physicians should use them only when other forms of analgesia have failed or when the patient is in severe, acute pain. Titration is the most effective way to dose opioids while minimizing risks of oversedation and respiratory depression. Morphine, fentanyl, and hydromorphone all appear to have the same analgesic effect at equipotent doses. Oxycodone, hydrocodone, and immediate-release morphine are also similarly effective, but morphine is the best choice at discharge because it is less addictive and, therefore, less likely to be abused. For patients with liver or kidney failure who need opioids for pain, fentanyl is the best choice.

REFERENCES

1. Rui P, Schappert SM. Opioids prescribed at discharge or given during emergency department visits among adults in the United States, 2016. Centers for Disease Control and Prevention. Reviewed May 31, 2019. https://www.cdc.gov/nchs/products/databriefs/db338.htm

2. Wide-ranging online data for epidemiologic research (WONDER). Centers for Disease Control and Prevention. Reviewed December 12, 2022. http://wonder.cdc.gov

3. American College of Emergency Physicians. *Optimizing the treatment of acute pain in the emergency department*; April 2017. https://www.acep.org/globalassets/new-pdfs/policy-statements/optimizing-the-treatment-of-acute-pain-in-the-ed.pdf

4. Chang AK, Bijur PE, Esses D, Barnaby DP, Baer J. Effect of a single dose of oral opioid and nonopioid analgesics on acute extremity pain in the emergency department: a randomized clinical trial. *JAMA*. 2017;318(17):1661-1667.

5. Bijur PE, Friedman BW, Irizarry E, Chang AK, Gallagher EJ. A randomized trial comparing the efficacy of five oral analgesics for treatment of acute musculoskeletal extremity pain in the emergency department. *Ann Emerg Med*. 2021 Mar;77(3):345-356.

6. Thomas SH, Silen W, Cheema F, et al. Effects of morphine analgesia on diagnostic accuracy in emergency department patients with abdominal pain: a prospective, randomized trial. *J Am Coll Surg*. 2003 Jan;196(1):18-31.

7. McCarthy DM, Engel KG, Cameron KA. Conversations about analgesics in the emergency department: a qualitative study. *Patient Educ Couns*. 2016 Jul;99(7):1130-1137.

■ **CASE ONE**

The emergency department became busy. When the physician returned, the patient was writhing in pain. The patient complained that the 4-mg dose of morphine did little to improve his severe pain. The physician administered another 4-mg dose of morphine. Thirty minutes elapsed, and the patient was still in significant pain.

The workup confirmed appendicitis, so surgery was consulted. While awaiting surgery, the patient's morphine doses were titrated in 4-mg increments, and pain control was finally achieved.

■ **CASE TWO**

A short while later, the patient became unresponsive and required bag-valve-mask ventilation. A quick assessment revealed agonal respirations and pinpoint pupils. The patient received 0.4 mg of naloxone, and her mental status quickly improved. To more safely manage her pain while awaiting surgery, she was given a nerve block.

■ **CASE THREE**

A few hours later, the patient became somnolent and confused. The inpatient workup showed increased ammonia levels. The appropriate treatment for hepatic encephalopathy was administered in addition to pneumonia treatment. Fortunately, the patient's mental status never declined to the point of his needing intubation. He was discharged home 1 week later.

8. Ducharme J. Acute pain management. In: Tintinalli JE, Ma OJ, Yealy DM, et al, eds. *Tintinalli's Emergency Medicine: A Comprehensive Study Guide.* 9th ed. McGraw-Hill Education; 2020:229-236.

9. Quigley C, Wiffen P. A systematic review of hydromorphone in acute and chronic pain. *J Pain Symptom Manage.* 2003 Feb;25(2):169-178.

10. Felden L, Walter C, Harder S, et al. Comparative clinical effects of hydromorphone and morphine: a meta-analysis. *Br J Anaesth.* 2011 Sep;107(3):319-328.

11. Chang AK, Bijur PE, Baccelieri A, Gallagher EJ. Efficacy and safety profile of a single dose of hydromorphone compared with morphine in older adults with acute, severe pain: a prospective, randomized, double-blind clinical trial. *Am J Geriatr Pharmacother.* 2009 Feb;7(1):1-10.

12. Häske D, Böttiger BW, Bouillon B, et al. Analgesia in patients with trauma in emergency medicine. *Dtsch Arztebl Int.* 2017 Nov 17;114(46):785-792.

13. Bijur PE, Kenny MK, Gallagher EJ. Intravenous morphine at 0.1 mg/kg is not effective for controlling severe acute pain in the majority of patients. *Ann Emerg Med.* 2005 Oct;46(4):362-367.

14. Lvovschi V, Aubrun F, Bonnet P, et al. Intravenous morphine titration to treat severe pain in the ED. *Am J Emerg Med.* 2008 Jul;26(6):676-682.

15. Miner JR, Kletti C, Herold M, Hubbard D, Biros MH. Randomized clinical trial of nebulized fentanyl citrate versus i.v. fentanyl citrate in children presenting to the emergency department with acute pain. *Acad Emerg Med.* 2007 Oct;14(10):895-898.

16. Chang AK, Bijur PE, Napolitano A, Lupow J, Gallagher EJ. Two milligrams i.v. hydromorphone is efficacious for treating pain but is associated with oxygen desaturation. *J Opioid Manag.* 2009 Mar-Apr;5(2):75-80.

17. Butler MM, Ancona RM, Beauchamp GA, et al. Emergency department prescription opioids as an initial exposure preceding addiction. *Ann Emerg Med.* 2016 Aug;68(2):202-208.

18. Chang AK, Bijur PE, Holden L, Gallagher EJ. Comparative analgesic efficacy of oxycodone/acetaminophen versus hydrocodone/acetaminophen for short-term pain management in adults following ED discharge. *Acad Emerg Med.* 2015 Nov;22(11):1254-1260.

19. Fassassi C, Dove D, Davis A, et al. Analgesic efficacy of morphine sulfate immediate release vs. oxycodone/acetaminophen for acute pain in the emergency department. *Am J Emerg Med.* 2021 Aug;46:579-584.

20. Marco CA, Plewa MC, Buderer N, Black C, Roberts A. Comparison of oxycodone and hydrocodone for the treatment of acute pain associated with fractures: a double-blind, randomized, controlled trial. *Acad Emerg Med.* 2005 Apr;12(4):282-288.

21. Wightman R, Perrone J, Portelli I, Nelson L. Likeability and abuse liability of commonly prescribed opioids. *J Med Toxicol.* 2012 Dec;8(4):335-340.

22. Surratt H, Kurtz S, Cicero T, Dart R, Baker G, Vorsanger G. Street prices of prescription opioids diverted to the illicit market: data from a national surveillance program. *J Pain.* 2013 Apr 1;14(4):S40.

23. Fassassi C, Dove D, Davis A, et al. Analgesic efficacy of morphine sulfate immediate release vs. oxycodone/acetaminophen for acute pain in the emergency department. *Am J Emerg Med.* 2021 Aug;46:579-584.

24. Graudins A, Meek R, Parkinson J, Egerton-Warburton D, Meyer A. A randomised controlled trial of paracetamol and ibuprofen with or without codeine or oxycodone as initial analgesia for adults with moderate pain from limb injury. *Emerg Med Australas.* 2016 Dec;28(6):666-672.

25. Zeng C, Dubreuil M, Larochelle MR, et al. Association of tramadol with all-cause mortality among patients with osteoarthritis. *JAMA.* 2019 Mar 12;321(10):969-982.

26. Verbeeck RK. Pharmacokinetics and dosage adjustment in patients with hepatic dysfunction. *Eur J Clin Pharmacol.* 2008 Dec;64(12):1147-1161.

27. Tegeder I, Lötsch J, Geisslinger G. Pharmacokinetics of opioids in liver disease. *Clin Pharmacokinet.* 1999 Jul;37(1):17-40.

28. Soleimanpour H, Safari S, Shahsavari Nia K, Sanaie S, Moayed Alavian S. Opioid drugs in patients with liver disease: a systematic review. *Hepat Mon.* 2016 Apr;16(4):e32636.

29. Bodd E, Jacobsen D, Lund E, Ripel Å, Mørland J, Wiik-Larsen E. Morphine-6-glucuronide might mediate the prolonged opioid effect of morphine in acute renal failure. *Hum Exp Toxicol.* 1990 Sep;9(5):317-321.

30. Dean M. Opioids in renal failure and dialysis patients. *J Pain Symptom Manage.* 2004 Nov;28(5):497-504.

31. Pham PC, Khaing K, Sievers TM, et al. 2017 update on pain management in patients with chronic kidney disease. *Clin Kidney J.* 2017 Oct;10(5):688-697.

32. Chau DL, Walker V, Pai L, Cho LM. Opiates and elderly: use and side effects. *Clin Interv Aging.* 2008;3(2):273-278.

33. Mehta V, Langford R. Acute pain management in opioid dependent patients. *Rev Pain.* 2009 Oct;3(2):10-14.

34. Culp C, Kim HK, Abdi S. Ketamine use for cancer and chronic pain management. *Front Pharmacol.* 2021 Feb 2;11:599721.

✖ Pitfalls

- Failing to treat acute pain with nonopioid analgesics like NSAIDs before administering opioids.
- Prescribing opioids to treat chronic pain conditions.
- Neglecting to reassess patients for adequate analgesia shortly after an initial opioid dose.
- Forgetting to treat patients with liver or kidney failure at lower doses of opioids.

The Critical ECG

Regular Narrow-Complex Tachycardia

By Jeremy Berberian, MD; William J. Brady, MD, FACEP; and
Amal Mattu, MD, FACEP

Dr. Berberian is the associate director of emergency medicine residency
education at ChristianaCare and assistant professor of emergency medicine
at Sidney Kimmel Medical College, Thomas Jefferson University in
Philadelphia, Pennsylvania. Dr. Brady is a professor of emergency medicine,
medicine, and nursing, and vice chair for faculty affairs in the Department
of Emergency Medicine at the University of Virginia School of Medicine
in Charlottesville. Dr. Mattu is a professor, vice chair, and codirector of
the Emergency Cardiology Fellowship in the Department of Emergency
Medicine at the University of Maryland School of Medicine in Baltimore.

Objectives

On completion of this article, you should be able to:

- List a differential diagnosis for a regular NCT.

- State the potential causes of supraventricular tachycardias with rates greater than 220 to 240 bpm.

- Formulate a differential diagnosis for the ECG pattern of STE in lead aVR with diffuse STD.

CASE PRESENTATION

A 39-year-old man with no past medical history presents with 3 days of palpitations and two episodes of syncope in the past 8 hours.

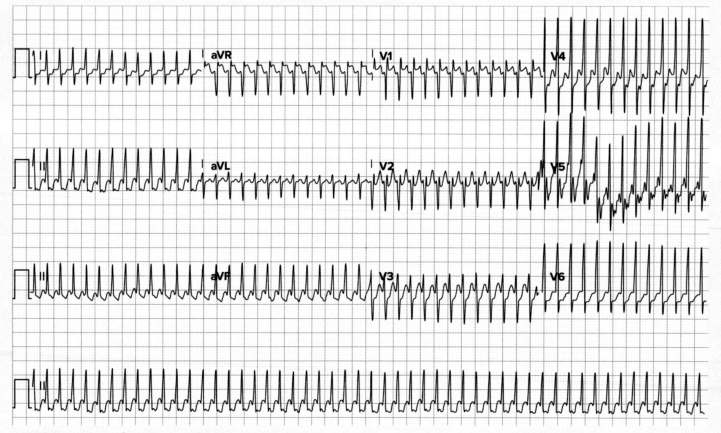

FIGURE 1. **ECG of a 39-year-old man.** *Credit:* EMRA.

Discussion

The patient's ECG shows a regular narrow-complex tachycardia (NCT) with a ventricular rate of 309 bpm, normal axis, ST-segment elevation (STE) in leads aVR and V_1, and ST-segment depression (STD) in leads I, II, III, aVF, and V_2 through V_6 (*Figure 1*).

The differential diagnosis for a regular NCT includes:

- Atrial flutter;

- Atrial tachycardia;

- Atrioventricular (AV) nodal re-entrant tachycardia (AVNRT);

- AV re-entry tachycardia (AVRT) (ie, Wolff-Parkinson-White syndrome) with orthodromic conduction;

- Junctional tachycardia;

- Narrow-complex ventricular tachycardia (VT); and

- Sinus tachycardia.

The absence of P waves on ECG rules out atrial tachycardia and sinus tachycardia. The heart rate is too fast for junctional tachycardia. The QRS complex duration is approximately 80 ms, so narrow-complex VT is unlikely. Without more history, it is impossible to tell whether the patient has AVNRT, orthodromic

AVRT (ie, retrograde conduction via the accessory pathway), or atrial flutter with 1:1 conduction.

The most impressive finding in this ECG is the ventricular rate of 309 bpm. NCT with ventricular rates this high are rarely seen in adults, even less so in patients who are walking and talking. The AV node's intrinsic refractory period prevents ventricular rates from exceeding 220 to 240 bpm in the absence of any extrinsic factors that increase conduction velocity. In such cases, successful termination of the tachydysrhythmia is often temporary, at best, until the underlying cause is identified and treated.

The differential diagnosis for causes of supraventricular tachycardias with rates greater than 220 to 240 bpm includes:

- Catecholamine surge;
- Sympathomimetic toxicity; and
- Hyperthyroidism or thyroid storm.

The differential diagnosis for the pattern of STE in lead aVR +/− lead V_1 with diffuse STD includes both acute coronary syndrome (ACS) and non-ACS etiologies.

ACS causes[1]:

- Left main coronary artery (LMCA) insufficiency (STE aVR > V_1 can be seen);
- Proximal left anterior descending artery (LAD) insufficiency (STE V_1 > aVR can be seen);
- Triple vessel disease;
- Global cardiac ischemia; and
- Prinzmetal angina.

Non-ACS causes[2]:

- Acute or severe anemia;
- Aortic dissection;
- Left bundle branch block and ventricular-paced rhythms;
- Left ventricular hypertrophy with strain pattern;
- Pulmonary embolism;
- Return of spontaneous circulation after epinephrine or defibrillation;
- Severe hypokalemia or hyperkalemia;
- Sodium channel blockade; and
- Supraventricular tachycardia (especially with rapid rates).

ACKNOWLEDGMENT

This case is reprinted from *Emergency ECGs: Case-Based Review and Interpretations*, available at www.emra.org/amazon or by scanning the QR code.

Although the pattern of STE in lead aVR +/− lead V_1 with diffuse STD is discussed in the cardiology literature, its clinical significance is somewhat controversial, likely because of the broad differential diagnosis associated with this pattern that includes both ACS and non-ACS causes. The 2018 Fourth Universal Definition of Myocardial Infarction states "ST-segment depression ≥1 mm in six or more leads, which may be associated with ST-segment elevation in leads aVR and/or V_1 and hemodynamic compromise, is suggestive of multivessel disease or left main disease" but does not provide specific management recommendations. Treatment should be guided by the underlying etiology, and both ACS and non-ACS causes should be considered. For patients suspected of having an ACS cause, this ECG pattern is highly suggestive of LMCA insufficiency, proximal LAD insufficiency, or triple vessel disease. Although this pattern does not meet traditional ST-elevation myocardial infarction criteria, it can represent high-risk ACS, including acute coronary occlusion, in the correct clinical context, and immediate angiography should be considered. Whether angiography is done by emergent cardiology consultation or activation of the cardiac catheterization lab depends on local practice preferences.

In the 39-year-old patient's ECG, the pattern of STE in leads aVR and V_1 with diffuse STD is likely due to the abnormal conduction associated with the supraventricular tachycardia. The ECG changes alone do not constitute a "failed stress test," and the decision to evaluate for ischemia as a cause, or consequence, of the tachydysrhythmia should be a clinical one.

REFERENCES

1. Thygesen K, Alpert JS, Jaffe AS, et al; Executive Group on behalf of the Joint European Society of Cardiology (ESC)/American College of Cardiology (ACC)/American Heart Association (AHA)/World Heart Federation (WHF) Task Force for the Universal Definition of Myocardial Infarction. Fourth universal definition of myocardial infarction (2018). *Circulation*. 2018 Nov 13;138(20):e618-e651.

2. Mattu A. ECG Weekly. https://ecgweekly.com

CASE RESOLUTION

The patient's emergency department workup was consistent with thyroid storm. He was chemically cardioverted with adenosine, after which he briefly went into sinus tachycardia before going into atrial fibrillation with a rapid ventricular rate at approximately 140 bpm. Atrial fibrillation is commonly seen with thyroid storm and often refractory to rate control or cardioversion until elevated thyroid hormones are treated.

This patient was treated with methimazole (propylthiouracil carries an FDA black box warning for risk of acute liver failure and should be reserved for patients who are in the first trimester of pregnancy or who are unable to tolerate any other treatment), potassium iodide, and steroids and was admitted to the ICU.

Treatment with a beta-blocker, specifically propranolol, was avoided due to concern for tachycardia-induced cardiomyopathy (TIC). The patient had been having palpitations for 3 days, and TIC is one of the severe complications of any untreated tachydysrhythmia. TIC is a dilated cardiomyopathy induced by a persistent tachydysrhythmia. It is often reversible, and after cessation of the tachydysrhythmia, ventricular function typically returns to normal. In this case, the patient's ejection fraction was severely reduced on bedside echocardiogram, so the tachycardic ventricular rates associated with the atrial fibrillation were likely necessary to maintain adequate cardiac output (note cardiac output = heart rate × stroke volume, or CO = HR × SV).

Anaphylaxis Caused by an Aspirated Foreign Body

By Dominic Nicacio, MD; and Lindsey Chaudoin, MD
Carolinas Medical Center in Charlotte, North Carolina

Reviewed by Sharon E. Mace, MD, FACEP

Objective

On completion of this article, you should be able to:

■ Recognize examination findings of foreign body aspiration.

CASE PRESENTATION

A 14-month-old boy presents via EMS for an allergic reaction. EMS reports that they were called to the child's home when his mother found him coughing, gagging, and having difficulty breathing after eating cashews. The patient had stridor, flushed skin, hives, and vomiting. His initial blood pressure was 63/46 mm Hg; SpO$_2$ was 80% on room air. He was given intramuscular epinephrine and diphenhydramine as well as an albuterol nebulizer. Afterward, his blood pressure improved to 106/76 mm Hg; SpO$_2$ was 99% on blow-by oxygen therapy.

On arrival, the patient is alert and has flushed, erythematous skin but normal vital signs on room air. He has no facial or intraoral edema but some nasal flaring. His lungs sound clear, but there is a faint biphasic noise that does not localize to the left or right lung and, thus, is concerning for stridor. No wheezing is heard.

The patient is given an additional dose of intramuscular epinephrine as well as intravenous steroids and famotidine due to ongoing respiratory symptoms and flushed skin that raise concern for persistent anaphylaxis. His flushed skin resolves, but the biphasic noise persists. To distinguish between the diagnoses of anaphylaxis-mediated upper airway obstruction and foreign body aspiration, the patient is sent to radiology for lateral decubitus x-rays and a posteroanterior chest x-ray. X-rays suggest air trapping in the right lung that is concerning for foreign body aspiration (*Figures 1, 2,* and *3*).

Surgery is consulted to discuss the findings and implications with the patient's parents; bronchoscopy is recommended. The mother is strongly against letting the child undergo the bronchoscopy, believing the noise is more likely from croup than a foreign body because the boy was sick recently and she thinks he coughed out all of the nut. After extensive conversations with the physicians, the mother and father agree to let the child undergo a CT scan to further evaluate for a foreign body. The CT shows a filling defect in the right main stem bronchus, consistent with an aspirated foreign body (*Figure 4*).

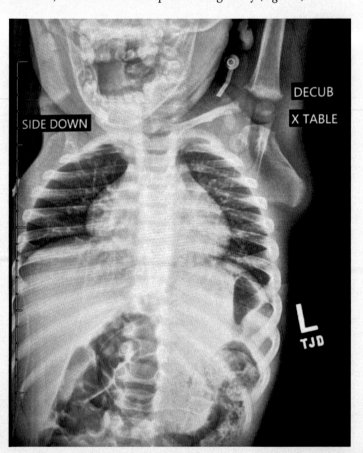

FIGURE 1. An upright posteroanterior chest x-ray showing subtle hyperinflation of the right lung. *Credit:* Dr. Dominic Nicacio and Dr. Lindsey Chaudoin.

FIGURE 2. A right lateral decubitus chest x-ray showing evidence of air trapping with little to no collapse of the right lung. *Credit:* Dr. Dominic Nicacio and Dr. Lindsey Chaudoin.

Discussion

This complicated case is an example of simultaneous foreign body aspiration into the lower airways and anaphylaxis. EMS promptly recognized the patient's anaphylaxis and gave lifesaving treatment. Even though the anaphylaxis appeared to be adequately addressed in the emergency department, the child continued to breathe abnormally in a way suggestive of persistent stridor. The differential diagnosis included an allergic reaction, wheezing induced by foreign body aspiration, and upper airway edema secondary to croup. Because the patient coughed after eating cashews before his symptoms started and most of his anaphylaxis symptoms resolved with epinephrine and antihistamines, foreign body aspiration was the most likely diagnosis. In cases of anaphylaxis secondary to foreign body aspiration, recurrent anaphylaxis is an ongoing risk, as long as the foreign body remains in the airway. This risk combined with the mother's initial refusal of medical recommendations could have justified the physician in taking emergency custody to make medical decisions. Fortunately, however, emergency custody was unnecessary after extensive conversations with the child's mother and father.

A review of the literature reveals which clinical examination and imaging modalities are most helpful for accurately diagnosing foreign body aspiration. Clinical examination findings of wheezing, coughing, stridor, and decreased air entry can raise clinical suspicion, but their absence does not rule out foreign body aspiration. According to some studies, up to 70% of children with foreign body aspiration have a normal clinical examination.[1] X-rays are also not especially sensitive or specific for foreign body aspiration. In a study of 28 pediatric patients undergoing bronchoscopy for suspected foreign body aspiration, decubitus chest x-rays had a sensitivity of only 27% and a specificity of 67%.[2] Another study showed that decubitus views do not increase sensitivity but may increase the false positivity rate.[3] Thus, the use of decubitus x-rays in foreign body aspiration is somewhat controversial. This same study suggests that obtaining expiratory views in a child (when able) may increase the true positivity rate without increasing the false positivity rate, but this method's overall accuracy is low and its clinical value uncertain.[3] Importantly, many patients are more likely to have an abnormal clinical examination or x-ray finding when they present 24 hours after the aspiration event.[1,4] Compared to x-rays, CT of the chest is a more accurate imaging modality for foreign body aspiration. It is highly reliable, with sensitivities of 100% and specificities from 81% to 100% in some studies.[5]

Despite this, a child with history and examination findings suggestive of foreign body aspiration should bypass the chest CT and undergo bronchoscopy, which is diagnostic and spares the child from radiation exposure. CT of the chest should be reserved for cases in which bronchoscopy is not a first option, such as when family refuses bronchoscopy or when bronchoscopy requires transfer to another facility. In some cases, physicians should also consider bronchoscopy regardless of x-ray results: Abnormal x-rays confirm the need for bronchoscopy, but normal x-rays do not rule it out when history and examination findings are concerning for foreign body aspiration.

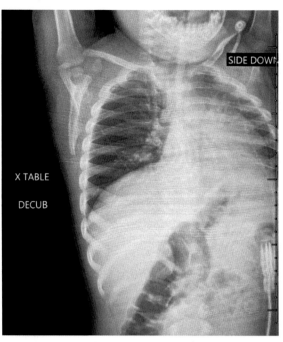

FIGURE 3. A left lateral decubitus chest x-ray showing appropriate collapse of the left lung. *Credit:* Dr. Dominic Nicacio and Dr. Lindsey Chaudoin.

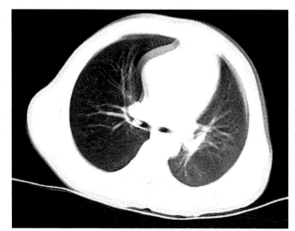

FIGURE 4. Axial cut of a noncontrasted chest CT showing a foreign body in the right main stem bronchus. *Credit:* Dr. Dominic Nicacio and Dr. Lindsey Chaudoin.

CASE RESOLUTION

After the child's CT was completed, his mother agreed to have him admitted to the hospital. The patient was observed overnight, with a bedside sitter available to alert staff of any elopement attempts by the mother. Elopement was not attempted, and the child had no episodes of recurrent anaphylaxis. Ultimately, pediatric surgery took the patient for a bronchoscopy the next morning. Rigid bronchoscopy showed an aspirated cashew, and the surgeon removed it with graspers. The patient tolerated the procedure well and was discharged home later that day with an epinephrine injection kit. He was seen for follow-up in the pediatrician's office 1 week later; he was doing well and had only a mild cough.

REFERENCES

1. Mu L, He P, Sun D. Inhalation of foreign bodies in Chinese children: a review of 400 cases. *Laryngoscope.* 1991 Jun;101(6):657-660.
2. Assefa D, Amin N, Stringel G, Dozor AJ. Use of decubitus radiographs in the diagnosis of foreign body aspiration in young children. *Pediatr Emerg Care.* 2007 Mar;23(3):154-157.
3. Brown JC, Chapman T, Klein EJ, et al. The utility of adding expiratory or decubitus chest radiographs to the radiographic evaluation of suspected pediatric airway foreign bodies. *Ann Emerg Med.* 2013 Jan;61(1):19-26.
4. Mu LC, Sun DQ, He P. Radiological diagnosis of aspirated foreign bodies in children: review of 343 cases. *J Laryngol Otol.* 1990 Oct;104(10):778-782.
5. Tseng HJ, Hanna TN, Shuaib W, Aized M, Khosa F, Linnau KF. Imaging foreign bodies: ingested, aspirated, and inserted. *Ann Emerg Med.* 2015 Dec;66(6):570-582.e5.

The Critical Procedure

Tendon Sheath Injections

By Steven J. Warrington, MD, MEd, MS
MercyOne Siouxland, Sioux City, Iowa

Objective

On completion of this article, you should be able to:
- Describe the steps for tendon sheath injections to manage tendinitis.

Introduction

Tendinitis management can be improved by using a local injection such as a corticosteroid or lidocaine as an adjunct to therapy. Importantly, however, tendon sheath injections are not intended to be the sole therapy for patients with tendinitis.

Contraindications

- Infection at the injection site (eg, overlying cellulitis)
- Bacteremia
- Significant coagulopathy
- Hypersensitivity or intolerance to medications used in the injection
- Poorly controlled diabetes
- Partial tendon rupture or significant tendon injury
- Recent or numerous injections at the same site

Benefits and Risks

The primary benefits of tendon sheath injections include pain reduction and increased tendon function. Patients' pain relief after the injections can also aid the diagnostic process. Tendon sheath injections increase the benefits gained from other treatments like physical therapy and exercise.

Risks of tendon sheath injections include those associated with any injection (eg, infection, bleeding, and pain) and side effects of the specific medications used in the injection (eg, allergic reactions, hyperglycemia, and nausea). Additional risks include intravascular or intraneural injection and damage to specific structures. The injection can cause tendon rupture along with atrophy or coloration changes to local tissue.

Alternatives

Patients with tendinitis have many treatment alternatives, including rest, physical or occupational therapy, and NSAIDs. Additionally, steroids can be administered orally and through routes other than tendon sheath injections.

TECHNIQUE

1. **Obtain** the patient's consent.
2. **Determine** the medications to be used and gather all required materials.
3. **Clean** and prepare the injection site.
4. **Consider** a superficial local injection and, if indicated, administer it first.
5. **Prepare** the medications by either mixing them into a single syringe or preparing two syringes. If using two syringes, consider if a stopcock is beneficial.
6. **Identify** landmarks and, if using an ultrasound for guidance, identify the tendon sheath target. Consider using a Z-track technique.
7. **Advance** the needle slowly. Question the patient on symptoms of paresthesias to avoid intraneural injection and aspirate when appropriate to avoid intravascular injection.
8. **Inject** the medication slowly. If pressure is met, consider withdrawing the needle somewhat or redirecting it.

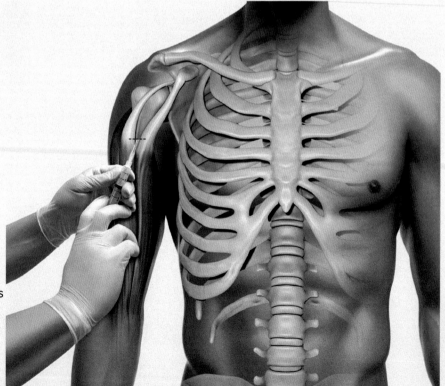

FIGURE 1. Tendon sheath injection. *Credit:* ACEP.

Reducing Side Effects

Like any injection, tendon sheath injections can be painful. To reduce the pain associated with injections, physicians can mix sodium bicarbonate with the anesthetic (eg, 9 mL anesthetic and 1 mL sodium bicarbonate). Warming the solution and injecting it slowly can each reduce the amount of pain associated with the procedure.

Side effects vary with the medications used in the solution. To reduce side effects, amide anesthetics like lidocaine can be chosen over ester anesthetics like procaine. Some medications like methylprednisolone are more commonly associated with acute synovitis when compared to others like triamcinolone; however, triamcinolone is more likely to cause facial flushing. For postprocedure pain, a long-acting anesthetic like bupivacaine can be beneficial.

Fistula formation can occur with tendon sheath injections but is less likely to occur if the Z-track method of injection is used. With the Z-track technique, physicians use an indirect path to inject the needle into the tendon. Two Z-track techniques are redirecting the needle once it is partially through the fatty layer of the tissue and creating tension on the skin prior to introducing the needle.

Special Considerations

Choosing the specific amount and mixture to be injected is somewhat arbitrary; many varied resources are available for aiding in the selection. Because most tendon sheath spaces are relatively small, a dose of 5 to 15 mg of methylprednisolone, or the equivalent of another steroid, is often suggested.

The frequency of repeat tendon sheath injections must also be taken into consideration. One suggestion is to refrain from administering injections at the same site more than once every 3 to 4 months. Another suggestion is to be wary of providing an additional injection at a site where there was little to no benefit from a prior injection. However, the tendon's location and each patient's situation must be considered when deciding whether to follow these suggestions.

A final consideration is whether to use one or multiple syringes for the injection. Mixing the anesthetic and corticosteroid together in the same syringe is common and may be beneficial because it reduces the number of movements associated with switching injections (also known as moving stopcocks). By contrast, two syringes are thought to be beneficial because they reduce the likelihood of precipitation or corticosteroid leakage near the surface of the skin.

Critical Cases in Orthopedics and Trauma

Charcot Neuroarthropathy of the Ankle

By Matthew Augusta; and John Kiel, DO, MPH, FACEP, CAQSM
University of New England College of Osteopathic Medicine, Biddeford, Maine; and the University of Florida College of Medicine – Jacksonville

Objective

On completion of this article, you should be able to:

■ Recall the presentation and management of Charcot neuroarthropathy.

CASE PRESENTATION

A 52-year-old man with a history of morbid obesity, hypertension, diabetes mellitus type 2, and osteomyelitis presents with an open right foot wound as well as edema and erythema that have worsened over the past week. He believes he may have broken his foot. He also reports nausea, vomiting, and chills. On examination, the dorsalis pedis and posterior tibial pulses are 1+, and sensation to light touch is reduced to the mid tibia. An ulceration with a granular base extends into the bone on the lateral plantar surface of his right foot. The tissue is necrotic with signs of crepitus. X-rays of the foot show near-total collapse of the ankle, talus fragmentation, and osteomyelitis of the midfoot (*Figure 1*).

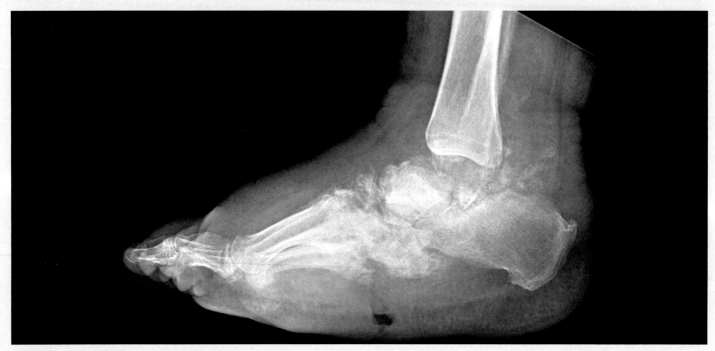

FIGURE 1. Initial lateral ankle x-ray demonstrating total collapse of the ankle with osteomyelitis of the midfoot. *Credit:* Dr. John Kiel.

Discussion

Charcot neuroarthropathy (CN) is a condition that most commonly affects the foot and ankle and increases the risk of fracture. CN occurs when insufficient vasomotor control in response to dysfunction of the autonomic nervous system leads to decreased bone strength.[1] Weight-bearing leads to repetitive fractures and subsequent deformity of the affected joint.[2] CN occurs most frequently in patients with diabetes complicated by neuropathy. One of the main complications of CN is wound ulcers. These ulcers increase the risk of osteomyelitis and, when persistent, have a 5-year mortality rate of up to 57%.[3]

Patients with CN classically present with an erythematous, warm, swollen foot and without a history of surgery or inciting trauma. Other physical examination findings include bony abnormalities, collapse of the plantar arch, and ulcerations. An elevated erythrocyte sedimentation rate is usually present. Prompt diagnosis is required to decrease the risk of joint deformity, ulceration, infection, and eventual limb loss.[4] Using the Sanders and Frykberg system, CN can be classified anatomically from class I to V based on joint involvement. Additionally, the modified Eichenholtz classification provides clinical and radiographic classification on a scale from 0 to III.[5]

X-rays should include weight-bearing lateral and anteroposterior views of both feet. Metabolic disturbances, bone deformation, debris, and joint distension are the x-ray findings most consistent with CN.[4]

The goals of management are to reduce inflammation, relieve pain, and preserve the architecture of the joint. Initial management should be nonoperative and includes total contact casting, weight off-loading, custom footwear, and patient education. Serial x-rays and observation follow, until all signs of inflammation disappear. Complications like skin ulcerations are managed with proper wound care. Patients with sepsis, acute osteomyelitis, or an ulceration in need of debridement should be admitted.[4] Alendronate and calcitonin have been shown to be beneficial medical adjuvants to recovery.[6,7] Chronic CN and CN with chronic osteomyelitis are managed with surgical debridement and internal or external fixation to restore joint alignment and stability. If simpler surgical interventions are unsuccessful, below-the-knee amputation is often necessary.[4]

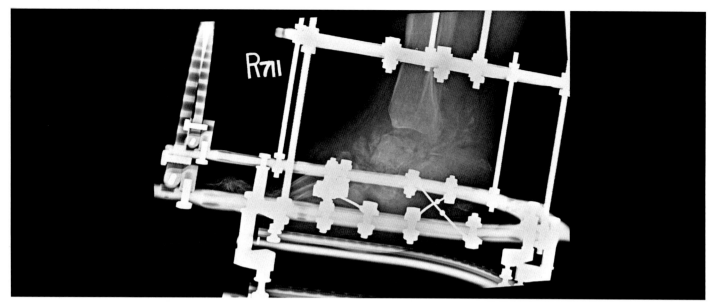

FIGURE 2. Lateral ankle x-ray following external fixation. *Credit:* Dr. John Kiel.

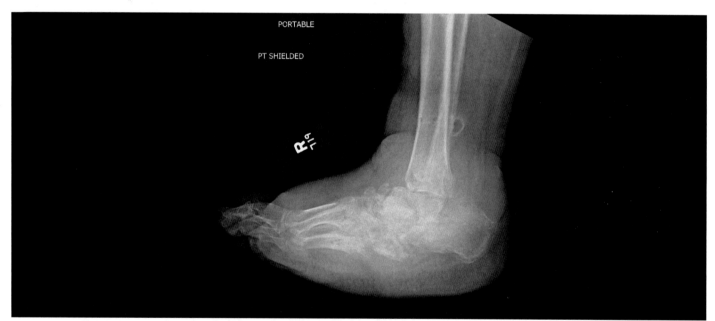

FIGURE 3. Lateral x-ray 3 months after external fixation showing no improvement. *Credit:* Dr. John Kiel.

CASE RESOLUTION

Because of the patient's chronic foot symptoms, he was treated surgically with multiplanar external fixation within days of his initial presentation (*Figure 2*). He was discharged on antibiotics and instructed to follow up with podiatry and wound care.

Although the patient's foot initially improved, he returned to the hospital 3 months later with fever, worsening pain, and advanced osteomyelitis that progressed proximally into the lateral malleolus. Repeat x-rays showed extensive midfoot debris and degenerative changes of the joint with bilateral subluxation (*Figure 3*). The patient was admitted, and a transtibial (below-the-knee) amputation was performed. At his 6-month follow-up with orthopedics, the patient was tolerating his prosthetic well and reported an improved quality of life.

REFERENCES

1. Hartemann-Heurtier A, Van GH, Grimaldi A. The Charcot foot. *Lancet.* 2002 Nov 30;360(9347):1776-1779.
2. Kaynak G, Birsel O, Güven MF, Öğüt T. An overview of the Charcot foot pathophysiology. *Diabet Foot Ankle.* 2013 Aug 2;4(1):21117.
3. Yammine K, Boulos K, Assi C, Hayek F. Amputation and mortality frequencies associated with diabetic Charcot foot arthropathy: a meta-analysis. *Foot Ankle Surg.* 2022 Dec;28(8):1170-1176.
4. Kavitha KV, Patil VS, Sanjeevi CB, Unnikrishnan AG. New concepts in the management of Charcot neuroarthropathy in diabetes. *Adv Exp Med Biol.* 2021;1307:391-415.
5. Rosenbaum AJ, DiPreta JA. Classifications in brief: Eichenholtz classification of Charcot arthropathy. *Clin Orthop Relat Res.* 2015 Mar;473(3):1168-1171.
6. Rogers LC, Frykberg RG, Armstrong DG, et al. The Charcot foot in diabetes. *Diabetes Care.* 2011 Sep;34(9):2123-2129.
7. Bem R, Jirkovská A, Fejfarová V, Skibová J, Jude EB. Intranasal calcitonin in the treatment of acute Charcot neuroosteoarthropathy: a randomized controlled trial. *Diabetes Care.* 2006 Jun;29(6):1392-1394.

The Critical Image

Leukocytosis and Fever in a Diabetic Patient

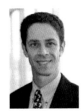

By Joshua S. Broder, MD, FACEP
Dr. Broder is a professor and the residency program director in the Department of Emergency Medicine at Duke University Medical Center in Durham, North Carolina.

Objectives

On completion of this article, you should be able to:

■ Describe x-ray findings of gas gangrene.

■ Manage gas gangrene appropriately, including not delaying surgery for imaging or laboratory tests and not relying on the LRINEC score in critically ill patients or when clinical suspicion is high.

CASE PRESENTATION

A 45-year-old woman with hypertension, heart failure, diabetes, and end-stage renal disease on hemodialysis presents with dyspnea. The patient states that she has had a cough and shortness of breath during exertion for the past week and a fever for the past 2 to 3 days. She denies vomiting, diarrhea, and chest and abdominal pain. She is anuric; has been receiving dialysis as usual, including a session the previous day; and is below her "dry weight." She reports that she has been compliant with prescribed medications. Her vital signs are BP 132/68, P 92, R 24, and T 38.2°C (100.7°F); SpO_2 is 100% on room air.

The patient is alert and in no significant distress. She has a regular cardiac rhythm and normal rate, with no accessory heart sounds. She is slightly tachypneic, with decreased breath sounds bilaterally. Her abdominal examination is normal, and she has no focal neurologic findings. Laboratory testing reveals the following:

- Glucose: 565 mg/dL
- Carbon dioxide (total): 21 mEq/L
- Beta-hydroxybutyrate: 0.33 mmol/L (normal <0.40 mmol/L)
- pH: 7.32
- WBC count: 29.1 x 10⁹/L; neutrophil count: 83%
- Hematocrit: 30.7%

- Hemoglobin: 10.2 g/dL
- Creatinine: 11.8 mg/dL
- Potassium: 5.7 mmol/L; sodium: 126 mEq/L
- Erythrocyte sedimentation rate: 125 mm/hr (normal <20 mm/hr)
- C-reactive protein: >38 mg/dL (normal ≤0.6 mg/dL)
- Lactate: 2.4 mmol/L (normal ≤2.2 mmol/L)

Her COVID-19 and influenza tests are negative. Anterior-posterior and lateral chest x-rays are ordered (*Figure 1*). The patient is admitted with a clinical diagnosis of community-acquired pneumonia and treated with ceftriaxone, azithromycin, and insulin. At the next shift change, another physician performs additional history and examination. The patient states that she stubbed her left foot 1 week ago and avulsed a toenail but has no pain from the incident. She has severe diabetic neuropathy, however. The lower extremities are examined in more detail, and x-rays of the foot are ordered (*Figures 2 and 3*).

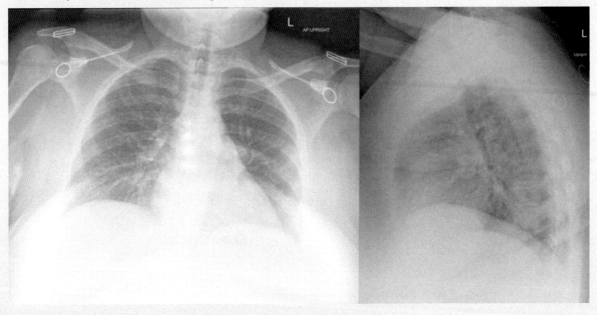

FIGURE 1. The patient's anteroposterior and lateral chest x-rays

Discussion

A thorough history and physical examination are the foundations for appropriate diagnosis and treatment, and physicians should be meticulous in performing these. As in this case, patients with complex medical histories can have multiple sources of fever, leukocytosis, and hyperglycemia.

Necrotizing soft tissue infections (NSTIs) are rare (annual incidence of 0.3-5 cases/100,000) but are life-threatening, with estimated mortality rates between 20% and 30%. Delays in surgical debridement are associated with higher mortality; therefore, consensus recommendations from both surgical and radiologic societies focus on rapid treatment, sometimes before diagnostic confirmation.[1,2] Although individual components of the physical examination have limited sensitivity, history and examination alone are sometimes sufficient for presumptive diagnosis and surgical treatment. Hemorrhagic bullae (sensitivity 25.2%, specificity 95.8%) and hypotension (sensitivity 21%, specificity 97.7%) are significant predictors of NSTI.

The American College of Radiology (ACR) recommends against delaying surgical treatment to obtain imaging in critically ill patients.[2] When imaging is performed, x-rays are usually appropriate. A meta-analysis of 23 studies found that soft tissue gas on x-ray is only 49% sensitive but 94% specific for necrotizing fasciitis, yielding a positive likelihood ratio of 8.17 and a negative likelihood ratio of 0.54.[1] As such, soft tissue emphysema strongly predicts NSTI, but its absence does not rule out NSTI. Rarely, gas can be introduced through an external wound rather than produced in situ by gas-forming organisms. Because half of all patients with NSTIs who undergo x-rays do not have soft tissue emphysema, additional *rapid* imaging may be necessary in uncertain cases. Soft tissue gas on CT is 89% sensitive and 93% specific for NSTI.[2] When obvious signs like soft tissue gas are absent, other CT findings such as fat stranding or fascial fluid are not specific for NSTI. One meta-analysis, taking into account multiple imaging findings, found that CT is 88.5% sensitive and 93.3% specific for NSTI.[1] The ACR states that CT and MRI are equivalent studies, with a rating of "usually indicated" for patients with initial normal x-rays or x-rays that show soft tissue gas but warrant further imaging. However, obtaining both CT and MRI imaging for diagnosis is usually unnecessary and could introduce dangerous delay.[2] Ultrasound (US) can also visualize soft tissue gas, fascial fluid, and fascial thickening and is rated as "may

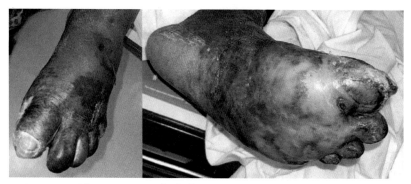

FIGURE 2. The patient's left foot demonstrating areas of ulceration and subcutaneous fluid collection. A foul odor is present.

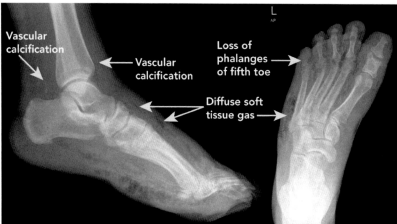

FIGURE 3. X-rays showing diffuse soft tissue gas strongly suggestive of gangrene with gas-forming organisms. Less critical findings include erosion of the phalanges consistent with osteomyelitis and extensive vascular calcifications of advanced peripheral arterial disease.

be appropriate" by the ACR. The sensitivity and specificity of US for NSTI vary widely in the literature.[2]

In clinically obvious cases, laboratory testing plays little role in diagnosis and should not delay surgery. For less certain presentations, a Laboratory Risk Indicator for Necrotizing Fasciitis (LRINEC) score of 6 or greater is 68.2% sensitive and 84.8% specific for NSTI, while a score of 8 or more is 40.8% sensitive and 94.9% specific.[1] The patient presented here had a LRINEC score of 13 — the maximum possible — and a compelling physical examination and x-ray.

CASE RESOLUTION

Antibiotic coverage for anaerobic, gram-positive, and gram-negative organisms, including *Pseudomonas*, was administered. The patient was taken emergently to the operating room for below-the-knee amputation of the left lower extremity. Blood cultures grew *Viridans steptococcus*.

REFERENCES

1. Fernando SM, Tran A, Cheng W, et al. Necrotizing soft tissue infection: diagnostic accuracy of physical examination, imaging, and LRINEC score: a systematic review and meta-analysis. *Ann Surg*. 2019 Jan;269(1):58-65.
2. Expert Panel on Musculoskeletal Imaging; Pierce JL, Perry MT, Wessel DE, et al. ACR Appropriateness Criteria® suspected osteomyelitis, septic arthritis, or soft tissue infection (excluding spine and diabetic foot): 2022 update. *J Am Coll Radiol*. 2022 Nov;19(11S):S473-S487.

Feature Editor: Joshua S. Broder, MD, FACEP. See also *Diagnostic Imaging for the Emergency Physician* (Winner of the 2011 Prose Award in Clinical Medicine, the American Publishers Award for Professional and Scholarly Excellence) and *Critical Images in Emergency Medicine* by Dr. Broder.

The LLSA Literature Review

Conservative Versus Interventional Treatment for Spontaneous Pneumothorax

By Aria C. Shi, MD; and
Andrew J. Eyre, MD, MS-HPEd
Harvard Affiliated Emergency Medicine Residency and
Brigham and Women's Hopsital, Boston, Massachusetts

Objective

On completion of this article, you should be able to:

■ Compare and contrast conservative and interventional management of spontaneous pneumothorax.

Brown SGA, Ball EL, Perrin K, et al; PSP Investigators. Conservative versus interventional treatment for spontaneous pneumothorax. *N Engl J Med.* 2020 Jan 30;382(5):405-415.

KEY POINTS

■ Conservative management with observation and watchful waiting may be reasonable for a subset of patients ages 14 to 50 years with a first-time unilateral spontaneous pneumothorax and who meet certain symptom and physiologic criteria.

■ A conservative approach to spontaneous pneumothorax likely spares many patients from unnecessary invasive procedures.

■ Conservative management for pneumothorax lowers the risk of serious adverse events and pneumothorax recurrence.

Management approaches for moderate to large primary spontaneous pneumothoraces vary widely. The most common approach includes insertion of a chest tube. However, more conservative approaches propose that a chest tube be placed only if conservative treatment fails or if patients meet certain symptomatic or physiologic criteria. Brown et al designed a nonblinded, multicenter, noninferiority trial to determine whether conservative management is an acceptable alternative to immediate intervention.

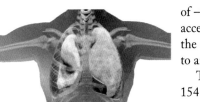

The trial included 316 participants, aged 14 to 50 years, who presented with a first-time unilateral, moderate to large primary spontaneous pneumothorax. They were randomized to either conservative or interventional management groups, and the rates of lung re-expansion within 8 weeks were compared between the two groups.

In the interventional group, a small-bore chest tube was inserted, and repeat chest x-rays were completed 1 and 5 hours post procedure; if patients in this group had a fully re-expanded lung without recurrence of the pneumothorax, the chest tube was removed, and they were discharged. Otherwise, they were admitted to the hospital.

Patients in the conservative arm were observed for a minimum of 4 hours before repeating a chest x-ray. Patients who did not need supplemental oxygen and were able to walk were discharged. Intervention was reserved for those patients with clinically significant symptoms despite adequate analgesia, chest pain or dyspnea that prevented mobilization, physiologic instability (systolic blood pressure <90 mm Hg, shock index value ≥1, or SpO_2 <90% on room air), an enlarging pneumothorax on repeat x-ray, or an unwillingness to continue with conservative treatment.

All study participants were reassessed at 2 weeks, 4 weeks, 8 weeks, 6 months, and 12 months. A noninferiority margin of −9 percentage points was used: Researchers accepted a successful re-expansion rate of 90% in the conservative management group compared to an anticipated 99% in the interventional group.

The interventional group consisted of 154 participants, and the conservative group consisted of 162 participants. Of the conservative participants, 137 (84.6%) did not undergo intervention, while 25 (15.4%) did. Lung re-expansion data were successfully collected on 131 of the interventional participants and 125 of the conservative participants. Successful lung re-expansion by 8 weeks occurred in 120/131 (98.5%) of the interventional group and 118/125 (94.4%) of the conservative group, which was considered noninferior. However, if all missing data were assumed to represent failed lung re-expansion, the results no longer met the noninferiority threshold.

Secondary outcomes demonstrated that the median time to radiographic resolution was 16 days in the interventional group versus 30 days in the conservative group; however, both groups had similar times to symptom resolution. Conservative management was associated with greater patient satisfaction; lower rates of serious adverse events, progression to surgery, and 12-month pneumothorax recurrence; and length of hospital stay.

Overall, conservative management spared 85% of patients from invasive intervention and had noninferior rates of successful lung re-expansion by 8 weeks. This trial showed modest but statistically fragile evidence that conservative management is noninferior to interventional management. Results support the idea that in patients with first-time spontaneous pneumothoraces who are hemodynamically stable and meet specific symptom criteria, emergency physicians should discuss with them both immediate intervention and more conservative watchful waiting management options.

Critical Decisions in Emergency Medicine's LLSA literature reviews features articles from ABEM's 2023 Lifelong Learning and Self-Assessment Reading List. Available online at acep.org/moc/llsa and on the ABEM website.

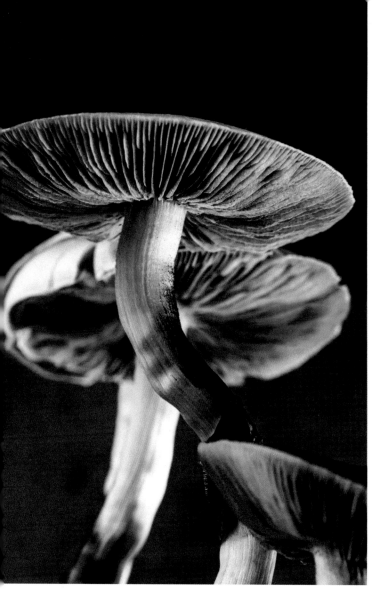

Poison Control

Pediatric Toxicology Considerations

LESSON 2

By Joseph Tagliaferro III, DO, FACEP; and
Jonathan Glauser, MD, MBA, FACEP
Dr. Tagliaferro and Dr. Glauser are professors of emergency
medicine at Case Western Reserve University and faculty
of emergency medicine at MetroHealth Medical Center in
Cleveland, Ohio.

Reviewed by Sharon E. Mace, MD, FACEP

Objectives

On completion of this lesson, you should be able to:

1. Identify signs and symptoms of lead toxicity.
2. Describe the stages of iron poisoning and indications for deferoxamine therapy.
3. Name selected plant poisonings and toxic mushroom syndromes.
4. Evaluate the management of insecticide and anticholinergic exposure.
5. Discuss common drugs of abuse and their presentations.
6. Distinguish and recognize toxic alcohol symptoms and treatment.
7. Recognize cardiac toxin signs and distinguish calcium channel from beta-blocker overdoses.

From the EM Model

17.0 Toxicologic Disorders
    17.1 Drug and Chemical Classes

▬ CRITICAL DECISIONS ▬

- How can lead and iron poisonings present, and how are they managed?
- How can plant and mushroom toxicities present, and how are they managed?
- What are the signs of insecticide toxicity?
- What are the clinical findings for drugs of abuse, and how are they managed?
- When should an acetaminophen overdose versus an aspirin overdose be suspected?
- How should household poisonings be diagnosed and managed?
- How can cardiac pharmaceuticals manifest as acute poisonings?

Children are apt to place nearly anything in their mouths, apart from healthy green vegetables. Ingestion of toxic substances or unintentional overdoses in children cause a variety of signs and symptoms and can be life-threatening, even when symptoms are slow to appear. Emergency physicians must be aware of the many presentations of toxic substance ingestions to accurately diagnose and manage these conditions in the pediatric population.

CASE PRESENTATION

■ CASE ONE
A 3-year-old girl is brought in by her mother after ingesting an unknown number of her grandfather's "heart pills." The bottle originally contained 100 pills and is now empty, but the girl's mother does not know how many pills had already been consumed; she did not bring in the pill bottle. The grandfather, who is hard of hearing, was at home during the incident. The child is lethargic with a blood pressure reading of 78 mm Hg systolic, a pulse of 48 bpm, and a blood glucose level of 317.

■ CASE TWO
A 30-month-old girl is brought in by her father following an episode of vomiting blood and appearing less active than usual. She was in the custody of her mother over the previous 4 days, and he does not know if the child got into her mother's medications. Her initial vital signs include BP 76/50 and P 135. She is quite irritable and seems to have diffuse abdominal discomfort.

■ CASE THREE
A 6-year-old boy was playing outside and fell into a 2-foot deep vat of malathion without submerging his head. He presents with drooling and is covered with vomit and liquid stool. He is arousable to speech. On arrival, his vital signs include BP 102/68 and P 40. The physical examination is notable for diffuse expiratory wheezing. His pupils are miotic, and bowel sounds are hyperactive.

Introduction
The management of the poisoned child may involve a certain amount of sleuthing to determine what was inhaled or ingested. Physicians should be familiar with toxidromes and their presentations, which can include pulmonary edema, high anion gap metabolic acidosis, hyperthermia, or GI findings (*Table 1*). Relatively few specific antidotes exist; supportive care is paramount until a diagnosis is made.

CRITICAL DECISION

How can lead and iron poisonings present, and how are they managed?

Evidence Currently Available
Although the frequency of elevated childhood blood lead levels (BLLs) is decreasing, there are still an estimated 500,000 children (aged 1-5 years) who have BLLs that are higher than the CDC's standard limit (3.5 µg/dL).[1,2] Lead exposure is one of the most dangerous types of environmental exposures, especially for children, in whom lead can affect a variety of organ systems and cause problems with mental and motor development.[3] A clinically significant proportion of children with abdominal pain may have elevated BLLs.[3]

Lead is a common element that humans have long utilized for waterproofing; electrical and radiation shielding; and manufacturing of ammunition, paints, plastics, ceramics, glass, and explosives.[4] Although certain sources of lead, such as decaying paint and lead waterworks, are well established and well publicized, others remain obscure. Bathtubs are one possible concealed source.[5] Additionally, there is an ecological link between greater soil lead levels and increased incidence of childhood BLLs.[2]

Iron is another element implicated in childhood poisonings. Most serious pediatric iron poisonings occur when children ingest maternal prenatal vitamins or ferrous sulfate tablets formulated for adults, which, unfortunately, frequently look like candy.[6] There is insufficient data to identify a safe lower limit for hazardous iron consumption.[6] Iron poisoning occurs as a result of the caustic impact of iron on the GI mucosa and the presence of free iron in the circulation.[6]

Clinical Manifestations
In cases of lead poisoning, children can present with stomach discomfort and should receive prompt treatment because of lead's ability to impair mental and physical development.[3] Physicians should submit blood tests for serum lead levels, obtain an abdominal x-ray, and keep patients under observation for 6 hours.

Iron poisoning is divided into four clinical phases. Phase one is typically 6 hours long and represents the consequences of immediate mucosal damage. Vomiting, diarrhea, and GI blood loss are significant early indications; if severe, the patient may slide into a coma or shock due to volume depletion and metabolic acidosis.[6] Phase two, which lasts between 6 and 24 hours after intake, is characterized by a decrease in GI symptoms. With adequate therapy to replenish fluid and blood losses, children can appear well and frequently recover completely without recurrence of symptoms. However, in some children, this remission is brief, and they progress to phase three, which is characterized by metabolic acidosis, coma, seizures, and persistent shock.[6] Phase three is thought to reflect hepatic damage and disruption of energy metabolism; patients in this phase have jaundice and increased transaminases, and in experimental iron poisonings, levels of lactic and citric acids increase prior to cardiac or respiratory failure. A phase four syndrome characterized by pyloric or duodenal stenosis caused by scarring and blockage is documented in survivors of severe iron poisoning.[6]

Patients who enter the emergency department with severe early symptoms such as vomiting, diarrhea, GI bleeding, depressed sensorium, or circulatory compromise require immediate intensive care. Severe iron poisoning is frequently linked with metabolic acidosis, leukocytosis, hyperglycemia, hyperbilirubinemia, elevated liver enzymes, and a prolonged prothrombin time. If there is considerable fluid loss, hemoconcentration and a high BUN level occur. The first order of business is to acquire venous access and draw blood for a CBC, liver function tests, blood type and cross-match analyses, and blood glucose, electrolyte, BUN, and serum iron levels all at the same time. Abdominal x-rays should also be obtained; they may reveal radiopaque iron in the stomach, but the absence of radiopaque iron does not imply a minor intake.[6] Abdominal x-rays should be repeated as soon as possible after decontaminating the GI tract to assess its efficacy and look for iron pill concretions.[6]

Iron levels in the serum often correlate poorly with clinical symptoms. When serum iron exceeds the iron-binding capacity of blood, this results in free-circulating iron.[6] Free-circulating iron levels less than 350 µg/dL when drawn 3 to 5 hours after ingestion, however, do usually indicate a benign course. Asymptomatic patients with these iron levels who also have a normal abdominal x-ray are considered low risk and can be released.[6] Children who are fully asymptomatic 6 hours after iron consumption are unlikely to develop systemic disease. Serious iron poisoning in children is defined as more than 20 mg/kg of elemental iron ingested; a serum iron level greater than 350 µg/dL; and symptoms of coma, shock, or acidosis. Patients with 350 to 500 µg/dL levels frequently exhibit moderate phase one symptoms but seldom develop major problems.[6] Iron levels greater than 500 µg/dL indicate that phase three symptoms are likely to develop; patients with these high iron levels or with acidosis, shock, or a positive x-ray (possibly) should be admitted for ongoing deferoxamine chelation treatment.[6] The serum iron determination cannot always be obtained immediately; total iron-binding capacity is seldom of value and no longer relevant in the acute treatment of iron poisoning.[6] For accurate calculation of elemental iron, emergency physicians must recall that ferrous gluconate is 12% iron and ferrous sulfate is 20% elemental iron.

Although serum iron levels are helpful, iron poisoning remains a clinical diagnosis. Patients who are ill require intensive hydration and assistance.[6] Among laboratory investigations, metabolic acidosis is probably the strongest predictor of toxicity. Additionally, radiopaque material on the abdominal x-ray can indicate that a considerable amount of iron was absorbed.

All pediatric patients suspected of ingesting iron are at high risk of developing life-threatening illnesses, but severe iron poisoning is relatively rare compared to the number of children who have very minor symptoms or are completely asymptomatic. Emergency physicians need a strategy that addresses both children who are seriously poisoned and those who will recover uneventfully after iron ingestion.[6]

Treatment Considerations

Lead poisoning is treated using chelation with edetate calcium disodium ($CaNa_2EDTA$) and dimercaprol, a method that reduces the mortality and morbidity of severe lead poisoning. Succimer, an oral chelator, has also been shown to be effective in lowering BLLs in asymptomatic children; however, the neurocognitive impact of this treatment is unknown.[6]

Toxin Ingested	Signs and Symptoms of Poisoning	Treatment
Lead	Abdominal pain, hypotension, metabolic acidosis, hypo- or hyperglycemia, stunted mental and motor development	Edetate calcium disodium chelation therapy, succimer
Iron	Vomiting, diarrhea, metabolic acidosis, seizures, shock, coma, cardiac or respiratory failure, pyloric or duodenal stenosis, leukocytosis, hyperglycemia, hyperbilirubinemia, elevated liver enzymes, prolonged prothrombin time	Whole bowel irrigation, deferoxamine chelation therapy
Plant toxins	GI irritation; digitalis; nicotinic, atropinic, epileptogenic, cyanogenic effects	Activated charcoal, observation, supportive care
Mushrooms	Muscarinic, anticholinergic, and hallucinogenic effects; GI effects; hepatic failure; renal failure	Activated charcoal, fluid and electrolyte management, atropine for muscarinic effects, hydration, supportive care, liver transplant
Insecticides	Muscarinic and nicotinic effects	Atropine, benzodiazepines (for seizures), pralidoxime
Dissociatives (PCP and dextromethorphan)	Inebriation, nystagmus, hypersalivation, pyrexia, repetitive movements, agitation, muscular rigidity, psychosis, seizures, coma, respiratory arrest	Stabilization of vitals, treatment of seizures
Hallucinogens	Pupillary dilation, hypertension, tachycardia, hyperreflexia, hyperpyrexia, dizziness, weakness, drowsiness, nausea, paresthesias	Isolation to a quiet area
Cannabis	Conjunctival injection, tachycardia, hypertension, agitation, hallucinations, anxiety, paranoia, vomiting, seizures, severe renal damage, supraventricular tachycardia	Drug discontinuation, benzodiazepines
Stimulants (amphetamines, cocaine, MDMA, and cathinones)	Alertness, restlessness, tremor, hypertension, tachycardia, myocardial ischemia, mydriasis, agitation, delirium, psychosis, hyperthermia, seizures, euphoria, disorientation, tremor, hyperactive reflexes, talkativeness, irritability, weakness, sleeplessness, fever, hallucinations, delusions. **MDMA:** Hyponatremia, serotonin syndrome, hepatotoxicity	Benzodiazepines, haloperidol, phentolamine, hydralazine, sodium nitroprusside
Sedative-hypnotics	Sluggishness, trouble thinking, dysarthria, ataxia, poor memory, poor judgment, emotional lability, limited attention span, lethargy or coma, respiratory depression	Intubation and ventilator support, flumazenil
Opioids	Respiratory depression, coma, miosis	Naloxone, buprenorphine
Inhalants	Sudden ventricular fibrillation, changes in mental status, coma, aspiration, respiratory arrest, sudden sniffing death syndrome	Beta-blockers, anti-arrhythmics, kidney function and vital signs monitoring
Alcohols (ethanol, isopropyl alcohol, methanol, and ethylene glycol)	Nausea, vomiting, stupor, ataxia, hypoglycemia, hypothermia, blindness, coma, metabolic acidosis or ketosis (depending on the alcohol type)	Supportive care, fomepizole (specifically for methanol and ethylene glycol toxicity), hemodialysis
Acetaminophen	Nausea, vomiting, anorexia, pallor, diaphoresis, malaise, stomach discomfort, liver failure	NAC therapy, fomepizole
Aspirin	Reye syndrome, fever, tachypnea, nausea, vomiting, lethargy, slurred speech, seizures, metabolic acidosis, respiratory alkalosis	GI decontamination, urine alkalinization, fluid resuscitation, hemodialysis, hemoperfusion
Household chemicals (acid caustics and alkaline caustics)	Airway edema, coagulation necrosis (acids), liquefaction necrosis (alkalis), esophageal perforation, vomiting, aspiration, CNS depression, stridor	GI endoscopy
Cardiac pharmaceuticals (beta-blockers, calcium channel blockers, clonidine, and digoxin)	Bradycardia, hypotension, hypo- or hyperglycemia, sedation, miosis, coma, seizures, respiratory depression, nausea and vomiting, vision abnormalities, lethargy and confusion, electrolyte problems, heart irregularities	Activated charcoal, atropine, insulin, fluid boluses, direct-acting vasopressors, calcium infusion, glucagon, lipid emulsion infusion, pacemaker, intra-aortic balloon pump, ECMO, naloxone, digoxin-specific antibodies

TABLE 1. Signs, symptoms, and treatments for toxicities encountered in the pediatric population

Acute iron poisoning is treated by minimizing absorption and increasing elimination.[6] The majority of children who are exposed to poisonous iron will vomit on their own. Activated charcoal cannot bind to iron salts and, therefore, offers no benefit. In patients who appear shortly after they have consumed liquid iron, stomach lavage with normal saline can be attempted to prevent leftover particulate matter from directly harming the mucosa and, perhaps, facilitate the breakdown of pill concretions (*Figure 1*).[3]

The early and intensive administration of whole bowel irrigation (WBI) is the basis of GI tract decontamination for iron-poisoned patients. This method is thought to reduce iron absorption and break up pill concretions that could cause direct mucosal damage. An abdominal x-ray, as previously stated, should be taken early in the evaluation of symptomatic individuals. If this investigation reveals considerable radiopaque material and the patient is able, WBI should be used for at least 4 to 6 hours. Even in symptomatic patients without clear signs of material on x-ray, a few hours of WBI, until rectal effluent is clear, may be required to expedite removal of leftover iron pill particles or "sludge," so long as there is no indication of peritonitis or perforation.[3]

Chelation treatment with parenteral deferoxamine increases the excretion of iron in the form of the ferrioxamine complex, which tints the urine orange or pink. Continuous intravenous infusion is the most effective approach, with a maximum suggested dosage of 15 mg/kg/hr (maximum daily dose 360 mg/kg and up to 6 g total). Although a greater infusion rate has been associated with hypotension, it may be necessary in severe ingestions. Crystalloid infusion should be administered for blood pressure management. Chelation is maintained until the serum iron level and urine color normalize, the metabolic acidosis resolves, and patients improve clinically. Deferoxamine doses can be titrated down as the clinical response improves and iron levels decrease. Notably, deferoxamine is thought to serve as a siderophore, promoting the development of specific bacteria such as *Yersinia enterocolitica*. Monitoring for *Yersinia* sepsis may be indicated.[3]

Once patients are stabilized, further complications that can occur are hypotension, severe metabolic acidosis, hypo- or hyperglycemia, anemia, colloid loss due to GI hemorrhage (after equilibration), renal failure due to shock, and hepatic failure with an accompanying bleeding diathesis. Maintaining a sufficient urine output is crucial to avoid renal failure and promote ferrioxamine-complex excretion. If renal failure progresses, chelation can be performed concurrently with dialysis because the ferrioxamine complex is dialyzable.[3]

CRITICAL DECISION

How can plant and mushroom toxicities present, and how are they managed?

Plant ingestions in the pediatric population are frequently reported as adventurous ingestions. The majority of these ingestions are of ordinary home and garden plants.[3] Fortunately, only a small percentage of these plants are a major hazard; most are low in toxicity when ingested in the small amounts emergency physicians normally encounter.[7]

Some examples of common nontoxic plants include: *Asparagus setaceus* (asparagus fern), *Begonia*, *Nephrolepis exaltata* (Boston ferns), *Cactaceae* (cactus), *Bellis perennis* (daisy), *Taraxacum* (dandelion), *Gardenia jasminoides* (gardenia), *Impatiens*, *Hemerocallis* (daylily), *Lilium longiflorum* (Easter lily), *Lilium lancifolium* (tiger lily), *Magnolia*, *Tagetes* (marigold), *Petunia*, *Rosa* (rose), *Viola* (violet), and *Salix babylonica* (weeping willow).

Specific toxic effects are caused by different plants:
- **GI irritation:** *Philodendron*, *Dieffenbachia*, *Phytolacca americana* (pokeweed), *Wisteria*, *Daphne laureola* (spurge laurel), *Ranunculus* (buttercup), *Narcissus* (daffodil), *Abrus precatorius* (rosary pea), and *Ricinus communis* (castor bean);
- **Digitalis effects:** *Convallaria majalis* (lily of the valley), *Digitalis* (foxglove), *Nerium oleander* (oleander), and *Taxus baccata* (yew);
- **Nicotinic effects:** *Nicotiana* (wild tobacco), *Laburnum* (golden chain tree), and *Conium maculatum* (poison hemlock);
- **Atropinic effects:** *Datura stramonium* (jimsonweed or thorn apple) and *Atropa belladonna* (deadly nightshade);
- **Epileptogenic effects:** *Cicuta* (water hemlock); and
- **Cyanogenic effects:** *Prunus* (plum), *Pyrus* (pear), *Malus* (apple), and *Malus sylvestris* (crab apple) seeds; *Hydrangea*; and *Sambucus* (elderberry) plants.

When pediatric patients present to the emergency department for plant ingestion, physicians should comprehensively assess these patients. Activated charcoal has been shown to be effective at adsorbing plant poisons. After a period of surveillance, if patients stay asymptomatic, they can be discharged and watched at home. Children should be hospitalized for further monitoring and particular or supportive treatment if they develop symptoms or are suspected or confirmed to have eaten a plant that causes dangerous intoxication.[3]

Wild mushrooms are another potential source of toxicity. Mushrooms are thought to be responsible for half of all plant- and fungal-poisoning deaths in the United States. Because of the difficulties in accurately identifying mushrooms, emergency physicians should not rely on a mushroom's identification for proper management of ingestions.[3]

In terms of how soon symptoms start after ingestion, mushrooms can be classified by two types: those with a quick symptom onset (ie, early-onset mushrooms) and those with a delayed onset. Regardless of the mushroom, the first line of defense for any suspected poisoning is activated charcoal and other GI decontamination techniques.[3]

If symptoms of mushroom poisoning appear within 6 hours of consumption, the prognosis is typically favorable with appropriate fluid and electrolyte management. Early-onset mushrooms can be further classified based on their toxicologic traits. Some early-onset mushrooms elicit muscarinic symptoms, such as perspiration, salivation, colic, and pulmonary edema, within 15 minutes.

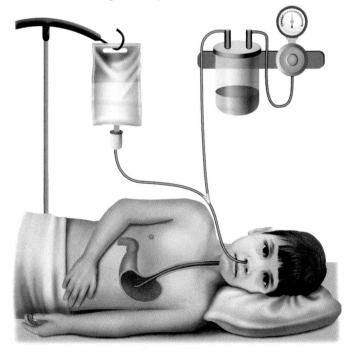

FIGURE 1. Gastric lavage. *Credit:* ACEP.

Atropine treatment effectively treats muscarinic symptoms. Other early-onset mushrooms produce anticholinergic effects such as sleepiness followed by mania and hallucinations. Another class of mushrooms with early-onset effects are hallucinogenic mushrooms, such as those containing psilocybin. In general, most mushrooms have GI effects, but early-onset mushroom subgroups can cause severe GI illness. When certain mushrooms are combined with alcohol, they cause a disulfiram-like adverse reaction to alcohol. All early-onset mushroom effects are managed with supportive care and careful hydration monitoring.[3]

The second type of mushroom causes serious symptoms to appear more than 6 hours after ingestion and accounts for 90% of mushroom-related deaths. *Amanita phalloides* (death cap mushroom) is the most lethal mushroom with delayed-symptom onset. After ingestion and a latent period, GI distress begins, followed by hepatic impairment approximately 24 hours after intake that can proceed to fulminant hepatic failure. Without a liver transplant, people in this condition usually die. Another *Amanita* mushroom, *A. smithiana*, causes symptoms to appear within 6 hours after consumption and can cause renal failure more than 24 hours later. Risk categorization based on delayed-onset symptoms has been unreliable in data from the Pacific Northwest, where *A. smithiana* grows.[3]

The poisonous effects of *A. phalloides* are caused by phallotoxin and amatoxin. First, phallotoxin causes nausea, vomiting, stomach discomfort, and diarrhea. Fever, tachycardia, and hyperglycemia are also possible during this phase. Later, amatoxin induces renal tubular and hepatic necrosis. Fluid and electrolyte supplementation are used to treat the gastroenteric phase. If renal failure develops, treatment with dialysis may be required. Early, repeated administration of activated charcoal after *A. phalloides* consumption appears to block enterohepatic recirculation of amatoxin, which can reduce hepatic damage.[3] Outcomes with additional therapy for *A. phalloides* toxicity are inconsistent. A regional poison control center can provide advice on experimental therapy, but numerous doses of activated charcoal and close attention to supportive care are still the mainstay treatment. Early referral for liver transplantation may be lifesaving for individuals with an otherwise dismal prognosis.[3] Liver transplantation is an effective therapy for acute liver failure from mushroom poisoning and can enhance the survival rate of patients with toxic liver failure.[8]

CRITICAL DECISION

What are the signs of insecticide toxicity?

Organophosphates are lipid-soluble insecticides often used in agricultural and household applications via sprayed dust or emulsion formulations. Some of these compounds are "systemic" insecticides, meaning they are absorbed by plant roots and distributed throughout the leaves, flowers, and fruits. These compounds can be absorbed by inhalation, ingestion, or skin penetration. They irreversibly phosphorylate the enzyme acetylcholinesterase in tissues, enabling acetylcholine buildup at cholinergic junctions in autonomic effector sites (causing muscarinic effects), skeletal muscle or autonomic ganglia (causing nicotinic effects), and the CNS.[3] Muscarinic receptor stimulation can cause bradycardia, bronchorrhea, bronchospasm, lacrimation, miosis, diaphoresis, profuse watery salivation, GI hyperactivity with vomiting, stomach pains, diarrhea, and involuntary urination, denoted by the acronym SLUDGE/BBB (salivation, lacrimation, urination, defection, GI cramps, emesis/bradycardia, bronchorrhea, bronchospasm). Nicotinic receptor activation can cause muscle fasciculations, flaccid paralysis, bradyarrhythmia, delirium, seizures, and coma.[9]

These clinical signs combined with a history of exposure to organophosphates are the greatest indicators of organophosphate toxicity. Children can also be exposed to acetylcholinesterase inhibitors if they consume an adult's Alzheimer or Parkinson disease medications (eg, rivastigmine, donepezil, tacrine, and galantamine).[3]

Because organophosphates are easily absorbed through the skin and mucous membranes, physicians and medical personnel must take measures against exposure to organophosphates from poisoned patients. To safeguard emergency responders, all contaminated clothes must be removed and kept in a plastic bag.[3]

The antidote for cholinergic poisoning is atropine. At the muscarinic receptors, atropine functions as a competitive antagonist of acetylcholine. Atropine, however, has no direct impact on nicotinic receptors and is ineffective for nicotinic-related symptoms such as muscle fasciculations or paralysis.[9] Atropine can also be used with a benzodiazepine to treat seizures in children with cholinergic overdose. The normal dosage for children is 0.01 to 0.03 mg/kg every 3 to 5 minutes, titrated according to clinical response. The maximum cumulative intravenous dosage is 1 mg in children and 2 mg in teenagers. Atropine can also be administered as a continuous infusion. Compared to typical bolus doses, quickly progressive atropine dosages, followed by infusion, lead to lower mortality, less need for respiratory support, and faster completion of atropinization. Atropine should be given in doubling doses to achieve atropinization before continuing as an infusion at patient-specific dosages. Using a dose-titrated doubling regimen, atropine should be dosed to resolve bronchorrhea produced by the muscarinic toxidrome.[4]

Pralidoxime is an antidote for organophosphate poisoning because it cleaves the organophosphate-acetylcholinesterase complex and releases the enzyme responsible for acetylcholine degradation. Pralidoxime works for both muscarinic and nicotinic symptoms. However, pralidoxime should only be taken alongside atropine because monotherapy can increase symptoms by transitory oxime-induced acetylcholinesterase inhibition. For children, the recommended intravenous dose of pralidoxime is 25 to 50 mg/kg (maximum 2 g/dose) given over 30 minutes. Continuous infusion can also be given and may produce better clinical results than bolus dosages. Adverse reactions to pralidoxime are uncommon in children but include hypertension, headache, blurred vision, nausea, and vomiting. Laryngospasm and muscle rigidity have also been documented in people who received rapid pralidoxime administration.[9] Because organophosphates are typically dissolved in hydrocarbon bases, physicians should be prepared to treat possible hydrocarbon pneumonitis.

Carbamate insecticides have a similar mode of action to organophosphate insecticides, but acetylcholinesterase inactivation in carbamate poisoning is reversible and transitory. Pralidoxime treatment is typically unnecessary following carbamate toxicity.[3]

CRITICAL DECISION

What are the clinical findings for drugs of abuse, and how are they managed?

Given the limits of history taking and laboratory testing in children, careful clinical assessment and detection of toxidromes are critical for proper management. Along with the more traditional illegal substances of abuse, prescription medications (particularly opioids and attention deficit hyperactivity disorder [ADHD] medication), over-the-counter medications, vitamins, herbal supplements, and synthetic compounds are all potential sources of toxicity in the pediatric population.[6] Patients with poisoning from drugs of abuse present after experiencing multiple trauma, accidental and deliberate overdoses, or sudden changes in mental status or behavior.[6] Children from resource-scarce environments report a high rate of lifetime drug use. The most frequently used drugs are inhalants, then cigarettes, alcohol, and marijuana.[10] Pediatric physicians should be aware of the following categories of drugs of abuse: psychoactive (dissociatives and hallucinogens), cannabis, stimulants (amphetamines and cocaine), sedative-hypnotics, opioids, inhalants, and alcohols.

Dissociatives

Phencyclidine's (PCP) clinical effects range from inebriation and nystagmus at low doses to psychosis, agitation, muscular rigidity, and seizures at high doses.[6] At moderate doses, PCP symptoms include hypersalivation, pyrexia, repetitive movements, and muscle rigidity.[6] Increased doses may result in convulsions, coma, or respiratory arrest. As a result of its sympathomimetic effects, PCP frequently causes hypertension and tachycardia. Dextromethorphan intoxication mimics the effects of low-dose PCP and can lead to a false-positive PCP urine test. Serum concentrations of PCP are rarely available and do not correspond with clinical symptoms.[6] As a result, management decisions are frequently based on exposure history or clinical suspicion. The initial treatment goal is to stabilize vital signs and address potentially life-threatening episodes such as seizures. Clinical evaluation of patients with severe intoxication should include a determination of renal function and the presence of rhabdomyolysis.[6]

Hallucinogens

Hallucinogens are psychoactive substances that can cause a variety of mental state alterations, including hallucinations, delusions, and paranoid ideation. Hallucinogens have sympathomimetic and serotonergic somatic effects, including pupillary dilation, hypertension, tachycardia, hyperreflexia, and hyperpyrexia.[6] After a single oral dose of 0.5 to 2 μg/kg of lysergic acid diethylamide (LSD), somatic symptoms such as dizziness, weakness, drowsiness, nausea, and paresthesias can occur.[6]

Because LSD is consumed in trace amounts and symptoms manifest hours after ingestion, GI decontamination is not recommended unless coingestion is suspected. Emergency physicians should consider laboratory tests for creatine kinase and renal function when clinical toxicity is substantial.[6] LSD and analogs are often not detected in routine urine toxicology screenings, and the continual evolution of new hallucinogens makes detection much more difficult. Thus, management is determined by exposure history, clinical suspicion of exposure based on assessment, and the severity of the clinical presentation.[6] Patients can experience major injuries from taking these drugs, so physicians should carefully assess them for secondary injuries. Clinical management includes moving patients to an isolated, quiet area. If possible, it is a good idea to have someone familiar to the pediatric patient attempt to calm and reassure them.[6]

Cannabis

Marijuana continues to be the second-most abused psychoactive substance after alcohol.[6] With the recent legalization of marijuana in some jurisdictions and the emergence of marijuana edibles, the incidence of young children's unintended exposures has increased, with edibles responsible for most pediatric cannabis toxicities.[6] In humans, cannabis poisoning most noticeably affects the CNS and cardiovascular system. Adolescents can experience toxicity if they are exposed to unusually powerful cannabis or if they consume multiple serving sizes of edibles too quickly.[6] In stabilized schizophrenics, marijuana can cause an acute exacerbation of symptoms. Some clinical findings of cannabis toxicity on examination are tachycardia,

hypertension, and prominent conjunctival injection. Infants and toddlers who consume edible cannabis or are passively exposed to marijuana smoke can experience profound lethargy or even coma, occasionally with tachycardia.[6] Synthetic cannabinoids are intrinsically more harmful than natural cannabinoids because of their unknown chemical composition and clinical consequences.[6] In most cases, the only treatment required is drug discontinuation. A benzodiazepine may be required in adolescents with a psychotic reaction or acute toxic delirium. These acute symptoms should improve after 4 to 6 hours of drug abstinence.[6]

Synthetic cannabinoids have a different toxicity profile than cannabis. Synthetic cannabinoids have a much higher affinity than tetrahydrocannabinol (THC) for cannabinoid receptors in the CNS and peripheral tissues.[6] Compared to THC, synthetic cannabinoids are associated with an increased risk of tachycardia, hypertension, agitation, hallucinations, anxiety, paranoia, and vomiting.[6] Synthetic cannabinoids have also been reported to be associated with seizures, severe renal damage, and supraventricular tachycardia.

Stimulants

Amphetamines (both prescribed and illicit methamphetamine), cocaine, and other newer compounds such as MDMA (ecstasy) and cathinones (bath salts) are all stimulants. The psychic effect of amphetamines is dose, mental-state, and personality dependent.[6] At low concentrations, these chemicals induce alertness and restlessness; at high concentrations, they generate a severe sympathomimetic toxidrome marked by hypertension, tachycardia, mydriasis, agitation, delirium, psychosis, hyperthermia, and seizures.[6] Symptoms of central effects include euphoria, restlessness, disorientation, tremor, hyperactive reflexes, talkativeness, irritability, weakness, sleeplessness, and fever.[6] The most frequent major adverse effect is a psychotic reaction characterized by intense hallucinations and paranoid delusions that is frequently misdiagnosed as schizophrenia.[6]

MDMA toxicity is distinct in that it manifests itself through hyponatremia, serotonin syndrome, and hepatotoxicity.[6] Use of a benzodiazepine or haloperidol (0.01 to 0.05 mg/kg IM) for severe agitation may be indicated. Severe hypertension that does not respond to benzodiazepines may require phentolamine, hydralazine, or intravenous sodium nitroprusside.[6]

Cocaine's most significant clinical effect is activation of the CNS. This results in sensations of well-being and euphoria that are frequently accompanied by gregariousness, restlessness, excitement, and a sense of clarity.[6] However, as the dose is increased, excessive stimulation can result in tremors, forced speech, agitation, and even tonic-clonic convulsions. Signs of CNS excitement in cocaine-exposed infants includes hyperactivity, dystonic posture, altered mental status, and outright seizures.[6] Apart from its stimulant properties, cocaine is a type IB antidysrhythmic with sodium channel–blocking activity in the heart. Toxicity can manifest as ECG abnormalities, seizures, or dysrhythmias and can cause myocardial ischemia.[6] Vital signs, especially core temperature, should be monitored immediately. Seizures necessitate rapid airway management and anticonvulsant medication. In cocaine toxicity, benzodiazepines are the preferred anticonvulsant because of their rapid start of action and their ability to decrease mortality when used to treat cocaine-induced seizures, as seen in animal studies.[6] Additionally, benzodiazepines should be liberally supplied to patients with mild to severe toxicity (agitation, hypertension, tachycardia) due to their ability to reverse a number of these clinical symptoms.[6]

Sedative-Hypnotics

Sedative-hypnotics have tranquilizing, euphoriant effects that can be similar to those of morphine.[6] After sedative-hypnotic use, adolescents can be sluggish, dysarthric, emotionally labile, and have trouble thinking, remembering, making judgments, and paying attention.[6] Lethargy or coma with relatively normal vital signs is the classic manifestation of an oral sedative-hypnotic overdose.[6] Respiratory depression can occur, particularly with administration of sedatives and hypnotics in combination (eg, benzodiazepines and ethanol). Toddlers who inadvertently use benzodiazepines may develop acute ataxia.[6] Continuous monitoring in an ICU, frequently with intubation and ventilator support, is the optimal treatment for substantial sedative overdose. Flumazenil, a benzodiazepine antagonist, can be used in certain situations when benzodiazepine intake is suspected; to reverse an observed, unintentional benzodiazepine overdose in a small child; or to avoid airway intubation after an iatrogenic overdose.[6] Flumazenil should not be administered empirically in unknown or deliberate overdoses because it can cause fatal convulsions.[6]

Opioids

Recreational use of insufflated heroin and ingested prescription opioid analgesics, particularly oxycodone and hydrocodone, has reached epidemic proportions in the United States over the last two decades and may be responsible for the first increase in overall drug-related mortality in a generation.[6] Opioids inevitably produce miosis, even after tolerance develops.[6] Another symptom of opioid poisoning is respiratory depression, owing in part to the brainstem respiratory center's lower sensitivity to increases in carbon dioxide tension, an effect frequently amplified during sleep.[6] If a patient's history of opioid use is unknown, the presence of coma, pinpoint pupils, and reduced respiration all suggest opioid toxicity.[6] The presence of track marks may indicate intravenous opioid use. The initial step in managing opioid overdose is to ensure adequate breathing and oxygenation. If there is severe respiratory depression or pulmonary edema, endotracheal intubation may be necessary. In individuals with opioid-induced respiratory depression, naloxone, an opioid antagonist, is the first line of therapy.[6] Doses as low as 0.2 to 0.4 mg/m² should be used cautiously in opioid-dependent patients. The initial dose of naloxone in opioid-naive children is 0.1 mg/kg.[6] Buprenorphine is a partial opioid agonist that is increasingly used to treat opioid use disorder in combination with other medications. Buprenorphine toxicity in children is comparable to that of full opioid agonists.[6]

Inhalants

The prevalence of inhalant abuse among young children and adolescents depends on how readily available they are.[6] Abuse patterns are highly regional, with the southwestern and southeastern United States having the highest abuse rates.[6] Three basic groups of psychotropic inhalants exist: hydrocarbons, nitrous oxide, and nitrites. Inebriation with inhalants can cause changes in mental status, such as coma, aspiration, or respiratory arrest. Each of the halogenated hydrocarbons is extremely carcinogenic to the heart and is linked to instances of sudden ventricular fibrillation in adolescents.[6] Sudden sniffing death syndrome has been described in adolescents who abuse inhalants and is most frequently associated with the use of halogenated hydrocarbons.[6]

Alcohols

Intoxication with ethanol (ethyl alcohol), isopropyl, methanol (methyl alcohol), and ethylene glycol alcohols can occur in the pediatric population. The volume of consumed liquid that is harmful depends on its alcohol concentration.[6] Alcohol is processed in the liver by the enzyme alcohol dehydrogenase and is eliminated at a dose-dependent rate.[6] The detoxification process takes longer when there is more alcohol in the blood because the body generates only so much alcohol dehydrogenase at a time (first-order metabolism). Physicians should strongly suspect toxic alcohol ingestions in any patient in a coma who has an unexplained osmolal gap (the difference between calculated and observed osmolality).[6]

Ethanol is the most frequently consumed alcohol. Children who consume ethanol may experience nausea, vomiting, stupor, and ataxia. In young children, ethanol consumption can result in hypoglycemia, hypothermia, and coma.[6] Children exposed to ethanol frequently exhibit a variety of clinical signs and symptoms that do not conform to the standard ethanol or sedative-hypnotic toxidrome. Pediatric ethanol poisonings are frequently treated supportively, with a typically swift recovery.[11]

Isopropyl alcohol can cause severe intoxication, including coma, when used to control fever in children.[6] Isopropyl alcohol poisoning typically manifests as ketosis without metabolic acidosis.[6] Most symptoms of isopropyl alcohol consumption are the same as those of ethanol consumption, except that isopropyl alcohol causes acute gastritis.

Although methanol itself is not harmful, it becomes toxic when its conversion to formaldehyde and formic acid by alcohol and aldehyde dehydrogenase produces poisonous toxic metabolites.[6] In the early stages of methanol intoxication, funduscopic examination may reveal hyperemia. If left untreated, methanol poisoning leads to blindness and a pale, avascular retina.[6] The most acute clinical risk associated with methanol use is severe metabolic acidosis, predominantly caused by formic acid generation.[6]

Ethylene glycol poisoning is uncommon but can cause substantial morbidity and, occasionally, death. Like methanol, ethylene glycol is virtually nontoxic in its pure form but becomes toxic as a product of drug metabolism. Alcohol dehydrogenase metabolizes ethylene glycol to form various hazardous intermediates, including glycolaldehyde, glycolic acid, and oxalate, which cause severe metabolic acidosis and calcium oxalate crystal deposition.[6] Physicians can recognize ethylene glycol poisoning based on patients' history of use or, when this is unknown and diabetic ketoacidosis has been ruled out, the presence of alcohol-like intoxication without the odor of alcohol, high anion gap metabolic acidosis, and an elevated osmolal gap in the absence of ethanol or methanol intake. Although a positive urinalysis for oxalate crystals is neither extremely sensitive nor specific for ethylene glycol intoxication, it can help corroborate the diagnosis.[6]

✔ Pearls

- Acid-base status is of critical importance. Physicians should be familiar with toxins associated with acidosis or ketosis.
- Careful attention should be given to vital signs. Toxidromes associated with abnormal vital signs can yield a clinical diagnosis.
- Management of intoxications still mainly rests on supportive care. Although rarely used, heroic measures, such as transplant, dialysis, or ECMO, must be considered in the pediatric population.
- In contrast to other harmful alcohols, isopropyl alcohol does not cause metabolic acidosis.

Methanol or ethylene glycol consumption can cause severe metabolic acidosis and should be treated with fomepizole, an alcohol dehydrogenase inhibitor that impedes the conversion of these chemicals to their hazardous metabolites.[6] Indications for fomepizole include a methanol or ethylene glycol level greater than 20 mg/dL, a serum ethanol level less than 100 mg/dL, a high anion gap, coma, or metabolic acidosis. Hemodialysis may be indicated in severe situations.

CRITICAL DECISION

When should an acetaminophen overdose versus an aspirin overdose be suspected?

Acetaminophen, also known as N-acetyl-p-aminophenol (APAP), is the most prescribed pediatric analgesic-antipyretic and one of the most frequently consumed medications by young children. APAP's major toxicity is hepatocellular injury. Signs and symptoms of APAP consumption are initially vague and nonspecific but can include nausea and vomiting, anorexia, pallor, and diaphoresis. These symptoms often subside within 12 to 24 hours, and patients can appear well for 1 to 4 days.[6] In this time, however, liver enzyme levels may rise, and jaundice with liver tenderness can develop. About 2% to 4% of children who are intoxicated and have toxic plasma levels of APAP will develop hepatic failure and die. Without receiving an antidote, children with APAP toxicity, in general, will die.[6] Anorexia, malaise, and stomach discomfort can develop into symptoms of fulminant liver failure, including hepatic encephalopathy, coagulopathy, and multisystem organ dysfunction.

The severity of an acute intoxication can be anticipated if the amount of APAP consumed and plasma APAP levels are known. The plasma APAP level, tested at least 4 hours after intake, is the most accurate indicator of liver injury severity.[6] In pediatric patients, a single acute overdose of less than 200 mg/kg of APAP is unlikely to cause substantial damage. For patients presenting to care within 24 hours of an acute overdose with a known time of intake, the Rumack-Matthew nomogram is available for predicting potential toxicity based on the plasma APAP level. Detectable APAP levels or signs of hepatotoxicity should prompt N-acetylcysteine (NAC) therapy.[6] NAC is most efficient at treating hepatotoxicity when administered intravenously or orally within 8 hours of APAP absorption. Additionally, past 8 hours of absorption, administering NAC still mitigates the degree of liver impairment.[6] The most common adverse response associated with intravenous NAC is an anaphylactoid reaction, which usually occurs during the comparatively higher-dose loading infusion. Fomepizole should be evaluated as an adjuvant in significant APAP overdoses because of NAC's known failure rate and fomepizole's safety profile.[12]

✖ Pitfalls

- Failing to consider toxic ingestions in children with predominantly GI symptoms such as vomiting, diarrhea, or hematemesis.
- Overlooking potential diagnostic modalities in poisoned children, including chest and abdominal x-rays and ECG.
- Neglecting to consider the specific indications for antidotes, such as deferoxamine, NAC, and fomepizole, because of their rarity.
- Overlooking clinical clues in cardiac medication overdoses.
- Failing to use blood gas measurements, including pH, in unknown ingestions.

Salicylates, most notably aspirin, are a significant cause of poisoning in children and teenagers. In the pediatric population, there is some evidence of probable interaction, synergism, and cotoxicity between aspirin and acetaminophen. Salicylates are well known and well documented for their toxicity in this group, most notably in the form of Reye syndrome.[13] Symptoms of salicylism include fever, tachypnea, nausea, vomiting, lethargy, slurred speech, and seizures. The combination of metabolic acidosis and respiratory alkalosis leads to a blood gas test result that almost always points to salicylism.[6] The severity of an acute aspirin poisoning is judged by the first signs and symptoms to appear, the amount of salicylate ingested, and the amount of salicylate found in the blood. Because aspirin overdose can cause a slow emptying of the stomach and formation of bezoars from ingested pills mixing, GI decontamination should be considered for children who ingested the drug in the last 4 to 6 hours.[6] Health care personnel should exercise caution when sedating or mechanically ventilating aspirin-poisoned patients because both can exacerbate acidosis and lead to more severe aspirin-induced neurotoxicity. Urine alkalinization should be coupled with fluid resuscitation in children and adolescents with symptomatic salicylate poisoning. By raising urine pH, sodium bicarbonate ionizes filtered aspirin, enhancing tubular secretion and preventing tubular reabsorption (ion trapping).[6] Hemodialysis or hemoperfusion can also be used to increase salicylate removal but is typically reserved for seriously ill patients.

CRITICAL DECISION

How should household poisonings be diagnosed and managed?

Although many household goods may not cause serious toxicity, consumption of acid and alkaline caustics can cause significant edema of the airways and esophageal and stomach damage. Acids cause coagulation necrosis, which typically results in superficial damage rather than deep, penetrating burns. Alkalis, by contrast, cause deep and penetrating liquefaction necrosis with serious consequences such as esophageal perforation.[6] Common household products that contain acid caustics are toilet bowl and drain cleaners. Household alkaline caustics include hair-relaxing gels and pastes; dishwasher and powdered laundry detergents (including laundry detergent pods); and oven and drain pipe cleaners that contain sodium hydroxide (lye), which comes in crystalline and liquid forms.[6] Alkaline caustics that are smeared on the face, lips, or tongue can cause severe lip swelling but rarely cause esophageal or systemic damage.[6] Some, such as laundry detergent pods, can cause vomiting, aspiration, and CNS depression.[6] Patients who experience vomiting, drooling, pain, or stridor after ingesting a caustic agent should be investigated further with upper GI endoscopy.[6] In cases of household poisonings, dilution or neutralization of the agent and GI decontamination should not be attempted because they can aggravate the injury.

CRITICAL DECISION

How can cardiac pharmaceuticals manifest as acute poisonings?

Beta-blockers, calcium channel blockers, clonidine, and digoxin can all be toxic even if taken in small amounts. The triad of bradycardia, hypotension, and *hypoglycemia* should raise suspicion for beta-blocker toxicity. The triad of bradycardia, hypotension, and *hyperglycemia* should raise suspicion for calcium channel blocker toxicity. Clues to clonidine toxicity include the triad of sedation, bradycardia, and pinpoint pupils, particularly in the absence of respiratory depression.[6]

CASE RESOLUTIONS

■ CASE ONE

It was unclear what the girl had ingested, but bradycardia and hyperglycemia strongly suggested calcium channel blocker ingestion. She was treated with hydration, atropine, and intravenous calcium, glucagon, and insulin. Lipid emulsion therapy was considered, but after these interventions, her blood pressure was 96/58 mm Hg and her pulse was 86 bpm. The next day, her mother brought an empty bottle of her grandfather's verapamil, confirming the diagnosis of calcium channel blocker poisoning.

■ CASE TWO

The girl was suspected to have ingested a large amount of her mother's prenatal vitamins. On arrival, her serum iron level was 534 µg/dL, and she had a venous pH of 7.21. She was given fluids and received 15 mg/kg/hr of deferoxamine over a 2-day ICU stay. Her blood pressure stabilized with intravenous hydration. She was discharged on hospital day 6 and will be followed for signs of GI obstruction and stricture.

■ CASE THREE

The patient exhibited muscarinic signs but never had a seizure. He remained awake and was managed with large doses of atropine for bronchorrhea. His airway was protected in the pediatric ICU, and he tolerated oral intake by hospital day 3. He was discharged home after a 5-day hospital stay.

After a large overdose, both beta-blockers and calcium channel blockers can cause severe cardiovascular and neurologic symptoms. Cardiovascular symptoms can include severe bradycardia and hypotension. CNS symptoms can include coma or convulsions and are more likely in beta-blocker than calcium channel blocker overdoses.[6] Metabolic acidosis can occur with calcium channel blockers. Management of significant ingestions of beta-blockers or calcium channel blockers should begin with aggressive gastric decontamination. Activated charcoal should be given to patients who present soon after ingestion if there are no contraindications.[6] Standard treatments such as atropine, insulin, fluid boluses, and direct-acting vasopressors (eg, norepinephrine) can improve bradycardia and hypotension, but many cases are resistant to these measures. Calcium infusion is an additional treatment that can be beneficial in these ingestions. Another treatment, glucagon, raises intracellular cyclic adenosine monophosphate (cAMP) via a mechanism separate from beta receptors and has normalized heart rate and blood pressure in beta-blocker overdoses.[6] Lipid emulsion infusion has been shown to be effective in animal studies and case reports of verapamil toxicity; it is often used when toxicity is resistant to standard therapy, including insulin, or if patients go into cardiac arrest. In severe situations, a pacemaker may be inserted, and an intra-aortic balloon pump or extracorporeal membrane oxygenation (ECMO) may be considered. Hemodialysis or hemoperfusion are unlikely to be beneficial in most situations.[6]

Clonidine, a centrally acting alpha-2–adrenergic agonist, has gained popularity for treating ADHD, agitation, and opiate withdrawal.[6] Even tiny doses, such as a single adult tablet, can substantially harm children. The first signs of toxicity are changes in mental state, ranging from lethargy to coma; hypothermia can also occur. Common presenting signs in severe intoxications can include coma, miosis, and respiratory depression.[6] Emergency endotracheal intubation may be indicated in severe intoxications. Activated charcoal is a useful treatment because it binds to clonidine. Naloxone is a proposed antidote for clonidine overdose, based on case reports of restored mental status and cardiorespiratory function following its administration.[6]

Digoxin is commonly used to treat congenital heart disease in newborns and congestive heart failure in the elderly.[6] Digoxin overdose symptoms include nausea, vomiting, and vision abnormalities. In more severe overdoses, digoxin can cause lethargy, confusion, electrolyte problems, and heart irregularities. Hyperkalemia is a defining feature of severe acute digoxin toxicity and is caused by a significant reduction of sodium-potassium ATPase activity.[6] The typical pattern of cardiac toxicity associated with digoxin overdose is prolonged atrioventricular dissociation manifested by first- to third-degree heart block. The first step in treating digoxin intoxication is to check patients' hemodynamic status. Digoxin-specific antibody fragments are a treatment used specifically to reverse the effects of digoxin.[6] In digoxin poisonings, these antibody fragments should be used when there are signs and symptoms of intoxication, life-threatening cardiac arrhythmias, or serum potassium levels of 5.5 mEq/L or more.[6]

Summary

Children may present in various ways after unintentional ingestions or toxic exposures. Few specific antibodies for counteracting these exposures exist in the acute setting. Emergency physicians must be prepared to recognize specific signs, symptoms, and toxidromes and manage them accordingly.

REFERENCES

1. CDC updates blood lead reference value to 3.5 µg/dL. Centers for Disease Control and Prevention. Updated March 25, 2022. https://www.cdc.gov/nceh/lead/news/cdc-updates-blood-lead-reference-value.html#:~:text=CDC%20uses%20a%20blood%20lead,dL%20to%203.5%20%CE%BCg%2FdL

2. Pavilonis B, Cheng Z, Johnson G, Maroko A. Lead, soils, and children: an ecological analysis of lead contamination in parks and elevated blood lead levels in Brooklyn, New York. *Arch Environ Contam Toxicol.* 2022 Jan;82(1):1-10.

3. Hosseini A, Fayaz A, Hassanian-Moghaddam H, et al. Blood lead concentrations among pediatric patients with abdominal pain: a prospective cross-sectional study. *BMC Gastroenterol.* 2021 Dec 20;21(1):493.

4. Nelson LS, Howland MA, Lewin NA, Smith SW, Goldfrank LR, Hoffman RS, eds. *Goldfrank's Toxicologic Emergencies.* 11th ed. McGraw-Hill Education; 2019.

5. Balza J. Hidden toxins: bathtubs as a potential source of lead exposure in children. *J Toxicol Environ Health A.* 2022 May;85(9):376-380.

6. Shaw KN, Bachur RG, eds. *Flesher and Ludwig's Textbook of Pediatric Emergency Medicine.* 8th ed. Wolters Kluwer; 2020.

7. Froberg B, Ibrahim D, Furbee RB. Plant poisoning. *Emerg Med Clin North Am.* 2007 May;25(2):375-433.

8. Wu J, Gong X, Hu Z, Sun Q. Acute liver failure caused by *Amanita verna*: a case series and review of the literature. *BMC Surg.* 2021 Dec 25;21(1):436.

9. Hon KL, Hui WF, Leung AK. Antidotes for childhood toxidromes. *Drugs Context.* 2021;10:2020-11-4.

10. Embleton L, Mwangi A, Vreeman R, Ayuku D, Braitstein P. The epidemiology of substance use among street children in resource-constrained settings: a systematic review and meta-analysis. *Addiction.* 2013 Oct;108(10):1722-1733.

11. Gaw CE, Osterhoudt KC. Ethanol intoxication of young children. *Pediatr Emerg Care.* 2019;35(10):722-730.

12. Link SL, Rampon G, Osmon S, Scalzo AJ, Rumack BH. Fomepizole as an adjunct in acetylcysteine treated acetaminophen overdose patients: a case series. *Clin Toxicol (Phila).* 2022;60(4):472-477.

13. Dinakaran D, Sergi CM. Co-ingestion of aspirin and acetaminophen promoting fulminant liver failure: a critical review of Reye syndrome in the current perspective at the dawn of the 21st century. *Clin Exp Pharmacol Physiol.* 2018;45(2):117-121.

CME Questions

Reviewed by Tareq Al-Salamah, MBBS, MPH, FACEP; and Sharon E. Mace, MD, FACEP

Qualified, paid subscribers to *Critical Decisions in Emergency Medicine* may receive CME certificates for up to 5 ACEP Category I credits, 5 *AMA PRA Category 1 Credits*™, and 5 AOA Category 2-B credits for completing this activity in its entirety. Submit your answers online at acep.org/cdem; a score of 75% or better is required. You may receive credit for completing the CME activity any time within 3 years of its publication date. Answers to this month's questions will be published in next month's issue.

1 **What is the correct dosing for morphine in an opioid-naive patient?**

A. 0.1 mg/kg
B. 0.1 mg/kg plus 0.05 mg/kg titrated to effect
C. 0.2 mg/kg
D. 0.2 mg/kg plus 0.1 mg/kg titrated to effect

2 **According to the American College of Emergency Physicians, which patient should receive an opioid in the emergency department?**

A. A patient with a chronic pain condition whose primary doctor is out of town
B. A patient with an acute traumatic femur fracture
C. A patient with dental pain
D. A patient with kidney stones

3 **Which opioid appears to be safest in patients with liver failure?**

A. Fentanyl
B. Hydromorphone
C. Morphine
D. Tramadol

4 **Which opioid can precipitate serotonin syndrome?**

A. Codeine
B. Hydromorphone
C. Morphine
D. Tramadol

5 **Which oral opioid is most expensive on the black market?**

A. Hydrocodone
B. Morphine sulfate
C. Oxycodone
D. Tramadol

6 **Which intravenous opioid is the best choice in patients with renal failure?**

A. Fentanyl
B. Hydrocodone
C. Hydromorphone
D. Morphine

7 **Which oral opioid is most addictive?**

A. Hydrocodone
B. Morphine sulfate
C. Oxycodone
D. Tramadol

8 **Which opioid has the shortest duration of action?**

A. Fentanyl
B. Hydrocodone
C. Morphine
D. Oxycodone

9 **Which morphine metabolite appears to cause respiratory depression in patients with renal failure?**

A. Hydromorphone
B. Morphine-3-glucuronide
C. Morphine-6-glucuronide
D. Oxycodone

10 **Which opioid analgesic causes the most euphoria?**

A. Codeine
B. Hydrocodone
C. Hydromorphone
D. Morphine

11 What is generally not indicated in the management of severe iron poisoning?

A. Abdominal x-rays
B. Activated charcoal
C. Gastric lavage
D. Whole bowel irrigation

12 Which laboratory value may indicate the use of deferoxamine for iron poisonings?

A. Decreased total iron-binding capacity
B. Elevated total iron-binding capacity
C. Serum iron level of 345 µg/dL
D. The presence of acidosis

13 In the management of *Amanita phalloides* poisoning, which therapy may be lifesaving?

A. Amatoxin antibodies
B. Chelation therapy
C. High-dose penicillin therapy
D. Liver transplant

14 Which symptom is a muscarinic effect, as opposed to a nicotinic effect?

A. Bronchorrhea
B. Delirium
C. Muscle fasciculations
D. Seizures

15 Which symptom is a side effect of pralidoxime?

A. Hydrocarbon pneumonitis
B. Laryngospasm
C. Muscle rigidity
D. All of these

16 In the laboratory evaluation of an agitated patient who has used PCP, what is most likely to be clinically useful?

A. Complete blood count
B. Serum LSD level
C. Serum PCP level
D. Total creatine kinase

17 In the management of agitation, tachycardia, hypertension, or seizures in the cocaine-intoxicated patient, which drug category would be the best choice?

A. Benzodiazepines
B. Beta-blockers
C. Calcium channel blockers
D. Haloperidol

18 The presence of coma, pinpoint pupils, and respiratory depression is suggestive of which toxicity?

A. Cocaine
B. Hallucinogens such as psilocybin mushrooms
C. Methamphetamine intoxication
D. Opioids such as morphine or heroin

19 Which alcohol is associated with gastritis and ketosis but not acidosis?

A. Ethyl alcohol
B. Ethylene glycol
C. Isopropyl alcohol
D. Methyl alcohol

20 Which toxic ingestion may be associated with calcium oxalate crystals in the urine?

A. Acetaminophen
B. Bath salts
C. Ethylene glycol
D. Methanol

ANSWER KEY FOR DECEMBER 2022, VOLUME 36, NUMBER 12

1	2	3	4	5	6	7	8	9	10	11	12	13	14	15	16	17	18	19	20
A	C	D	B	B	A	C	D	B	C	D	B	D	C	B	C	D	D	A	C

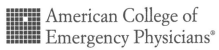

American College of Emergency Physicians®

ADVANCING EMERGENCY CARE

Post Office Box 619911
Dallas, Texas 75261-9911

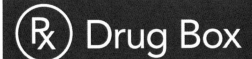

Drug Box

Doxycycline Postexposure Prophylaxis

By Micaela Simon, FNP-C, AAHIVS; and Frank LoVecchio, DO, MPH, FACEP
Be Well Family Care, Tempe, and Valleywise Health and ASU, Phoenix, Arizona

Objective
On completion of this column, you should be able to:
- Explain the recommendations for doxyPEP in bacterial STI prevention.

Background
A 2022 study revealed that significant proportions of bacterial STIs, such as gonorrhea, chlamydia, and syphilis, are prevented with a single dose of doxycycline administered within 3 days of unprotected sex. The clinical trial was terminated early after the treatment was shown to be statistically effective for men who have sex with men (MSM) and transgender women; both groups were either living with HIV or on HIV pre-exposure prophylaxis (HIV PrEP).

Research
The study compared two groups of approximately 1,200 total patients in San Francisco and Seattle. One group received 200 mg of doxycycline postexposure prophylaxis (doxyPEP) within 3 days of having unprotected sex; the other group received the current standard of care (ie, no doxyPEP). Randomization between the doxyPEP and non-doxyPEP groups was 2:1. STI testing was completed at enrollment, quarterly, and when patients were symptomatic. Patients had a median number of nine sex partners in the 3 months prior to treatment. During the past year, 67% of the participants had gonorrhea, 58% had *Chlamydia trachomatis*, and 20% had syphilis. At enrollment, 18% of the participants had gonorrhea, 10% had *C. trachomatis*, and 2% had syphilis.

An interim analysis revealed a 66% and 62% reduction in STIs in patients on HIV PrEP and patients with HIV, respectively, who received doxyPEP compared to patients who did not receive doxyPEP. Gonorrhea, chlamydia, and syphilis were each reduced. Doxycycline was considered safe and well tolerated in these patients, with no reports of serious drug-related adverse events.

Among 360 participants on HIV PrEP, 65 STI endpoints (29.5%) occurred in controls, and 47 STI endpoints (9.6%) occurred in doxyPEP recipients (RR 0.33; 95% CI, 0.23-0.47; P <0.0001). Among 194 participants with HIV, 30 STI endpoints (27.8%) occurred in controls, and 31 STI endpoints (11.7%) occurred in doxyPEP recipients (RR 0.42; 95% CI, 0.25-0.75; P = 0.0014).

Results from this study suggest doxyPEP taken within 3 days of unprotected sex by patients at high risk for STIs can decrease the likelihood of developing gonorrhea, chlamydia, and syphilis. Although doxycycline's efficacy in preventing these STIs in lower-risk groups is unknown, physicians may consider prescribing it for similar situations of unprotected sex in lower-risk patients as well. Doxycycline's effectiveness in preventing other bacterial STIs is also unknown. DoxyPEP does not prevent HIV, mpox, or other viral STIs such as human papillomavirus and herpes simplex virus.

REFERENCE
Luetkemeyer A, Dombrowski J, Cohen S, et al. Doxycycline post-exposure prophylaxis for STI prevention among MSM and transgender women on HIV PrEP or living with HIV: high efficacy to reduce incident STI's in a randomized trial. AIDS 2022. https://programme.aids2022.org/Abstract/Abstract/?abstractid=13231

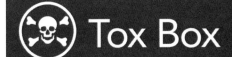

Tox Box

Acute Arsenic Ingestion

By Christian A. Tomaszewski, MD, MS, MBA, FACEP
University of California San Diego Health

Objective
On completion of this column, you should be able to:
- Recognize and treat acute arsenic poisoning.

Arsenic compounds are typically used as pesticides and in ceramic and semiconductor manufacturing and often have a distinct garlicky odor. Acute arsenic poisoning usually occurs through ingestion but can also occur through inhalation or skin absorption.

Toxicokinetics
- Readily absorbed in the GI tract
- Potentially lethal at doses >120-200 mg in adults and >2 mg/kg in children
- More toxic in inorganic trivalent and pentavalent forms than in organic forms
- Disruptive to oxidative phosphorylation and inhibitive to gluconeogenesis and glutathione metabolism

Clinical Manifestations
- ***Dermatologic:*** Irritation and mucosal burning
- ***GI:*** Abdominal pain, nausea, vomiting, and watery diarrhea
- ***Cardiac:*** Hypotension, tachycardia, and QTc prolongation
- ***Neurologic:*** Delayed motor and sensory neuropathies
- ***Renal:*** Renal failure
- ***Hepatic:*** Hepatitis

Diagnostics
- If symptomatic:
  - CBC and comprehensive metabolic panel
  - Tests for arsenic concentration
- Arsenic concentration:
  - 24-hour urinary arsenic (>100 μg is abnormal)
  - May need to speciate if elevated from seafood
- ECG — check QTc interval
- Abdominal x-ray — arsenic compounds are radiopaque

Treatment
- IV fluids for rehydration
- Antidote if symptomatic:
  - Dimercaprol 3-5 mg/kg IM every 4-6 hours for severe poisoning
  - Dimercaptosuccinic acid (ie, succimer) 10 mg/kg PO every 8 hours for 5 days
- Hemodialysis is usually ineffective.

Critical decisions
in emergency medicine

Volume 37 Number 2: **February 2023**

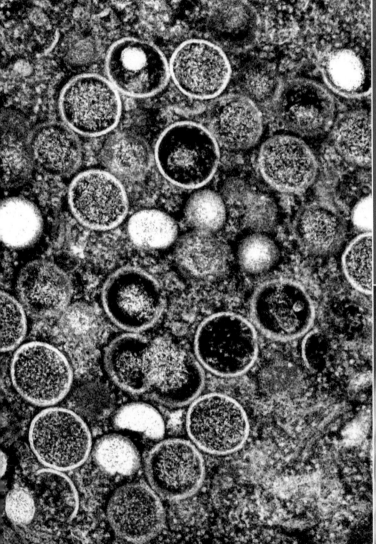

Skin Deep

The mpox outbreak of 2022 was declared a public health emergency by the WHO and proved to be a diagnostic challenge for emergency physicians worldwide. Mpox can vary in its presentation, and its lesions can appear like those of other illnesses. Emergency physicians must be familiar with the signs, symptoms, and diagnostic process to properly mitigate this viral infection.

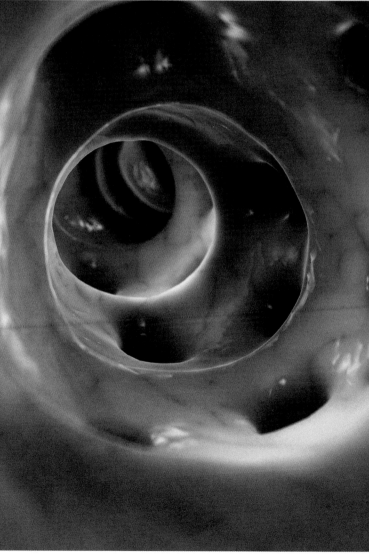

Gut Feeling

Emergency department visits for inflammatory bowel disease, including Crohn disease and ulcerative colitis, are trending upward. Presentations can be similar to diverticular disease. Emergency physicians must be able to differentiate between these GI diseases for accurate treatment of their potentially life-threatening complications.

THE OFFICIAL CME PUBLICATION OF THE AMERICAN COLLEGE OF EMERGENCY PHYSICIANS

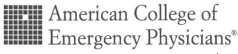

American College of Emergency Physicians®

ADVANCING EMERGENCY CARE

Critical decisions
in emergency medicine

Critical Decisions in Emergency Medicine is the official CME publication of the American College of Emergency Physicians. Additional volumes are available.

EDITOR-IN-CHIEF

Michael S. Beeson, MD, MBA, FACEP
Northeastern Ohio Universities,
Rootstown, OH

SECTION EDITORS

Joshua S. Broder, MD, FACEP
Duke University, Durham, NC

Andrew J. Eyre, MD, MS-HPEd
Brigham and Women's Hospital/
Harvard Medical School, Boston, MA

John Kiel, DO, MPH, FACEP, CAQSM
University of Florida College of Medicine,
Jacksonville, FL

Frank LoVecchio, DO, MPH, FACEP
Valleywise, Arizona State University, University of Arizona, and Creighton Colleges of Medicine, Phoenix, AZ

Sharon E. Mace, MD, FACEP
Cleveland Clinic Lerner College of Medicine/
Case Western Reserve University, Cleveland, OH

Amal Mattu, MD, FACEP
University of Maryland, Baltimore, MD

Christian A. Tomaszewski, MD, MS, MBA, FACEP
University of California Health Sciences,
San Diego, CA

Steven J. Warrington, MD, MEd, MS
MercyOne Siouxland, Sioux City, IA

ASSOCIATE EDITORS

Tareq Al-Salamah, MBBS, MPH, FACEP
King Saud University, Riyadh, Saudi Arabia/
University of Maryland, Baltimore, MD

Wan-Tsu Chang, MD
University of Maryland, Baltimore, MD

Ann M. Dietrich, MD, FAAP, FACEP
University of South Carolina College of Medicine,
Greenville, SC

Kelsey Drake, MD, MPH, FACEP
St. Anthony Hospital, Lakewood, CO

Walter L. Green, MD, FACEP
UT Southwestern Medical Center, Dallas, TX

John C. Greenwood, MD
University of Pennsylvania, Philadelphia, PA

Danya Khoujah, MBBS, MEHP, FACEP
University of Maryland, Baltimore, MD

Nathaniel Mann, MD
Greenville Health System, Greenville, SC

George Sternbach, MD, FACEP
Stanford University Medical Center, Stanford, CA

EDITORIAL STAFF

Suzannah Alexander, Editorial Director
salexander@acep.org

Joy Carrico, JD
Managing Editor

Alex Bass
Assistant Editor

Kyle Powell
Graphic Artist

ISSN2325-0186 (Print)   ISSN2325-8365 (Online)

Contents

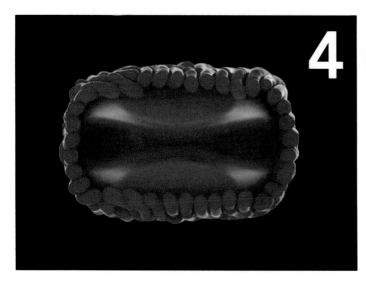

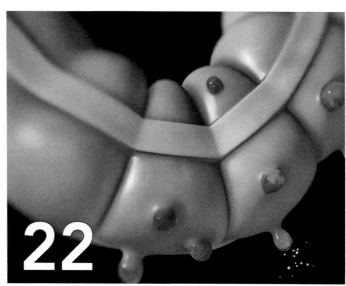

FEATURES

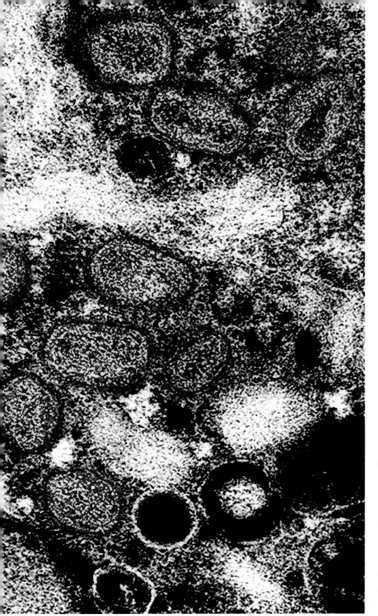

Skin Deep

Managing Mpox

LESSON 3

 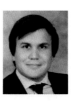

By Jacob A. Gianuzzi, DO; Ernesto Weisson, MD; Brandon Wisinski, DO, MBA, MS; John Downing, DO, FACEP; Alexis Borrelli; and Jonathan Martin, DO

Dr. Gianuzzi and Dr. Weisson are emergency medicine residents and Dr. Wisinski is an attending physician at Franciscan Health Olympia Fields, Illinois. Dr. Downing is an attending physician and medical director at Franciscan Health Munster in Munster, Indiana, and faculty for the Franciscan Health Emergency Medicine Residency in Olympia Fields. Ms. Borrelli is at Midwestern University in Chicago, Illinois. Dr. Martin is an infectious disease attending physician for Cook County Health and an associate professor of medicine at Rush University in Chicago.

Reviewed by Michael S. Beeson, MD, MBA, FACEP

Objectives

On completion of this lesson, you should be able to:

1. State the risk factors for mpox and identify high-risk populations.
2. Describe the three phases of mpox and the accompanying signs and symptoms.
3. Distinguish the characteristics of mpox lesions from lesions of other dermatologic diseases.
4. Explain the diagnostic process and treatment options for mpox.

From the EM Model

10.0 Systemic Infectious Disorders
    10.6 Viral
    10.7 Emerging Infections/Pandemics

■ CRITICAL DECISIONS ■

- What epidemiologic features led the mpox outbreak to be declared a global health emergency?
- What are the three phases of mpox, and how do symptoms differ by phase?
- How are mpox lesions differentiated from similar dermatologic infections like chickenpox, scabies, and smallpox?
- How is mpox diagnosed?
- What prevention and treatment options exist for mpox, and which patients are candidates?
- What are the common complications of mpox, and when do they occur?

The mpox outbreak of 2022 was declared a public health emergency by the WHO and proved to be a diagnostic challenge for emergency physicians worldwide. Mpox can vary in its presentation, and its lesions can appear similar to those of other illnesses. Emergency physicians must be familiar with the signs, symptoms, and diagnostic process to properly mitigate this propagating viral infection.

CASE ONE

A 34-year-old man presents with generalized fatigue, a headache, and a sore throat that has lasted 2 days. He states that he recently traveled from California and denies having received COVID-19 or influenza vaccines this season. He reports that acetaminophen has not relieved his symptoms. His initial vital signs include BP 133/67, P 93, and T 38.1°C (100.6°F); SpO_2 is 97% on room air. On examination, he appears comfortable with no significant findings; his oropharynx is clear, and he has no rash or nuchal rigidity.

CASE TWO

A 2-year-old girl presents with a rash and decreased appetite for the past 3 days. She has had low-grade fevers and nasal congestion. A rash extends primarily across her hands, feet, and face. She attends day care and is up to date on vaccinations. Her vital signs include BP 113/57, P 104, and T 38.3°C (100.9°F); SpO_2 is 99% on room air. During examination, the girl is fussy and has mild rhinorrhea and several white papular lesions along her palms and feet.

CASE THREE

A 22-year-old man presents with a penile rash. He has also been fatigued over the last 3 to 4 days and has had a backache, chills, and swollen lymph nodes in the groin area. Approximately 1 week prior to symptoms, he spent 3 days at a rave, where he danced and used drugs with other young men. Hydrocortisone cream has not helped his rash despite multiple applications over the last 3 days. His vital signs include BP 121/73, P 83, and T 37.2°C (98.9°F); SpO_2 is 96% on room air. Multiple pustule-like lesions on his penis and groin area are seen during examination along with several prominent inguinal lymph nodes. No penile discharge is noted.

Introduction

Mpox (previously monkeypox) is a zoonotic infection caused by the *Monkeypox virus*, a large, enveloped, and linear double-stranded DNA poxvirus of the genus *Orthopoxvirus* — the same genus as the *Variola virus* (smallpox virus) and the *Vaccinia virus* (used in the smallpox vaccine) (*Figure 1*). The *Monkeypox virus* is endemic to Central and West Africa, but 2022 saw a concerning increase in cases in nonendemic areas of Europe and the Americas (*Figure 2*).[1] Initial signs and symptoms of mpox are nonspecific and systemic, such as fever, fatigue, headaches, myalgia, and lymphadenopathy. These systemic symptoms are followed by the development of mucocutaneous lesions that often last from 2 to 3 weeks. Infection spreads from human to human or animal to human through direct contact with lesions and bodily fluids.[2] Although cases of mpox have been reported since the 1970s, the recent 2022 outbreak highlights the challenges emergency physicians face in successfully diagnosing a previously uncommon disease that presents with nonspecific, variable symptoms and that is misconceived as being contracted only through sexual activity. Mpox is not exclusively a sexually transmitted infection (STI); it can infect anyone who has been in close, prolonged physical contact with an infected person's active lesions, including family members or caregivers. Several infections have been described in people who did not have traditional risk factors.

CRITICAL DECISION

What epidemiologic features led the mpox outbreak to be declared a global health emergency?

The *Monkeypox virus* was first identified in 1958 when a pox-like disease broke out in colonies of research monkeys. The first human cases were recorded in the Democratic Republic of the Congo in 1970; in the decades since, the *Monkeypox virus* has been endemic to regions of Central and West Africa. It spreads from animals to humans mainly through direct contact with lesions on animal reservoirs, which are predominantly small rodents, such as tree squirrels, Gambian rats, and prairie dogs. In 2022, increased numbers of mpox cases in nonendemic regions led the WHO to begin closely monitoring the spread and burden of the virus. When the WHO received reports of 3,040 mpox cases in 47 countries by June 2022, the International Health Regulations Emergency Committee met to assess whether this mpox outbreak constituted a public health emergency of international concern (PHEIC). The WHO's criteria for the PHEIC designation include:

- A serious, sudden, unusual, or unexpected emergence;

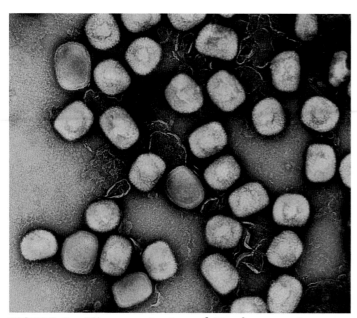

FIGURE 1. **Microscopic view of *Monkeypox virus*.** *Credit:* CDC. https://phil.cdc.gov/Details.aspx?pid=26499

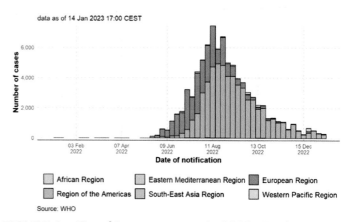

FIGURE 2. **Trend in mpox cases in 2022.** *Credit:* WHO. https://worldhealthorg.shinyapps.io/mpx_global/

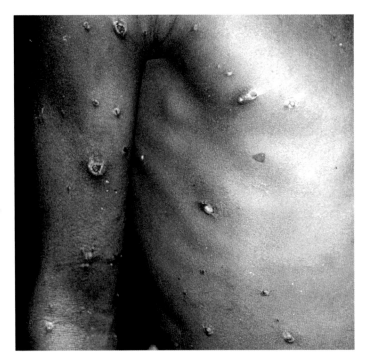

FIGURE 3. Mpox lesions on a chest. *Credit:* CDC.
https://phil.cdc.gov/Details.aspx?pid=12779

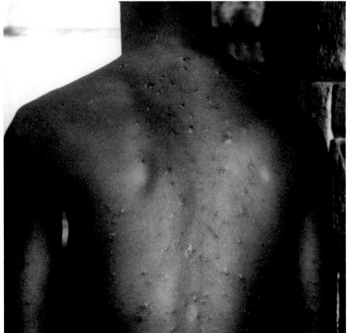

FIGURE 4. Chickenpox lesions on a back.
Credit: CDC. https://phil.cdc.gov/Details.aspx?pid=4367

- Implications for public health beyond the affected region's national border; and
- The potential need for immediate international action.

Although not considered a PHEIC at this initial meeting, 4 weeks later (after cases rose to 16,000 in 75 countries and territories, including 5 deaths) the committee reconvened and declared the mpox outbreak a PHEIC.

In August 2022, the United States followed suit, as did many other countries affected by mpox, and declared the mpox outbreak a public health emergency (PHE). The PHE declaration allows the Department of Health and Human Services (HHS) to expedite actions for addressing the outbreak, including increased resource flexibility and reduced restrictions on data sharing. The HHS renewed mpox as a PHE on November 2, 2022. However, it has since announced that it will not renew mpox's PHE status after its expiration on January 31, 2023, due to a low number of cases.[3,4] In November 2022, the WHO announced a name change for the condition from monkeypox to mpox, to reduce stigma associated with the name.[5]

Currently, patients who are most at risk of mpox include men who have sex with men (MSM), persons living with HIV, commercial sex workers, and people who are taking HIV pre- or postexposure prophylaxis (PrEP and PEP, respectively) or who are candidates for PrEP or PEP.

CRITICAL DECISION

What are the three phases of mpox, and how do symptoms differ by phase?

Clinical manifestations of an infection of the classic *Monkeypox virus* strain differ from those of the new, epidemic *Monkeypox virus* variant. The classic form of an mpox infection consists of three phases: the incubation, prodrome, and eruptive phases. The incubation period lasts anywhere from 3 to 34 days, with a mean of 13 days. The subsequent prodromal phase ranges in duration from 1 to 4 days and consists of fatigue, fever, headache, and cervical and maxillary lymphadenopathy. The final eruptive phase lasts

from 14 to 28 days and consists of a viral exanthem in a centrifugal distribution, concentrated on the face and extremities. The rash appears as macules that progress to papules, vesicles, and pustules; they eventually desquamate to form areas of hypopigmentation followed by hyperpigmentation. The lesions typically progress together through the stages of development, tend to be firm with an umbilicated center, and are associated with pruritis and myalgia (*Figure 3*). Children and young adults are more commonly affected by the classic form of mpox, further complicating its differentiation from another infection that predominates in this age group, the varicella infection (ie, chickenpox).

By contrast, an infection with the epidemic variant of mpox often presents without a prodromal phase; unlike the classic form's lesions that progress together, each lesion in the epidemic form can progress at a different rate, leading to a clinical presentation of lesions in various stages of healing, similar to that of chickenpox. It is not uncommon for patients infected with the epidemic variant to present in a fulminant eruptive phase characterized by varying stages of macules and papules, umbilicated vesicles, pustules, and desquamation with varying degrees of hypo- and hyperpigmentation. Epidemic mpox's lesions are often described as painful or pruritic and are fewer in number and associated with less prominent lymphadenopathy than those of the classic form.[6] Lesions from the epidemic variant also occur primarily in the perianal and genital region, followed by the face and mouth, and less commonly, the hands, feet, and chest.

CRITICAL DECISION

How are mpox lesions differentiated from similar dermatologic infections like chickenpox, scabies, and smallpox?

An important clinical skill is the ability to differentiate between dermatologic lesions. This skill is often neglected in emergency medicine, however, because of the rarity of life-threatening dermatologic diseases and, before the recent mpox outbreak, the rarity of having more than one pox disease circulating in the same geographic region at the same time. Notably, several unique features of mpox lesions distinguish them from similar dermatologic infections like chickenpox, scabies, and smallpox.

Chickenpox infections manifest primarily as fragile, thin-walled, clear fluid–filled blisters that are polymorphous in nature, meaning they appear in waves and at various stages of healing (*Figure 4*). Although mpox lesions can also be polymorphous, they are larger, deeper, firmer, and more rubbery than the superficial, fragile lesions of chickenpox. Mpox lesions' hardier texture is attributed to the cell debris, rather than fluid or pus, that fills them. Childhood chickenpox usually lacks a prodrome phase. In adolescents and adults with chickenpox — the most-affected mpox demographic by far — the prodrome phase is more common, but its presence cannot definitively differentiate chickenpox from mpox. Also, although chickenpox lesions develop diffusely, they rarely involve the palms and soles like mpox lesions can. The timeline of lesions is also helpful: Chickenpox lesions heal within 14 days — usually within 5 to 7 days in most cases — while mpox lesions usually persist longer at 14 to 28 days. Importantly, mpox lesions can persist for months in immunosuppressed patients.

Mpox infections have also been commonly mistaken for scabies, a dermatologic disease caused by infestation with a mite called *Sarcoptes scabiei*. While in their papular or vesicular phase, mpox lesions can appear very similar to scabies. Lesion distribution can also be similar between mpox infections and scabies, but scabies lesions tend to occur in skin folds such as the wrist, interdigital spaces, beltline, and gluteal sulcus, where the mites prefer to live (*Figure 5*). Both diseases can have a similarly longer duration because scabies infections usually persist until appropriate medical treatment is administered.

Smallpox, whose infecting organism is also a member of the genus *Orthopoxvirus*, is the most similar in presentation to mpox. However, naturally occurring smallpox was declared eradicated by the WHO in 1980; herd immunity was achieved in the late 1970s, and no further natural outbreaks occurred after 1978.[7] Although the dermal lesions of smallpox are nearly indistinguishable from mpox, smallpox lesions appear more abruptly and diffusely, occurring within a 36-hour period — after which no new lesions form — and involve both the skin and mucous membranes. Smallpox is also accompanied by a prodrome phase of flu-like and GI symptoms that have not been described in mpox. Furthermore, following smallpox's dermatologic manifestation, the disease can take four distinct clinical courses — ordinary, modified, malignant, or hemorrhagic — all of which are readily distinguishable from mpox, in which cutaneous lesions are its end stage.

If the suspected mode of mpox transmission is sexual activity, physicians must consider other STIs as part of mpox's differential diagnosis because multiple infections can be transmitted during sexual activity. Coinfections with HIV, herpes, syphilis, and other STIs have been widely reported.[8,9] Many STIs present similarly to mpox and can be overlooked, especially in high-risk populations. Lesions associated with genital herpesvirus infections are typically more vesicular. They are also clustered in and largely limited to the genitals and mucosal surfaces in immunocompetent patients. Primary syphilis typically presents as a round, firm, painless chancre at the point of inoculation. The rash of secondary syphilis is disseminated and associated with constitutional symptoms like fever and malaise, which are similar to those of the classic form of mpox. Ulcers associated with secondary syphilis, however, are rare, and secondary syphilis' rash is usually more macular, papular, or maculopapular than that of mpox.

CRITICAL DECISION

How is mpox diagnosed?

Rapid identification and diagnosis of mpox is critical to limiting its spread; infected persons remain contagious until the lesions crust over and fall off. Specimens for evaluation are collected by swabbing the lesions or exudate and transporting them to a laboratory according to individual lab requirements. Alternatively, skin biopsies may be obtained and sent for pathologic evaluation. Specimens are evaluated through electron microscopy, viral culture, or molecular identification using nucleic acid amplification tests such as polymerase chain reaction (PCR) and DNA sequencing. The WHO currently recommends PCR testing that targets various viral genomes of mpox.[10] Serologic testing can also evaluate for MPXV-specific immunoglobulin M within 5 days of presentation or immunoglobulin G after 8 days of presentation but is rarely used in clinical practice.[11]

CRITICAL DECISION

What prevention and treatment options exist for mpox, and which patients are candidates?

Mpox Treatment and Indications

The vast majority of mpox infections are self-limiting and best managed supportively. For example, in patients with significant pain from mpox lesions, especially in those with mpox tonsillitis or proctitis, analgesic therapy with NSAIDs and acetaminophen may be indicated.

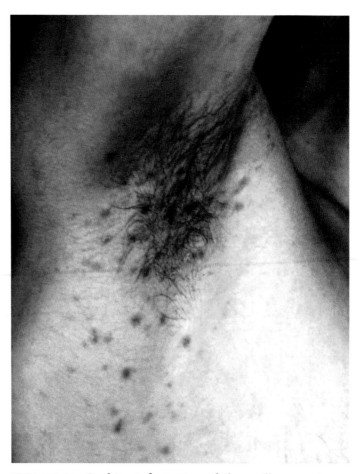

FIGURE 5. Scabies infestation of the axillary region. *Credit:* CDC. https://phil.cdc.gov/Details.aspx?pid=15345

In patients who develop mpox proctitis, other supportive therapies such as stool softeners and sitz baths may be beneficial. Dehydration secondary to tonsillitis-induced dysphagia or persistent vomiting can be treated with antiemetics. Intravenous fluid hydration may also be administered, depending on the clinical assessment of volume status.

For patients with or at high risk of severe mpox, several antiviral therapies exist to minimize disease severity, mitigate pain and swelling, and reduce the sequelae of abscesses and scarring. Indications for antiviral treatment include severe disease; involvement of sensitive anatomical sites such as the oropharynx, rectum, anus, eye, or CNS; a severely compromised immune system; young age, especially patients younger than 8 years; pregnancy and breastfeeding; and comorbidities of chronic skin diseases such as atopic dermatitis or psoriasis.[12]

Tecovirimat is an antiviral drug originally developed to treat smallpox and is now utilized in both the United States and Europe as a first-line antiviral treatment for mpox. Tecovirimat reduces the duration and amount of viral shedding by blocking the *Orthopoxvirus* envelope protein vp37. Blocking this protein inhibits cell-to-cell viral transmission by preventing viral maturation and release from its host cell.[6] Tecovirimat exists in both oral and intravenous forms, and side effects include headaches, abdominal pain, nausea, and vomiting. Tecovirimat's use is currently limited to physicians enrolled in the open trial network authorized under the CDC's Investigational New Drug protocol.[12]

Brincidofovir is an alternative mpox antiviral agent utilized in the United States and originally developed to treat smallpox. Brincidofovir inhibits *Orthopoxvirus'* DNA polymerase. Patients who use brincidofovir must complete liver function tests before and during treatment because this medication can elevate transaminases and bilirubin. Other side effects include abdominal pain, nausea, vomiting, and diarrhea. Brincidofovir is taken orally, but an intravenous equivalent known as cidofovir also exists. Cidofovir has the same mechanism of action as brincidofvir but has greater potential for kidney damage. Other side effects of cidofovir include fever, decreased serum bicarbonate, proteinuria, neutropenia, iritis, and uveitis. The utilization of these medications is limited to patients who have taken tecovirimat and still have severe mpox or are at a higher risk of progression to severe mpox.

Vaccinia immune globulin is an FDA-licensed intravenous treatment for complications from the smallpox vaccine and is now utilized to treat severe mpox infections in patients with an impaired antibody response who continue to have severe symptoms after receiving other mpox treatments. Vaccinia immune globulin provides passive immunity to mpox by using antibodies from people vaccinated against smallpox. Side effects include headache, nausea, rigors, and dizziness.[13]

Mpox Prevention, Vaccinations, and Candidacy

Because most mpox cases are mild and self-limiting, community-level public health measures are the preferred approach for reducing its transmission. This approach recommends that infected and likely infected people isolate at home, avoid individuals at high risk of developing serious infections, avoid public transport, cover their skin lesions (to limit contact), and follow strict hand hygiene.

Potential vaccines are being evaluated for mpox. The smallpox vaccination has sufficient cross-reactivity among orthopoxviruses to protect against mpox infection. However, this vaccine's routine use as a prevention strategy was discontinued in the 1980s when smallpox was eradicated. Currently, the two FDA-licensed smallpox vaccines

being evaluated for their efficacy against the current epidemic mpox are the smallpox (live attenuated vaccinia virus) vaccine and the smallpox and mpox (replication-deficient live vaccinia virus) vaccine (*Table 1*). The smallpox (vaccinia) vaccine is a live attenuated vaccine utilized both before and after mpox exposure to prevent disease.[6] It is a second-generation smallpox vaccine with a similar safety profile to the first generation.[14] Only one dose is required, and it is administered using the scarification technique, in which multiple puncture wounds are made in the skin when giving the vaccine. If vaccinated successfully, a "take," or open sore with localized infection, develops at the injection site; immunity is then achieved 28 days after successful vaccine administration. The smallpox and monkeypox vaccine is a third-generation, replication-deficient live vaccine used to prevent smallpox in Europe and the United States. The US Food and Drug Administration has authorized the vaccine for emergency use as an mpox PrEP in adults considered at high risk of severe disease. It is administered subcutaneously in two doses 28 days apart; immunity is achieved 2 weeks after the second dose is administered.[15]

Recommendations

Each smallpox vaccine is recommended for different groups of people. Currently, the smallpox and mpox vaccine is indicated for sex workers, MSM, anyone with recent (<14 days) skin-to-skin or close contact with someone diagnosed with mpox, people with HIV (especially those who do not regularly take their antiviral medications) or who are eligible for or currently taking HIV PrEP, and anyone who anticipates having these risk factors. The Advisory Committee on Immunization Practices currently recommends the smallpox vaccine or the smallpox and mpox vaccine for any person at risk of occupational exposure to orthopoxviruses, including mpox. Additionally, individuals who administer the smallpox vaccine or care for patients infected with mpox should be offered either vaccine. Booster vaccination doses are recommended every 3 years with the smallpox vaccine or every 4 years with the smallpox and mpox vaccine for workers who will have long-term exposure to mpox and other virulent orthopoxviruses. Other candidates for vaccination include certain military personnel and laboratory workers.[16]

✔ Pearls

- Mpox should be suspected in patients presenting with a diffuse ulcerative rash, especially when those patients are considered high risk, including MSM, commercial sex workers, patients with HIV, or people taking HIV PrEP or PEP.

- Patients suspected of having contracted mpox through sexual activity should be tested for other STIs including gonorrhea, chlamydia, syphilis, and HIV. Many patients with mpox have a concurrent STI.

- Antiviral treatment with tecovirimat is recommended for anyone with mpox who has severe disease, has lesions in a sensitive anatomic site, is immunocompromised, is pregnant or breastfeeding, or is younger than 8 years old.

- Mpox vaccinations can be considered for anyone in a high-risk group.

Vaccine	Type	Indications	Contraindications	Side Effects	Special Considerations
Smallpox Vaccine	Live attenuated vaccinia virus	PrEP and PEP • Individuals with occupational exposure to mpox and other orthopoxviruses • Individuals who administer mpox vaccines • Medical professionals caring for patients with mpox • Certain military personnel and laboratory workers	• Hypersensitivity to any vaccine component • Immunocompromised • History of exfoliative dermatitis, including atopy • History of ischemic heart disease • Pregnant or breastfeeding • Living with anyone with a contraindication	• **Cardiac (rare):** pericarditis, myocarditis, dilated cardiomyopathy, and ischemia • **CNS (rare):** encephalopathy, encephalitis, Guillain-Barré syndrome, Bell palsy, and keratitis • **Dermatologic (rare):** Stevens-Johnson syndrome, erythema multiforme, and eczema • **Other side effects:** local vaccine reaction, nausea, diarrhea, lymphadenopathy, fatigue, headache, and myalgias	• Single-dose vaccine • Immunity at 28 days post vaccine • Benefit must outweigh risk in patients with ischemic cardiac disease • Booster every 3 years if viral exposure is chronic
Smallpox and Mpox Vaccine	Replication-deficient live vaccinia virus	PrEP only • Individuals with occupational exposure to mpox and other orthopoxviruses • Individuals who administer mpox vaccines • Medical professionals caring for patients with mpox • Certain military personnel and laboratory workers	• Hypersensitivity to any vaccine component • Immunocompromised • History of exfoliative dermatitis, including atopy • History of ischemic heart disease • Pregnant or breastfeeding	• **Cardiac (rare):** ST- or T-wave anomalies, palpitations, tachycardia, and asymptomatic, mild troponin elevations <2x upper limit of normal • **GI:** appetite changes and nausea • **Other side effects:** local vaccine reaction, fatigue, and headache	• Two-dose vaccine • Immunity at 14 days post series • Booster every 4 years if viral exposure is chronic

TABLE 1. Comparison of the smallpox vaccine and smallpox and monkeypox vaccine

Vaccine Adverse Effects

Complications of the smallpox vaccine include cardiac effects such as myocarditis.[14] As a nonreplicating vaccine, the smallpox and mpox vaccine is thought to have less risk of adverse effects than the smallpox vaccine. However, the risk of myocarditis in individuals who receive the smallpox and mpox vaccine is currently unknown.[16]

Special Considerations

Both vaccinations are contraindicated in individuals with significant allergies to any of the vaccine components. The smallpox vaccine is contraindicated as a primary vaccine in individuals who are immunocompromised, are pregnant or breastfeeding, have a history of exfoliative skin conditions such as atopic dermatitis, or have a known underlying heart disease such as coronary artery disease or cardiomyopathy. Immunocompromising conditions include, but are not limited to, malignancy, HIV or AIDS, and transplant organ recipients. The smallpox vaccine is also contraindicated in individuals who live with anyone with these conditions. Individuals who cannot receive the smallpox vaccine for any of these reasons may be able to receive the smallpox and mpox vaccine but may still be at risk of severe disease and, therefore, should attempt to avoid exposure to orthopoxviruses for the duration of their condition if possible (eg, breastfeeding and pregnancy).[17]

CRITICAL DECISION

What are the common complications of mpox, and when do they occur?

The most common complication of mpox is a superimposed cutaneous bacterial infection, or cellulitis. Pneumonitis and keratitis, the latter of which can lead to vision loss, are also possible.[18] Mpox is associated with neurologic complications, including mood disturbances and neuralgia (nerve pain described as burning or electric sensations). Although rare, mpox invasion of the nervous system can cause encephalitis and seizures, particularly in immunosuppressed patients — a sequelae in these patients also seen with other viruses, most notably herpes and varicella-zoster.[19] Guillain-Barré syndrome, transverse myelitis, and acute disseminated encephalomyelitis (historically seen after smallpox infections) are also theoretical neurologic complications of mpox but have not yet been documented.[20]

Summary

Mpox is a zoonotic viral infection that spreads between humans through close physical contact. Previously endemic to Central and West Africa, recent mpox outbreaks have occurred in other parts of the world, causing the WHO to declare it a PHEIC.

Mpox presents as a diffuse or localized ulcerative rash that is sometimes associated with fevers and lymphadenopathy. The rash starts as papular and progresses to pustular with central umbilication. The lesions are painful; have a firm and rubbery texture; take multiple weeks to heal; and in the most recent outbreak, present in various stages of healing — all important features that can help differentiate mpox from other clinical diagnoses like genital herpes, syphilis, and chickenpox. Groups most at risk of the 2022 epidemic mpox infection are MSM, people with or at risk of contracting HIV, and commercial sex workers.

The disease is often self-limiting and treated with supportive care, but antiviral treatment may benefit people with severe cases of mpox, weakened immune systems, or lesions in sensitive areas. The most common mpox antiviral agent is tecovirimat. Vaccination either as PrEP or early PEP is indicated for high-risk groups.

CASE RESOLUTIONS

■ CASE ONE

This patient recently traveled from a state with more cases of viral illness, including mpox. His clinical presentation was similar to other viral syndromes, including COVID-19 and influenza, but because of his recent travel, mpox was included in the differential diagnosis. His symptoms had recently started, without evidence of a rash. The patient was evaluated for sepsis given his fever and elevated heart rate (>90 bpm). His workup was negative for influenza and COVID-19. His laboratory results, chest x-ray, and urinalysis were unremarkable. He was discharged home with supportive care but returned a day later with a prevalent rash across his upper back. An mpox viral panel was positive on day 7 of symptoms. He continued with supportive care and had almost complete symptom resolution 15 days after symptom onset.

■ CASE TWO

The otherwise healthy 2-year-old patient had a rash that was concerning for mpox, several pediatric viruses including coxsackievirus, and tick-borne illnesses. However, her rash did not fit the description of most of the common viruses in children. Viral swabs were negative for COVID-19 and influenza. She was treated conservatively with ibuprofen for her fever, and her family was given reassurance. Viral swabs for mpox were positive on day 7 of symptoms. Continued supportive care at home led to complete resolution of symptoms approximately 16 days from symptom onset.

■ CASE THREE

Several high-risk behaviors and symptoms for mpox, including a genital rash, were revealed after obtaining this patient's history and conducting his physical examination. His workup was unremarkable, and mpox swabs were negative. He was discharged home with recommendations for supportive care. Two days later, he returned with a worsened rash that had spread to his anus, a high fever of 39.2°C (102.6°F), and tachycardia (120 bpm). He also had shortness of breath and increased work of breathing. Several of his lesions had merged and begun bleeding mildly. Viral swabs collected earlier were positive at this time. Intravenous fluids were administered along with antipyretics. Given his significant worsening, tecovirimat was prescribed, and he was hospitalized for 2 days. On day 8 of symptoms, his fever improved, and he was discharged home for outpatient management. His symptoms almost completely resolved 2 weeks later.

REFERENCES

1. Soheili M, Nasseri S, Afraie M, et al. Monkeypox: virology, pathophysiology, clinical characteristics, epidemiology, vaccines, diagnosis, and treatments. *J Pharm Pharm Sci.* 2022;25:297-322.

2. Kaler J, Hussain A, Flores G, Kheiri S, Desrosiers D. Monkeypox: a comprehensive review of transmission, pathogenesis, and manifestation. *Cureus.* 2022 Jul 3;14(7):e26531.

3. Statement from HHS Secretary Becerra on mpox. US Department of Health and Human Services. Published Dec. 2, 2022. https://www.hhs.gov/about/news/2022/12/02/statement-from-hhs-secretary-becerra-on-mpox.html

4. Mpox. Centers for Disease Control and Prevention. Reviewed January 6, 2023. https://www.cdc.gov/poxvirus/monkeypox/index.html

5. WHO recommends new name for monkeypox disease. World Health Organization. Published November 28, 2022. https://www.who.int/news/item/28-11-2022-who-recommends-new-name-for-monkeypox-disease

6. Thornhill JP, Barkati S, Walmsley S, et al. Monkeypox virus infection in humans across 16 countries — April-June 2022. *N Engl J Med.* 2022 Aug 25;387(8):679-691.

7. Fenner F, Henderson DA, Arita I, Jezek Z, Ladnyi ID. *Smallpox and Its Eradication.* World Health Organization; 1988. https://apps.who.int/iris/handle/10665/39485

8. Hussain A, Kaler J, Lau G, Maxwell T. Clinical conundrums: differentiating monkeypox from similarly presenting infections. *Cureus.* 2022 Oct 4;14(10):e29929.

9. Curran KG, Eberly K, Russell OO, et al. HIV and sexually transmitted infections among persons with monkeypox — eight U.S. jurisdictions, May 17-July 22, 2022. *MMWR Morb Mortal Wkly Rep.* 2022 Sep 9;71(36):1141-1147.

10. Rizk JG, Lippi G, Henry BM, Forthal DN, Rizk Y. Prevention and treatment of monkeypox. *Drugs.* 2022 Jun;82(9):957-963.

11. Poland GA, Kennedy RB, Tosh PK. Prevention of monkeypox with vaccines: a rapid review. *Lancet Infect Dis.* 2022 Dec;22(12):e349-e358.

12. Gessain A, Nakoune E, Yazdanpanah Y. Monkeypox. *N Engl J Med.* 2022 Nov 10;387(19):1783-1793.

13. Jiang Z, Sun J, Zhang L, et al. Laboratory diagnostics for monkeypox: an overview of sensitivities from various published tests. *Travel Med Infect Dis.* 2022 Sep-Oct;49:102425.

14. Petersen E, Kantele A, Koopmans M, et al. Human monkeypox: epidemiologic and clinical characteristics, diagnosis, and prevention. *Infect Dis Clin North Am.* 2019 Dec;33(4):1027-1043.

15. Rao AK, Petersen BW, Whitehill F, et al. Use of JYNNEOS (smallpox and monkeypox vaccine, live, nonreplicating) for preexposure vaccination of persons at risk for occupational exposure to orthopoxviruses: recommendations of the advisory committee on immunization practices — United States, 2022. *MMWR Morb and Mortal Wkly Rep.* 2022 Jun 3;71(22):734-742.

16. Guidance for tecovirimat use. Centers for Disease Control and Prevention. Reviewed September 15, 2022. https://www.cdc.gov/poxvirus/monkeypox/clinicians/Tecovirimat.html

17. Monkeypox. In: Organization of Teratology Information Specialists (OTIS). *Mother To Baby.* 2022 Jul. https://www.ncbi.nlm.nih.gov/books/NBK583256/

18. Saxena SK, Ansari S, Maurya VK, et al. Re-emerging human monkeypox: a major public-health debacle. *J Med Virol.* 2023 Jan;95(1):e27902.

19. Badenoch JB, Conti I, Rengasamy ER, et al. Neurological and psychiatric presentations associated with human *monkeypox virus* infection: a systematic review and meta-analysis. *EClinicalMedicine.* 2022 Oct;52:101644.

20. Billioux BJ, Mbaya OT, Sejvar J, Nath A. Potential complications of monkeypox. *Lancet Neurol.* 2022 Oct;21(10):872.

✖ Pitfalls

- Assuming mpox is transmitted only sexually and failing to test for the illness in symptomatic patients without traditional risk factors.
- Expecting mpox lesions to heal within 14 to 28 days for all patients. Lesions in patients with immunosuppression may take months to heal. Patients with lesions should be educated to avoid physical contact with others until all lesions have completely healed.
- Failing to recognize that the epidemic *Monkeypox virus* strain responsible for the latest outbreak presents differently from the classic form of mpox.

The LLSA Literature Review
End-of-Life Care

By Mobolaji Fowose, MD, MPH; and Michael E. Abboud, MD, MSEd

Department of Emergency Medicine, University of Pennsylvania in Philadelphia

Reviewed by Andrew J. Eyre, MD, MS-HPEd

Objective

On completion of this article, you should be able to:

■ Explain how to appropriately deliver EOL care in the emergency department.

Long DA, Koyfman A, Long B. Oncologic emergencies: palliative care in the emergency department setting. *J Emerg Med.* 2021 Feb;60(2):175-191.

KEY POINTS

■ EOL care is an important and common part of health care in the emergency department.

■ Advance directives and goals of care should be confirmed for each patient. When plans are not already documented, physicians should empathetically discuss developing EOL plans with patients and their health care proxies.

■ Dyspnea is the EOL symptom that distresses patients the most but can be managed with opioids.

■ Pain at EOL can be managed with opioids, but nonopioid alternatives should also be considered.

■ The WHO estimates that by 2050 the worldwide number of people older than 60 years will increase by 10%. Unfortunately, many of these individuals will develop terminal illnesses that require emergency care, so emergency physicians must be competent in EOL matters. EOL care aims to provide quality care by maximizing comfort and alleviating distress while respecting patients' wishes to avoid aggressive, life-sustaining treatment.

Advance Directives

Many patients with terminal illnesses document their medical care goals in an advance directive. Common orders that go along with an advance directive include a do-not-resuscitate (DNR) or a do-not-intubate (DNI) order. A more specific type of advance directive is the physician orders for life-sustaining treatment (POLST) form that specifies medical orders for interventions like noninvasive ventilation and intravenous fluids. Emergency physicians use these documents to provide quality end-of-life (EOL) care according to patients' wishes.

One of emergency physicians' biggest challenges in caring for EOL patients is accessing their advance directives in a timely manner before managing their condition. Even in patients with clearly written and obtainable directives, it is often still difficult to decide how aggressive treatment should be when patients become critically ill. Thoughtful communication between emergency physicians, patients, and their health care proxies is crucial to building a therapeutic alliance that ensures medical decisions are made according to patients' wishes. Emergency physicians should educate patients and their proxies about the available medical therapies and expectations of EOL care and then should collaborate on a care plan and clearly document it in the medical record.

Symptom Management

Patients with terminal illnesses display signs and symptoms that life is near its end. Symptoms that suggest a short survival time include anorexia, asthenia (lack of energy), dry mouth, and confusion. In patients with advanced malignancy, symptoms of dyspnea, anorexia, tachycardia, or low systolic blood pressure are associated with being near the end. Distressing symptoms along with symptoms that are less severe, but still uncomfortable, must be treated. Nausea is treated with antiemetics. The "death rattle" — noisy breathing caused by the pooling of secretions in the airway — can be treated with glycopyrrolate.

Although dyspnea can be managed in multiple ways, studies suggest that intubation and mechanical ventilation increase suffering. Noninvasive therapies for dyspnea should be considered in patients with a DNI status; however, the masks in noninvasive, bilevel ventilation are often uncomfortable and can also increase suffering. Additionally, oxygen therapy has not been shown to relieve EOL dyspnea. The best-studied therapy for EOL dyspnea is opioid therapy. Opioids reduce the chemoreceptor response to hypercapnia and decrease anxiety and the sensation of breathlessness. Physicians may fear that the utilization of narcotics may hasten death, but the literature does not support this belief when low-dose opioids are used — the dose needed to relieve EOL dyspnea is lower than that for pain control. Starting with intravenous morphine at 1 to 2 mg or with intravenous hydromorphone at 0.2 to 0.4 mg, with redosing as needed, can be sufficient.

Benzodiazepine use for EOL dyspnea is more controversial. Although benzodiazepines can relieve the anxiety associated with dyspnea, they can also increase sedation. Some studies encourage low-dose benzodiazepines in combination with other agents in some patient populations.

Pain is another common, distressing symptom in terminally ill patients; it can be nociceptive, neuropathic, or bone related. Nociceptive pain is caused by the stretching of organs, usually from malignancy; neuropathic and bone-related pain are from pathologic fractures or metastatic disease. Opioids are the first-line therapy for severe pain. When selecting the type and quantity of opioids, physicians must consider the duration of effect, potential side effects, and patient tolerance.

Nonopioid alternatives should be considered for mild to severe pain. Nociceptive and bone-related pain can be treated with NSAIDs, acetaminophen, or low-dose intravenous ketamine (0.1-0.3 mg/kg). Gabapentin, anticonvulsants, or antidepressants can be effective for neuropathic pain.

Critical Decisions in Emergency Medicine's LLSA literature reviews features articles from ABEM's 2023 Lifelong Learning and Self-Assessment Reading List. Available online at acep.org/moc/llsa and on the ABEM website.

Volume 37 Number 2: **February 2023**   11

The Critical ECG

Wellens Syndrome

By Jeremy Berberian, MD; William J. Brady, MD, FACEP; and Amal Mattu, MD, FACEP

Dr. Berberian is the associate director of emergency medicine residency education at ChristianaCare and assistant professor of emergency medicine at Sidney Kimmel Medical College, Thomas Jefferson University in Philadelphia, Pennsylvania. Dr. Brady is a professor of emergency medicine, medicine, and nursing, and vice chair for faculty affairs in the Department of Emergency Medicine at the University of Virginia School of Medicine in Charlottesville. Dr. Mattu is a professor, vice chair, and codirector of the Emergency Cardiology Fellowship in the Department of Emergency Medicine at the University of Maryland School of Medicine in Baltimore.

Objectives

On completion of this article, you should be able to:

- Define the ECG diagnostic criteria and historical features of Wellens syndrome.
- Explain the clinical significance of Wellens syndrome.
- Describe the common ECG criteria for poor R-wave progression.

CASE PRESENTATION

A 76-year-old man presents for exertional chest pain that resolved immediately prior to arrival. His ECG shows sinus bradycardia at 58 bpm; normal axis; normal QRS complex duration; T-wave inversion (TWI) in leads I, aVL, V_4, and V_5; and biphasic T-waves in V_2 and V_3. The TWI and biphasic T waves are new since his ECG from 6 months ago (*Figures 1* and *2*).

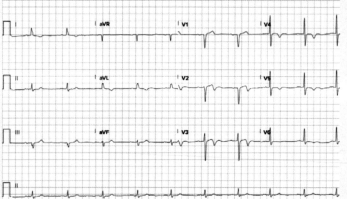

FIGURE 1. ECG of a 76-year-old man. *Credit:* EMRA.

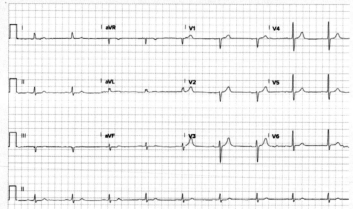

FIGURE 2. ECG 6 months previously. *Credit:* EMRA.

Discussion

The morphology of the precordial TWI is typically seen in Wellens syndrome — also called left anterior descending artery (LAD) coronary T-wave syndrome — which describes an abnormal T-wave pattern seen in patients in a pain-free state after a recent history of anginal symptoms. These characteristic ECG findings were first described in 1982 by Dr. Hein JJ Wellens, a Dutch cardiologist who found that 75% of patients with this syndrome developed an anterior myocardial infarction (MI) within a few weeks of hospital admission if no intervention was performed.[1] The diagnostic criteria include the following:

- Biphasic (type A, as seen in the case presentation) or deeply inverted (type B) T waves in the midprecordial leads, typically V_2 and V_3 (*Figures 3* and *4*);
- Isoelectric or minimally elevated ST segment (<1 mm);
- No precordial Q waves;
- Preserved precordial R-wave progression; and
- Normal or minimally elevated troponins.

There is no universal definition for a preserved precordial R-wave progression, but common criteria include the following:

- R wave greater than 2 to 4 mm in lead V_3 or V_4;
- R wave in lead V_4 greater than lead V_3 or in lead V_3 greater than lead V_2; or
- R wave in lead V_3 greater than or equal to 3 mm.

The patient's ECG pattern is concerning for a critical stenosis or lesion of the proximal LAD, and the T-wave abnormalities are thought to represent reperfusion after an ischemic event. Biphasic T waves, also called Wellens type A, are an early finding, while deeply inverted T waves, also called Wellens type B, are a later, more common finding (up to 75% of cases). Patients with these ECG findings in the appropriate clinical context have a high likelihood of developing an anterior MI within a short time frame and should be admitted for cardiac catheterization.[1] Coronary angiography

ACKNOWLEDGMENT

This case is reprinted from *Emergency ECGs: Case-Based Review and Interpretations*, available at www.emra.org/amazon or by scanning the QR code.

is required to evaluate the need for early angioplasty or coronary bypass surgery; provocative testing, especially exercise stress testing, should be avoided because it could precipitate an acute MI or cardiac arrest.[2,3,4]

Importantly, these ECG findings were originally described in patients in a pain-free state. In fact, these ECG changes can persist from the painful presentation into the pain-free state — the ECG changes do not resolve until the LAD lesion is successfully managed with either percutaneous coronary intervention or a coronary artery bypass graft.

The term Wellens waves is sometimes used to describe these ECG findings in symptomatic patients. In these cases, the ECG changes are due to active ischemia. The term pseudo-Wellens is commonly used to describe these ECG findings when associated with causes other than LAD stenosis, such as left ventricular hypertrophy, pulmonary embolism, hypertrophic cardiomyopathy, intracranial hemorrhage, and right bundle branch block. ECG changes from these causes are due to repolarization abnormalities.

LEARNING POINTS

- Wellens syndrome describes an abnormal T-wave pattern seen in the midprecordial leads, typically V_2 to V_3, in a pain-free state with recent history of anginal symptoms.
  - Type A: biphasic T waves seen immediately upon reperfusion
  - Type B: deeply inverted T waves, later finding
- These findings represent critical stenosis of the proximal LAD and warrant admission for cardiac catheterization.
  - Provocative testing should be avoided because it could precipitate an MI.
- Wellens syndrome is associated with a high risk of an anterior MI if left untreated.

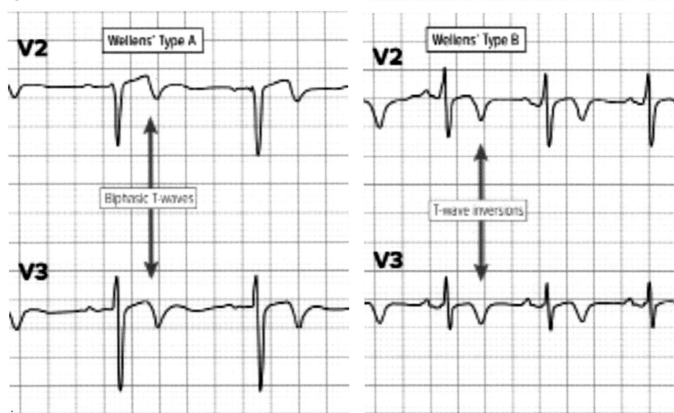

FIGURE 3. Biphasic T waves, as seen in Wellens type A (from this case presentation). *Credit:* EMRA.

FIGURE 4. TWI, as seen in Wellens type B (from a different case presentation). *Credit:* EMRA.

CASE RESOLUTION

This patient presented in the middle of the night and was ultimately admitted for an urgent, but not emergent, cardiac catheterization later that morning. He was found to have a 95% occlusion of the proximal LAD, which was successfully treated with a stent.

REFERENCES

1. de Zwaan C, Bär FW, Wellens HJ. Characteristic electrocardiographic pattern indicating a critical stenosis high in left anterior descending coronary artery in patients admitted because of impending myocardial infarction. *Am Heart J.* 1982 Apr;103(4)(part 2):730-736.
2. de Zwaan C, Bär FW, Janssen JH, et al. Angiographic and clinical characteristics of patients with unstable angina showing an ECG pattern indicating critical narrowing of the proximal LAD coronary artery. *Am Heart J.* 1989 Mar;117(3):657-665.
3. Rhinehardt J, Brady WJ, Perron AD, Mattu A. Electrocardiographic manifestations of Wellens' syndrome. *Am J Emerg Med.* 2002 Nov;20(7):638-643.
4. Patel K, Alattar F, Koneru J, Shamoon F. ST-elevation myocardial infarction after pharmacologic persantine stress test in a patient with wellens syndrome. *Case Rep Emerg Med.* 2014;2014:530451.

Splenic Laceration

By Jordan Griep, MD; and
Mark Pittman, MD, FACEP, FAWM
Prisma Health — Upstate, Greenville, South Carolina
Reviewed by Ann M Dietrich, MD, FAAP, FACEP

Objective

On completion of this article, you should be able to:

■ Identify the appropriate steps for definitive management of splenic lacerations in pediatric patients.

CASE PRESENTATION

A 13-year-old girl without a significant medical history presents via EMS after a motor vehicle collision. The patient was seated at the rear passenger side and was wearing a seat belt when her vehicle was struck head on by another vehicle that was traveling approximately 30 mph. The patient denies loss of consciousness and was able to extricate herself from the vehicle and ambulate on scene. She noticed abrasions across her chest and shortness of breath immediately after the collision. On arrival, the patient has a cervical collar in place and an intact airway with bilateral breath sounds present. Initial vital signs are BP 122/75, P 109, R 17, and T 36.9°C (98.4°F); SpO_2 is 99% on room air. The patient complains of pain in her left lower thorax and left upper abdominal quadrant. Her Glasgow Coma Scale (GCS) score is 15. The physical examination is significant for tachycardia, seat belt sign to the upper abdomen and sternum, and mild tenderness to palpation of the left upper abdominal quadrant without rebound or guarding. FAST examination is performed (*Figure 1*).

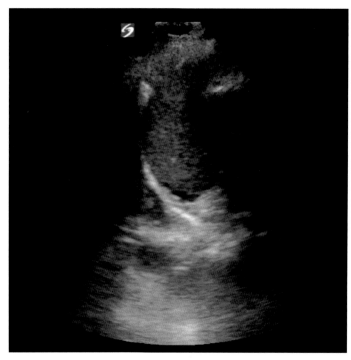

FIGURE 1. FAST examination revealing free fluid in the left upper quadrant of the abdomen.
Credit: Dr. Mark Pittman.

Pediatric Abdominal Imaging by the Numbers[7,11]			
Imaging Modality	Ionizing Radiation Exposure (mSv)	Sensitivity (%)	Specificity (%)
Abdominal CT	10	98	85
Ultrasound	0	35	96

TABLE 1. Comparison of CT and ultrasound for pediatric abdominal imaging

Overview

Blunt abdominal trauma is a major cause of morbidity and mortality in the pediatric population. Often, this trauma occurs from falls, sports injuries, surgical complications, and motor vehicle collisions.[1] Although falls are the most frequent cause of injury, the most severe injuries come from motor vehicle collisions.[2] Pediatric patients are often better than adults at physiologically compensating for injuries, which can make timely diagnosis difficult. Children can lose almost half of their circulating volume before hypotension is reliably detected; therefore, tachycardia is often the only presenting sign of intra-abdominal trauma.[2]

The spleen is the most commonly injured organ in pediatric abdominal injuries.[3] Between 2007 and 2015, the National Trauma Data Bank recorded that there were 26,694 pediatric patients with isolated splenic injury.[4] Unlike in adults, the pediatric ribcage does not fully protect the spleen, explaining the finding of splenic pathology in up to 25% of pediatric trauma cases.[1] How well the spleen is protected in children varies with growth of the thorax. A recent study showed that, on average, taller children have a larger spleen, but their overall risk of splenic trauma decreases as they grow because their spleen takes up less of their abdominal cavity.[5,6] Boys also appear to be at higher risk of splenic trauma than girls.[4] When evaluating pediatric patients for splenic laceration, the risk will vary depending on age and body habitus. In most pediatric trauma cases, physical examinations are difficult because patients are distraught and their history is limited. Considering the prevalence of splenic trauma in children, a good understanding of its diagnostic management, including the benefits and limitations of imaging modalities, is critical to reduce pediatric morbidity and mortality.

Diagnosis

Millisieverts (mSv) are an issue of concern; the risk of radiation exposure must be considered when evaluating for pediatric splenic lacerations. To minimize exposure, many emergency physicians prefer ultrasound over CT for initial imaging (*Table 1*). A recent study estimated that the average radiation exposure

FAST Examination		
Choice of Probe	Windows	Limitations
• Curvilinear • Phased array	• Hepatorenal • Splenorenal • Suprapubic • Subxiphoid	• Bowel gas may obstruct view • Inability to penetrate bone • Body habitus can make obtaining certain views difficult • Difficult to obtain in uncooperative patients

TABLE 2. Probes, windows, and limitations of the FAST examination

from a CT of the abdomen and pelvis is 20 mSv (10 mSv from each separately).[7] For comparison, yearly background radiation exposure averages around 2 to 3 mSv, a chest x-ray averages 0.02 mSv, and an abdominal x-ray averages 0.7 mSv.[8] Additionally, the risk of radiation is often considered higher in the pediatric population because earlier exposure is thought to allow more time for radiation's adverse effects, such as malignancy, to develop. Although CT can provide more detail than ultrasound in evaluating intra-abdominal injury, ultrasound is a useful tool to evaluate blunt abdominal trauma and is often the first imaging choice in a busy emergency department. A child's total blood volume is estimated to be 75 to 80 mL/kg; although not specific to children, a study showed that as little as 100 mL of fluid can be detected on a focused assessment with sonography in trauma (FAST) examination, which could help detect injury in children (*Table 2*).[9,10] Other benefits of ultrasound in the clinical setting include the ability for dynamic bedside reassessment, zero exposure to ionizing radiation, and the overall ease of use.

A recent meta-analysis by Tian et al found that pediatric abdominal ultrasound has "a pooled sensitivity of 35% and specificity of 96%," while CT with contrast yields a sensitivity of 98% and specificity of 85%.[11] This same study also

Categorization of Splenic Lacerations Based on the American Association for the Surgery of Trauma Guidelines[12]	
Laceration Grade	Characteristics
I	Tear of the splenic capsule <1 cm in parenchymal depth
II	Tear of the splenic capsule 1-3 cm in parenchymal depth without involvement of a trabecular vessel
III	Tear of the splenic capsule >3 cm in depth or with involvement of the trabecular vessels
IV	Splenic laceration involving segmental or hilar vessels, which results in major devascularization of >25% of the spleen
V	Complete splenic shatter

TABLE 3. Grading of splenic lacerations

found that although a positive point-of-care ultrasound (POCUS) FAST examination is predictive of an intra-abdominal injury, a negative test is often unreliable and leads to further workup. Current recommendations state that stable patients with a positive FAST examination should undergo CT prior to intervention, while unstable patients with a positive FAST examination may need expedited intervention. In a subset of low-risk patients — GCS scores of 14 or 15, a normal abdominal examination, and a negative FAST examination — observation with serial POCUS FAST examinations is recommended before determining if further diagnostic workup is needed; however, these observation plans should be discussed and coordinated with surgical colleagues should transition of care become necessary.[11] Ultimately, a positive FAST examination during evaluation for intra-abdominal injury in the pediatric population can expedite care, but a single negative POCUS FAST examination leaves too much uncertainty and requires further workup for definitive management.

CASE RESOLUTION

FAST examination revealed free fluid in the left upper quadrant of the abdomen. Pediatric surgery was consulted, and the patient was stable enough for a CT. CT of the abdomen and pelvis with intravenous contrast revealed a left lower lung pulmonary contusion, left eighth- and ninth-rib fractures, and a grade II splenic laceration with hemoperitoneum but without evidence of active arterial extravasation (*Table 3*).[4] Pediatric surgery admitted the patient for observation, serial abdominal examinations, and frequent vital sign checks. The patient remained in stable condition overnight and had reassuring repeat laboratory results the following morning. The patient was ultimately discharged with scheduled pediatric surgery follow-up in 2 weeks.

REFERENCES

1. Di Serafino M, Verde F, Ferro F, et al. Ultrasonography of the pediatric spleen: a pictorial essay. *J Ultrasound*. 2019 Dec;22(4):503-512.
2. Gaines BA. Intra-abdominal solid organ injury in children: diagnosis and treatment. *J Trauma*. 2009 Aug;67(2)(suppl):S135-S139.
3. Lynch T, Kilgar J, Al Shibli A. Pediatric abdominal trauma. *Curr Pediatr Rev*. 2018;14(1):59-63.
4. Chahine AH, Gilyard S, Hanna TN, et al. Management of splenic trauma in contemporary clinical practice: a National Trauma Data Bank study. *Acad Radiol*. 2021 Nov;28(suppl 1):S138-S147.
5. Mohtasib RS, Alshamiri K, Jobeir A, et al. Sonographic measurements for spleen size in healthy Saudi children and correlation with body parameters. *Ann Saudi Med*. 2021 Jan-Feb;41(1):14-23.
6. Pelizzo G, Guazzotti M, Klersy C, et al. Spleen size evaluation in children: time to define splenomegaly for pediatric surgeons and pediatricians. *PLoS One*. 2018 Aug 23;13(8):e0202741.
7. Ogbole GI. Radiation dose in pædiatric computed tomography: risks and benefits. *Ann Ib Postgrad Med*. 2010 Dec;8(2):118-126.
8. Chawla A, Peh WCG. Abdominal radiographs in the emergency department: current status and controversies. *J Med Radiat Sci*. 2018 Dec;65(4):250-251.
9. Howie SRC. Blood sample volumes in child health research: review of safe limits. *Bull World Health Organ*. 2011 Jan 1;89(1):46-53.
10. Richards JR, McGahan JP. Focused assessment with sonography in trauma (FAST) in 2017: what radiologists can learn. *Radiology*. 2017 Apr;283(1):30-48.
11. Liang T, Roseman E, Gao M, Sinert R. The utility of the focused assessment with sonography in trauma examination in pediatric blunt abdominal trauma: a systematic review and meta-analysis. *Pediatr Emerg Care*. 2021 Feb 1;37(2):108-118.
12. Lynn KN, Werder GM, Callaghan RM, Sullivan AN, Jafri ZH, Bloom DA. Pediatric blunt splenic trauma: a comprehensive review. *Pediatr Radiol*. 2009 Sep;39(9):904-916.

Reduction of a Nursemaid's Elbow

By Steven J. Warrington, MD, MEd, MS
MercyOne Siouxland, Sioux City, Iowa

Objective

On completion of this article, you should be able to:
- Explain two reduction approaches for subluxation of the radial head, or nursemaid's elbow.

Introduction

Subluxation of the radial head, better known as a nursemaid's elbow, is fairly common in pediatric patients and requires reduction. However, sometimes one reduction technique does not resolve the issue.

Contraindications
- Nursemaid's elbow secondary to trauma or a fall
- Nursemaid's elbow with an associated fracture

Benefits and Risks

Reducing this type of subluxation allows for a return of elbow function and resolves any pain that may occur with the condition. Current medical literature states that there are minimal to no risks with the procedure. However, reductions can be unsuccessful. A number of patients do not have a successful reduction on the first attempt and need additional attempts and, potentially, additional techniques. The potential for an unsuccessful reduction should be discussed with patients' caregivers.

Alternatives

The supination-flexion technique is anecdotally the most common approach to reduction, but the hyperpronation technique, with flexion as needed, can also be used to reduce a nursemaid's elbow. The hyperpronation technique can be used on the initial attempt instead of as a second-attempt technique. Although studies are limited, the hyperpronation approach may have a higher initial success rate and may cause less discomfort.

Reducing Side Effects

Pain and anxiety can occur in patients with a nursemaid's elbow if the dislocation has existed for a long time or if patients are sensitive. In these cases, adjunct medication through oral or nasal routes can be beneficial. Additionally, anxiety can be reduced by allowing caregivers to hold patients during the process.

Special Considerations

Because a nursemaid's elbow is an orthopedic issue, evaluation with x-rays can be considered, although their role in the classic presentation of a nursemaid's elbow is limited. X-rays should be considered if trauma (accidental or nonaccidental) is a suspected cause or if there is local bruising and swelling around the elbow. Typically, x-rays are performed if the procedure repeatedly fails or if the elbow has not returned to its normal level of function prior to discharge from the emergency department. Some physicians do not recommend radiographic evaluation for classic presentations at the first visit and instead advocate waiting 24 hours after a perceived successful reduction to re-evaluate function and decide if x-rays are warranted.

TECHNIQUES

1. **Obtain** consent after diagnosing subluxation of the radial head; discuss the potential need for repeat attempts, and explain that transient discomfort may be experienced during the procedure. Additionally, consider anxiolytics or analgesics as needed and instruct the patient's caregiver on how to hold the child during the reduction.

2. **Attempt** the hyperpronation technique first (*Figure 1*).

   - **Direct** the caregiver to hold the child on the caregiver's lap with the affected elbow easily accessible.

   - **Hold** the child's elbow at a 90° angle with one hand.

   - **Quickly** hyperpronate the patient's wrist using the other hand, with the speed and force normally used for the supination-flexion technique.

   - **Consider** flexion of the patient's elbow afterward, as is done with the standard supination-flexion technique.

   - **Assess** neurovascular status and function. Importantly, function may not return for 15 to 30 minutes or longer after the procedure.

3. **Consider** a second reduction using hyperpronation or an alternative technique if normal function does not return or if the reduction appears to be unsuccessful.

4. **Attempt** the second technique of supination-flexion, if needed (*Figure 2*).

   - **Direct** the caregiver to hold the child on the caregiver's lap with the affected elbow easily accessible.

   - **Hold** the child's elbow at a 90° angle with one hand.

   - **Quickly** supinate the patient's wrist.

   - **Flex** the patient's elbow so that their wrist closely approaches their shoulder.

   - **Assess** neurovascular status and function. Function may not return for 15 to 30 minutes or longer after the procedure.

5. **Order** imaging of the patient's elbow if it has not improved or returned to baseline function.

6. **Discuss** the results with a specialist if available or, as the literature suggests, splint the elbow at a 90° angle if no abnormalities are found on x-ray or during examination.

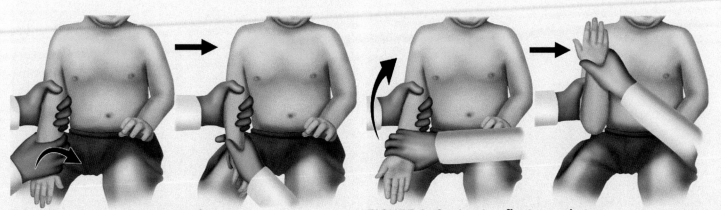

FIGURE 1. Hyperpronation technique

FIGURE 2. Supination-flexion technique

Critical Cases in Orthopedics and Trauma

Isolated Subtalar Dislocation

By Eric Lakey, MD; and Ian Storch, MD
University of Florida College of Medicine — Jacksonville
Reviewed by John Kiel, DO, MPH, FACEP, CAQSM

Objective

On completion of this article, you should be able to:

■ Discuss how to manage isolated subtalar dislocations.

CASE PRESENTATION

A 21-year-old man with a history of cystic fibrosis presents with left ankle pain after a single-vehicle motorcycle crash. He states that he was accelerating onto the freeway when he hit a patch of gravel and lost control of his back wheel. He attempted to plant his left foot on the ground to stabilize the motorcycle and immediately felt pain in his foot. In the field, he was splinted by EMS without reduction before being transferred to the trauma center. On arrival, he has a left ankle deformity with pulses present and no open wound. His physical examination is notable for a closed deformity of the left hindfoot with medial foot displacement and lateral skin tenting over the distal fibula. No additional injuries are identified on primary and secondary surveys. Left foot and ankle x-rays are notable for a left medial subtalar joint dislocation with fractures at the left posterior talar process and base of the fifth metatarsal (*Figures 1* and *2*).

Discussion

Subtalar dislocation is a rare injury, accounting for only 1% to 2% of all dislocations.[1] The injury is associated with a high-energy mechanism on a plantar-flexed foot. Young men are most affected, with a 6:1 ratio of men to women. Patients with a subtalar dislocation present with deformity and tenderness at the ankle and hindfoot. Because of its association with high-energy mechanisms, patients suspected of having a subtalar dislocation should undergo a full advanced trauma life support survey to evaluate for additional injuries.

Diagnosis is confirmed by plain x-rays of the foot and ankle that demonstrate dislocation of the subtalar joint. Approximately 85% of subtalar dislocations are medial, 15% are lateral, and a small fraction are posterior or anterior.[2] Once a subtalar dislocation is confirmed, physicians should assess for neurovascular status, evaluate for additional injuries in the foot and ankle, and reduce the dislocation.

Concomitant injuries of the malleoli, fifth metatarsal, and talus are almost always found; there are only a few case reports in the literature of subtalar dislocations without an associated fracture.[3,4] Approximately 25% of subtalar dislocations are open, and up to 32% require open reduction.[2,5] Lateral dislocations are more likely to be open and more likely to have soft-tissue entrapment that necessitates open reduction. Given the high rate of concomitant injuries, expert opinion recommends obtaining a postreduction CT, which in one case series was shown to change injury management in 44% of cases.[6,7]

Procedure

Closed reduction is achieved by flexing the hips and knees (to release tension on the gastrocnemius and accentuate the deformity under traction) and then applying direct pressure on the talar head to correct the deformity. Patients are then typically placed on non–weight-bearing restrictions with immobilization of the foot for 4 to 6 weeks. There is a high rate of complication — 50% to 80% of patients develop post-traumatic arthritis. Only 20% of patients regain full range of motion.[8]

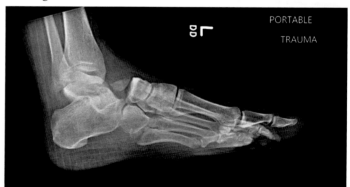

FIGURE 1. Anterior-posterior x-ray of the left ankle showing dislocation of the left medial subtalar joint and fractures of the left posterior talar process and base of the fifth metatarsal

FIGURE 2. Lateral x-ray of the left ankle showing dislocation of the left medial subtalar joint and fractures of the left posterior talar process and base of the fifth metatarsal

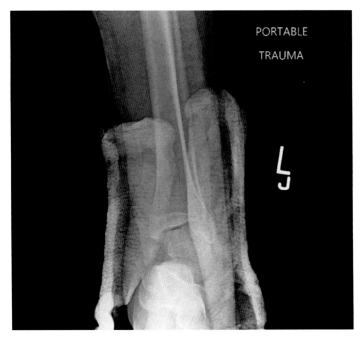

FIGURE 3. Anterior-posterior x-ray of the left ankle post reduction

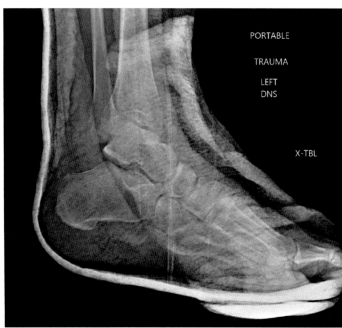

FIGURE 4. Lateral x-ray of the left foot post reduction

CASE RESOLUTION

The patient was sedated with propofol, and podiatry performed a closed reduction of both the subtalar and talonavicular joints (*Figures 3* and *4*). The next day, the patient was seen by physical and occupational therapy and was cleared to discharge home as non–weight-bearing with crutches; plans were made for outpatient podiatry follow-up.

The patient followed up with outpatient podiatry 19 days after his initial injury. He was compliant with his non–weight-bearing status and reported significant improvement with both pain and swelling. Repeat left foot x-rays demonstrated a healing base of the fifth metatarsal fracture, persistent inferomedial subluxation of the talonavicular joint, a large osseous fragment within the subtalar joint, and a nondisplaced cuboid fracture that was not found on initial x-rays (*Figures 5* and *6*). Unfortunately, a CT scan was not obtained at the time of injury but may have led to earlier detection and treatment of the persistent talonavicular subluxation and cuboid fracture. An MRI of the left foot was ordered to aid with surgical planning, and his splint was exchanged for a controlled ankle movement boot. He returned 29 days post injury for open reduction and internal fixation of the residual talonavicular subluxation and talar fracture as well as for a deltoid ligament repair.

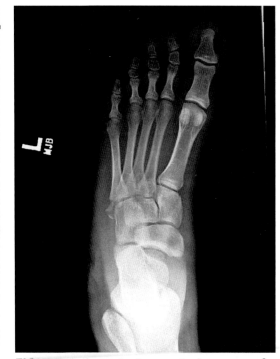

FIGURE 5. An anterior-posterior x-ray of the left foot 19 days post injury

REFERENCES

1. Perugia D, Basile A, Massoni C, Gumina S, Rossi F, Ferretti A. Conservative treatment of subtalar dislocations. *Int Orthop*. 2002;26(1):56-60.
2. Lugani G, Rigoni M, Puddu L, et al. Subtalar dislocation: a narrative review. *Musculoskelet Surg*. 2022 Dec;106(4):337-344.
3. Inokuchi S, Hashimoto T, Usami N. Posterior subtalar dislocation. *J Trauma*. 1997 Feb;42(2):310-313.
4. Giannoulis D, Papadopoulos D, Lykissas M, Koulouvaris P, Gkiatas I, Mavrodontidis A. Subtalar dislocation without associated fractures: case report and review of the literature. *World J Orthop*. 2015 Apr 18;6(3):374-379.
5. Bibbo C, Anderson RB, Davis WH. Injury characteristics and the clinical outcome of subtalar dislocations: a clinical and radiographic analysis of 25 cases. *Foot Ankle Int*. 2003 Feb;24(2):158-163.
6. Yoder W, Nelson P, Bowen M, Frania S. Talocalcaneal navicular dislocations: a review. In: *Podiatry Institute Update 2011*. The Podiatry Insitute, Inc. 49-55. https://www.podiatryinstitute.com/pdfs/Update_2011/2011_11.pdf
7. Bibbo C, Lin SS, Abidi N, et al. Missed and associated injuries after subtalar dislocation: the role of CT. *Foot Ankle Int*. 2001 Apr;22(4):324-328.
8. Horning J, DiPreta J. Subtalar dislocation. *Orthopedics*. 2009 Dec;32(12):904.

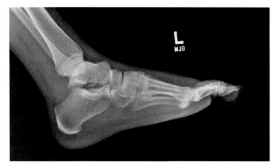

FIGURE 6. A lateral x-ray of the left foot 19 days post injury

The Critical Image

A Vomiting Infant

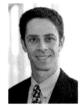

By Joshua S. Broder, MD, FACEP
Dr. Broder is a professor and the residency program director in the Department of Emergency Medicine at Duke University Medical Center in Durham, North Carolina.
Case contributors: Emily Sterrett, MD; and Carmen Estrada Huerta, MD

Objectives

On completion of this article, you should be able to:

- Describe the presentation of malrotation and midgut volvulus in infants.
- Identify imaging modalities for diagnosing malrotation and midgut volvulus.

CASE PRESENTATION

A 6-day-old, full-term female infant presents with bright yellow-green vomiting after feeding. The patient has been afebrile and has continued to breastfeed, urinate, and pass stools. Her parents deny that the infant has been more irritable than usual. The infant's vital signs include P 136, R 46, and T 37°C (98.6 °F); SpO$_2$ is 99% on room air. On examination, the child appears to be sleeping. Her fontanelles are normal, and there is no scleral icterus or jaundice. Her mucous membranes are moist, with some yellow discoloration of the tongue. Heart and lung examinations are normal, and her abdomen is not distended. Capillary refill time is less than 3 seconds. The patient's glucose level is 52 mg/dL, so she is treated for hypoglycemia. While in the emergency department, she vomits yellow-green liquid three more times. Abdominal x-rays followed by an upper GI (UGI) series are obtained (*Figures 1* and *2*).

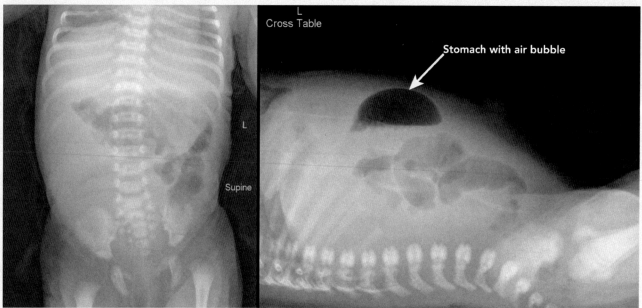

FIGURE 1. Anterior-posterior (*left*) and lateral (*right*) abdominal x-rays showing a nonobstructive gas pattern. No pneumatosis or free air is seen (although the latter can be difficult to identify on supine anterior-posterior images). The gastric air bubble is prominent, with an air-fluid level seen on the lateral image.

Discussion

Vomiting in neonates can be an ominous presentation — serious congenital anatomic abnormalities as well as metabolic causes must be considered. Intestinal atresias and stenosis in newborns usually present as vomiting or inadequate feeding within the first 2 days of life. Midgut volvulus in the setting of malrotation often occurs in the early neonatal period (>50% in the first month of life) but also may present with declining frequency at any time in life.[1] The condition is marked by bilious emesis, which suggests intestinal obstruction distal to the ampulla of Vater. Hypertrophic pyloric stenosis commonly presents with nonbilious emesis between 2 weeks and 3 months of life and is appropriately evaluated with ultrasound as the initial imaging test.[2]

For vomiting within the first 2 days of life, the American College of Radiology (ACR) recommends using abdominal x-rays as the initial imaging study.[2] These x-rays may show the double bubble sign without distal gas, indicating duodenal obstruction — usually from duodenal atresia (91% of the time) but occasionally from midgut volvulus (6% of the time).[3] A triple bubble sign without distal gas suggests jejunal obstruction, also most commonly from atresia. Importantly, a normal bowel gas pattern *does not rule out* malrotation or volvulus with incomplete obstruction.[2] If diagnostic uncertainty persists after plain x-rays, a fluoroscopic UGI series is indicated when a proximal obstruction is suspected, and a fluoroscopic contrast enema is indicated when a distal obstruction is suspected.[2]

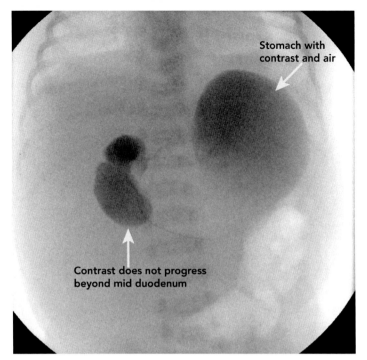

FIGURE 2. UGI series, patient consumed 10 ml of the oral contrast agent Iopamidol from a bottle. The contrast is filling the stomach to reach the proximal duodenum but not progessing beyond the mid duodenum, even after 30 minutes. This indicates a high-grade duodenal obstruction. The patient had bilious emesis during the procedure.

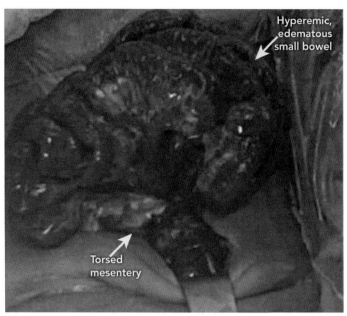

FIGURE 3. An intraoperative photo confirming midgut volvulus with malrotation and a very small vascular pedicle. The small bowel appears hyperemic and edematous but still viable. The cecum was found fixed to the right upper quadrant retroperitoneum. Peritoneal fibrous bands (Ladd bands) were divided, and the bowel was detorsed. Because of the abnormal location of the cecum, an appendectomy was also performed to avoid future difficulty with diagnosing appendicitis, should it develop. The Ladd procedure describes these steps.

Midgut volvulus requires rapid evaluation and treatment because of high reported mortality rates (20% to 40%).[4] In the first 72 hours of life, 1 in 5 patients with bilious vomiting has midgut volvulus.[5] If malrotation and volvulus are strongly suspected, particularly beyond the first 2 days of life, the ACR recommends initial testing with a fluoroscopic UGI series, even though no literature exists to support using this imaging prior to plain x-rays.[2] A UGI series evaluates for malrotation by visualizing the position of the duodenal-jejunal junction (ligament of Treitz). It can also identify an intestinal obstruction — marked by the failure of ingested contrast to progress through the GI tract — caused by volvulus, atresia, or other conditions. UGI has a reported sensitivity of 96% for malrotation and 79% for volvulus.[6]

In uncertain cases of volvulus or malrotation, ultrasound can be a useful adjunct imaging modality, although it also has limited literature support.[2] Ultrasound can identify abnormal relative positions of the superior mesenteric artery (SMA) and vein (SMV) as well as the third portion of the duodenum, all of which are findings seen in malrotation. According to a small prospective study, the presence of a Doppler whirlpool sign — a clockwise rotation of the SMV and mesentery around the SMA — is 95% sensitive and 89% specific for midgut volvulus.[7]

CASE RESOLUTION

The infant was taken directly from the radiology suite to the operating room for an exploratory laparotomy, which confirmed intestinal malrotation with midgut volvulus (*Figure 3*). The patient underwent the Ladd procedure and recovered without the need for a bowel resection.

REFERENCES

1. Adams SD, Stanton MP. Malrotation and intestinal atresias. *Early Hum Dev.* 2014 Dec;90(12):921-925.
2. Alazraki AL, Rigsby CK, Iyer RS, et al; Expert Panel on Pediatric Imaging. ACR Appropriateness Criteria® vomiting in infants. *J Am Coll Radiol.* 2020 Nov;17(11)(suppl):S505-S515.
3. Chandrasekaran S, Asokaraju A. Clinical profile and predictors of outcome in congenital duodenal obstruction. *Int Surg J.* 2017;4(8):2605-2611.
4. Maya-Enero S, Prat-Ortells J, Martín-Solé O, De Haro-Jorge I, Pertierra-Cortada A, Iriondo-Sanz M. Distinguishing outcomes of neonatal intestinal volvulus: review of our experience over the last 20 years. *Acta Paediatr.* 2022 Feb;111(2):284-290.
5. Lilien LD, Srinivasan G, Pyati SP, Yeh TF, Pildes RS. Green vomiting in the first 72 hours in normal infants. *Am J Dis Child.* 1986 Jul;140(7):662-664.
6. Sizemore AW, Rabbani KZ, Ladd A, Applegate KE. Diagnostic performance of the upper gastrointestinal series in the evaluation of children with clinically suspected malrotation. *Pediatr Radiol.* 2008 May;38(5):518-528.
7. Zhang W, Sun H, Luo F. The efficiency of sonography in diagnosing volvulus in neonates with suspected intestinal malrotation. *Medicine (Baltimore).* 2017 Oct;96(42):e8287.

Feature Editor: Joshua S. Broder, MD, FACEP. See also *Diagnostic Imaging for the Emergency Physician* (Winner of the 2011 Prose Award in Clinical Medicine, the American Publishers Award for Professional and Scholarly Excellence) and *Critical Images in Emergency Medicine* by Dr. Broder.

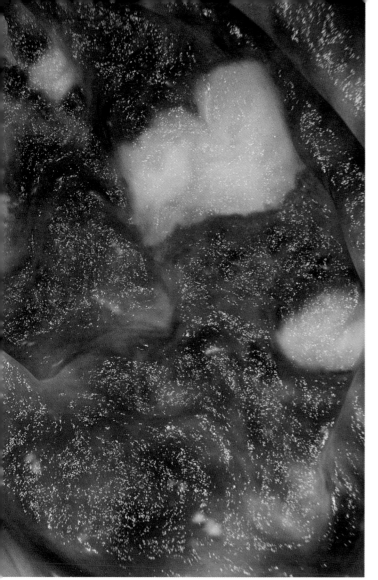

Gut Feeling

Emergency Presentations of Inflammatory Bowel and Diverticular Diseases

LESSON 4

By Alexander Kleinmann, MD; Monica Lopez-Islas, MD; Shruti Chandra, MD, MEHP; and Bernard Lopez, MD, MS, CPE, FACEP
Dr. Kleinmann is a clinical assistant professor; Dr. Lopez-Islas is a resident; Dr. Chandra is an associate professor in the Department of Emergency Medicine, director of phase three (expanded fourth year), and program director for the master of education program; and Dr. Lopez is a professor and executive vice chair in the Department of Emergency Medicine and senior associate dean of diversity and community engagement at Sidney Kimmel Medical College at Thomas Jefferson University in Philadelphia, Pennsylvania.

Reviewed by Walter L. Green, MD, FACEP

Objectives

On completion of this lesson, you should be able to:

1. Identify the pathophysiology of IBD.
2. List the important extraintestinal manifestations found in IBD.
3. Discuss the presentation and clinical findings in toxic megacolon.
4. Describe the diagnosis and management of IBD.
5. Explain the etiology and pathophysiology of diverticular disease.
6. Restate the diagnosis and management of diverticulitis and diverticular bleeding.

From the EM Model

2.0 Abdominal and Gastrointestinal Disorders
    2.8 Small Bowel
        2.8.2 Inflammatory Disorders
            2.8.2.1 Regional Enteritis/Crohn Disease
    2.9 Large Bowel
        2.9.2 Inflammatory Disorders
            2.9.2.4 Ulcerative Colitis
        2.9.4 Structural Disorders
            2.9.4.2 Diverticula

▬ CRITICAL DECISIONS ▬

- What are the unique clinical presentations of IBD?

- How is toxic megacolon diagnosed?

- What emergency department testing should be obtained for patients with IBD?

- How is IBD best managed in the emergency department?

- What tests should be ordered for patients with diverticular disease?

- How is diverticular disease risk stratified?

Approximately 3.1 million Americans, more than 1% of the population in the United States, have inflammatory bowel disease, which includes Crohn disease and ulcerative colitis. Emergency department visits for inflammatory bowel disease are trending upward. Presentations can be similar to the more common diverticular disease. Emergency physicians must be able to differentiate between these GI diseases for accurate treatment of their potentially life-threatening complications.

CASE PRESENTATIONS

CASE ONE

A 38-year-old woman with a history of CD presents with abdominal pain, fever, and bloody diarrhea that has been ongoing for the past month. Over the past 5 days, her symptoms significantly worsened, and she has lost 10 pounds. Her other medical history includes anemia, psoriasis, and kidney stones. Her surgical history is notable for a small bowel resection. She takes adalimumab, methotrexate, folate, and hydrocodone-acetaminophen. On examination, she is lying in bed and appears mildly uncomfortable. Her vital signs include BP 99/50, P 96, R 14, and T 38.4°C (101.1°F). She appears slightly dehydrated, with dry mucous membranes. No icterus is present. Her abdomen is soft and nondistended but diffusely tender, without guarding or rebound. The rest of her examination is unremarkable. The patient states that she is on maximal medical therapy and wonders if there is anything else that can be done for her condition. Laboratory tests and CT of the abdomen and pelvis are ordered.

CASE TWO

A 33-year-old man with a history of UC presents with 4 days of worsening nausea, vomiting, bloody diarrhea, and abdominal pain. Two weeks ago, he developed symptoms typical of a UC flare but did not have relief or improvement of symptoms after a trial of prednisone prescribed by his gastroenterologist. He has not been able to eat or drink and has noticed that his abdomen is bloated. Physical examination reveals an ill-appearing man in moderate discomfort. His vital signs include BP 92/64, P 131, R 22, and T 38.9°C (102°F). He has dry mucous membranes and poor skin turgor. His abdomen is distended, with absent bowel sounds, and is diffusely tender to palpation. The rectal examination is trace positive for occult blood. An intravenous line is started, and an obstruction series of x-rays is ordered.

CASE THREE

A 72-year-old man presents with 3 days of abdominal pain. He has had similar pain in the past but not to such a degree. He has been able to eat normally. On the day of presentation, he noticed an increase in the severity of his pain and described it as a sharp, constant pain in his left side. He denies fever or chills. On examination, the patient appears uncomfortable but not toxic. His vital signs include BP 155/82, P 86, R 16, and T 38.3°C (100.9°F). He has no icterus, and his lungs are clear. His abdominal examination reveals moderate tenderness with guarding and rebound in the left lower quadrant. There also appears to be a mass in the area. His rectal examination elicits discomfort in the left perirectal area, and a stool guaiac test is negative. Genital examination is unremarkable. The patient undergoes laboratory tests and a CT of the abdomen and pelvis. He asks if he can go home because he does not like hospitals. He says he is hungry and could take oral medications at home.

Introduction

Crohn Disease

Crohn disease (CD) is an inflammatory bowel disease (IBD) that can affect the entire GI tract. Most commonly, it involves the terminal ileum (33% of cases) and colon; however, the esophagus, stomach, and proximal small bowel can also be involved. The inflammation found in CD involves all layers of the bowel with characteristic discontinuity ("skip lesions"). Inflammation leads to the formation of ulcerations, the hallmark pathologic finding. These ulcerations develop over lymphoid aggregates and can combine to form even larger ulcerations. Multiple, distinct islands of ulceration are scattered among patches of mucosa, giving an endoscopic appearance known as "cobblestoning." The most severe manifestation of CD is complete ulceration through all layers of the bowel wall, leading to fistulas, sinuses, abscesses, or frank perforation. Chronic fibrotic changes over time can cause strictures.[1] The etiology of CD is not entirely understood and is thought to be due to genetic, environmental, infectious, and immunologic factors. Studies of twins have shown greater concordance of CD in identical twins; smoking has been associated with an increased number of CD attacks ("flares"); multiple bacteria have been proposed as part of the inflammatory cascade; and studies have indicated that CD may be initiated through helper T cells.[2] The worldwide prevalence of CD ranges from 3 to 20 cases per 100,000 people.[3] There is a slight female predominance. CD has a bimodal distribution of incidence: an initial peak in the third decade of life (20s) and a later peak in the sixth (50s).[4,5] Evidence still supports increased prevalence in northern latitudes versus southern latitudes.

Ulcerative Colitis

Ulcerative colitis (UC), like CD, is an inflammatory condition that affects the GI tract but, unlike CD, is typically limited to the rectum and colon and affects only the mucosa and submucosa. UC is also continuous (rather than the skip lesions of CD), with no areas of normal mucosa within the inflamed area. The inflammation of UC has a slow onset that waxes and wanes in intensity over time. The mucosa is erythematous and friable, and superficial ulcers are often present. Chronic changes are marked by areas of fibrosis and loss of haustra and mucosal folds.[2] UC's prevalence in the United States ranges from 37.5 to 238 cases per 100,000 people. From 7,000 to 43,000 new cases of UC are estimated to occur each year in the United States. UC has a slight male predominance.[1,4,6] As with CD, the etiology and development of UC are multifactorial and are thought to include environmental, infectious, and immunologic factors. In contrast to CD, the role of genetics in UC is likely insignificant. UC is classified by anatomic location as follows: proctitis (limited to the rectum), proctosigmoiditis (rectum to sigmoid), left-sided colitis (rectum to splenic flexure), and pancolitis (rectum to beyond the splenic flexure). Most adult patients with UC present with proctitis, followed by left-sided colitis. Only 15% present with pancolitis.[7] In some cases, UC can involve the terminal ileum, making it difficult without past history to distinguish from CD. In general, significant overlap

Clinical	Ulcerative Colitis	Crohn Disease
Abdominal pain	Common	Common
Diarrhea	Common	Common
Hematochezia	Common	Uncommon
Mucus or pus in stools	Common	Rare
Anemia	Common	Uncommon
Any bowel obstruction	Rare	Common
Malnutrition	Uncommon	Common
Location and Type of Involvement		
Upper GI involvement	Never	Uncommon
Small bowel involvement*	Never	Common
Large bowel	Always	Common
Rectal involvement	Always	Rare
Anal involvement	Rare	Common
Continuous	Always	Uncommon
Complications		
Primary sclerosing cholangitis	Rare	Very rare
Toxic megacolon	Rare	Very rare
Strictures	Rare	Uncommon
Fistulas	Never	Uncommon
Abscesses	Rare	Uncommon

* Except backwash ileitis, which is secondary inflammation due to the backwash of contents into the small bowel

TABLE 1. Comparison of characteristics in CD and UC

Urgencies and Emergencies
Scleritis
Uveitis
Thrombosis
Nonurgent or Nonemergent
Ophthalmologic • Episcleritis
Renal • Nephrolithiasis
GI • Primary sclerosing cholangitis • Aphthous stomatitis • Gallstones • Pancreatitis • Malabsorption (malnutrition)
Hematologic • Anemia (blood loss, chronic disease)

Musculoskeletal
• Arthritis
  • Medication induced
  • Axial (ankylosing spondylitis)
  • Peripheral
• Tendinitis
• Osteoporosis

Integumentary • Erythema nodosum • Pyoderma gangrenosum • Other

TABLE 2. Extraintestinal manifestations of IBD

in clinical presentation exists between UC and CD — only 9% to 20% of new IBD cases are diagnosed correctly between the two conditions (*Table 1*).[8]

According to the CDC, 3.1 million people in the United States have IBD.[9] IBD has the highest incidence in White people, particularly those of Ashkenazi Jewish descent; however, in the United States and United Kingdom, people of African descent have begun to manifest similar incidence rates. IBD contributes to almost 0.1% of emergency department visits each year. Studies indicate a rise over time. Between 2006 and 2013, annual IBD emergency department visits increased from 30/100,000 to 42/100,000; inpatient admission rates, however, have remained relatively stable.[4]

Diverticular Disease

Diverticular disease is quite common in the United States and is thought to occur because of the low-fiber diet of developed countries.[10] This diet can lead to small stools and, therefore, straining and increased pressure during bowel movements that can cause the condition diverticulosis. Diverticulosis, specifically, is a condition in which the large-bowel submucosa herniates through the muscular layer and existing paths of small blood vessels. The pouches formed in diverticulosis, known as diverticula, commonly develop as people age. Diverticulosis is painless but can cause bleeding when the local blood supply is eroded. When undigested food and stool get trapped in these diverticula and lead to inflammation, diverticulitis occurs. Diverticulitis typically

presents with left lower quadrant pain but can also present with bleeding and abscess formation.[11] Diverticular bleeding is a common cause of lower GI bleeding — nearly 25% of acute lower GI bleeds are from diverticular disease — and can be life-threatening. Overall, diverticular disease accounts for an estimated 130,000 hospitalizations yearly in the United States.[12] Its prevalence is similar in men and women and increases with age, ranging from approximately 10% in adults younger than 40 years to 50% to 70% among those 80 years or older.[13] In general, the diagnosis of diverticular disease is not difficult to make and can often be made on clinical grounds alone. As with IBD, the emergency physician must be concerned about potential complications.

CRITICAL DECISION

What are the unique clinical presentations of IBD?

The typical presentation of patients with either CD or UC is crampy abdominal pain and diarrhea. The location of pain varies by the area of inflammation. Additionally, patients may experience tenesmus and rectal urgency. The diarrhea is often bloody and can be mixed with pus or mucus. Systemic symptoms can include malaise, fever, and weight loss.[7] Because these diseases are chronic, patients typically report a history of CD or UC, stating they are having another flare of their disease. The necessary physical examination depends on the severity of the attack and should include identifying distension and locating tenderness. Pain, dehydration due to decreased oral intake, and anemia from GI bleeding are the typical concerns for IBD patients. In addition to the usual presentation, patients with IBD can have unique GI or extraintestinal findings. Emergency physicians should be familiar with these manifestations because they aid in diagnosing first-time presentations of IBD and can prevent further morbidity. Notably, CD has a long clinical prodrome (average of 7 years), and most patients present with long-standing complaints.[14] Thus, some patients with chronic abdominal pain evaluated by emergency physicians may actually have CD, and further testing may be warranted to reveal the diagnosis.

Extraintestinal manifestations affect up to 25% of patients with IBD and include skin, eye, blood, and liver dysfunctions (*Table 2*).[15] Skin manifestations are common and include erythema nodosum and pyoderma gangrenosum. The three most common ocular complications, which affect 0.5% to 3% of patients with IBD, are episcleritis, scleritis, and uveitis. Episcleritis is an inflammation of superficial scleral blood vessels that will blanch when exposed to phenylephrine to help determine the diagnosis. Episcleritis is usually unilateral and relatively benign and painless. Scleritis and uveitis, by contrast, cause severe eye pain and can be associated with an abnormal pupillary response and permanent vision loss. They are treated with higher-dose topical steroids and cycloplegics and, in certain cases, systemic steroids, systemic NSAIDs, and immunosuppressant medications.[16,17] Any painful red eye complaint in patients with IBD requires an urgent ophthalmology consultation.

The risk of venous thromboembolic disease is also increased with IBD. In one study, IBD patients were 4.3 times more likely to have deep vein thrombosis or pulmonary embolism than controls and 15.8 times more likely when having an active flare. IBD patients are especially more at risk of developing a venous thromboembolism while hospitalized.[18] The reasons for this are likely multifactorial. First, IBD patients often have multiple risk factors for venous thromboembolism, including surgery, steroid use, fluid depletion, central catheter use, and immobilization due to severe disease. Second, inflammatory responses are mediated by factors like interleukin-6 that activate coagulation. Furthermore, inflammatory states also lead to decreased fibrinolysis, which leads to a prothrombotic state. Overall, abnormalities in coagulation, platelets, fibrinolysis, and endothelial function have been documented in patients with IBD.[19]

Primary sclerosing cholangitis is a disease associated with IBD that inevitably leads to cirrhosis and liver failure and has a mean survival of 12 years from diagnosis. Primary sclerosing cholangitis presents with fatigue, pruritus, fever, chills, night sweats, and right upper quadrant pain. The condition is estimated to occur in 2.5% to 7.5% of patients with UC. Any IBD patient with elevated alkaline phosphatase levels should be suspected of having primary sclerosing cholangitis or cholecystitis or cholelithiasis, which are also associated with IBD. An elevated bilirubin may be found and is indicative of cholestasis from strictures in the biliary tree.

Two other causes of abdominal pain not directly related to bowel wall inflammation in patients with CD are gallstones (cholelithiasis) and kidney stones. The ileitis commonly found in CD affects the absorption of bile salts and can lead to gallstone formation. The incidence of gallbladder disease in patients with CD is doubled compared to controls.[20] Kidney stones can be composed of either calcium oxalate or uric acid. Steatorrhea (found in both CD and UC), due to inadequate bile secretion, leads to increased oxalate absorption and increased oxaluria as well as dehydration and metabolic acidosis. This combination leads to increased formation of both calcium oxalate and uric acid stones.[21]

Patients with IBD are also at an increased risk of opportunistic infections because of the immunosuppressive medications (azathioprine, cyclosporine, 6-mercaptopurine, infliximab, and tumor necrosis factor α) commonly used to treat their condition. Additionally, cyclosporine can cause myelosuppression, electrolyte disturbances, hepatotoxicity, and nephrotoxicity. Azathioprine and 6-mercaptopurine can cause bone marrow suppression and pancreatitis. Infliximab can lead to tuberculosis and fungal infections. Emergency physicians should be aware of these side effects.

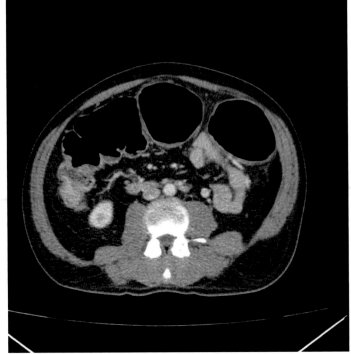

FIGURE 1. CT scan of UC with toxic megacolon.
Credit: Copyright 2023 Dr. David Puyó. Image courtesy of Dr. David Puyó, radiopaedia.org, rID: 65739. Used under license.

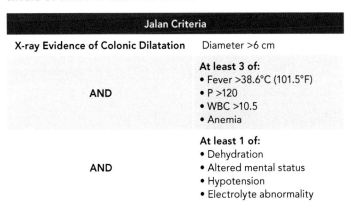

Jalan Criteria	
X-ray Evidence of Colonic Dilatation	Diameter >6 cm
AND	**At least 3 of:** • Fever >38.6°C (101.5°F) • P >120 • WBC >10.5 • Anemia
AND	**At least 1 of:** • Dehydration • Altered mental status • Hypotension • Electrolyte abnormality

TABLE 3. Jalan criteria for toxic megacolon[25]

Disease in Remission	Asymptomatic without the use of steroids (CD activity index [CDAI] score <150)
Mild to Moderate Disease	Ambulatory; able to eat; well hydrated; without systemic toxicity, abdominal tenderness, painful mass, intestinal obstruction, or more than 10% weight loss (CDAI score 150-220)
Moderate to Severe Disease	Failure to respond to treatment for mild to moderate disease, or more prominent symptoms of fever, significant weight loss, abdominal pain or tenderness, intermittent nausea or vomiting, or significant anemia (CDAI score 220-450)
Severe to Fulminant Disease	Persistent symptoms despite the introduction of conventional corticosteroids or biologic agents as outpatients, or individuals presenting with high fevers, persistent vomiting, evidence of intestinal obstruction, significant peritoneal signs, cachexia, or evidence of an abscess (CDAI score >450)

TABLE 4. Working definition of CD severity[28]

CRITICAL DECISION

How is toxic megacolon diagnosed?

Toxic megacolon is a life-threatening complication of IBD, defined by acute colonic dilatation of the transverse colon to more than 6 cm in diameter. Different types of colonic inflammation can lead to toxic megacolon, but most cases occur in patients with IBD.[22]

IBD patients are at risk of developing toxic megacolon because of inflammation of the bowel's smooth muscle layer. Toxic megacolon typically presents after several days of IBD symptoms and is found in 2.3% of CD patients and 10% of UC patients. The mortality rate for patients developing toxic megacolon is 19%, with perforation significantly increasing the risk of death.[23,24] Symptoms include abdominal pain, fever, chills, and diarrhea. Obstipation is a particularly ominous sign. Physical findings include abdominal distension and tenderness, tachycardia, and signs of dehydration. Adjunctive imaging is helpful, and plain x-rays may show dilatation of the transverse or ascending colon of more than 6 cm. CT will demonstrate diffuse colonic wall thickening, submucosal edema, pericolic stranding, or dilatation of the transverse colon with an abnormal haustral pattern (*Figure 1*). The Jalan criteria can be used as a guide for the diagnosis of toxic megacolon (*Table 3*).[25] The diagnosis requires:
- Evidence of colonic dilatation (transverse colon >6 cm);
- Any three of the following: fever above 38.6°C (101.5°F), tachycardia greater than 120 bpm, WBC count greater than 10.5×10^9/L, and anemia; and
- Any one of the following: dehydration, mental status changes, electrolyte disturbances, and hypotension.[24]

CRITICAL DECISION

What emergency department testing should be obtained for patients with IBD?

The diagnosis and treatment of IBD are guided by clinical presentation; there is no specific laboratory test that will diagnose either condition. Despite the unique features of

Mild Disease	Less than four stools daily, with or without blood; no systemic signs of toxicity; and a normal erythrocyte sedimentation rate
Moderate Disease	More than four stools daily but with minimal signs of toxicity
Severe Disease	More than six bloody stools daily and evidence of toxicity as demonstrated by fever, tachycardia, anemia, or an elevated erythrocyte sedimentation rate
Fulminant Disease	More than 10 bowel movements daily, continuous bleeding, toxicity, abdominal tenderness and distension, blood transfusion requirement, and colonic dilatation on abdominal x-rays

TABLE 5. Clinical severity of UC[29]

IBD, the diagnosis depends on clinical findings, laboratory data, and imaging. Ultimately, colonoscopy is used to make the definitive diagnosis in first-time presentations and may be useful in guiding treatment in patients with known disease. Furthermore, the differential diagnosis of diarrhea with abdominal pain includes other types of colitis, such as infectious colitis. A CBC may be useful to detect infection or significant blood loss. Electrolyte levels can help determine the degree of dehydration from vomiting or diarrhea. Stool cultures should be ordered on all admitted patients because they are helpful in ruling out infectious causes. *Clostridioides difficile* (formerly *Clostridium difficile*) toxin assay is important for any patient on antibiotics to rule out the possibility of *C. difficile* enterocolitis. An obstruction series of x-rays can provide early clues in diagnosing complications such as obstruction, perforation, and toxic megacolon. CT with intravenous and oral contrast is the preferred method of imaging because it is both sensitive and specific.[26] The CT can demonstrate the changes typical of CD and UC as well as perforation, pneumatosis, toxic megacolon, mural thickening, and luminal narrowing. Axial imaging can demonstrate a target or halo appearance. In this finding, the lumen of the bowel is surrounded by a ring of soft-tissue density that represents mucosa, lamina propria, and muscularis mucosa, followed by a low-density ring that represents fatty infiltrate of the submucosa, and then another soft-tissue density ring that represents the muscularis propria. Patients may have homogeneous bowel wall thickening suggestive of fibrosis. CT is particularly useful in the diagnosis of abscesses and fistulas. Abscesses are common in CD and appear on CT as a fluid collection with ring enhancement. Fistulas affect 20% to 40% of patients with CD and appear as contrast communicating to any hollow viscus.[27]

CRITICAL DECISION

How is IBD best managed in the emergency department?

Treatment of CD and UC is largely supportive. Definitive treatment should be made in conjunction with a gastroenterologist as often as possible. Patients who are having a flare because of an uncomplicated mild to moderate exacerbation from medication noncompliance may need only to restart their maintenance therapy. Patients with a mild to moderate flare who have been compliant with maintenance therapy may require added corticosteroids, typically 40 to 60 mg of prednisone (or an equivalent dose) daily. In general, if suspicion is strong for a first episode of IBD, patients should be admitted for further workup, treatment, and counseling. However, in patients with mild symptoms and perceived reliable follow-up, discharge with clear return precautions and recommendations for prompt gastroenterology re-evaluation is an acceptable alternative to admission. Patients with severe disease that is unresponsive to oral corticosteroids need admission for intravenous steroids. Fulminant colitis requires consultation with a gastroenterologist and surgeon to evaluate for emergent colectomy (*Tables 4* and *5*).[15,28,29] Lastly, patients with toxic megacolon, abscess, obstruction, or significant pain should be admitted for inpatient therapy. Admitted patients should be started on intravenous corticosteroids, and broad-spectrum antibiotics can be considered if abscesses are present. Acute surgical management is needed for patients with bowel perforation, toxic megacolon, significant hemorrhage, or obstruction. Management of toxic megacolon consists of bowel rest, intravenous fluid rehydration, correction of electrolyte disturbances, intravenous corticosteroids, and broad-spectrum antibiotics. Narcotics and anticholinergics should be avoided because they can exacerbate colonic dilatation. Patients may require decompression with a nasogastric tube and rectal tube.

Diverticular Disease

Among patients with diverticulosis, 10% to 25% will develop diverticulitis. Diverticulitis results from inflammation or infection of diverticula. The progression of diverticulitis can lead to localized microperforation or free perforation into the peritoneum. Although the cause of diverticular rupture is unknown, inflammation and increasing intraluminal pressure are thought to be key factors; stasis, alteration in local bacterial microflora, and local ischemia have also been implicated.[30] Diverticular disease is typically found in the descending colon. Patients classically present with left lower quadrant abdominal pain, obstipation, and low-grade fever. Seventy percent of patients with severe complications from acute diverticulitis have never had a prior episode.[30] The mortality rate has been reported as 1% among patients admitted for acute diverticulitis and 5.5% among those admitted for diverticular perforation.[31] Complications include abscess, perforation, fistula, bleeding, and stricture.

Notably, right-sided diverticulitis is common in Asia and rare in western countries, with a reported incidence of 76% in Asian countries and 1% to 5% in western populations.[32-34] Patients with right-sided diverticulitis tend to be younger with fewer comorbidities and tend to do better than patients with left-sided diverticulitis. Right-sided diverticulitis is often diagnosed incidentally during the workup of appendicitis.

Diverticular bleeding is caused when a penetrating artery running adjacent to a diverticulum ruptures. These arteries sustain insults over time, causing asymmetric changes within the vessel that eventually lead to the vessel's rupture into the lumen of the bowel. Inflammation is usually not associated with diverticular bleeding.[35] Diverticular bleeding is common, accounting for 23% of acute lower GI bleeds.[36] Severe diverticular bleeding can occur in 3% to 5% of patients with diverticulosis, and most bleeding occurs in patients older than 50 years.[37,38] Interestingly, although most diverticula are in the left colon, at least 50% of diverticular bleeds occur in patients with right-sided diverticulitis, probably because right-sided diverticula usually have a narrower base and larger dome that make them more prone to bleeding.[38]

Diverticular bleeding typically presents painlessly, with copious amounts of red or maroon blood with clots. Rarely, melena can occur from right-sided bleeding. Hemorrhage is self-contained in 70% to 80% of patients; however, rebleeds occur in 22% to 38% of patients. A small percentage of patients have uncontrolled GI bleeding that requires surgery. In these cases, identification of the bleeding source is essential and requires specialty consultation for definitive diagnosis and treatment.

CRITICAL DECISION

What tests should be ordered for patients with diverticular disease?

In uncomplicated diverticulitis (focal left lower quadrant pain, absence of peritoneal irritation, nontoxic appearance of the patient, no evidence of alternative disease), no studies are required, and the patient may be treated empirically. Ancillary testing should be obtained when the diagnosis is in question or if evidence suggests peritoneal inflammation, systemic illness, abscess formation, or perforation. Although laboratory testing is typically ordered, CT is the most useful test. CT can demonstrate inflammation, abscess formation, and perforation and can delineate the extent of disease. CT can also help make an alternative diagnosis when findings of diverticulitis are absent.

For diverticular bleeding, emergency physicians may need to initiate studies that can localize the bleeding, such as CT angiography or tagged RBC studies. Angiography can detect a bleeding rate of 1 mL/minute, and technetium scanning can detect a bleeding rate of 0.5 mL/minute. CT angiography has the added benefit of therapeutic intervention through intra-arterial vasopressin or subsegmental embolism.

CRITICAL DECISION

How is diverticular disease risk stratified?

Uncomplicated diverticulitis has been traditionally treated in the outpatient setting with oral antibiotics. New guidelines suggest that antibiotics should be used more selectively in patients with acute uncomplicated diverticulitis.[39] Antibiotics have not been proven to shorten disease duration or prevent recurrence. Immunosuppressed patients, pregnant patients, septic patients, or patients with significant comorbidities should receive antibiotics. Antibiotics should cover gram-negative aerobic and anaerobic bacteria. Analgesics and follow-up should be arranged. Hospitalization should be considered for patients with comorbidities, advanced age, an inability to take oral liquids, poor social support, or poor follow-up. Patients with peritonitis, systemic illness, bowel obstruction, and small (<5 cm in diameter) abscesses should be admitted for intravenous antibiotics and analgesia. In addition to intravenous antibiotics and analgesia, patients with larger abscesses, evidence of perforation, fistulas, or colonic dilatation require surgical consultation and further definitive care, which may include drainage of abscesses and removal of fistulas. Those with diverticular bleeding generally require admission for supportive care, such as intravascular volume replacement and blood products, and definitive diagnosis and treatment.

Summary

IBD is relatively common and has a complex clinical presentation. It can affect almost every organ system and, therefore, can present with a multitude of symptoms. Recognizing extraintestinal signs can lead to earlier diagnosis. Management of patients with an initial presentation of disease differs from management of patients with chronic disease. The differential diagnosis is broad for patients with undiagnosed disease and includes etiologies that require a more specialized workup than is typically available in emergency departments. By contrast, a patient with known disease is likely already taking immunosuppressive therapy or chronic antibiotics, placing them at risk of opportunistic infections and *C. difficile*. Both patients with new-onset and chronic IBD are at risk of toxic megacolon and extraintestinal emergencies.

Diverticulitis is a very common disease that can have potentially deadly outcomes in patients with perforated diverticula and diverticular bleeds. Physicians must differentiate diverticular disease from IBD and other diseases in the broad differential diagnosis, especially in older patients who are more at risk of other serious illnesses with a similar presentation to diverticular disease.

REFERENCES

1. Kappelman MD, Rifas-Shiman SL, Kleinman K, et al. The prevalence and geographic distribution of Crohn's disease and ulcerative colitis in the United States. *Clin Gastroenterol Hepatol.* 2007 Dec;5(12):1424-1429.

2. Thoreson R, Cullen JJ. Pathophysiology of inflammatory bowel disease: an overview. *Surg Clin North Am.* 2007 Jun;87(3):575-585.

3. Molodecky NA, Soon IS, Rabi DM, et al. Increasing incidence and prevalence of the inflammatory bowel diseases with time, based on systematic review. *Gastroenterology.* 2012 Jan;142(1):46-54.e42.

4. Ding Z, Patel A, Izanec J, Pericone CD, Lin JH, Baugh CW. Trends in US emergency department visits and subsequent hospital admission among patients with inflammatory bowel disease presenting with abdominal pain: a real-world study from a national emergency department sample database. *J Mark Access Health Policy.* 2021 Apr 19;9(1):1912924.

5. Feuerstein JD, Cheifetz AS. Crohn disease: epidemiology, diagnosis, and management. *Mayo Clin Proc.* 2017 Jul;92(7):1088-1103.

6. Loftus EV Jr, Sandborn WJ. Epidemiology of inflammatory bowel disease. *Gastroenterol Clin North Am.* 2002 Mar;31(1):1-20.

7. Ghosh S, Shand A, Ferguson A. Ulcerative colitis. *BMJ.* 2000 Apr 22;320(7242):1119-1123.

8. Mitchell PJ, Rabau MY, Haboubi NY. Indeterminate colitis. *Tech Coloproctol.* 2007 Jun;11(2):91-96.

9. Inflammatory bowel disease. Centers for Disease Control and Prevention. Reviewed April 15, 2022. https://www.cdc.gov/ibd/features/IBD-more-chronic-diseases.html

10. Burkitt DP, Walker AR, Painter NS. Effect of dietary fibre on stools and transit-times, and its role in the causation of disease. *Lancet.* 1972 Dec 30;2(7792):1408-1411.

11. Salem TA, Molloy RG, O'Dwyer PJ. Prospective study on the management of patients with complicated diverticular disease. *Colorectal Dis.* 2006 Mar;8(3):173-176.

12. Munson KD, Hensien MA, Jacob LN, Robinson AM, Liston WA. Diverticulitis. A comprehensive follow-up. *Dis Colon Rectum.* 1996 Mar;39(3):318-322.

13. Ferzoco LB, Raptopoulos V, Silen W. Acute diverticulitis. *N Engl J Med.* 1998 May 21;338(21):1521-1526.

14. Pimentel M, Chang M, Chow EJ, et al. Identification of a prodromal period in Crohn's disease but not ulcerative colitis. *Am J Gastroenterol.* 2000;95(12):3458-3462.

15. Baumgart DC, Sandborn WJ. Inflammatory bowel disease: clinical aspects and established and evolving therapies. *Lancet.* 2007 May 12;369(9573):1641-1657.

16. Mintz R, Feller ER, Bahr RL, Shah SA. Ocular manifestations of inflammatory bowel disease. *Inflamm Bowel Dis.* 2004 Mar;10(2):135-139.

17. Lyons JL, Rosenbaum JT. Uveitis associated with inflammatory bowel disease compared with uveitis associated with spondyloarthropathy. *Arch Ophthalmol.* 1997 Jan;115(1):61-64.

18. Grainge MJ, West J, Card TR. Venous thromboembolism during active disease and remission in inflammatory bowel disease: a cohort study. *Lancet.* 2010 Feb;375(9715):657-663.

✔ Pearls

- CD can affect the entire GI tract, while UC tends to affect the rectum and colon.

- Extraintestinal manifestations of IBD are fistulas, abscesses, anemia, and ocular disturbances; they provide emergency physicians with significant clues for diagnosing a first-time presentation of IBD.

- In IBD patients with abdominal pain, suspect primary sclerosing cholangitis, cholecystitis, or cholelithiasis if alkaline phosphatase levels are elevated.

- Toxic megacolon should be considered in IBD patients with systemic illness, obstipation, and a significantly dilated colon on x-ray.

- In consultation with a gastroenterologist, physicians should administer steroids to treat IBD patients who are unresponsive to their usual therapy.

- Although most IBD patients who present with abdominal symptoms have a history of IBD, only 30% of acute diverticulitis patients who present with severe complications have a history of diverticulitis.

- Diverticular bleeding is common, accounting for nearly 25% of acute lower GI bleeds.

- Uncomplicated diverticulitis — defined as left lower quadrant pain, usually in a relatively younger patient who is nontoxic appearing — can be diagnosed clinically.

CASE RESOLUTIONS

■ CASE ONE

The young woman had an exacerbation of her CD. Laboratory test results were at baseline. CT of the abdomen and pelvis showed extensive wall thickening and pericolonic hyperemia involving the rectum, sigmoid colon, descending colon, and scattered portions of the transverse colon. No abscesses or fistulous communications were visualized. She was admitted to a medical service and started on intravenous methylprednisolone, ciprofloxacin, and metronidazole. She was gradually transitioned to a low-residue oral diet and was placed on oral antibiotics. She was discharged home after a 4-day stay.

■ CASE TWO

The 33-year-old man's obstruction series demonstrated a markedly enlarged colon with a transverse colonic diameter of 8 cm. This finding, along with the fever, tachycardia, and hypotension, raised suspicion for toxic megacolon. A CT scan was obtained and confirmed the diagnosis. A nasogastric tube was placed while the patient was in the emergency department.

He was admitted to the gastroenterology service with a surgery team consult. After 1 week of supportive care and aggressive management, his symptoms resolved without the need for surgical intervention.

■ CASE THREE

The 72-year-old man's laboratory results showed an elevated WBC count; his CT scan showed a rim-enhancing hypodensity adjacent to the sigmoid colon with stranding and numerous diverticula, consistent with an abscess. He was informed that an abscess put him at an increased risk of mortality, and he agreed to stay at the hospital. He was started on intravenous ampicillin-sulbactam. The interventional radiologist thought that the abscess was too small to drain and recommended observation. Three days later, a repeat CT scan showed resolution of the abscess with decreased stranding. The patient was started on a high-fiber diet and was placed on oral cephalosporin and metronidazole therapy. On the fourth hospital day, he was discharged home with close gastroenterology follow-up.

19. Danese S, Papa A, Saibeni S, Repici A, Malesci A, Vecchi M. Inflammation and coagulation in inflammatory bowel disease: the clot thickens. *Am J Gastroenterol.* 2007 Jan;102(1):174-186.

20. Parente F, Pastore L, Bargiggia S, et al. Incidence and risk factors for gallstones in patients with inflammatory bowel disease: a large case-control study. *Hepatology.* 2007 May;45(5):1267-1274.

21. Obialo CI, Clayman RV, Matts JP, et al. Pathogenesis of nephrolithiasis post-partial ileal bypass surgery: case-control study. The POSCH Group. *Kidney Int.* 1991;39(6):1249-1254.

22. Desai J, Elnaggar M, Hanfy AA, Doshi R. Toxic megacolon: background, pathophysiology, management challenges and solutions. *Clin Exp Gastroenterol.* 2020 May 19;13:203-210.

23. Strauss RJ, Flint GW, Platt N, Levin L, Wise L. The surgical management of toxic dilatation of the colon: a report of 28 cases and review of the literature. *Ann Surg.* 1976 Dec;184(6): 682-688.

24. Gan SI, Beck PL. A new look at toxic megacolon: an update and review of incidence, etiology, pathogenesis, and management. *Am J Gastroenterol.* 2003 Nov;98(11):2363-2371.

25. Jalan KN, Sircus W, Card WI, et al. An experience of ulcerative colitis. I. Toxic dilation in 55 cases. *Gastroenterology.* 1969 Jul;57(1):68-82.

26. Hill BC, Johnson SC, Owens EK, Gerber JL, Senagore AJ. CT scan for suspected acute abdominal process: impact of combinations of IV, oral, and rectal contrast. *World J Surg.* 2010 Apr;34(4):699-703.

27. Gore RM, Balthazar EJ, Ghahremani GG, Miller FH. CT features of ulcerative colitis and Crohn's disease. *AJR Am J Roentgenol.* 1996 Jul;167(1):3-15.

28. Lichtenstein GR, Hanauer SB, Sandborn WJ; Practice Parameters Committee of American College of Gastroenterology. The management of Crohn's disease in adults. *Am J Gastroenterol.* 2009 Feb;104(2):465-483.

29. Kornbluth A, Sachar DB; Practice Parameters Committee of the American College of Gastroenterology. Ulcerative colitis practice guidelines in adults: American College of Gastroenterology, Practice Parameters Committee. *Am J Gastroenterol.* 2010;105(3):501-523.

30. Touzios JG, Dozois EJ. Diverticulosis and acute diverticulitis. *Gastroenterol Clin North Am.* 2009 Sep;38(3):513-525.

31. Mäkelä JT, Kiviniemi HO, Laitinen ST. Spectrum of disease and outcome among patients with acute diverticulitis. *Dig Surg.* 2010 Aug;27(3):190-196.

32. Graham SM, Ballantyne GH. Cecal diverticulitis. A review of the American experience. *Dis Colon Rectum.* 1987 Oct;30(10):821-826.

33. Hughes LE. Postmortem survey of diverticular disease of the colon. I. Diverticulosis and diverticulitis. *Gut.* 1969 May;10(5):336-344

34. Markham NI, Li AK. Diverticulitis of the right colon — experience from Hong Kong. *Gut.* 1992 Apr;33(4):547-549.

35. Meyers MA, Alonso DR, Gray GF, Baer JW. Pathogenesis of bleeding colonic diverticulosis. *Gastroenterology.* 1976 Oct;71(4):577-583.

36. Machicado GA, Jensen DM. Acute and chronic management of lower gastrointestinal bleeding: cost-effective approaches. *Gastroenterologist.* 1997 Sep;5(3):189-201.

37. Stollman N, Raskin JB. Diverticular disease of the colon. *Lancet.* 2004 Feb 21;363(9409):631-639.

38. Lewis M; NDSG. Bleeding colonic diverticula. *J Clin Gastroenterol.* 2008 Nov-Dec;42(10):1156-1158.

39. Mora-López L, Ruiz-Edo N, Estrada-Ferrer O, et al. Efficacy and safety of nonantibiotic outpatient treatment in mild acute diverticulitis (DINAMO-study): a multicentre, randomized, open-label, noninferiority trial. *Ann Surg.* 2021 Nov 1;274(5):e435-e442.

✖ Pitfalls

- Neglecting to perform a complete physical examination that includes examining for extraintestinal manifestations of IBD.

- Failing to diagnose scleritis and initiate treatment with systemic steroids, systemic NSAIDs, and possibly systemic immunosuppressants.

- Forgetting to consider toxic megacolon in patients with IBD who complain of obstipation.

- Disregarding the admission of patients with uncomplicated diverticulitis when they have comorbidities, are of an advanced age, cannot take oral liquids, have poor social support, or are unreliable for follow-up.

CME Questions

Reviewed by Michael S. Beeson, MD, MBA, FACEP; and Walter L. Green, MD, FACEP

Qualified, paid subscribers to *Critical Decisions in Emergency Medicine* may receive CME certificates for up to 5 ACEP Category I credits, 5 *AMA PRA Category 1 Credits™*, and 5 AOA Category 2-B credits for completing this activity in its entirety. Submit your answers online at acep.org/cdem; a score of 75% or better is required. You may receive credit for completing the CME activity any time within 3 years of its publication date. Answers to this month's questions will be published in next month's issue.

1 **Which is a known reservoir of *Monkeypox virus*?**
   A. Amphibians
   B. Birds
   C. Reptiles
   D. Small mammals

2 **A 32-year-old man presents with the chief complaint of an itchy and painful rash that was preceded by fatigue and fever for the past 2 to 3 days. The patient is on HIV pre-exposure prophylaxis. On examination, he has a rash that consists of a few lesions in the perianal region that are in various stages, from macules to papules, and are rubbery when palpated. His vital signs are BP 139/84, P 87, R 17, and T 38.2°C (100.8°F); SpO$_2$ is 98% on room air. What is the most likely diagnosis?**
   A. Herpes
   B. Mpox
   C. Scabies
   D. Varicella

3 **What is an indicator for mpox antiviral treatment?**
   A. Being middle-aged at the time of infection
   B. HIV pre-exposure prophylaxis use
   C. Lesions near the anus
   D. Moderate symptoms of infection

4 **Before treatment with brincidofovir, what test must be obtained?**
   A. HIV testing
   B. Liver function testing
   C. Renal function testing
   D. Syphilis testing

5 **A 43-year-old man presents for an STI evaluation. He reports he is homeless and has sex with men. His medical history includes type 2 diabetes mellitus. During the patient encounter, he reports that he heard about the mpox vaccine on the news and has a friend who contracted mpox; he asks if he can receive the vaccine. The physician is concerned about this man's reliability for follow-up. What is the most appropriate vaccination to recommend?**
   A. Smallpox vaccine
   B. Smallpox and mpox vaccine
   C. Vaccinia immune globulin
   D. Varicella vaccine

6 **A 7-year-old girl was recently diagnosed with mpox and presents for further evaluation of developing symptoms. She has had decreased oral intake secondary to painful lesions and lymphadenopathy. Her urine specific-gravity measurement is 1.030. What should be the first-line therapy for this patient?**
   A. Intravenous fluids, pain medication, and cidofovir
   B. Intravenous fluids, pain medication, and tecovirimat
   C. Oral hydration and vaccinia immune globulin
   D. Oral hydration, pain medication, and brincidofovir

7 **Differentiating mpox from smallpox is often difficult because of the similarities in their dermal lesions. However, the rate of skin-lesion onset is more rapid with smallpox. What is the average rate of lesion onset in smallpox infections?**
   A. 12 to 18 hours
   B. 24 to 36 hours
   C. 48 to 72 hours
   D. 72 to 96 hours

8 **What side effects are associated with tecovirimat?**
   A. Abdominal pain, nausea, and vomiting
   B. Elevated transaminases and bilirubin
   C. Iritis and uveitis
   D. Neutropenia and proteinuria

9 **What is the most common agent used to treat mpox?**
   A. Brincidofovir
   B. Cidofovir
   C. Tecovirimat
   D. Vaccinia immune globulin

10 **The WHO defines a public health emergency of international concern as "an extraordinary event which is determined to constitute a public health risk to other States through the international spread of disease and to potentially require a coordinated international response." Which criterion is not used to determine if a situation is a public health emergency of international concern?**
   A. It carries implications for public health beyond the affected State's national border
   B. It involves extensive disease burden and economic consequences
   C. It is serious, sudden, unusual, or unexpected
   D. It may require immediate international action

11 **A patient presents with diffuse abdominal pain, fever, and an elevated WBC count. CT imaging is notable for pericolic stranding and continuous inflammation from the splenic flexure to the rectum. What conclusion can be reached about the definitive diagnosis?**

   A. More information is needed to diagnose this patient's condition
   B. The patient has Crohn disease
   C. The patient has diverticulitis
   D. The patient has infectious colitis

12 **A patient with ulcerative colitis presents with complaints of several weeks of fatigue, pruritus, fever, chills, night sweats, and right upper quadrant pain. The patient likely has which condition?**

   A. Cholecystitis
   B. Diverticulitis
   C. Primary sclerosing cholangitis
   D. Renal colic

13 **What percentage of patients with inflammatory bowel disease have extraintestinal manifestations?**

   A. 5%
   B. 10%
   C. 25%
   D. 50%

14 **The Jalan criteria for identifying toxic megacolon include evidence of a transverse colon diameter of more than 6 cm plus how many of the following: fever above 38.6°C (101.5°F), heart rate faster than 120 bpm, WBC count above 10.5×10^9/L, and anemia?**

   A. 1
   B. 2
   C. 3
   D. 4

15 **What is the most serious extraintestinal finding in inflammatory bowel disease?**

   A. Episcleritis
   B. Erythema nodosum
   C. Pyoderma gangrenosum
   D. Uveitis

16 **What is the cause of diverticulitis?**

   A. Allergies to ingested foods
   B. Fecalith that blocks the diverticular mouth and causes stasis, inflammation, and eventually perforation
   C. High-fiber diets
   D. Inflammation or infection within the diverticula

17 **What is more typical of patients with right-sided diverticulitis?**

   A. They are more likely to be of Asian descent
   B. They have worse medical outcomes
   C. They tend to be older
   D. They tend to eat more fiber

18 **Which patient with diverticulitis can be safely discharged home?**

   A. A 35-year-old woman with no peritoneal findings and no abscess or perforation on her CT scan
   B. An 80-year-old patient with arthritis and nausea
   C. A patient with a 2-cm diameter diverticular abscess on the CT scan
   D. A patient with diabetes and moderate pain

19 **A 60-year-old woman with a history of diverticula presents with bright red blood through the rectum. What is true about this patient's diverticular bleeding?**

   A. The patient's bleed is from a venous source in the GI tract
   B. The patient's bleed is most likely from diverticula in the left colon
   C. The patient's bleed is uncommon because diverticular bleeds are more likely in younger adults
   D. The patient's bleed will most likely self-resolve

20 **A patient presents with a flare of ulcerative colitis that he states is worse than previous flares. What specifically should the patient be examined for?**

   A. Anal involvement
   B. Esophageal involvement
   C. Fistula
   D. Toxic megacolon

ANSWER KEY FOR JANUARY 2023, VOLUME 37, NUMBER 1

1	2	3	4	5	6	7	8	9	10	11	12	13	14	15	16	17	18	19	20
B	B	A	D	C	A	C	A	C	C	B	D	D	A	D	D	A	D	C	C

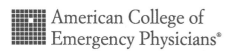

American College of
Emergency Physicians®

ADVANCING EMERGENCY CARE ___/_
Post Office Box 619911
Dallas, Texas 75261-9911

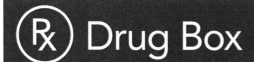

Drug Box

CDC's New Guidelines for Opioid Prescriptions

By Frank LoVecchio, DO, MPH, FACEP
Valleywise Health and ASU, Phoenix, Arizona

Objective
On completion of this column, you should be able to:
- State the CDC's new recommendations for opioid prescriptions.

Background
In 2016, to help physicians weigh the risks and benefits of treatment, the CDC updated its guidelines for prescribing opioids for chronic pain.[1] The guidelines led to an overall decrease in opioid prescriptions and increase in nonopioid prescriptions for pain. However, the 2016 guidelines also led to policies, regulations, and legislation that many physicians thought were inconsistent with and went beyond these guidelines.[2] In 2022, the CDC released new guidelines to clarify how emergency physicians and physicians in outpatient settings should prescribe opioids for adults with pain "in situations other than those of sickle cell disease, cancer-related pain, palliative care, and end-of-life care."[3]

2022 Guidelines
The new guidelines relevant to emergency physicians are as follows:
- Nonopioid therapies are as effective as opioids for common types of acute pain. Physicians should use nonpharmacologic and nonopioid pharmacologic therapies when possible and should consider opioid therapy for acute pain only when benefits outweigh risks.
- Nonopioid therapies are preferred for subacute and chronic pain.
- Opioid therapy for acute, subacute, or chronic pain should be prescribed as immediate release instead of extended release and long acting.
- Physicians should be especially cautious when prescribing opioids with benzodiazepines.
- Before and periodically during opioid therapy, physicians should evaluate for and discuss opioid-related risks with patients and mitigate risks during treatment, including offering naloxone.
- When prescribing opioids for acute pain, physicians should give the minimum quantity needed for the expected duration of treatment.
- Physicians should offer or arrange for treatment with evidence-based medications for patients with opioid use disorder (OUD). Detoxification without OUD medications is not recommended because it increases the risks of resuming drug use, overdose, and death from overdose.
- When opioids are used continuously for more than a few days, they should be tapered before discontinuing. Tapering doses by 10% or less per month in patients with chronic opioid use (≥1 year) will most likely be tolerated better than more rapid tapers.
- To discourage misapplication of thresholds, the new recommendations avoid giving specific dosage thresholds and instead give general advice, such as avoiding dosage increases above levels with diminishing returns.

REFERENCES
1. Dowell D, Haegerich TM, Chou R. CDC guideline for prescribing opioids for chronic pain — United States, 2016. *MMWR Recomm Rep.* 2016 Mar 18;65(1):1-49.
2. Dowell D, Haegerich T, Chou R. No shortcuts to safer opioid prescribing. *N Engl J Med.* 2019 Jun 13;380(24):2285-2287.
3. Dowell D, Ragan KR, Jones CM, Baldwin GT, Chou R. CDC clinical practice guideline for prescribing opioids for pain — United States, 2022. *MMWR Recomm Rep.* 2022 Nov 4;71(3):1-95.

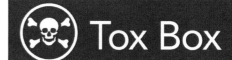

Tox Box

Potassium Chlorate Poisoning

By Christian A. Tomaszewski, MD, MS, MBA, FACEP
University of California San Diego Health

Objective
On completion of this column, you should be able to:
- Discuss how to identify and treat $KClO_3$ poisoning.

Introduction
Severe potassium chlorate ($KClO_3$) poisoning can occur from the ingestion of laboratory or herbicidal solutions. Match heads also contain $KClO_3$ and can cause toxicity if ingested in excess (>20 heads), especially in young children. $KClO_3$ is also found in dyes, fireworks, and disinfectants.

Pharmacology
- Potentially lethal dose
  - >1 g in infants (>20 match heads)
  - >5 g in adults
- Kinetics
  - Readily absorbed in the GI tract, but inhaling can also lead to poisoning
  - Slowly excreted by the kidneys
- Strong oxidizer
  - Hemolysis with methemoglobinemia
  - Renal toxicity with direct proximal tubular necrosis

Clinical Manifestations
- **GI:** Mucosal irritation, nausea, vomiting
- **Hematologic:** Methemoglobinemia (resistant), hemolysis
- **Renal:** Renal failure with acute tubular necrosis
- **Hepatic:** Hyperbilirubinemia

Laboratory
- CBC and comprehensive metabolic panel if symptomatic (vomiting, diarrhea)
- Methemoglobin level if cyanotic
- Coagulation studies if hemolysis is present

Treatment
- Intravenous fluids for rehydration and oxygen as needed
- Methylene blue 1 mg/kg for methemoglobinemia
  - Can repeat after 1 hr
  - Avoid in cases of G6PD deficiency
- Hemodialysis to treat renal failure
- Exchange transfusion for severe poisoning

Disposition
- Can discharge if asymptomatic 6 hr post ingestion
- Trend CBC and methemoglobin levels if symptomatic

Critical decisions
in emergency medicine

Volume 37 Number 3: **March 2023**

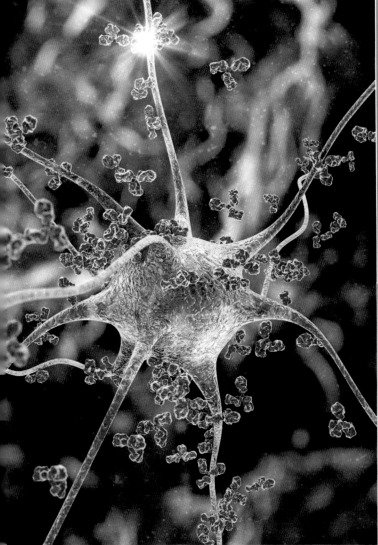

Bundle of Nerves

Rapid progression of transverse myelitis and Guillain-Barré syndrome can lead to life-threatening complications, such as spinal shock or respiratory failure. Emergency physicians must be familiar with the clinical presentations, workup, monitoring, and management of these neurologic disorders to improve the overall prognosis of each patient.

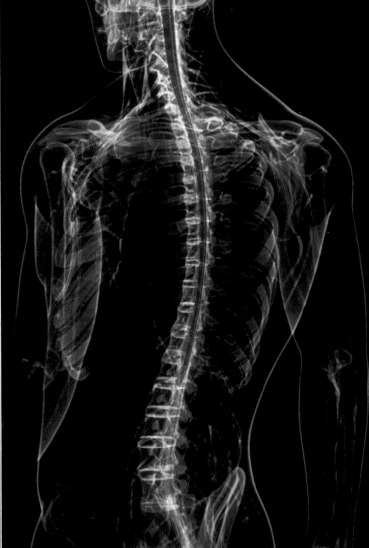

Show Some Backbone

Traumatic spinal injury is a common occurrence in the United States and can have potentially devastating consequences. Emergency physicians are often the first clinicians to evaluate these patients. Recognizing these cases early and managing them appropriately provides spinal injury patients with their best chance to avoid secondary neurologic injury.

THE OFFICIAL CME PUBLICATION OF THE AMERICAN COLLEGE OF EMERGENCY PHYSICIANS

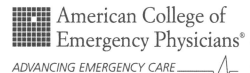

American College of Emergency Physicians®

ADVANCING EMERGENCY CARE

Critical decisions
in emergency medicine

Critical Decisions in Emergency Medicine is the official CME publication of the American College of Emergency Physicians. Additional volumes are available.

EDITOR-IN-CHIEF

Michael S. Beeson, MD, MBA, FACEP
Northeastern Ohio Universities,
Rootstown, OH

SECTION EDITORS

Joshua S. Broder, MD, FACEP
Duke University, Durham, NC

Andrew J. Eyre, MD, MS-HPEd
Brigham and Women's Hospital/
Harvard Medical School, Boston, MA

John Kiel, DO, MPH, FACEP, CAQSM
University of Florida College of Medicine,
Jacksonville, FL

Frank LoVecchio, DO, MPH, FACEP
Valleywise, Arizona State University, University of Arizona,
and Creighton Colleges of Medicine, Phoenix, AZ

Sharon E. Mace, MD, FACEP
Cleveland Clinic Lerner College of Medicine/
Case Western Reserve University, Cleveland, OH

Amal Mattu, MD, FACEP
University of Maryland, Baltimore, MD

Christian A. Tomaszewski, MD, MS, MBA, FACEP
University of California Health Sciences,
San Diego, CA

Steven J. Warrington, MD, MEd, MS
MercyOne Siouxland, Sioux City, IA

ASSOCIATE EDITORS

Tareq Al-Salamah, MBBS, MPH, FACEP
King Saud University, Riyadh, Saudi Arabia/
University of Maryland, Baltimore, MD

Wan-Tsu Chang, MD
University of Maryland, Baltimore, MD

Ann M. Dietrich, MD, FAAP, FACEP
University of South Carolina College of Medicine,
Greenville, SC

Kelsey Drake, MD, MPH, FACEP
St. Anthony Hospital, Lakewood, CO

Walter L. Green, MD, FACEP
UT Southwestern Medical Center, Dallas, TX

John C. Greenwood, MD
University of Pennsylvania, Philadelphia, PA

Danya Khoujah, MBBS, MEHP, FACEP
University of Maryland, Baltimore, MD

Nathaniel Mann, MD
Greenville Health System, Greenville, SC

George Sternbach, MD, FACEP
Stanford University Medical Center, Stanford, CA

EDITORIAL STAFF

Suzannah Alexander, Editorial Director
salexander@acep.org

Joy Carrico, JD
Managing Editor

Alex Bass
Assistant Editor

Kyle Powell
Graphic Artist

ISSN2325-0186 (Print)   ISSN2325-8365 (Online)

Contents

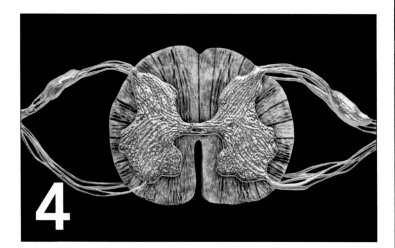

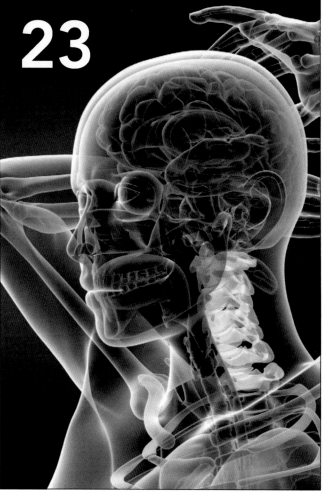

FEATURES

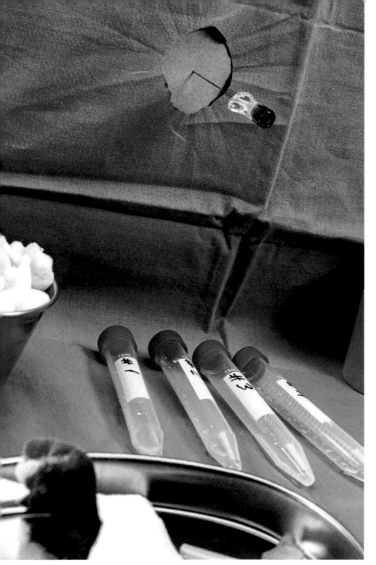

Bundle of Nerves

Transverse Myelitis and Guillain-Barré Syndrome

LESSON 5

By Taylor Lindquist, DO; and Kathleen Stephanos, MD
Dr. Lindquist is an emergency medicine and pediatric resident at the University of Maryland Medical Center in Baltimore. Dr. Stephanos is an assistant professor and assistant clerkship director in the Departments of Emergency Medicine and Pediatrics at the University of Maryland School of Medicine.

Reviewed by Amal Mattu, MD, FACEP

Objectives

On completion of this lesson, you should be able to:
1. Recognize typical and atypical presentations of transverse myelitis and GBS.
2. Define the diagnostic criteria for transverse myelitis and GBS.
3. Discuss the steps to a thorough evaluation of pediatric and adult patients with suspected transverse myelitis or GBS.
4. Propose appropriate treatments for transverse myelitis and GBS.
5. Describe the clinical course and prognosis of transverse myelitis and GBS.

From the EM Model

12.0 Nervous System Disorders
    12.5 Infections/Inflammatory Disorders
        12.5.4 Myelitis
    12.7 Neuromuscular Disorders
        12.7.1 Guillain-Barré Syndrome

■ CRITICAL DECISIONS ■

- What are transverse myelitis and GBS, and how do they present?
- What are the diagnostic criteria for transverse myelitis and GBS?
- What is an appropriate emergency department workup for transverse myelitis and GBS?
- Should treatment for transverse myelitis or GBS start in the emergency department?
- Are transverse myelitis and GBS found in pediatric patients?
- Is an emergency neurology consultation or transfer to a tertiary care facility recommended for patients with transverse myelitis or GBS?
- What is the recovery period for patients with transverse myelitis or GBS, and do symptoms recur?

Rapid progression of transverse myelitis and Guillain-Barré syndrome (GBS) can lead to life-threatening complications, such as spinal shock or respiratory failure. GBS can also cause autonomic instability and life-threatening dysrhythmias. Emergency physicians must be familiar with the clinical presentations, workup, monitoring, and management of these neurologic disorders to improve the overall prognosis of each patient.

CASE ONE

A 17-year-old boy arrives for an evaluation of weakness in his legs. His mother reports that he has had weakness in both lower legs that has grown progressively worse for the last 9 days. She decided to bring him in because he was unable to stand or get out of bed. The patient describes a recent tingling and burning sensation from the waist down as well as an increased sensation to urinate over the last several days. During the review of systems, the physician finds that the patient's pediatrician diagnosed him with a viral upper respiratory infection 2 weeks ago. During examination, the patient has 3/5 ankle dorsiflexion, knee extension, and hip flexion as well as hyperesthesia to light touch below the umbilicus.

CASE TWO

A 53-year-old man with a history of diabetes mellitis presents with progressive tingling in all extremities. This is his third physician visit in 2 weeks for the same complaint. What was

initially believed to be diabetic neuropathy has now developed into worsening tingling in the hands and tingling and weakness in the legs and feet. During the review of systems, the physician learns that the patient had a self-resolved diarrheal illness approximately 4 weeks ago. On examination, the patient has decreased sensation symmetrically throughout all extremities with absent patellar and Achilles reflexes and decreased bicep and tricep reflexes.

CASE THREE

A 22-year-old man arrives via EMS with acute-onset ophthalmoplegia suspected to be secondary to a stroke. The patient has no preexisting medical conditions but had a viral illness that was diagnosed as mononucleosis several weeks ago. He reports seeing double, blurred vision, difficulty speaking, and tingling in his extremities. His overall examination is normal, other than neurologic findings of symmetric facial paresis, fixed mydriatic pupils, ataxia, distal hyporeflexia, and decreased sensation in the hands and feet.

Introduction

For emergency physicians, patients' chief complaint of weakness or numbness gives way to a broad differential diagnosis. Among the many potential diagnoses are the neurologic disorders transverse myelitis and GBS. With only 1,400 new cases per year of transverse myelitis and 1.54 to 2.66 GBS cases per 100,000 people older than 50 years in the United States, these disorders are relatively rare and, therefore, challenging to diagnose.[1-3] Understanding their etiology, clinical presentations, workup, and management can help emergency physicians diagnose and treat these disorders early in their course to improve the overall prognosis and prevent rapid progression to life-threatening symptoms like spinal shock, respiratory failure, or dysrhythmias.

CRITICAL DECISION

What are transverse myelitis and GBS, and how do they present?

Transverse Myelitis

Transverse myelitis is a rare mixed inflammatory disorder of the spinal cord that leads to motor, sensory, and autonomic dysfunction.[4] Lymphocytes and monocytes are involved in the inflammation, demyelination, and axonal injury of the spinal cord that ultimately disrupt ascending and descending neuroanatomic pathways.[5] Transverse myelitis has a bimodal distribution: The first peak affects people between the ages of 10 and 19 years, and the second peak affects those between 30 and 39 years.[1,2] There is no sex or familial predisposition.[4] Transverse myelitis can be idiopathic or secondary to a systemic disorder. Some causes include systemic inflammatory autoimmune disorders (eg, systemic lupus erythematosus or Sjögren syndrome), parainfectious diseases, paraneoplastic syndromes, and toxins or drugs (eg, venom of a brown recluse spider or heroin).[4,6] Transverse myelitis is part of a spectrum of neuroinflammatory disorders and can be the initial presentation of multiple sclerosis (MS), neuromyelitis optica spectrum disorder (NMOSD), or myelin oligodendrocyte glycoprotein antibody disease.[7]

Although patients' presentations vary by the etiology, transverse myelitis is recognized from its combination of motor, sensory, and autonomic dysfunctions. Not all patients

with transverse myelitis present with all three dysfunctions — especially in the beginning of the disease course — but they eventually develop the triad as the disease progresses. Motor dysfunction in these patients often involves the lower extremities and presents as weakness and diminished muscle tone.[8] Once the disease has progressed, approximately 50% of patients are unable to move their legs.[4] Patients can present in the acute phase with signs of spinal shock such as flaccid limb tone and absent reflexes, which can lead to a misdiagnosis of GBS.[6] As the clinical course evolves, patients may have upper motor signs of hyperreflexia, the Babinski sign, and increased muscle tone.[5,8] Patients with sensory dysfunction report numbness, paresthesia, or band-like dysesthesias.[4] These symptoms can follow a dermatomal distribution and can be similar to neuropathic pain (eg, burning or aching sensations) (*Figure 1*).[5] Chief complaints from autonomic dysfunction in transverse myelitis include urinary or bowel incontinence, urinary urgency or retention, sexual dysfunction, tenesmus, and constipation.[4,9]

The history of symptom onset is critical to diagnosing transverse myelitis — the Transverse Myelitis Consortium Working Group's diagnostic criteria for idiopathic acute transverse myelitis emphasizes the importance of the symptomatic time line. The criteria include progression to nadir between 4 hours and 21 days after symptom onset. For patients whose symptoms reach maximal severity in less than 4 hours after onset, a rapidly evolving vascular myelopathy and ischemia should be considered instead (eg, thrombosis of the anterior spinal artery).[4] Patients outside of the 21-day time frame should be evaluated for myelopathy secondary to arteriovenous fistulas, the chronic progressive form of MS, or other slowly progressive myelopathies.[4]

Transverse myelitis can have atypical presentations. For example, in one case report, a patient with transverse myelitis presented with left upper quadrant abdominal pain, left-sided flank pain, and left lower-extremity weakness.[10] Although a presentation of abdominal pain with neurologic deficits is more typical of aortic pathology, this patient was ultimately diagnosed with transverse myelitis after the unilateral extremity weakness became bilateral and sensory changes developed during the course of the visit.[10] Patients can also present with acute partial transverse myelitis, which includes asymmetric neurologic impairments that are attributable to a specific anatomic tract.[6] Specific tract involvement can cause hemicord (ie, Brown-Séquard syndrome) or central cord clinical manifestations.[6] Patients with acute partial transverse myelitis are at an increased risk of recurrence and transition to MS.[6]

GBS

GBS shares some characteristics with transverse myelitis but also has its own distinguishing features (*Table 1*). All subtypes of GBS have a male predominance, distinguishing the condition from nearly all other forms of autoimmune disease, which are more common in women.[11] Often, women who develop GBS have a history of other immune disorders, rheumatologic disorders, preeclampsia, or prior blood or blood product transfusions.[12] GBS can occur in any age group but is more common in adults older than 50 years. Now that people are routinely vaccinated against polio, GBS is the most common cause of acute flaccid paralysis worldwide.[13] A 2008 study estimated the annual cost of GBS to be $1.7 billion, $200 million of which was purely medical costs (adjusting for inflation, total impact was estimated to be $2 billion with $270 million in medical costs).[14]

In 1916, three doctors, Georges Guillain, Jean-Alexandre Barré, and André Strohl, identified GBS and described the myelin of patients with the condition as "pulverized and in many instances completely dissolved."[15] GBS is an acute polyradiculopathy that is often considered to be one entity but can be subcategorized into several different typical presentations. The most common subtype is acute inflammatory demyelinating polyneuropathy (AIDP). It often has the classic presentation of ascending, tingling paresthesia; weakness; and accompanying areflexia.[13] Back pain is common in these patients because of inflammatory changes in the nerve roots. Limb pain and headache can occur as well, albeit rarely.[16] This classic form of GBS makes up approximately 95% of cases in North America.[13]

The axonal subtype of GBS is less common overall, although it makes up 30% to 60% of cases in China, Japan, South America, and Bangladesh. Axonal forms can be divided into sensory and motor forms. Acute motor axonal neuropathy is the second most common form of GBS and presents with similar symptoms to classic GBS but without the sensory component. Patients have acute motor weakness and progress to develop areflexia, ataxia, and oculomotor symptoms.[17] Acute sensory axonal neuropathy, by contrast, is exceptionally rare, with fewer than 10 cases reported in the literature.[18] This form presents with sensory symptoms alongside areflexia but without any associated motor deficits. Complete loss of sensation without motor deficits, however, can still lead to unsteady ambulation.[18]

Miller Fisher syndrome, discovered as its own entity in 1932 but later categorized as being within the GBS spectrum, presents with acute ophthalmoplegia, ataxia, and areflexia. It makes up about 5% of all GBS cases in Western countries and up to 25% of cases in Asian populations. Patients with Miller Fisher syndrome have at least two of the three symptoms of ophthalmoplegia, ataxia, and areflexia. It can affect nearly any cranial nerve, but cranial nerves III, IV, and VI are usually involved.[19] Bickerstaff brainstem encephalitis is the least common variant of GBS and presents with ataxia, encephalopathy, and ophthalmoplegia. The median age of onset is around 35 years, and it is more common in Asian than Western countries.[20]

Many patients with GBS had an illness 1 to 6 weeks before symptom onset, usually either gastroenteritis or an upper respiratory illness — up to 71% of patients can identify a recent,

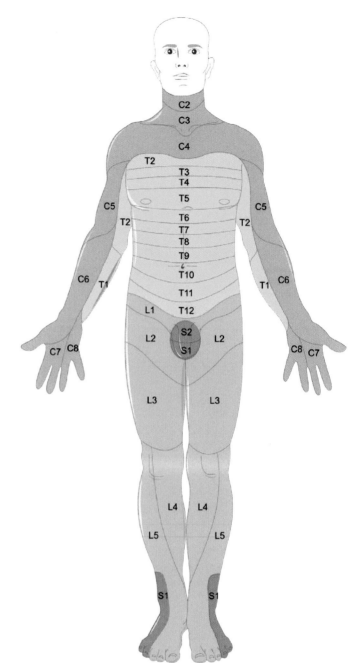

FIGURE 1. Dermatomes. *Credit:* Copyright Servier Medical Art, CC BY 2.0, Flickr.com. https://www.flickr.com/photos/serviermedicalart/9948080234

	Transverse Myelitis	GBS
Incidence	1,400 people/yr	2/100,000 people/yr
Age	Bimodal 10-19 yr and 30-39 yr	All, more common >50 yr
Sex	Male = female	Male > female
Reflexes	Decreased then increased	Decreased or absent
Strength	Decreased	Decreased
Sensation	Increased or decreased	Decreased
Progression to Nadir	>4 hr, <3 wk	>12 hr, <4 wk
Autonomic Instability	Rare	Common

TABLE 1. A review and comparison of the classic presentations of transverse myelitis and GBS. Not all patients fall into these typical presentations.

often viral, infection.[21] Infection with *Campylobacter jejuni* is the most common inciting illness, while cytomegalovirus (CMV) is the second-most common. The lipooligosaccharides of *C. jejuni* are thought to resemble the gangliosides of the human peripheral membrane, inciting an autoimmune mimicry response that causes peripheral membrane destruction.[22] Other infections associated with GBS are Epstein-Barr virus (EBV) and mycoplasma. Trauma, medications, and vaccines (most notably the 1976 influenza vaccine) have also been associated with the onset of GBS. Rituximab, alemtuzumab, and efalizumab are specific medications implicated in the disease.[13] COVID-19 vaccines are also correlated with GBS, most commonly AIDP.[23]

Patients with GBS often have an indolent course and present multiple times for vague complaints of paresthesia or weakness. It sometimes takes several medical visits before a diagnosis is made. Gradual disease progression occurs before symptoms reach their nadir at around 4 weeks from disease onset. By the time their symptoms peak, all GBS patients have areflexia; the prevalence of all other symptoms can be harder to classify. Approximately 93% of patients have all-limb involvement, 6% have isolated leg involvement, and 1% have isolated arm involvement.[13]

CRITICAL DECISION

What are the diagnostic criteria for transverse myelitis and GBS?

Transverse Myelitis

The Transverse Myelitis Consortium Working Group's diagnostic criteria can aid in the diagnosis of idiopathic transverse myelitis (*Table 2*). Diagnostic criteria include the time it takes to progress to nadir; development of sensory, motor, or autonomic symptoms; bilateral signs and symptoms; and a clearly defined sensory level. Additional criteria include findings from imaging and the workup. First, extra-axial compressive etiologies must be excluded by neuroimaging with MRI or myelography. Importantly, CT of the spine is inadequate for diagnosis. In patients with transverse myelitis, MRI reveals gadolinium enhancement of the spine. Lumbar puncture (LP) is recommended for analysis of CSF and often demonstrates inflammation in the spinal cord through pleocytosis or elevated IgG index. Diagnosis of transverse myelitis requires gadolinium enhancement, evidence of pleocytosis, or evidence of elevated IgG index; however, all three findings strengthen the diagnosis. If none of the criteria are met but transverse myelitis is still high on the differential diagnosis, patients should undergo repeat LP and MRI of the spinal cord between 2 and 7 days after symptom onset.[4]

GBS

The diagnosis of GBS requires only two clinical criteria: distal areflexia and weakness or sensory deficits that are progressive and symmetric in more than one limb. Additional testing supports the diagnosis, but not all testing is positive at symptom onset. Additional supportive findings include albuminocytologic dissociation, which leads to elevated protein within the CSF; abnormal nerve conduction testing; progression of the disease; cranial nerve involvement; and autonomic dysfunction. Because of its predominantly clinical nature, diagnosing GBS is a challenge. The Brighton criteria was developed to help support the diagnosis. It is a scoring system based on several factors: the absence of alternative diagnoses, decreased or areflexic limbs associated with

Inclusion Criteria	Exclusion Criteria
• Development of sensory, motor, or autonomic dysfunction attributable to the spinal cord	• History of previous radiation to the spine within the last 10 yr
• Bilateral signs and symptoms (not necessarily symmetric)	• Clear arterial distribution clinical deficit consistent with thrombosis of the anterior spinal artery
• Clearly defined sensory level	• Abnormal flow voids on the surface of the spinal cord consistent with arteriovenous malformation
• Exclusion of extra-axial compressive etiology by neuroimaging (MRI or myelography; CT of the spine is not adequate)	• Serologic or clinical evidence of connective tissue disease (eg, sarcoidosis, Behçet disease, Sjögren syndrome, systemic lupus erythematosus, or mixed connective tissue disorder)*
• Inflammation within the spinal cord demonstrated by CSF pleocytosis *or* elevated IgG index *or* gadolinium enhancement. If none of the inflammatory criteria is met at symptom onset, repeat MRI and LP evaluation between 2 and 7 d after symptom onset.	• CNS manifestations of syphilis, Lyme disease, HIV, human T-lymphotrophic virus 1, *Mycoplasma*, other viral infection (eg, HSV-1, HSV-2, VZV, EBV, CMV, human herpesvirus-6, enteroviruses)*
• Progression to nadir between 4 hr and 21 d following onset of symptoms (if patient awakens with symptoms, symptoms must become more pronounced from the point of awakening)	• Brain MRI abnormalities suggestive of MS*
	• History of clinically apparent optic neuritis

* Do not exclude disease-associated acute transverse myelitis

TABLE 2. Transverse Myelitis Consortium Working Group's inclusion and exclusion diagnostic criteria for idiopathic acute transverse myelitis[4]

weakness, a monophasic development of symptoms that peak between 12 hours and 28 days, bilateral and flaccid weakness of the limbs, a CSF cell count of less than 50 cells/µL, a CSF protein concentration higher than normal, and nerve conduction testing that supports a GBS subtype.[24] Although the results from these criteria can increase the likelihood of an accurate GBS diagnosis on initial presentation, many of the tests needed for these results cannot be completed in the emergency department, making them of limited use to emergency physicians. Additionally, this tool has not been validated in pediatric patients.[25] For Miller Fisher syndrome, the classic presentation is the triad of ophthalmoplegia, areflexia, and ataxia, with symptoms usually peaking in less than 4 weeks.[19]

CRITICAL DECISION

What is an appropriate emergency department workup for transverse myelitis and GBS?

Transverse Myelitis

Imaging or CSF evaluation is required to diagnose acute transverse myelitis. In the emergency department, urgent spinal imaging is warranted to rule out compressive etiologies that may require neurosurgical management. Although not easily attainable, MRI of the cervical, thoracic, and lumbar spine with gadolinium enhancement is the gold standard for evaluating and diagnosing transverse myelitis. If an MRI is unfeasible, a spinal CT or CT myelogram can be performed to rule out compressive etiologies with the understanding that a normal CT does not rule out intrinsic spinal cord injury or disease.[9] If CT is negative for a compressive etiology, further workup with an MRI is necessary, even if it requires transfer to another facility.[4] To avoid false negatives with MRIs, the entire spine should be imaged. For example, in some cases, patients can present with misleading localizing signs such as a thoracic sensory level caused by cervical lesions, which would not be visualized on a thoracic spine MRI.[5] On T2-weighted MRI, transverse myelitis presents as a high-signal intensity (*Figure 2*).[9] Its lesions span at least two vertebral segments. This helps differentiate the disease from MS, which typically spans fewer than two vertebral segments and NMOSD, which typically spans three or more vertebral segments.[5] Nevertheless, not all patients fit this textbook definition, with many reported to have longitudinally extensive transverse myelitis that extends across three or more vertebral segments.[6] MRI of the brain is also commonly performed with MRI of the spine to rule out other demyelinating diseases. In patients with transverse myelitis, results from an MRI of the brain are normal.

In addition to MRI, LP for CSF evaluation is a critical part of diagnosing transverse myelitis. Transverse myelitis patients often demonstrate CSF pleocytosis, defined as greater than 5 cells/µL; approximately 50% of transverse myelitis patients have findings of more than 100 cells/µL.[7] In addition to pleocytosis, an elevated IgG index is often seen in transverse myelitis. Physicians should obtain routine CSF laboratory tests such as protein levels, glucose levels, and bacterial cultures and additional tests such as cytology tests, the venereal disease research laboratory test, oligoclonal banding, and viral panels (polymerase chain reaction tests for herpes simplex virus [HSV], varicella zoster virus [VZV], and CMV).[7]

Although blood work is often normal in patients with idiopathic transverse myelitis, it should be done to rule out potential secondary or treatable causes of myelopathy. Routine blood tests to perform include vitamin B_{12} levels, methylmalonic acid levels, thyroid function tests, syphilis tests, HIV serology, and any relevant antibody titers for infections associated with transverse myelitis, like *Mycoplasma*.[6] Even though results for many of these laboratory tests will not return while patients are in the emergency department, once received they can be used by hospitalists and neurologists to tailor and expedite care. Neurology consultants may also recommend laboratory tests for antinuclear antibody, neuromyelitis optica–specific immune globulin, and myelin oligodendrocyte protein levels.

GBS

For diagnosing and distinguishing GBS from transverse myelitis, the main tool is the clinical examination. Obtaining a history to assess for any recent illness that could have contributed to the onset of GBS is especially important. Also inquiring about alcohol use, tick exposure, or HIV infection can rule out other potential causes of symptoms. HIV seroconversion can mimic GBS, so rapid HIV testing should be ordered.[26] Other testing is also done to exclude other causes and support a GBS diagnosis. Importantly, although some test results support a GBS diagnosis, absence of these results does not exclude the diagnosis; no laboratory test can confirm or exclude the diagnosis of GBS.[13]

Blood antibody testing should be considered, keeping in mind that results will not return during the emergency department visit and that patients without any positive antibodies can still have GBS. Many antibodies, however, have been implicated in GBS. Of the GBS subtypes, Miller Fisher syndrome has the highest rate of positive antibodies, reading positive in around 62% of cases. Antibody testing can also be useful in predicting

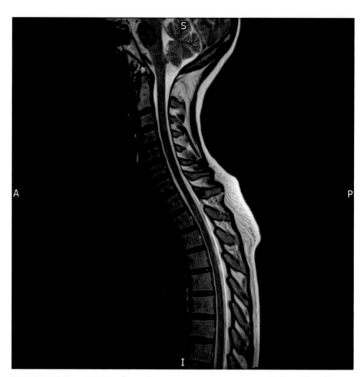

FIGURE 2. MRI showing transverse myelitis. *Credit: Copyright Anil Geetha Virupakshappa. Image courtesy of Anil Geetha Virupakshappa and Radiopaedia.org, rID: 155860. Used under license.*

patient outcomes. For example, patients with anti–ganglioside-monosialic acid IgG antibodies have lower recovery rates and worse prognoses for recovering their ability to walk.[27]

LP is the primary emergency department test for GBS. Patients with GBS classically have elevated protein levels without significant elevations in WBC counts; WBC counts should be less than 50 cells/µL in GBS patients. If they are greater than 50 cells/µL, other causes of symptoms such as meningitis or transverse myelitis should be considered instead. Unfortunately, LP results are not reliably abnormal in GBS patients, especially in the early stages of symptoms. The classic GBS finding of albuminocytologic dissociation is present in only 44% to 81% of patients, with higher rates occurring later in the clinical course.[28,29] Additionally, false-positive tests occur and are thought to be related to age-associated rises in normal CSF protein levels, which are often not considered when setting normal laboratory values.[30] Imaging in suspected cases of GBS can exclude other diagnoses but does not usually detect findings that confirm GBS. MRI, however, may show inflammation of the nerve roots to suggest GBS but more often will be normal (*Figure 3*). Needle electromyography (EMG) is of little use in the early days of symptoms but, as the disease progresses, can help distinguish between different GBS subtypes. A needle EMG should be obtained after 10 to 14 days of symptoms, although irregularities can present as early as day 3.[22] In the first 4 days of symptoms, nerve conduction studies appropriately classify GBS by subtype in fewer than 30% of patients.[31]

The differential diagnosis for GBS is broad and includes other polyradiculopathies that are infectious, environmental, toxicologic, and metabolic in origin. The more common GBS mimics are Wernicke encephalopathy, myasthenia gravis, botulism, tick paralysis, and HIV seroconversion. Less common mimics include Lambert-Eaton syndrome, acute intermittent porphyria, and sensory neuropathies from diabetes or other autoimmune disorders.[26] Because the polio vaccination rate has declined, poliomyelitis should also be considered in the differential diagnosis.[32] Polio is most common in children younger than 5 years and presents with a hyperacute onset of symptoms, including total paralysis within a few hours in some cases.[33] Several symptoms suggest that GBS is not the correct diagnosis. Other than the GBS subtype of Bickerstaff brainstem encephalitis, changes in mental status do not occur in GBS patients. Symptoms of GBS are also symmetric by the time they peak at 4 weeks, and they gradually improve. If symptoms worsen after 8 weeks or are something other than monophasic, other diagnoses are more likely.

CRITICAL DECISION

Should treatment for transverse myelitis or GBS start in the emergency department?

Emergency physicians must treat patients with transverse myelitis or GBS like any other critical patient — by running through the steps of airway, breathing, and circulation. Patients with severe presentations may require respiratory and oropharyngeal support. Those with dyspnea, accessory muscle use, hypercarbia, or poor oxygenation may require emergent intubation. Because of the potential for aspiration, patients with dysarthria or dysphagia should not be allowed to eat or drink anything (nothing by mouth) or should have a nasogastric or orogastric tube placed. Patients with urinary retention from autonomic dysfunction may need a urinary catheter.

Transverse Myelitis

After stabilizing patients, physicians should not delay treatment for MRI or LP results in suspected transverse myelitis cases.[34] Treatment should be started right away to halt progression and shorten the recovery period.[5] High-dose corticosteroids are the first-line treatment for transverse myelitis and aim to resolve spinal cord inflammation. There are no randomized controlled trials to support the use of corticosteroids in transverse myelitis patients, but retrospective data from case studies and extrapolated data from randomized controlled studies of MS have shown that early treatment with steroids improves neurologic outcomes and increases the likelihood of a full recovery.[5,8] Physicians should start with high-dose intravenous regimens such as methylprednisolone 1,000 mg daily. Evidence is lacking to say which corticosteroids, routes, and doses are superior.[5] Typically, patients are treated with intravenous methylprednisolone for 3 to 5 days. For patients with steroid contraindications or life-threatening symptoms (eg, severe respiratory compromise), physicians should consider plasma exchange as an alternative or additive treatment.[8] Patients with transverse myelitis often undergo 5 to 7 exchanges every other day over the course of 10 to 14 days.[8] Plasma exchange is also recommended for patients who do not respond to corticosteroids.[5] Neurologists may also recommend intravenous immune globulin (IVIG) as an adjunct to steroids or as a second-line option. IVIG is usually dosed at 2 g/kg for 2 to 5 days. Ultimately, patients diagnosed with transverse myelitis require hospital admission for continued treatment and observation.[5]

GBS

For GBS patients in the emergency department, the primary concern is supportive care. Like patients with transverse myelitis, GBS patients require early evaluation of their respiratory status.

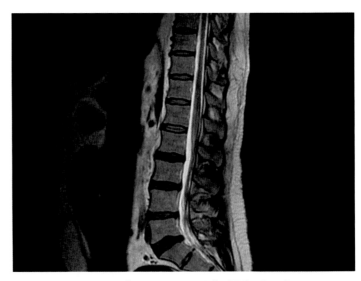

FIGURE 3. MRI of a patient with GBS. *Credit:* Copyright Ammar Haouimi. Image courtesy of Ammar Haouimi and Radiopaedia.org, rID: 70759. Used under license.

A negative inspiratory force (NIF) value can be measured on a bedside manometer when patients inhale deeply. Patients with an NIF value of less than −20 to −30 cm H_2O should be monitored closely for respiratory decompensation and, if necessary, should be intubated; nearly 30% of GBS patients require intubation. GBS patients in whom intubation is delayed experience a high rate of ventilator-associated pneumonia.[35] Emergency physicians should not hesitate to intubate patients with an NIF value outside of the normal range or with a noticeable decline in their respiratory status while in the emergency department.

Autonomic dysfunction is also high in GBS patients, affecting nearly 70%. The most common symptoms of autonomic dysfunction are constipation (22%) and diarrhea (21%), but autonomic dysfunction can also cause fatal dysrhythmias. Urinary retention and blood pressure variability are other symptoms.[36] All GBS patients with autonomic dysfunction should be placed on continuous cardiopulmonary monitoring and should remain on telemetry, and all symptoms of autonomic dysfunction should be treated in the emergency department.

Treatment options for GBS include plasma exchange and IVIG. IVIG is administered at a standard dose of 2 g/kg. Both treatments are equally effective in adults, and no evidence suggests that administering both treatments together or in sequence improves outcomes compared to monotherapy.[13] IVIG is often preferred because it requires less equipment, costs less, is more available, and has similar outcomes to plasma exchange. Ideally, IVIG or plasma exchange should be started within the first 2 weeks of symptoms in any patient with GBS or up to 4 weeks in patients with GBS who cannot ambulate. Some studies report that these treatments have some efficacy if given within the first 4 weeks of symptoms in GBS patients in general.[37] Importantly, steroids are not used to treat GBS, making GBS a relatively unique autoimmune disorder. In fact, steroids in GBS patients have been associated with worse long-term outcomes in some randomized controlled trials.[37,38]

All GBS patients require admission for monitoring. While in the emergency department, patients should have regular NIF testing, close telemetry, and blood pressure monitoring. Patients' conditions can progress rapidly and require intubation in the short amount of time they are in the emergency department.

CRITICAL DECISION

Are transverse myelitis and GBS found in pediatric patients?

Transverse Myelitis

Transverse myelitis affects approximately 0.2 out of 100,000 children per year and accounts for approximately 20% of acute demyelinating syndromes in children.[9] Pediatric presentations also follow a bimodal distribution: Cases peak in children younger than 3 years and in children between 5 and 17 years.[6] Approximately 60% of pediatric transverse myelitis cases are thought to be triggered by a recent vaccination or viral illness.[5] However, vaccines and viral illnesses often precede other demyelinating syndromes as well, so a recent history of either one of these events cannot establish a transverse myelitis diagnosis. Like in adults, the characteristic triad of autonomic, motor, and sensory deficits is seen in pediatric patients. Pediatric patients also require a spinal MRI or LP for diagnosis. Recommended treatment is high-dose corticosteroids, with plasma exchange or IVIG as second-line treatments for refractory patients or patients with incomplete recovery. Because most pediatric patients present with postinfectious, postvaccination, or idiopathic transverse myelitis, most cases are monophasic.[5] When gathering history, emergency physicians should ask if similar symptoms occurred earlier in life; any recurrence of deficits should raise suspicion for relapsing demyelinating syndromes. Compared to adults, functional recovery is often better in pediatric patients.[6]

GBS

GBS affects people of all ages and is also the most common cause of acute flaccid paralysis in children. In the pediatric population, GBS typically affects children younger than 5 years. The duration of illness is shorter in children, and recovery is quicker than in adults. Progression of symptoms occurs within hours to days, typically reaching a nadir within 4 weeks. Symptoms of autonomic dysfunction are prevalent in children. GBS has a similar mortality rate in children and adults — 3% to 5% — but, overall rates of complete recovery seem to be higher in children. The male predominance of GBS applies to the pediatric population as well.[25] The subtype Miller Fisher syndrome is rarer in children than in adults.[39]

Current treatment recommendations for children with GBS are similar to those for adults: rapid initiation of IVIG or plasma exchange. Plasma exchange is less available, more expensive, and requires close monitoring, but some studies suggest that it may decrease the length of stay for pediatric patients, which could offset its higher cost.[40] Other studies have recommended using plasma exchange alongside IVIG if IVIG is not tolerated well or if GBS symptoms are severe and progressive despite IVIG treatment; however, some studies suggest that combining the two therapies in children is not beneficial.[41] Given the small size of these studies, there is no definitive evidence for one treatment over the other.

CRITICAL DECISION

Is an emergency neurology consultation or transfer to a tertiary care facility recommended for patients with transverse myelitis or GBS?

Transverse Myelitis

Neurologic consultations for transverse myelitis are usually urgent rather than emergent. When transverse myelitis is suspected, early communication with neurologists can expedite final treatment recommendations and provide insight into additional serum or CSF testing for ruling out alternative diagnoses. Although transfer to a tertiary care facility is usually unnecessary, it may be appropriate in some cases when access is needed to MRI or neurologists with more experience treating transverse myelitis.

GBS

Similarly, involvement of neurology specialists for emergency management of GBS is likely unnecessary but will be required during patient care at the urgent level. All GBS patients require admission, typically at the intermediate care level (at a minimum) for continuous cardiopulmonary monitoring and regular NIF testing. Patients are at high risk of decompensating because of progressive respiratory muscle weakness, which in GBS patients does not present with the typical symptoms of respiratory distress. Many require care in the ICU for respiratory monitoring.[35,36] EMG is often needed to evaluate for GBS and, if unavailable, requires transfer to a facility where it is available.

CRITICAL DECISION

What is the recovery period for patients with transverse myelitis or GBS, and do symptoms recur?

Transverse Myelitis

Diagnosing the specific type of transverse myelitis — that is, distinguishing between idiopathic and secondary cases and, for secondary cases, distinguishing between causes — is important because they have different prognoses. Patients with idiopathic transverse myelitis usually recover gradually over the course of approximately 3 months after onset, but improvement may continue for a year or longer.[5] Approximately 50% to 70% of patients with idiopathic transverse myelitis recover partially or completely and can ambulate with or without aid.[5]

Patients with transverse myelitis from secondary causes have more variable outcomes depending on the underlying etiology. For example, patients with transverse myelitis associated with NMOSD are more likely to have clinically significant residual neurologic deficits, while those with transverse myelitis associated with MS are more likely to recover substantially, if not completely.[5] Although overall outcomes are difficult to

✔ Pearls

- Idiopathic, postinfectious, and postvaccination transverse myelitis are usually monophasic. Once pseudoexacerbation is ruled out, patients who present with repeat attacks should be evaluated for relapsing diseases such as MS or NMOSD.
- Emergency physicians should always rule out compressive etiologies with spinal imaging before evaluating for transverse myelitis.
- Patients with GBS who have an NIF value of less than −20 to −30 cm H_2O should be closely monitored for respiratory decompensation; intubation may be necessary.
- Patients who present with bulbar symptoms and weakness should be evaluated for Miller Fisher syndrome.

predict, severe weakness, hypotonia, areflexia, and spinal shock are recognized as poor prognostic signs.[6]

Etiologies of transverse myelitis are also somewhat predictive of patients' clinical courses. Idiopathic, postinfectious, and postvaccination forms of transverse myelitis are usually monophasic syndromes. By contrast, MS and NMOSD are relapsing diseases, so patients with transverse myelitis secondary to these two diseases are at high risk of future attacks.[5]

Pseudoexacerbation should also be considered when evaluating patients with a history of transverse myelitis who again present with neurologic deficits. Pseudoexacerbation is a transient worsening of symptoms caused by infections and metabolic or physiologic derangements (eg, hyperglycemia), rather than a recurrence of transverse myelitis.[6] Treatment of pseudoexacerbation is aimed at the underlying cause (eg, antibiotics for urinary tract infections) and usually also improves neurologic symptoms. Triggers of pseudoexacerbation should always be ruled out first before attributing symptoms to recurrent transverse myelitis. If the workup is negative for triggers of pseudoexacerbation, physicians should then explore a diagnosis for relapsing-remitting diseases like MS or NMOSD.

GBS

GBS is classically monophasic. Symptoms usually peak around week 4 of the illness but, in rare cases, may progress until week 8 before gradually improving. If symptoms continue to worsen after 8 weeks, alternative etiologies should be considered. The degree of symptom resolution varies depending on the patient. GBS has a 2.5% to 5% mortality rate, usually due to autonomic dysfunction or ventilator-associated pneumonia (if patients are intubated). Of the surviving patients, 75% recover completely and return to baseline by 12 months after symptom onset. The average recovery time is 10.1 weeks. Approximately 25% of patients have residual deficits, and around 10% to 20% are unable to walk without assistance.[13] Pediatric patients have a higher rate of complete recovery and a faster return to baseline. Approximately 6% of children with GBS have residual deficits that prevent them from walking.[42]

The overall recurrence rate for GBS is low, less than 5%. Vaccinations have been associated with GBS onset, but these associations seem to be predominantly temporal. Nevertheless, out of fear of recurrence, many patients opt out of future vaccinations, which puts them at risk of other diseases.[43] GBS recurrence seems to be more common in women and pediatric patients and typically occurs at a mean interval of 7 years after initial presentation. Patients with a recurrence typically have more severe symptoms with each repeat event.[44] Although it is rare, GBS recurrence should be strongly considered in patients with a history of GBS who present again with similar symptoms.

Summary

Transverse myelitis and GBS are two immune-mediated polyneuropathies that require early recognition and diagnosis to avoid progression to life-threatening complications. Understanding the common and atypical presentations of these diseases in adult and pediatric patients helps expedite an appropriate workup. Physicians must also recognize when to request an urgent neurology consultation or transfer patients to a higher level of care. Once a diagnosis for one of these conditions is made (or highly suspected for some cases), treatment should be initiated in the emergency department, and patients should be admitted to the hospital for close observation and further management.

REFERENCES

1. Jeffery DR, Mandler RN, Davis LE. Transverse myelitis. Retrospective analysis of 33 cases, with differentiation of cases associated with multiple sclerosis and parainfectious events. *Arch Neurol.* 1993 May;50(5):532-535.
2. Christensen PB, Wermuth L, Hinge HH, Bømers K. Clinical course and long-term prognosis of acute transverse myelopathy. *Acta Neurol Scand.* 1990 May;81(5):431-435.
3. Sejvar JJ, Baughman AL, Wise M, Morgan OW. Population incidence of Guillain-Barré syndrome: a systematic review and meta-analysis. *Neuroepidemiology.* 2011;36(2):123-133.
4. Transverse Myelitis Consortium Working Group. Proposed diagnostic criteria and nosology of acute transverse myelitis. *Neurology.* 2002 Aug 27;59(4):499-505.
5. Frohman EM, Wingerchuk DM. Transverse myelitis. *N Engl J Med.* 2010 Aug 5;363(6):564-572.
6. Beh SC, Greenberg BM, Frohman T, Frohman EM. Transverse myelitis. *Neurol Clin.* 2013 Feb;31(1):79-138.
7. Greenburg B. Transverse myelitis. UpToDate. Updated February 14, 2023. https://www.uptodate.com/contents/transverse-myelitis
8. Theroux LM, Brenton JN. Acute transverse and flaccid myelitis in children. *Curr Treat Options Neurol.* 2019 Dec 3;21(12):64.
9. Huh Y, Park E-J, Jung J-W, Oh S, Choi S-C. Clinical insights for early detection of acute transverse myelitis in the emergency department. *Clin Exp Emerg Med.* 2015 Mar 31;2(1):44-50.
10. Pavesi-Krieger C, Rech MA, Lovett S. Atypical presentation of transverse myelitis in the emergency department. *Am J Emerg Med.* 2021 Dec;50:813.e5-813.e6.
11. McCombe PA, Hardy TA, Nona RJ, Greer JM. Sex differences in Guillain Barré syndrome, chronic inflammatory demyelinating polyradiculoneuropathy and experimental autoimmune neuritis. *Front Immunol.* 2022 Dec 9;13:1038411.
12. Auger N, Quach C, Healy-Profitós J, Dinh T, Chassé M. Early predictors of Guillain-Barré syndrome in the life course of women. *Int J Epidemiol.* 2018 Feb 1;47(1):280-288.
13. Lehmann HC, Hughes RAC, Kieseier BC, Hartung H-P. Recent developments and future directions in Guillain-Barré syndrome. *J Peripher Nerv Syst.* 2012 Dec;17(suppl 3):57-70.
14. Frenzen PD. Economic cost of Guillain-Barré syndrome in the United States. *Neurology.* 2008 Jul 1;71(1):21-27.
15. Schott B. History of Guillain-Barré syndrome. *Rev Neurol (Paris).* 1982;138(12):931-938.
16. Farmakidis C, Inan S, Milstein M, Herskovitz S. Headache and pain in Guillain-Barré syndrome. *Curr Pain Headache Rep.* 2015 Aug;19(8):40.
17. McGrogan A, Madle GC, Seaman HE, de Vries CS. The epidemiology of Guillain-Barré syndrome worldwide. A systematic literature review. *Neuroepidemiology.* 2009;32(2):150-163.

✖ Pitfalls

- Ordering imaging for only a certain area of the spine based on patients' sensory-level deficits, rather than ordering a whole-spine MRI.
- Waiting to treat suspected cases of transverse myelitis with high-dose intravenous corticosteroids until LP or MRI results are obtained.
- Relying on results from LP rather than the clinical examination to diagnose GBS.
- Overlooking symptoms of autonomic instability in GBS patients and failing to monitor these symptoms appropriately.

■ CASE ONE

The emergency physician suspected a diagnosis of transverse myelitis based on symptoms of bilateral lower-extremity motor deficits, the well-defined level of sensory deficits, and the urinary urgency that was concerning for autonomic dysfunction. To rule out compressive etiologies and provide further diagnostic clues, a whole-spine MRI with contrast was obtained; it revealed a gadolinium-enhancing signal abnormality that spanned from T3 to T4. A brain MRI was normal. In addition to routine laboratory tests, the patient received an LP, which returned with a WBC count of 18 cells/μL, normal protein and glucose levels, negative cell culture and Gram stain, and negative oligoclonal banding. The patient met diagnostic criteria for transverse myelitis, likely secondary to a recent viral illness. He was initiated on intravenous methylprednisolone and admitted to the neurology service for further monitoring and management.

■ CASE TWO

After a complete evaluation, GBS was suspected based on clinical findings and symptom progression. The patient was immediately placed on continuous pulse oximetry, and an NIF test was conducted.

The NIF value was –25 cm H_2O on presentation, but a repeat reading 1 hour later showed a decline to –15 cm H_2O. Because of rapid symptom progression, the patient was urgently intubated. LP was performed and showed an elevated protein level and normal WBC count of 10 cells/μL, supporting the diagnosis of GBS. Neurology was consulted for nerve conduction studies, and the patient was admitted to the ICU for IVIG initiation. Several weeks later, the patient's symptoms improved, with a gradual return to baseline neurologic status.

■ CASE THREE

The immediate evaluation of the patient was concerning for cerebellar stroke; however, because of the symptom of areflexia, the emergency physician began to suspect Miller Fisher syndrome. LP in the emergency department showed a WBC count of 40 cells/μL and elevated protein levels. MRI showed no focal findings. The patient had a normal NIF value and was admitted to intermediate care for monitoring. Inpatient nerve conduction studies were consistent with the Miller Fisher syndrome subtype of GBS. Plasma exchange was performed, with subsequent gradual improvement of symptoms. The patient was eventually discharged.

18. Yang J, Huan M, Jiang H, Song C, Zhong L, Liang Z. Pure sensory Guillain-Barré syndrome: a case report and review of the literature. *Exp Ther Med.* 2014 Nov;8(5):1397-1401.

19. Rocha Cabrero F, Morrison EH. Miller Fisher syndrome. *StatPearls [Internet].* StatPearls Publishing LLC; 2022. Updated September 22, 2022. https://www.ncbi.nlm.nih.gov/books/NBK507717/

20. Ito M, Kuwabara S, Odaka M, et al. Bickerstaff's brainstem encephalitis and Fisher syndrome form a continuous spectrum: clinical analysis of 581 cases. *J Neurol.* 2008 May;255(5):674-682.

21. Berlit P, Rakicky J. The Miller Fisher syndrome. Review of the literature. *J Clin Neuroophthalmol.* 1992 Mar;12(1):57-63.

22. Nguyen TP, Taylor RS. Guillain Barre syndrome. *StatPearls [Internet].* StatPearls Publishing LLC; 2022. Updated July 4, 2022. https://www.ncbi.nlm.nih.gov/books/NBK532254/

23. Shao SC, Wang C-H, Chang K-C, Hung M-J, Chen H-Y, Liao S-C. Guillain-Barré syndrome associated with COVID-19 vaccination. *Emerg Infect Dis.* 2021 Dec;27(12):3175-3178.

24. Fokke C, van den Berg B, Drenthen J, Walgaard C, van Doorn PA, Jacobs BC. Diagnosis of Guillain-Barré syndrome and validation of Brighton criteria. *Brain.* 2014 Jan;137(pt 1):33-43.

25. Roodbol J, de Wit M-CY, van den Berg B, et al. Diagnosis of Guillain-Barré syndrome in children and validation of the Brighton criteria. *J Neurol.* 2017 May;264(5):856-861.

26. Tham SL, Prasad K, Umapathi T. Guillain-Barré syndrome mimics. *Brain Behav.* 2018 Apr 10;8(5):e00960.

27. Lleixà C, Martín-Aguilar L, Pascual-Goñi E, et al. Autoantibody screening in Guillain-Barré syndrome. *J Neuroinflammation.* 2021 Nov 1;18(1):251.

28. Majed B, Zephir H, Pichonnier-Cassagne V, et al. Lumbar punctures: use and diagnostic efficiency in emergency medical departments. *Int J Emerg Med.* 2009 Nov 19;2(4):227-235.

29. Rath J, Zulehner G, Schober B, et al. Cerebrospinal fluid analysis in Guillain-Barré syndrome: value of albumin quotients. *J Neurol.* 2021 Sep;268(9):3294-3300.

30. Hegen H, Ladstätter F, Bsteh G, et al. Cerebrospinal fluid protein in Guillain-Barré syndrome: need for age-dependent interpretation. *Eur J Neurol.* 2021 Mar;28(3):965-973.

31. Rath J, Schober B, Zulehner G, et al. Nerve conduction studies in Guillain-Barré syndrome: influence of timing and value of repeated measurements. *J Neurol Sci.* 2021 Jan 15;420:117267.

32. Seither R, Laury J, Mugerwa-Kasujja A, Knighton CL, Black CL. Vaccination coverage with selected vaccines and exemption rates among children in kindergarten — United States, 2020–21 school year. *MMWR Morb Mortal Wkly Rep.* 2022 Apr 22;71(16):561-568.

33. Wolbert JG, Higginbotham K. Poliomyelitis. *StatPearls [Internet].* StatPearls Publishing LLC; 2022. Updated June 21, 2022. https://www.ncbi.nlm.nih.gov/books/NBK558944/

34. Simone CG, Emmady PD. Transverse myelitis. *StatPearls [Internet].* StatPearls Publishing LLC; 2022. Updated November 15, 2022. https://www.ncbi.nlm.nih.gov/books/NBK559302/

35. Melone MA, Heming N, Meng P, et al. Early mechanical ventilation in patients with Guillain-Barré syndrome at high risk of respiratory failure: a randomized trial. *Ann Intensive Care.* 2020 Sep 30;10(1):128.

36. Singh J, Raja V Sr, Irfan M, Hashmat O, Syed M, Shahbaz NN. Frequency of autonomic dysfunction in patients of Guillain Barre syndrome in a tertiary care hospital. *Cureus.* 2020 Dec 15;12(12):e12101.

37. Liu S, Dong C, Ubogu EE. Immunotherapy of Guillain-Barré syndrome. *Hum Vaccin Immunother.* 2018;14(11):2568-2579.

38. Hughes RA, Brassington R, Gunn AA, van Doorn PA. Corticosteroids for Guillain-Barre syndrome. *Cochrane Database Syst Rev.* 2016 Oct 24;10(10):CD001446.

39. Khiri N, Lazreg M, Bkiyar H, Diyas S, Housni B. Miller Fischer syndrome: about a paediatric case. *Pan Afr Med J.* 2018 May 17;30:37.

40. Saad K, Mohamad IL, Abd El-Hamed MA, et al. A comparison between plasmapheresis and intravenous immunoglobulin in children with Guillain-Barré syndrome in Upper Egypt. *Ther Adv Neurol Disord.* 2016 Jan;9(1):3-8.

41. Korinthenberg R, Trollmann R, Felderhoff-Müser U, et al. Diagnosis and treatment of Guillain-Barré syndrome in childhood and adolescence: an evidence- and consensus-based guideline. *Eur J Paediatr Neurol.* 2020 Mar;25:5-16.

42. Salehiomran MR, Nikkhah A, Mahdavi M. Prognosis of Guillain-Barré syndrome in children. *Iran J Child Neurol.* 2016 Spring;10(2):38-41.

43. Haber P, Sejvar J, Mikaeloff Y, DeStefano F. Vaccines and Guillain-Barré syndrome. *Drug Saf.* 2009;32(4):309-323.

44. Kuitwaard K, van Koningsveld R, Ruts L, Jacobs BC, van Doorn PA. Recurrent Guillain-Barré syndrome. *J Neurol Neurosurg Psychiatry.* 2009 Jan;80(1):56-59.

The LLSA Literature Review
Management of Acute Ischemic Strokes

By Jamie Aron, MD; and Andrew J. Eyre, MD, MS-HPEd
Harvard Affiliated Emergency Medicine Residency and
Brigham and Women's Hospital/Harvard Medical School,
Boston, Massachussetts

Objective

On completion of this article, you should be able to:

■ Discuss the timing of acute ischemic stroke treatment options.

Powers WJ. Acute ischemic stroke. *N Engl J Med.* 2020 Jul 16;383(3):252-260.

KEY POINTS

■ Intravenous alteplase should be considered in patients who present within 4.5 hours of symptom onset regardless of the hospital setting.

■ Mechanical thrombectomy can be considered up to 24 hours from the time of onset.

■ No evidence currently suggests that either alteplase or tenecteplase is superior to the other.

Acute ischemic strokes can be life-altering, if not fatal. Signs and symptoms of a stroke must be promptly recognized to initiate treatment as soon as possible. With ongoing research and improving technology, stroke guidelines and therapeutic options continue to evolve. Treatment for patients with acute ischemic strokes largely depends on symptom duration, symptom severity, medical history, and imaging findings. Physicians should inquire about the time of onset (ie, the last time the patient was known to be well), and patients should undergo a rapid neurologic examination and noncontrast head CT to rule out an intracranial hemorrhage, a mass, or an alternative diagnosis. Although noncontrast head CT is the recommended initial imaging modality, additional advanced imaging such as CT angiography (CTA) or MRI may be needed for further management. The team should also obtain a point-of-care glucose reading and standard blood tests to evaluate for metabolic or toxicologic causes of altered mental status or acute neurologic deficits.

Although emergency physicians should follow institutional protocols and collaborate with stroke experts, the evidence-based guidelines offered by Powers regarding stroke treatment options at different times from symptom onset are useful.

From Time of Onset to 4.5 Hours After Onset

Guidelines recommend administering intravenous thrombolytics for patients who meet imaging, stroke severity, and other inclusion criteria. The thrombolytic agent used in treatment will likely depend on the hospital. Alteplase and tenecteplase are both tissue plasminogen activators (tPA) that are widely available and have their own eligibility criteria. Alteplase is better studied, but tenecteplase has a longer half-life and can be given as a single bolus, making it easier to administer. Currently, these two thrombolytics demonstrate no difference in effectiveness.

If available, a subsequent CTA or MR angiography (MRA) should be performed, and a mechanical thrombectomy should be considered in eligible patients.

From 4.5 to 9 Hours After Onset

A CTA or MRA should be obtained, and a mechanical thrombectomy should be considered in eligible patients. If patients are ineligible for a mechanical thrombectomy or transfer to a thrombectomy center for the procedure is unfeasible, administer intravenous alteplase, if appropriate.

From 9 to 24 Hours After Onset

A CTA or MRA should be performed; in eligible patients, a mechanical thrombectomy or transfer to a thrombectomy center where one can be performed should be considered. After administration of intravenous alteplase or completion of a mechanical thrombectomy, patients should be admitted to the ICU for careful monitoring of blood pressure, temperature, blood glucose levels, and signs of brain herniation, cerebral edema, or a rapid change in neurologic status.

By 24 Hours After Onset

Patients should be evaluated for dual antiplatelet treatment eligibility. A combination of clopidogrel and aspirin for 21 days after an acute ischemic stroke has been shown to lower the risk of a subsequent ischemic or hemorrhagic stroke.

By 48 Hours After Onset

Aspirin should be considered for patients not already on dual antithrombotic therapy

Summary

Although each health care institution varies greatly in its capabilities, intravenous tPA is broadly available, and eligibility criteria exist. If the patient is not in a hospital where a mechanical thrombectomy can be performed, transfer to a mechanical thrombectomy–capable center should be considered within 24 hours of symptom onset. If a patient presents to a hospital with mechanical thrombectomy capabilities and is eligible for intravenous alteplase at 4.5 hours or less since symptom onset, they should continue to be treated with intravenous alteplase even if they may also receive a mechanical thrombectomy.

Critical Decisions in Emergency Medicine's LLSA literature reviews features articles from ABEM's 2023 Lifelong Learning and Self-Assessment Reading List. Available online at acep.org/moc/llsa and on the ABEM website.

The Critical ECG
Atrial Flutter With Variable Block

By Jeremy Berberian, MD; William J. Brady, MD, FACEP;
and Amal Mattu, MD, FACEP

Dr. Berberian is the associate director of emergency medicine residency education at ChristianaCare and assistant professor of emergency medicine at Sidney Kimmel Medical College, Thomas Jefferson University in Philadelphia, Pennsylvania. Dr. Brady is a professor of emergency medicine, medicine, and nursing, and vice chair for faculty affairs in the Department of Emergency Medicine at the University of Virginia School of Medicine in Charlottesville. Dr. Mattu is a professor, vice chair, and codirector of the Emergency Cardiology Fellowship in the Department of Emergency Medicine at the University of Maryland School of Medicine in Baltimore.

Objectives

On completion of this article, you should be able to:

- Describe the ECG findings seen with atrial flutter.
- Identify the ratio of flutter waves to QRS complexes in an ECG with atrial flutter.
- Define the ECG characteristics of an RBBB.

CASE PRESENTATION

A 66-year-old man with a history of only hypertension presents with exertional near-syncope. His ECG shows atrial flutter with variable block and an average ventricular rate of 57 bpm, a normal axis, and a prolonged QRS complex duration with a right bundle branch block (RBBB) (*Figure 1*).

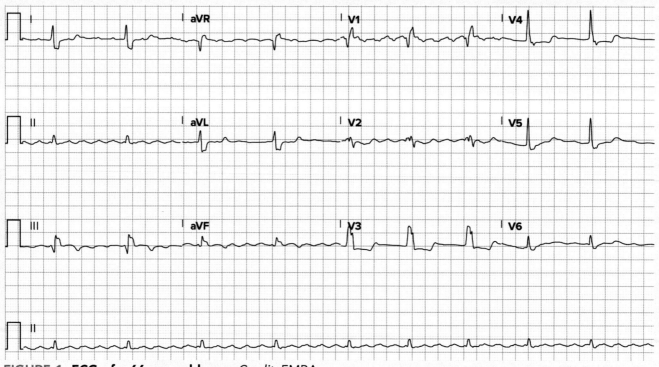

FIGURE 1. ECG of a 66-year-old man. *Credit:* EMRA.

Discussion

Flutter waves on ECG, also called F waves, are diagnostic of atrial flutter and are best seen in the inferior leads. Atrial flutter typically occurs because of a right atrial reentry circuit around the tricuspid ring. It is classified as a macro-reentry tachycardia because it revolves around a large obstacle, the right atrium, as opposed to a small obstacle like the atrioventricular (AV) node.

The patient's ECG shows atrial flutter with both a 5:1 and 4:1 conduction (*Figure 2*). His flutter waves have a consistent FF interval of 230 ms, which equates to approximately 260 bpm. Beats 1 through 4 and beat 9 show a 5:1 flutter. Using beats 1 and 2 as an example, the RR interval is 1,150 ms, which is exactly 5 times the FF interval of 230 ms (*Figure 3*). This is consistent with

the 5:1 flutter (ie, 5 flutter waves for every 1 QRS complex). Beats 5 through 8 show an RR interval of 920 ms, which is exactly 4 times the FF interval and consistent with the 4:1 flutter (*Figure 4*).

An RBBB is also seen in the patient's ECG. Characteristic findings in an RBBB include the following:

- QRS complex duration ≥120 ms;
- rsr', rsR', or rSR' pattern in lead V_1 +/− V_2 (*Figure 5*);
- Variations in lead V_1 include a qR pattern or broad R wave that is often notched;
- In lead V_1, the initial upward deflection should always be smaller than the second upward deflection (see *Figure 5*);
- S-wave duration greater than R-wave duration or greater than 40 ms in leads I and V_6 (*Figures 6* and *7*);

This patient had new-onset atrial flutter that was likely rate controlled by his use of metoprolol for hypertension. The time of onset was unclear, and the patient remained hemodynamically stable. As such, there was no indication for immediate cardioversion. The patient was admitted to the cardiology service and spontaneously converted to sinus rhythm.

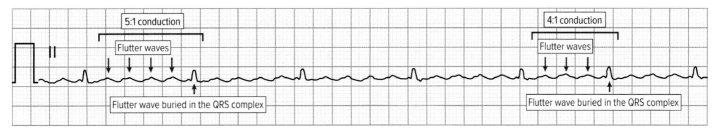

FIGURE 2. The lead II rhythm strip shows atrial flutter with both a 5:1 and 4:1 conduction. *Credit:* EMRA.

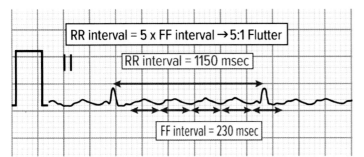

FIGURE 3. The atrial rate is exactly five times the ventricular rate, as seen here in the initial portion of the lead II rhythm strip, consistent with atrial flutter with a 5:1 conduction. *Credit:* EMRA.

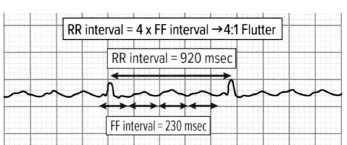

FIGURE 4. The atrial rate is exactly four times the ventricular rate between the fifth and seventh QRS complexes (the fifth and sixth QRS complexes from the lead II rhythm strip are shown here), consistent with atrial flutter with a 4:1 conduction. *Credit:* EMRA.

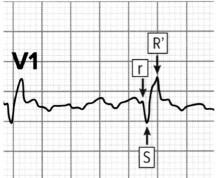

FIGURE 5. The rSR' pattern in lead V_1 is consistent with an RBBB. *Credit:* EMRA.

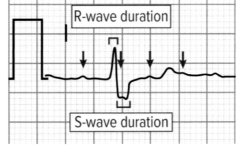

FIGURE 6. The S-wave duration is greater than the R-wave duration in lead I, consistent with an RBBB, and flutter waves (*purple arrows*) appear similar to P waves. *Credit:* EMRA.

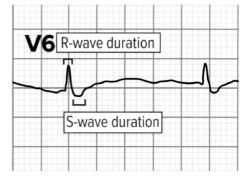

FIGURE 7. The S-wave duration is greater than the R-wave duration in lead V_6, consistent with an RBBB. *Credit:* EMRA.

- Normal R-wave peak time in leads V_5 and V_6 but greater than 50 ms in lead V_1 (only required if a broad R wave +/− a notch is present in lead V_1); and
- Repolarization abnormalities include ST-segment depression (STD) and T-wave inversion (TWI) in lead V_1 +/− leads V_2 and V_3 if they have an rsR' pattern; ST-segment elevation (STE) or upright T waves in those leads are concerning for ischemia.

An RBBB will typically have STD and TWI in lead V_1, and if leads V_2 and V_3 have an rsR' pattern present, they will also typically have STD and TWI. Consequently, upright T waves or STE in those leads with an rsR' pattern is concerning for ischemia, and even isoelectric or minimally elevated ST segments can be a subtle indicator of early acute myocardial

infarction. Otherwise, the presence of an RBBB does not confound the ECG evaluation of acute coronary syndrome like a left bundle branch block does. This patient's ECG shows an STD in lead V_4, but this is unlikely to be clinically significant in this case (*Figures 4, 5,* and *6*).

ACKNOWLEDGMENT

This case is reprinted from *Emergency ECGs: Case-Based Review and Interpretations*, available at www.emra.org/amazon or by scanning the QR code.

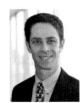

The Critical Image

A Brain Lesion in a Pediatric Patient

By Joshua S. Broder, MD, FACEP
Dr. Broder is a professor and the residency program director in the Department of Emergency Medicine at Duke University Medical Center in Durham, North Carolina.

Objectives

On completion of this article, you should be able to:

- Describe the differential diagnosis for brain lesions seen on MRI.
- Identify the role of gadolinium contrast in MRI.

CASE PRESENTATION

A 17-year-old girl presents after a possible focal seizure at home. The patient describes having had uncontrolled flapping movements of her right hand that lasted minutes. She has been experiencing intermittent headaches for several weeks, and a recent outpatient MRI of her brain showed a left temporal mass. She was referred to a neurosurgeon who recommended a brain biopsy. During the review of systems, the patient reports migratory joint pain, an intermittent subjective fever, and transient rashes over the past month. She has no history of drug or alcohol use.

Her vital signs are BP 110/70, P 83, R 17, and T 36.8°C (98.3°F); SpO_2 is 100% on room air. She is in no distress and is neurologically intact. The patient's cardiac examination is notable for a grade 2/6 systolic murmur at the left sternal border, which her mother states has been present since early childhood. The patient's joints are not swollen and have normal range of motion. Her mother shows a photo of a rash on the patient's heel from 2 weeks earlier (*Figure 1*).

The emergency physician reviews the MRI images and orders additional laboratory testing. Blood cultures are obtained. Laboratory testing reveals:

- Erythrocyte sedimentation rate of greater than 130 mm/hr (normal is 0-13 mm/hr);
- C-reactive protein level of 7.48 mg/dL (normal is ≤0.60 mg/dL); and
- Normal WBC count.

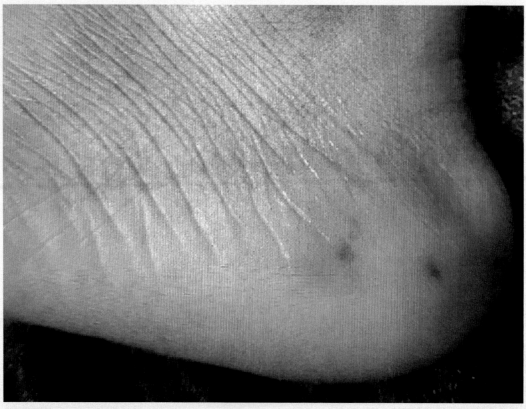

FIGURE 1. Patient's heel showing a painful rash that has occurred intermittently over the past month

Discussion

Clinically significant neuroimaging findings occur in only about 1% of pediatric patients who have headaches without neurologic abnormalities; thus, the American College of Radiology designates neuroimaging in this population as usually not appropriate.[1] When the history and physical examination suggest that a headache is secondary to another condition, such as a brain mass, MRI is usually appropriate. MRI of the brain is usually indicated in pediatric patients with abnormal neurologic examinations (eg, focal neurologic abnormalities, evidence of increased intracranial pressure, or an altered level of consciousness), seizures (including focal seizures), or suspected intracranial infection.[1,2]

MRI without contrast reveals structural abnormalities, such as hydrocephalus or mass effect, and is therefore usually the initial imaging test of choice for seizures. Abnormal noncontrast findings may prompt gadolinium-enhanced imaging, which is more sensitive for suspected malignancy, infection, and inflammation (*Figure 2*).[1] If an infection such as meningitis, encephalitis, or a brain abscess is suspected, MRI without and with contrast is usually appropriate and may reveal meningeal or parenchymal enhancement.[1]

Contrast-enhancing lesions on MRI have a differential diagnosis that includes neoplasm, infection, and inflammatory conditions (eg, multiple sclerosis). Multiple lesions can indicate metastatic disease, demyelinating disorders, inflammation, or infection, whereas solitary lesions are more likely primary brain neoplasms.[3] Infections, however, can masquerade as neoplasia.[4] Certain tumor types may favor specific anatomic locations, and the location of lesions within white matter can indicate demyelinating processes like multiple sclerosis. Imaging alone does not always provide a definitive diagnosis, reinforcing the importance of a careful history and physical examination for context.

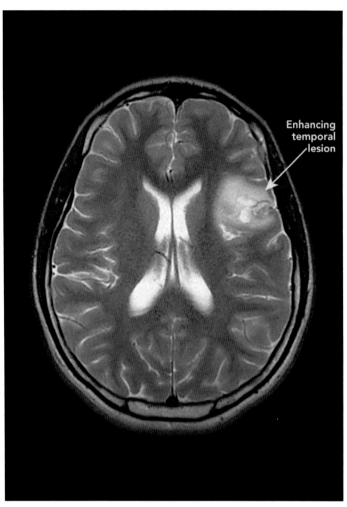

Enhancing temporal lesion

FIGURE 2. T2-weighted MRI with gadolinium contrast showing an enhancing lesion in the cortical grey matter of the temporal lobe

CASE RESOLUTION

The patient was admitted to the hospital; three of her peripheral blood cultures grew *Streptococcus oralis*, which is an oral commensal bacterium sometimes seen in native valve endocarditis. A transesophageal echocardiogram showed a thickened mitral valve, possibly a vegetation or a congenital anomaly. The patient met multiple modified Duke criteria for infective endocarditis, including positive blood cultures, valvular abnormality, fever, and immunologic phenomena, including Osler nodes (see *Figure 1*).[5] She was treated for subacute bacterial endocarditis with a brain abscess. Her *Streptococcus* isolate was highly susceptible to penicillin, which has excellent CNS distribution. Her blood cultures cleared after 24 hours of antibiotic therapy. After discharge, the patient completed a 2-week course of synergistic gentamicin and a 6-week course of intravenous penicillin G. At follow-up, her symptoms, laboratory findings, and imaging had all improved.

REFERENCES

1. Hayes LL, Palasis S, Bartel TB, et al; Expert Panel on Pediatric Imaging. ACR Appropriateness Criteria® Headache-Child. *J Am Coll Radiol.* 2018 May;15(5)(suppl):S78-S90.

2. Trofimova A, Milla SS, Ryan ME, et al; Expert Panel on Pediatric Imaging. ACR Appropriateness Criteria® Seizures-Child. *J Am Coll Radiol.* 2021 May;18(5)(suppl):S199-S211.

3. Villanueva-Meyer JE, Mabray MC, Cha S. Current clinical brain tumor imaging. *Neurosurgery.* 2017 Sep 1;81(3):397-415.

4. Ruderman B, Thoureen T, Broder J. Viridans streptococci intracranial abscess masquerading as metastatic disease. *JETem.* 2018 Jan 15;3(1):V7-V8. https://jetem.org/intracranial_abscess/

5. Li JS, Sexton DJ, Mick N, et al. Proposed modifications to the Duke criteria for the diagnosis of infective endocarditis. *Clin Infect Dis.* 2000 Apr;30(4):633-638.

Feature Editor: Joshua S. Broder, MD, FACEP. See also *Diagnostic Imaging for the Emergency Physician* (Winner of the 2011 Prose Award in Clinical Medicine, the American Publishers Award for Professional and Scholarly Excellence) and *Critical Images in Emergency Medicine* by Dr. Broder.

Pediatric Diphenhydramine Overdose

By Samantha (Gabby) Lacey, MD;
and Ann M. Dietrich, MD, FAAP, FACEP

Prisma Health — Upstate, Greenville, South Carolina

Reviewed by Sharon E. Mace, MD, FACEP

Objective

On completion of this article, you should be able to:

■ Discuss how to recognize and manage diphenhydramine overdoses.

CASE PRESENTATION

A 15-year-old boy presents after an intentional 500-mg ingestion of diphenhydramine approximately 1 hour prior to arrival. On arrival, he is hemodynamically stable, his initial pulse is 85 bpm, and his ECG shows a QRS interval of 109 ms and QTc interval of 445 ms (*Figure 1*). He denies having hallucinations and does not appear agitated on examination. Other than a cannabinoid-positive urine drug screen, urine toxicology results and aspirin and acetaminophen levels are normal.

After discussing the case with poison control, the physician gives the patient activated charcoal and an initial dose of sodium bicarbonate (0.5 mg/kg). Repeat ECG reveals a QRS interval of 113 ms, QTc interval of 446 ms, and a pulse of 78 bpm. Because his QRS interval remains longer than 100 ms, the patient is given an additional ampoule of sodium bicarbonate.

After this second dose, another ECG is collected and reveals a pulse of 91 bpm, QRS interval of 110 ms, and QTc interval of 474 ms (*Figure 2*). The patient is given a sodium bicarbonate infusion (sodium bicarbonate in dextrose 5% maintenance fluids) because his QTc interval remains prolonged after taking 2 ampoules of sodium bicarbonate. He is admitted to the pediatric ICU for continued cardiac monitoring. He does not require benzodiazepines for agitation at any time during his emergency department stay.

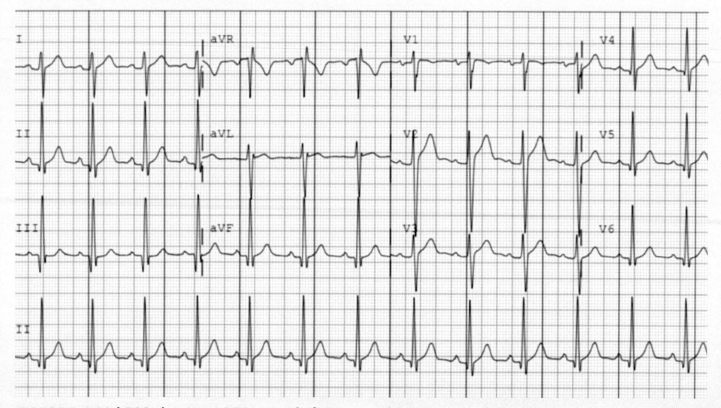

FIGURE 1. Initial ECG showing a QRS interval of 109 ms and QTc interval of 445 ms.
Credit: Dr. Samantha Lacey.

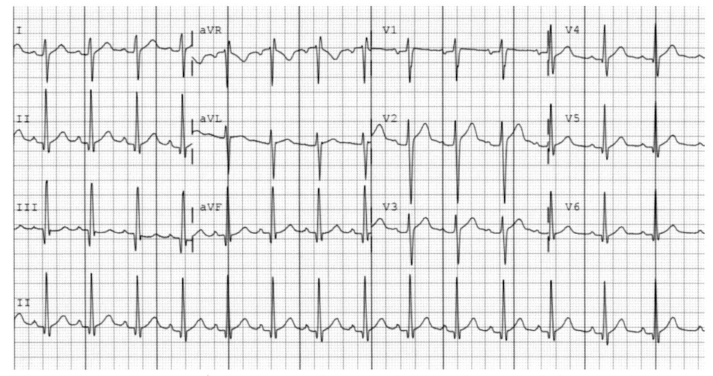

FIGURE 2. Repeat ECG showing a QRS interval of 110 ms and prolonged QTc interval of 474 ms.
Credit: Dr. Samantha Lacey.

Discussion

Diphenhydramine is a first-generation antihistamine. It is also one of the top 15 drugs involved in overdose deaths, accounting for 3.2% of drug overdose deaths in the United States.[1] Diphenhydramine overdoses can occur secondary to oral, topical, or intravenous exposures. Symptoms of mild diphenhydramine overdose generally include sedation and the classic antimuscarinic toxidrome of mydriasis, dry mucous membranes, tachycardia, and decreased bowel sounds.[2] Severe ingestions are more likely to cause agitation, delirium, hallucinations, seizures, or coma.[3] Diphenhydramine blocks sodium and potassium channels in the myocardium, which leads to findings of widened QRS and QTc intervals on ECG.[4]

A thorough history is needed to diagnose diphenhydramine overdose. If patients are altered or unable to give a history, the history should be obtained from family. Patients should be assessed for anticholinergic signs and symptoms, and if there is concern for overdose, physicians should perform an ECG, urine drug screen, and full toxicology screen that tests for levels of acetaminophen, salicylate, and alcohol. Management of diphenhydramine overdose includes using activated charcoal in patients who have ingested diphenhydramine within the past 2 hours and who are alert and able to protect their airway. Agitation or seizures in diphenhydramine overdose are treated with benzodiazepines. QRS intervals longer than 100 ms and prolonged QTc intervals (>460 ms in pediatrics) should be treated with 1 mEq/kg of sodium bicarbonate, with repeated doses as needed if no improvement occurs or ECG worsens.[5] Once a patient has received two or more doses of sodium bicarbonate, starting an intravenous infusion is appropriate. Ultimate disposition requires continued cardiac monitoring and sodium bicarbonate infusions, often in the ICU.

CASE RESOLUTION

The patient's sodium bicarbonate infusion was discontinued in the ICU because he was not having hallucinations or tachycardia. The following morning, another ECG was obtained and showed normal QRS and QTc intervals. The patient was ultimately discharged to inpatient psychiatric hospitalization.

REFERENCES

1. Hedegaard H, Bastian BA, Trinidad JP, Spencer M, Warner M. Drugs most frequently involved in drug overdose deaths: United States, 2011-2016. *Natl Vital Stat Rep.* 2018 Dec;67(9):1-14.
2. Abdi A, Rose E, Levine M. Diphenhydramine overdose with intraventricular conduction delay treated with hypertonic sodium bicarbonate and i.v. lipid emulsion. *West J Emerg Med.* 2014 Nov;15(7):855-888.
3. Levine M, Brooks DE, Truitt CA, Wolk BJ, Boyer EW, Ruha A-M. Toxicology in the ICU: part 1: general overview and approach to treatment. *Chest.* 2011 Sep 1;140(3):795-806.
4. Zareba W, Moss AJ, Rosero SZ, Hajj-Ali R, Konecki J, Andrews M. Electrocardiographic findings in patients with diphenhydramine overdose. *Am J Cardiol.* 1997 Nov 1;80(9):1168-1173.
5. Dickinson DF. The normal ECG in childhood and adolescence. *Heart.* 2005 Dec;91(12):1626-1630.

Open Achilles Tendon Laceration

By Jacob Feldsher, MD
University of Florida College of Medicine — Jacksonville

Reviewed by John Kiel, DO, MPH, FACEP, CAQSM

Objective

On completion of this article, you should be able to:

- Explain how to diagnose an Achilles tendon rupture or laceration.

CASE PRESENTATION

A 44-year-old man with no significant medical or surgical history presents with right ankle pain. He reports that 8 days ago he cut the back of his right ankle on a piece of metal fencing. That same day, he went to an urgent care center where his laceration was repaired with sutures. His physical examination findings and diagnostic imaging results (if completed) from the urgent care center are unknown. On examination, there is a ball-like deformity proximal to his laceration. The laceration is approximately 5 cm in length, is located just proximal to the calcaneus, and appears to be healing well. He has limited plantar flexion and reports pain with passive dorsiflexion of his right foot.

Discussion

This patient presents with a full-thickness Achilles tendon laceration that was missed during his initial evaluation at the urgent care center. Bedside ultrasonography confirmed the diagnosis without the need for further imaging (*Figure 1*).

The Achilles tendon forms a common tendon where the gastrocnemius and soleus muscles meet. It arises in the middle of the calf and inserts onto the calcaneus. Although many studies exist on acute Achilles tendon rupture, the literature on open Achilles tendon injuries is scarce.[1] Approximately 62% to 75% of spontaneous ruptures are associated with sports. People with sedentary lifestyles are most at risk for spontaneous ruptures when sudden or repetitive movements stress the tendon, although these ruptures also occur during sports activities where remarkably high forces are generated, such as the high jump.[2]

According to the American Academy of Orthopedic Surgery's consensus opinion, a ruptured Achilles tendon can be diagnosed clinically.[3] No consensus exists on whether imaging should be obtained to support a diagnosis of an Achilles tendon rupture; however, when imaging is used to support the diagnosis, ultrasound is an excellent option. In a recent meta-analysis of patients with full Achilles tendon ruptures that were treated surgically, ultrasound had a sensitivity of 94.8% and specificity of 98.7% for detecting the condition.[4] In a single-center, retrospective analysis from a hospital in Nigeria, primary repair was used to manage open Achilles injuries from motor vehicle and farming accidents in patients who presented early and did not have significant tissue loss or comorbidity.[1]

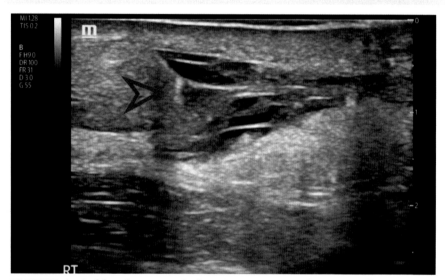

FIGURE 1. Ankle ultrasound showing a torn and proximally retracted Achilles tendon (*red arrow*) in long axis

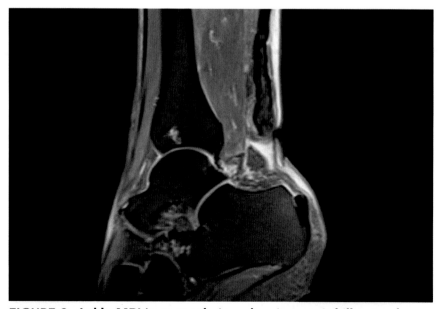

FIGURE 2. Ankle MRI in coronal view showing an Achilles tendon tear with an approximately 4-cm retraction from the calcaneus

CASE RESOLUTION

The patient was placed in a posterior short leg splint while in plantar flexion and was provided crutches. He was advised to follow up with an outpatient orthopedist for further management. The patient was seen by an orthopedic specialist 1 month later. MRI of the right ankle showed a full-thickness tear of the Achilles tendon at the calcaneal insertion with a 4-cm retraction (*Figure 2*). The patient underwent primary Achilles tendon repair with reattachment to the calcaneus (*Figure 3*). No immediate complications were seen following surgery. Postoperatively, the patient was initially non–weight-bearing but at his 2-month follow-up visit transitioned to a controlled-ankle-movement (CAM) boot with weight-bearing as tolerated. At the patient's last follow-up visit, he still used his CAM boot and was weight-bearing as tolerated but planned to transition out of his boot after a physical therapy evaluation. His right ankle's active range of motion was still limited. The patient was subsequently lost to follow-up.

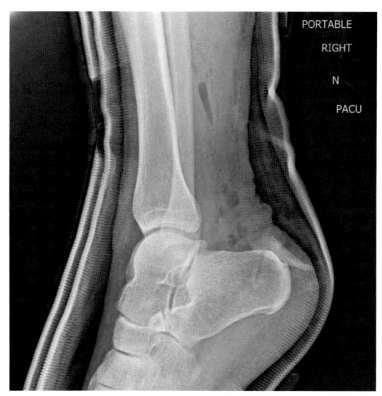

FIGURE 3. Postoperative ankle x-ray showing an ankle splinted in plantar flexion with subcutaneous emphysema

REFERENCES

1. Awe AA, Esezobor EE, Aigbonoga QO. Experience with managing open Achilles tendon injuries in a tertiary hospital in Southern Nigeria. *J West Afr Coll Surg.* 2015 Oct-Dec;5(4):30-40.
2. Järvinen TAH, Kannus P, Maffulli N, Khan KM. Achilles tendon disorders: etiology and epidemiology. *Foot Ankle Clin.* 2005 Jun;10(2):255-266.
3. Chiodo CP, Glazebrook M, Bluman EM, et al; American Academy of Orthopedic Surgeons. Diagnosis and treatment of acute Achilles tendon rupture. *J Am Acad Orthop Surg.* 2010 Aug;18(8):503-510.
4. Aminlari A, Stone J, McKee R, et al. Diagnosing Achilles tendon rupture with ultrasound in patients treated surgically: a systematic review and meta-analysis. *J Emerg Med.* 2021 Nov;61(5):558-567.

Mallet Finger Splint

By Steven J. Warrington, MD, MEd, MS
MercyOne Siouxland, Sioux City, Iowa

Objective

On completion of this article, you should be able to:

■ Explain how to splint a mallet finger.

Introduction

Patients can develop a mallet finger from a tendon rupture or an avulsion fracture. Although some cases of mallet finger involve a laceration or open component, short-term management for many cases is done with a splint in extension or slight hyperextension. If a prefabricated mallet finger splint is unavailable, physicians can form and apply their own splint.

Contraindications

■ No complete contraindication
■ Untreated associated open wounds

Benefits and Risks

Splinting is the recommended initial therapy for most cases of mallet finger, even in patients who need surgical management, and provides definitive care in some cases. Continued splinting, however, is not recommended if distal interphalangeal (DIP) joint subluxation occurs from a poorly reduced avulsion fracture.

Primary risks of splinting are skin and nail complications, including maceration, ulceration, infection, and nail dystrophy. Deformities and dysfunction at the DIP joint, such as swan-neck deformities and extension lag, are also risks. Splint therapy can fail if patients do not follow instructions for wearing their splint and caring for their injury.

Alternatives

Commercial finger splints are available as alternatives to the ones made in the emergency department. The current literature suggests similar outcomes regardless of the splint used. Surgical care is another alternative to splinting, but many patients who need surgery still need initial splinting in the emergency department while awaiting surgical care.

Reducing Side Effects

Proper patient education can reduce the risks of skin complications and treatment failure. Patients should be instructed on how to care for the affected digit, including keeping the DIP joint in continual extension for a full 6 to 8 weeks, even when cleaning the area. They should be instructed to avoid intermittently bending the finger to check functionality.

Special Considerations

Despite the many splinting techniques available — commercially available splints, dorsal finger splints, volar finger splints, and combined dorsal and volar finger splints — the literature suggests similar outcomes. The literature also states that only the DIP joint requires immobilization; the proximal interphalangeal (PIP) joint can remain free. Lastly, the ideal degree of slight hyperextension (<10°) at the DIP joint when forming the splint is unclear from the literature.

▬ TECHNIQUE ▬

1. **Clean** and repair any associated wounds. Consult a specialist if needed (eg, open fracture).

2. **Consider** imaging to evaluate for an avulsion fracture.

3. **Measure** a splint that goes from the fingertip to the middle phalanx so that it immobilizes the DIP joint without immobilizing the PIP joint.

4. **Smooth** out cut edges of the splint to ensure they will not damage tissue when the PIP joint is flexed.

5. **Form** the splint to create slight hyperextension (5°-10°) at the DIP joint.

6. **Apply** the splint to the digit and secure it with tape. Some application styles place the splint on the dorsal aspect, while others place it on the volar aspect.

7. **Assess** for ongoing subluxation at the DIP joint after splinting. If ongoing subluxation is seen, close follow-up for surgical therapy may be indicated.

8. **Educate** the patient on proper care and the need to maintain continual extension for a full 6 weeks, including during cleaning. Emphasize that even brief

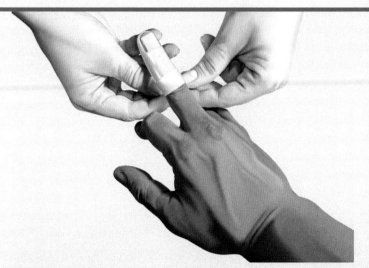

FIGURE 1. Mallet finger splint. *Credit:* ACEP.

self-assessment of DIP joint flexion and extension can increase healing time and risk treatment failure.

9. **Instruct** the patient on follow-up recommendations based on the specific injury.

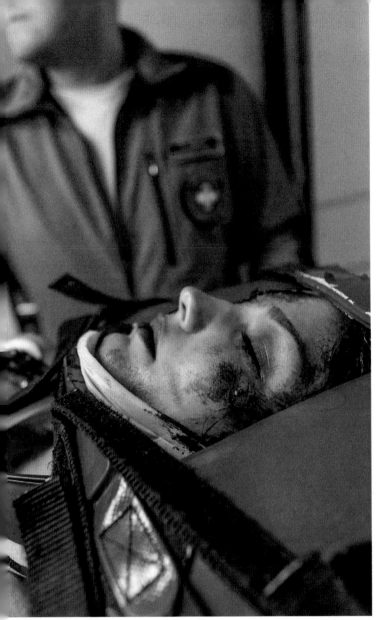

Show Some Backbone

Traumatic Spinal Cord Injury

LESSON **6**

By Carlos Rodriguez, MD; Allan Winger, MD; Ryan Poulo, MD; and Andrew Glunk, MD

Dr. Rodriguez is the assistant program director at Thomas Jefferson University in Philadelphia, Pennsylvania. Dr. Winger, Dr. Poulo, and Dr. Glunk are emergency medicine residents at Thomas Jefferson University.

Reviewed by Danya Khoujah, MBBS, MEHP, FACEP

Objectives

On completion of this lesson, you should be able to:

1. Discuss the different patterns of incomplete SCIs.
2. Describe the risks and benefits of spinal motion restriction and identify when continued immobilization is necessary.
3. Select the appropriate imaging modalities for the evaluation of spinal trauma.
4. Distinguish stable from unstable vertebral fractures using evidence-based decision tools and state the management for each.
5. Differentiate between spinal shock and neurogenic shock and describe the management of neurogenic shock in trauma patients.

From the EM Model

18.0 Traumatic Disorders
    18.1 Trauma
        18.1.7 Spine Trauma

CRITICAL DECISIONS

- What are the categories of incomplete SCIs?

- When is cervical spine imaging required?

- When is a cervical collar or spine board needed?

- What imaging modality is most appropriate for evaluating spinal trauma?

- How do emergency physicians determine if spinal fractures are stable or unstable?

- What is neurogenic shock, and how is it managed?

Traumatic spinal injury is a common occurrence in the United States and can have potentially devastating consequences. Emergency physicians are often the first to evaluate these patients. Recognizing these cases early and managing them appropriately provides spinal injury patients with their best chance to avoid secondary neurologic injury.

■ CASE ONE

An 84-year-old man arrives via EMS. He is in a cervical collar. The patient has a history of atrial fibrillation and takes warfarin. EMTs report that the patient was walking on a sidewalk when he lost his footing on an ice patch. He fell forward and hit the front of his head. He felt his neck bend backward following the impact. His vital signs include BP 172/90, P 94, R 16, and T 37.2 °C (98.9°F). He is alert and oriented and denies loss of consciousness; however, he states that he is experiencing new weakness bilaterally in his upper extremities.

■ CASE TWO

A 27-year-old man with no past medical history is brought in by police after being stabbed. The patient is found to also have an injury to the spine at the level of the T8 vertebra. His vital signs include BP 152/85,

P 97, R 20, and T 37.0°C (98.6°F). He has no other traumatic injuries. Examination reveals weakness in his left lower extremity and an inability to feel pain in his right lower extremity.

■ CASE THREE

A 40-year-old woman with an unknown past medical history is brought in by EMS following a high-speed motor vehicle collision. On examination, the patient has lacerations to the face and a step-off deformity at the level of the C5 vertebra; no other traumatic injuries are noted. The patient is obtunded, and the decision is made to intubate her. Her vital signs prior to intubation include BP 72/40, P 40, R 20, and T 37.0 °C (98.6°F). Because of the significant mechanism of injury, massive transfusion protocol is ordered. The patient's blood pressure does not respond to volume resuscitation.

Introduction

Approximately 17,000 cases of spinal cord injury (SCI) occur in the United States annually.[1] These injury patterns can severely impact the physical and emotional well-being of individuals and have been found to significantly increase the risk of mortality.[2] Additionally, because patients with SCIs often require complex follow-up care, these injuries come at significant cost. It is estimated that a patient with an SCI will require $1.1 to $4.6 million in follow-up care, making early recognition of SCIs monumentally important in mitigating patients' follow-up needs.[3] Initial stabilization with a cervical spine collar can prevent worsening injury. The early identification of neurogenic shock and appropriate treatment can preserve penumbra. When SCI is identified, the appropriate surgeons can be consulted, and the appropriate care can be expedited.

CRITICAL DECISION

What are the categories of incomplete SCIs?

The three categories of incomplete SCI are central cord syndrome, anterior cord syndrome, and Brown-Séquard syndrome.[4] History and physical examination findings differentiate these injury patterns.

Central Cord Syndrome

Of the incomplete SCIs, central cord syndrome is the most common (*Figure 1*).[5] This syndrome often arises from hyperextension of the cervical spine. Hyperextension causes damage to the central fibers of the corticospinal and spinothalamic tracts, which are responsible for voluntary motor function and nociception, temperature, touch, and pressure, respectively (*Figure 2*).[4]

Within the corticospinal tract, motor neurons of the upper extremities are centrally located, while those of the lower extremities are situated laterally.[4] Because of this, motor function of the upper extremities is more predominately affected than that of the lower extremities.

Management of this injury begins in the field with rigid immobilization of the spine.[6] For emergency physicians, hemodynamic management is a key aspect of treatment.[7] Although controversial, the suggested mean arterial pressure (MAP) goal lies between 85 to 90 mm Hg, which ensures adequate blood supply to the injured spinal cord and preserves penumbra.[8]

An inflammatory cascade is often triggered in this setting. Inflammation can cause expansion of the area of injury, causing further compression.[9,10] The use of steroids has been studied to mitigate this inflammation.[11] Methylprednisolone use was found to increase the risks of mortality, infection, longer ICU stays, and gastric ulcers.[12,13] In 2013, the Congress of Neurosurgeons released a level 1 advisory *against* the use of steroids.[11] The choice between surgery or conservative management is dependent on the injury and should be made in collaboration with a surgical team.

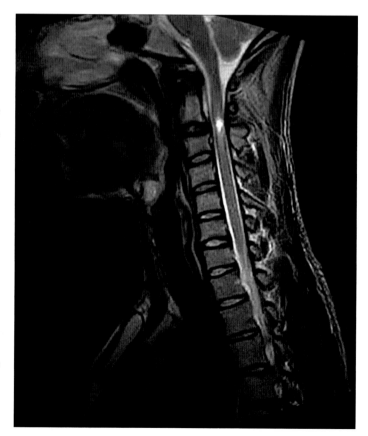

FIGURE 1. MRI showing central cord syndrome.
Credit: Copyright 2023 Dr. Arthur Daire. Image courtesy of Dr. Arthur Daire and Radiopaedia.org, rID: 30935. Used under license.

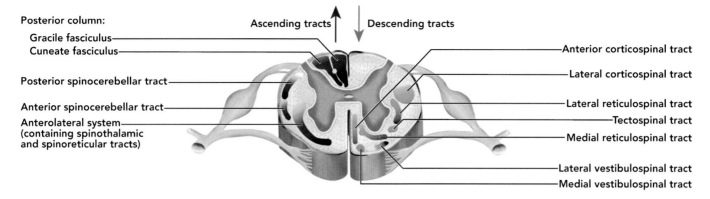

FIGURE 2. Spinal cord tracts. *Credit:* ACEP.

Anterior Cord Syndrome

Anterior cord syndrome occurs from damage to the anterior two-thirds of the spinal cord. This syndrome often results from injury to the anterior spinal artery, most commonly from aortic surgery.[14] However, it can also occur from trauma, often from direct anterior injury to or a flexion injury of the neck.[4] This injury causes damage to both the spinothalamic and corticospinal tracts, which leads to loss of motor function and sensation, pain, and temperature perception distal to the injury.[4] The posterior spinal columns remain intact, so vibration and tactile sensations are preserved.

Management of this condition relies heavily on physical and occupational therapy to help patients recover motor function. The prognosis depends on numerous factors, primarily the severity of the initial injury.[14]

Brown-Séquard Syndrome

Brown-Séquard syndrome represents approximately 4% of SCI cases annually in the United States.[15] This injury occurs secondary to hemisection of the posterior spinal cord, often due to penetrating trauma. It can also result from lateral cord compression from a spinal fracture.[4] Brown-Séquard syndrome is characterized by ipsilateral loss of motor function, vibration, and proprioception with contralateral loss of pain and temperature sensation. Management should be done in conjunction with a neurosurgical team, including the possibility of decompressive surgery.[15] The use of steroids remains controversial and has been found to have no role in this injury.[15] The overall prognosis for Brown-Séquard syndrome is good.[4] In the setting of traumatic injury, motor function is recovered in the majority of cases.[15]

CRITICAL DECISION

When is cervical spine imaging required?

It can be difficult to decide when to opt for imaging in patients with trauma to the cervical spine and when it is appropriate to defer. Two validated clinical decision-making tools are available to aid clinicians in this determination.

NEXUS Criteria

One clinical decision-making tool used is the NEXUS (**N**ational **E**mergency **X**-radiography **U**tilization **S**tudy) criteria for cervical spine imaging. This tool is a well-validated clinical aid that can guide physicians to safely rule out cervical spine injury (CSI) without imaging in alert, stable trauma patients. Detection of clinically significant CSI is 99.6% sensitive.[16] To defer imaging, patients must meet all five criteria: absence of midline tenderness, absence of focal neurologic deficit, normal level of alertness and consciousness, no evidence of intoxication, and no distracting injuries. If patients meet all criteria, imaging can be deferred.[16]

CCR

The Canadian cervical spine rule (CCR) is 100% sensitive for detecting medically significant CSIs.[17] For this tool, physicians must go through three assessments in sequential order.[17] The first assessment requires that patients have no high-risk factors, including age older than 65 years, a dangerous mechanism of injury (eg, a fall from >3 ft [0.9 m] or 5 stairs; an axial load injury; a high speed motor vehicle collision, rollover, or ejection; a bicycle collision; or a motorized recreational vehicle injury), or paraesthesias in the extremities. If the risk-factors assessment is negative, physicians should move on to the second assessment, which focuses on low-risk factors. These factors include a simple rear-end motor vehicle collision, sitting position in the emergency department, ambulation at any time following the accident, delayed onset of neck pain, and absence of midline cervical spine tenderness. If patients have no low-risk factors, then they do not meet the low-risk criteria, and imaging is required. If at least one of these low-risk factors is positive, physicians can continue to the third assessment. This assessment evaluates patients' ability to rotate their cervical spine. If patients can rotate their neck, imaging can be deferred.[17]

Imaging Decisions for Older Patients

Older patients warrant special consideration. As the US population ages, the proportion of geriatric patients seen in the emergency department continues to increase. This population's decreased mobility is accompanied by a greater prevalence of CSIs. This raises the question of whether bedside history and examination can exclude a CSI in older patients, thereby decreasing length of stay and improving patient flow.

The joint policy statement put out by ACEP largely follows NEXUS criteria for ruling out cervical spine imaging. Although some studies have found the CCR to be superior to the NEXUS low-risk criteria in excluding clinically significant CSI, CCR automatically calls for imaging if patients are older than 65 years. In an attempt to reduce the need for unnecessary spinal imaging in geriatric patients, Williams et al conducted a study in 2021 that excluded CSI in older patients if they had no external evidence of trauma above the clavicles, did not suffer from altered mental status, and exhibited no tenderness on palpation of the cervical spine; this combination of factors had a sensitivity of 100%.[18] Although these findings have yet to be validated in prospective studies, emergency physicians can use their clinical discretion to apply these rules and potentially forego imaging in older patients.

CRITICAL DECISION

When is a cervical collar or spine board needed?

Cervical Collars

Traumatic injury is a frequent cause for presentation to the emergency department. In 2020, motor vehicle collisions accounted for almost 1.6 million injuries and resulted in over 35,000 deaths in the United States.[19] Other causes of trauma include falls, assaults, or sports injuries. Any of these patients can present with a traumatic spinal injury. Many patients are brought in by EMS and have a rigid collar applied in the field, and emergency physicians must determine when the collar can be cleared, or if continued immobilization is necessary. Some patients present as walk-ins and have no cervical collar applied; it then becomes incumbent on the physicians to determine the mechanism and details surrounding the injury to decide if cervical immobilization is warranted.

Although spinal immobilization has become a mainstay of prehospital care, it has drawbacks. Patients in cervical collars can often face long stays, with delays in collar clearance due to the unavailability of CT equipment, the responsiveness of the trauma team, or the acuity of other patients. Use of rigid collars results in patient discomfort and dissatisfaction. Its use also complicates airway management and intubation and obscures other traumatic injuries to the neck. These risks must be weighed against the benefits of preventing neurologic injury and the probability of an unstable spine; therefore, routine or indiscriminate use of cervical collars is not recommended.

Because of the devastating consequences of missing an unstable spine and the risk of causing permanent neurologic damage, recognizing the need for immobilization is essential; however, the topic can be controversial. A Cochrane review in 2001 aimed at examining the effect of different immobilization techniques on neurologic disability and mortality found no randomized controlled trials of immobilization in trauma patients, thus calling the benefit of immobilization techniques into question.[20] This result is partially because many studies that were conducted to measure the efficacy of immobilization were performed with healthy volunteers or cadavers, and these findings were extrapolated to trauma patients. Some studies went as far as to suggest that cervical collars are not beneficial at all. Using cadavers to create an unstable cervical spine and measuring displacement between C1 and C2, Ben-Galim et al found that using cervical collars in blunt traumatic injury can sometimes cause, rather than prevent, secondary spinal injury.[21]

With the uncertainty surrounding the use of cervical collars, it is imperative to distinguish instances that call for immobilization from circumstances where collar application is unnecessary. In conjunction with the American College of Surgeons Committee on Trauma and the National Association of EMS Physicians, ACEP approved a policy statement in 2018 regarding spinal motion restriction in trauma patients (*Table 1*).[22] Of note, the joint statement points out that spine restriction has no role in penetrating trauma cases.

Spine Boards

While the literature may appear ambiguous on the net benefits of cervical collars, the same cannot be said for long spine boards. Spine boards and cervical collars have been employed in tandem since the 1960s to fully immobilize the spine in the setting of traumatic injury; however, a body of literature has been growing that describes the disadvantages of spine board use and advocates for early discontinuation, if not total abandonment.[23,24] The consensus on complications from prolonged spine board use is clear. Development of pressure ulcers, increased pain, pain for longer duration, restriction

Criteria	Clarification
Acutely altered level of consciousness	Glasgow Coma Scale score <15 or evidence of intoxication
Midline neck or back pain or tenderness	N/A
Focal neurologic deficits	Numbness or motor weakness
Anatomic deformity of spine	N/A
Distracting injuries	Long-bone fracture, crush injuries, burns, etc.

TABLE 1. Indications for spine restriction in blunt trauma[21]

of pulmonary expansion, and worsening respiratory function are all complications that have been described. Spine board use has also been shown to alter a physical examination, resulting in increased use of imaging. By contrast, the benefits of spine board use remain largely unproven, and its continuation stems mostly from historical use.[24]

If EMS transports a patient to the emergency department on a spine board, the patient should be removed from the board as soon as feasibly possible. Doing so may involve removing the patient from the spine board after completing the primary survey, during the log roll, or immediately on arrival. The ACEP joint policy from 2018 does not discourage spine board use in prehospital immobilization, but it does advocate for inhospital removal as soon as possible (see *Table 1*).[22] As with cervical collar immobilization, spine board use for thoracic or lumbar immobilization in the setting of penetrating trauma is unwarranted.

CRITICAL DECISION

What imaging modality is most appropriate for evaluating spinal trauma?

Spinal imaging can be somewhat of a contentious topic. In a busy emergency department, imaging can act as the bottleneck that impedes patient flow, especially in cases with low-impact or unclear mechanisms of injury and when imaging is not prioritized through protocol. If sufficient concern exists for a potential spinal injury, the key consideration to pursuing imaging involves selecting the most appropriate modality to effectively rule out the pathology with respect to the patient's age.

X-ray Versus CT

X-rays have the advantage of being rapidly obtained and exposing the patient to minimal radiation. In pediatric and young adult populations, x-rays may be preferred to reduce lifetime exposure to radiation and potential malignancy later in life, but the question remains whether x-ray alone is an adequate imaging modality for spinal trauma. Although CT has been shown to be superior to x-ray in adult trauma patients, several studies examining pediatric patients have yielded nebulous and conflicting results. Some have argued that the best approach would be to screen with x-ray and proceed with CT if concern still exists. Others have found x-ray sufficiently sensitive and add that CT imaging yields little additional clinical value. While the Pediatric Emergency Care Applied Research Network has a dedicated decision-making tool for obtaining a head CT, no such aid exists for cervical or thoracolumbar spinal injury; thus, it is often left to the discretion of emergency physicians. Adding to the difficulty is that different studies report different sensitivities for x-ray and CT, depending on how "significant spinal injuries" is defined.[25] Using NEXUS definitions of clinically significant and nonsignificant injuries, Hale et al identified 75 pediatric patients with CSIs who underwent both CT and cervical x-ray at the time of initial evaluation and found that x-ray failed to identify 32% of clinically significant CSIs.[25] Although it does not specifically address pediatric or adult patients, the Eastern Association for the Surgery of Trauma Practice Management Guidelines recommend CT for the evaluation of CSIs and state that x-rays should not be used.[26] Likewise, their recommendations for thoracolumbar evaluation following blunt trauma call for CT, noting that multidetector CT allows for the reformatting of the thoracolumbar spine in chest and abdomen studies without additional radiation and declaring x-rays inadequate for detection of traumatic injury.[27] Additionally, the American College of Surgeons Best Practice Guidelines, published as recently as March 2022, state that multidetector CT sensitivity for CSI approaches 98%, while sensitivity for thoracolumbar injury approaches 100%.[28] They add that reconstruction of the thoracic and lumbar spine in chest/abdomen/pelvis studies provides sufficient sensitivity to exclude thoracolumbar injury.

On the other end of the age spectrum, geriatric patients also present unique challenges. Older patients are particularly vulnerable to spinal injury, owing to their decreased mobility, decreased reaction time, and often-numerous comorbidities. The spine also becomes more susceptible to fractures as it stiffens and becomes more osteoporotic with age.[28] Older patients require more liberal use of CT imaging to exclude serious pathology, even in instances of low-energy mechanisms of injury. This becomes especially true in patients who cannot offer a good history and examination due to delirium, dementia, or other conditions with altered mental status.

Indications for MRI

MRI offers the greatest detail in imaging and can detect ligamentous and spinal cord insults in addition to bony injury. This greater detail is offset by the prolonged time of imaging, availability, and patient tolerance. With the high degree of sensitivity of multidetector CT for detecting clinically significant bony spinal injury, the utility of MRI for the detection of bony spinal injury is negligible. Whether patients are awake and alert or obtunded and unevaluable, multidetector CT has been shown to be sufficiently sensitive to rule out unstable spinal injuries, and MRI adds little additional benefit in this situation. Various studies have examined the utility of MRI in the evaluation of SCI in patients with negative CT scans and persistent neurologic symptoms. Although MRI is more sensitive at detecting CSI, the rate of capturing clinically significant injury is low. One meta-analysis of 23 studies found 16 missed unstable CSI injuries on MRI in 5,286 cases with negative CTs, a miss rate of 0.3%.[28] When MRI did capture an injury that was missed on CT, it was rarely found to change management. If significant spinal injury is found on CT, MRI should be considered as a complementary study to assess spinal cord or nerve root involvement and to aid in preoperative planning. If CT evaluation is unremarkable and concern remains for occult unstable spinal injury, physicians must balance the need for greater detail against the challenges of obtaining MRI imaging. In addition to the aforementioned challenges, MRI requires patients to remain motionless, which can be difficult in altered or anxious patients. Additionally, secondary equipment, such as a ventilator or multiple intravenous lines, can make MRI unfeasible.

CRITICAL DECISION

How do emergency physicians determine if spinal fractures are stable or unstable?

Numerous attempts have been made to classify whether a traumatic injury to the vertebral spine constitutes a stable or unstable injury.[29,30] This delineation is significant because unstable spinal injuries pose the risk of irritation or damage to the spinal cord or nerve roots, which can lead to permanent neurologic dysfunction if left unstable. This classification can also determine the likelihood that patients will need immediate operative intervention. Evaluation of the spine can often be difficult in the acute setting due to polytrauma, pain, altered mental status, or obtundation. As a rule, it is best to assume that spinal injuries are unstable in trauma patients until definitively ruled out.

CSIs

The cervical spine is especially vulnerable to injury given its high degree of flexibility.[31] Traditionally, the mnemonic to recall unstable CSIs is "Jefferson Bit Off a Hangman's Thumb" (*Table 2*). The majority of the unstable fractures described by this mnemonic involve the atlantoaxial joint; thus, it does not provide a comprehensive overview of unstable CSIs. Recognition of these fractures should prompt emergency physicians to immediately involve a spine specialist because injuries to the subaxial cervical spine are at high risk of secondary neurologic injury.

In one attempt to standardize injury classification, Vaccaro et al in 2007 developed the subaxial injury classification scale (SLIC), a tool that is available on MDCalc.[29,32] The SLIC scoring system is based on fracture morphology, involvement of the posterior ligament, and neurologic findings on examination to determine if CSI requires immediate operative decompression and stabilization (*Table 3*). For injuries where operative management is deemed unnecessary, patients can be discharged with hard cervical collars to prevent secondary injury, outpatient MRI imaging, and follow-up with a spine specialist.[30] Patients with unstable fractures require admission for operative management by a spine service or transfer to a higher level of care if a spine surgeon is unavailable.

Thoracolumbar Injuries

Much of the literature groups injuries to the thoracic and lumbar spines together. The thoracic spine is relatively immobile, given its small intervertebral discs and connection to ribs whose cartilages articulate directly with the sternum. By contrast, the lumbar spine is more flexible, and because of this difference in flexibility, the majority of thoracolumbar spinal injuries (TLSI) occur at the thoracolumbar junction, T10 to L2.[30] Much like the SLIC tool for CSI, a classification tool is available to determine stability following TLSI. The thoracolumbar injury classification scale, or TLICS, is also available on MDCalc (see *Table 3*).[29,30] TLSIs that are determined to be stable for outpatient management can be discharged with a thoracolumbosacral orthosis brace, MRI, and spine specialist follow-up.

✔ Pearls

- Steroid use in incomplete SCIs is currently controversial, and the decision to use them should be made with the aid of a spine surgery team.
- Motion restriction in spinal injuries due to penetrating trauma is unwarranted.
- Validated decision-making tools can aid in determining if an SCI is stable or unstable.
- Early engagement of specialists is a must if any concern exists for SCI.

What is neurogenic shock, and how is it managed?

Neurogenic shock and spinal shock are separate pathologies on the same spectrum. Spinal shock describes the sudden change in physiology immediately after SCIs, including loss of spinal cord function distal to the level of injury, anesthesia, loss of bladder and bowel control, loss of reflexes, and flaccid paralysis. Neurogenic shock is a component of spinal shock and specifically refers to the resulting hypotension, bradycardia, and hypothermia that result from loss of sympathetic innervation.[33]

Hypotension related to traumatic injuries, including those affecting the spinal cord, is most frequently a result of acute blood loss and subsequent hypovolemia and should be treated with blood administration per trauma guidelines. The differential diagnosis for trauma-related shock should remain broad and include cardiac injury, tension pneumothorax, pericardial tamponade, and neurogenic shock. Neurogenic shock in the setting of SCI is a diagnosis of exclusion. It is a form of distributive shock with diffuse loss of sympathetic vascular tone and bradycardia causing hypotension. On examination, patients may feel warm; however, an inability to shunt blood to the core makes them more prone to hypothermia.[4]

Managing neurogenic shock in the acute phase includes vasopressor support, reversal of bradycardia, maintaining normothermia, and possibly, use of high-dose steroids.[4,10,33] Many experts suggest treating hypotension with a MAP goal of 85 mm Hg or greater to maintain adequate spinal perfusion and prevent further ischemic injury.[34] No clear evidence exists to support the prioritization of one vasopressor over another; however, the reflex bradycardia from α-receptor agonists, such as phenylephrine, can worsen bradycardia from interruption of sympathetic signals.[33,35] Bradycardia can be treated with atropine or glycopyrrolate.[36] Evidence is mixed regarding the use of intravenous steroids to improve neurologic outcomes, and this decision should be made in conjunction with a spinal surgeon.[10]

Summary

Traumatic SCI is a disease process with significant morbidity and mortality. Early recognition is crucial to prevent further complications. Injury can be quickly identified with physical examination and history. Early immobilization of the spine helps prevent further damage in appropriate patients. Physicians should have a high index of suspicion for neurogenic shock in the setting of trauma and persistent hypotension; however, it is important to remember that neurogenic shock is a diagnosis of exclusion. Appropriate management of neurogenic shock is essential to maintain perfusion to the spine during injury. A surgical consult should be sought early for definitive treatment of these patients. Multidisciplinary teams, including physical and occupational therapy, are needed to aid these patients in their recovery.

REFERENCES

1. Spinal cord injury (SCI) 2016 facts and figures at a glance. *J Spinal Cord Med.* 2016 Jul;39(4):493-494.
2. Krause JS, Sternberb M, Lottes S, Maides J. Mortality after spinal cord injury: an 11-year prospective study. *Arch Phys Med Rehabil.* 1997 Aug;78(8):815-821.
3. Ahuja CS, Wilson JR, Nori S, et al. Traumatic spinal cord injury. *Nat Rev Dis Primers.* 2017 Apr 27;3:17018.
4. Go S. Spine trauma. In: Tintinalli JE, Ma OJ, Yealy DM, et al, eds. *Tintinalli's Emergency Medicine: A Comprehensive Study Guide.* 9th ed. McGraw-Hill Education; 2020:1696-1714.

Mnemonic	Fracture	Mechanism
Jefferson	Jefferson or C1 burst fracture	Axial loading
Bit	Bilateral facet dislocation	Flexion
Off	Odontoid type II and III fractures (type I is stable)	Flexion
A	Atlantoaxial dislocation Atlanto-occipital dislocation	Flexion
Hangman's	Hangman's or bilateral C2 pedicle fracture	Extension
Thumb	Teardrop fracture	Extension or flexion

TABLE 2. **Mnemonic for unstable spine injuries**

Category	TLICS Score	SLIC Score
Morphology		
No abnormality	0	0
Compression	1	1
Burst	2	2
Translation or rotation	3	3
Distraction	4	4
Posterior ligamentous complex (TLICS) and Discoligamentous complex (SLIC)		
Intact	0	0
Indeterminate	2	1
Disrupted	3	2
Neurologic Status		
Intact	0	0
Nerve root injury	2	1
Complete cord injury	2	2
Incomplete cord injury	3	3
Cauda equina injury	3	N/A

TABLE 3. **TLICS and SLIC scales.** A score greater than 4 indicates operative management.

5. Brodell DW, Jain A, Elfar JC, Mesfin A. National trends in the management of central cord syndrome: an analysis of 16,134 patients. *Spine J.* 2015 Mar 1;15(3):435-442.
6. Resnick DK. Updated guidelines for the management of acute cervical spine and spinal cord injury. *Neurosurgery.* 2013 Mar;72(suppl 2):1.
7. Martin ND, Kepler C, Zubair M, Sayadipour A, Cohen M, Weinstein M. Increased mean arterial pressure goals after spinal cord injury and functional outcome. *J Emerg Trauma Shock.* 2015 Apr-Jun;8(2):94-98.
8. Walters BC, Hadley MN, Hurlbert RJ, et al. Guidelines for the management of acute cervical spine and spinal cord injuries: 2013 update. *Neurosurgery.* 2013 Aug;60:82-91.
9. Bydon M, Lin J, Macki M, Gokaslan ZL, Bydon A. The current role of steroids in acute spinal cord injury. *World Neurosurg.* 2014 Nov;82(5):848-854.
10. Bracken MB. Steroids for acute spinal cord injury. *Cochrane Database Syst Rev.* 2012 Jan 18;1(1):CD001046.
11. Divi SN, Schroeder GD, Mangan JJ, et al. Management of acute traumatic central cord syndrome: a narrative teview. *Global Spine J.* 2019 May;9(1)(suppl):89S-97S.
12. Gerndt SJ, Rodriguez JL, Pawlik JW, et al. Consequences of high-dose steroid therapy for acute spinal cord injury. *J Trauma.* 1997 Feb;42(2):279-284.
13. Roberts I, Yates D, Sandercock P, et al; CRASH Trial Collaborators. Effect of intravenous corticosteroids on death within 14 days in 10,008 adults with clinically significant head injury (MRC CRASH trial): randomised placebo-controlled trial. *Lancet.* 2004 Oct;364(9442):1321-1328.
14. Pearl NA, Dubensky L. Anterior Cord Syndrome. In: *StatPearls [Internet].* StatPearls Publishing; 2022. Updated August 22, 2022. https://www.ncbi.nlm.nih.gov/books/NBK559117/
15. Shams S, Arain A. Brown Sequard syndrome. In: *StatPearls [Internet].* StatPearls Publishing; 2022. Updated September 12, 2022. https://www.ncbi.nlm.nih.gov/books/NBK538135/

■ CASE ONE

The patient was further examined and found to have 4/5 strength in the upper extremities, with preserved motor function in the lower extremities. CT of the cervical spine demonstrated no acute fracture; however, CT did show cervical stenosis. MRI of the spine was obtained. On the T2-weighted sequence, there was increased signal centrally in the cord at the level of C3 and C4. A neurosurgeon was consulted, and the patient was admitted to the surgical ICU for neurologic checks. Because there was no fracture, the patient received conservative management. He was eventually sent to a rehabilitation facility. Following 6 weeks of intensive physical and occupational therapy, the patient regained function in his upper extremities.

■ CASE TWO

A neurosurgeon was consulted. CT of the spine was obtained, which demonstrated no fracture but did show air tracking at the level of T8. MRI demonstrated no foreign body at the level of injury; however, it showed edema at the level of T8. The decision was made to treat the patient conservatively. The patient worked with both physical and occupational therapy and, after 2 years, regained some function in his left lower extremity.

■ CASE THREE

The patient was started on norepinephrine to aid in blood pressure support. With the addition of pressors, the patient maintained a MAP of 85 mm Hg. The patient received a pan CT, which demonstrated no intrathoracic or intra-abdominal trauma. However, CT cervical spine demonstrated a dislocation of C6 to C7. MRI demonstrated edema and contusion at the level of C7. The patient was taken to the operating room for open reduction and surgical stabilization. She was admitted to the ICU. With correction of the hypotension, the patient began to have an improved mental status and was extubated. She required 4 weeks of pressors but was eventually weaned from them and sent to a rehabilitation facility for further strength training and management.

16. Hoffman JR, Mower WR, Wolfson AB, Todd KH, Zucker MI. Validity of a set of clinical criteria to rule out injury to the cervical spine in patients with blunt trauma. National Emergency X-Radiography Utilization Study Group. *N Engl J Med.* 2000 Jul 13;343(2):94-99.

17. Stiell IG, Wells GA, Vandemheen KL, et al. The Canadian c-spine rule for radiography in alert and stable trauma patients. *JAMA.* 2001 Oct 17;286(15):1841-1848.

18. Williams JR, Muesch AJ, Svenson JE, Clegg AW, Patterson BW, Ward MA. Utility of bedside assessment to evaluate for cervical-spine fracture post ground-level fall for patients 65 years and older. *Am J Emerg Med.* 2022 Mar;53:208-214.

19. United States Department of Transportatioin. Traffic safety facts annual report. National Highway Traffic Safety Administration. Published June 2022. https://cdan.nhtsa.gov/tsftables/National%20Statistics.pdf

20. Kwan I, Bunn F, Roberts IG. Spinal immobilisation for trauma patients. *Cochrane Database Syst Rev.* 2001;2001(2):CD002803.

21. Ben-Galim P, Dreiangel N, Mattox KL, Reitman CA, Babak Kalantar S, Hipp JA. Extrication collars can result in abnormal separation between vertebrae in the presence of a dissociative injury. *J Trauma.* 2010 Aug;69(2):447-450.

22. Fischer PE, Perina DG, Delbridge TR, et al. Spinal motion restriction in the trauma patient — a joint position statement. *Prehosp Emerg Care.* 2018 Nov-Dec;22(6):659-661.

23. Feld FX. Removal of the long spine board from clinical practice: A historical perspective. *J of Athl Train.* 2018 Aug;53(8):752-755.

24. White CC IV, Domeier RM, Millin MG; Standards and Clinical Practice Committee; National Association of EMS Physicians. EMS spinal precautions and the use of the long backboard — resource document to the position statement of the National Association of EMS Physicians and the American College of Surgeons Committee on Trauma. *Prehosp Emerg Care.* 2014 Apr-Jun;18(2):306-314.

25. Hale AT, Alvarado A, Bey AK, et al. X-ray vs. CT in identifying significant c-spine injuries in the pediatric population. *Childs Nerv Syst.* 2017 Nov;33(11):1977-1983.

26. Como JJ, Diaz JJ, Dunham CM, et al. Practice management guidelines for identification of cervical spine injuries following trauma: update from the Eastern Asociation for the Surgery of Trauma Practice Management Guidelines Committee. *J Trauma.* 2009 Sep;67(3):651-659.

27. Sixta S, Moore FO, Ditillo MF, et al. Screening for thoracolumbar spinal injuries in blunt trauma: an Eastern Association for the Surgery of Trauma practice management guideline. *J Trauma Acute Care Surg.* 2012 Nov;73(5)(suppl 4):S326-S332.

28. Malhotra A, Wu X, Kalra VB, et al. Utility of MRI for cervical spine clearance after blunt traumatic injury: a meta-analysis. *Eur Radiol.* 2017 Mar;27(3):1148-1160.

29. American College of Surgeons. Best Practice Guidelines: Spine Injury. American College of Surgeons. Published March 2022. https://www.facs.org/media/k45gikqv/spine_injury_guidelines.pdf

30. Rajasekaran S, Kanna RM, Shetty AP. Management of thoracolumbar spine trauma: an overview. *Indian J Orthop.* 2015 Jan-Feb;49(1):72-82.

31. DiPompeo CM, Das JM. Subaxial cervical spine fractures. In: *StatPearls [Internet].* StatPearls Publishing; 2022. Updated April 9, 2022. https://www.ncbi.nlm.nih.gov/books/NBK546617/

32. Patel AA, Dailey A, Brodke DS, et al. Subaxial cervical spine trauma classification: the subaxial injury classification system and case examples. *Neurosurg Focus.* 2008;25(5):E8.

33. Ziu E, Mesfin FB. Spinal shock. In: *StatPearls [Internet].* StatPearls Publishing; 2022. Updated March 3, 2022. https://www.ncbi.nlm.nih.gov/books/NBK448163/

34. Hadley MN, Walters BC, Grabb PA, et al. Blood pressure management after acute spinal cord injury. *Neurosurgery.* 2002 Mar;50(3)(suppl):S58-S62.

35. Yue JK, Tsolinas RE, Burke JF, et al. Vasopressor support in managing acute spinal cord injury: current knowledge. *J Neurosurg Sci.* 2019 Jun;63(3):308-317.

36. Brady WJ, Glass GF III. Cardiac rhythm disturbances. In: Tintinalli JE, Ma OJ, Yealy DM, et al, eds. *Tintinalli's Emergency Medicine: A Comprehensive Study Guide.* 9th ed. McGraw-Hill Education; 2020:99-123.

✖ Pitfalls

- Keeping patients on a spinal board in the emergency department.
- Screening for spinal injury with x-rays only.
- Assuming neurogenic shock is the cause of hypotension in trauma patients.

MDCALC

Canadian Cervical Spine Rule. https://www.mdcalc.com/calc/696/canadian-c-spine-rule

NEXUS Criteria for Cervical Spine Imaging. https://www.mdcalc.com/calc/703/nexus-criteria-c-spine-imaging

Subaxial Injury Classification and Severity Scale. https://www.mdcalc.com/calc/10085/subaxial-injury-classification-severity-scale-slics

Thoracolumbar Injury Classification and Severity Scale. https://www.mdcalc.com/calc/10126/thoracolumbar-injury-classification-severity-scale-tlics

CME Questions

Reviewed by **Amal Mattu, MD, FACEP; and Danya Khoujah, MBBS, MEHP, FACEP**

Qualified, paid subscribers to *Critical Decisions in Emergency Medicine* may receive CME certificates for up to 5 ACEP Category I credits, 5 *AMA PRA Category 1 Credits™*, and 5 AOA Category 2-B credits for completing this activity in its entirety. Submit your answers online at acep.org/cdem; a score of 75% or better is required. You may receive credit for completing the CME activity any time within 3 years of its publication date. Answers to this month's questions will be published in next month's issue.

1 A physician is concerned a patient may have transverse myelitis. Which finding warrants exploring an alternative diagnosis?

- A. Bilateral signs and symptoms
- B. Development of sensory, motor, or autonomic dysfunction attributable to the spinal cord
- C. Inflammation within the spinal cord demonstrated by CSF pleocytosis, elevated IgG index, or gadolinium enhancement
- D. Progression to nadir of symptoms within less than 4 hours

2 A patient presents with signs and symptoms concerning for transverse myelitis and localized to the lumbar region. Which imaging modality is the gold standard for assessing this patient for transverse myelitis?

- A. Brain and lumbar spine MRI with gadolinium contrast
- B. Cervical, thoracic, and lumbar spine MRI with gadolinium contrast
- C. Cervical, thoracic, and lumbar spine MRI without contrast
- D. Lumbar spine CT with contrast

3 Which patient presentation is concerning for transverse myelitis?

- A. 18-year-old woman with radicular pain, painful bilateral vision loss, and lower-extremity weakness
- B. 38-year-old woman with areflexia, bilateral hand paresthesia, and bilateral lower-extremity weakness
- C. 65-year-old man with numbness, bilateral lower-extremity weakness, and urinary incontinence that have developed over the past 7 days
- D. 83-year-old man with bilateral lower-extremity weakness and loss of pain and temperature sensation that have developed over the last 2 hours but spared proprioception and vibratory sense

4 A 48-year-old woman who was diagnosed with transverse myelitis approximately 4 months ago presents for evaluation of lower-extremity weakness and tingling that began 2 days ago. She reports these are similar to the symptoms she had when she was diagnosed with transverse myelitis. A review of systems is positive for fever, chills, dysuria, and hematuria for the last 6 days. Workup reveals a urinary tract infection. How should this patient be treated?

- A. Antibiotics for the urinary tract infection
- B. Intravenous corticosteroids
- C. Intravenous immune globulin therapy
- D. Plasma exchange

5 A patient presents with symptoms that are concerning for transverse myelitis. He reports feeling short of breath. A physical examination reveals he has a weak cough and is tachypneic and using accessory muscles to breathe; his SpO_2 is 87% on 5 L/min of oxygen through a nasal cannula. What is the most appropriate next step in management?

- A. Blood work and MRI
- B. Immediate neurology consultation
- C. Intravenous high-dose corticosteroids
- D. Rapid sequence intubation

6 How is the diagnosis of Guillain-Barré syndrome established in the emergency department?

- A. Examination findings of areflexia with symmetric weakness
- B. Lumbar puncture revealing elevated glucose levels
- C. Lumbar puncture revealing leukocytosis
- D. MRI showing hyperdense lesions on T2 sequence

7 Which lumbar puncture results would most likely confirm Guillain-Barré syndrome?

- A. WBC count of 3 cells/μL, normal protein and glucose levels, negative Gram stain and culture
- B. WBC count of 25 cells/μL, elevated protein levels, normal glucose levels, negative Gram stain and culture
- C. WBC count of 55 cells/μL, elevated protein levels, normal glucose levels, negative Gram stain and culture
- D. WBC count of 55 cells/μL, low protein levels, normal glucose levels, negative Gram stain and culture

8 What is indicated in the emergent evaluation of a patient suspected to have Guillain-Barré syndrome?

- A. CT of the head
- B. Lumbar puncture
- C. MRI for nerve root inflammation
- D. Nerve conduction studies

9 A patient presents with progressive extremity paresthesia and areflexia on examination. Unfortunately, bad weather prohibits transfer to another facility that can initiate proper treatment. What is the best treatment that can be initiated in the emergency department?

- A. Intravenous immune globulin
- B. Intravenous immune globulin with plasma exchange
- C. Intravenous methylprednisolone
- D. Intubation for an NIF value of –15 cm H_2O

10 A 15-year-old boy presents with acute-onset diplopia, difficulty walking, and bilateral hand and foot paresthesia. On examination, he has limited extraocular movements, ataxia, and decreased reflexes. Miller Fisher syndrome is suspected. What is most likely associated with this patient's history?

- A. A distant history of varicella infection
- B. A history of chronic alcohol use
- C. A recent diagnosis of cytomegalovirus infection
- D. A recent diagnosis of HIV infection

11 **A 94-year-old woman presents following a fall with hyperextension of the neck. She is complaining of weakness in the upper extremities. What incomplete spinal cord injury does she most likely have?**

A. Anterior cord syndrome
B. Brown-Séquard syndrome
C. Central cord syndrome
D. None of these

12 **What are the examination findings of Brown-Séquard syndrome?**

A. Complete loss of motor function and sensation below the injury
B. Contralateral loss of motor function, vibration, and proprioception with ipsilateral loss of pain and temperature sensation
C. Ipsilateral loss of motor function, vibration, and proprioception with contralateral loss of pain and temperature sensation
D. Motor deficits, with upper extremities more affected than lower extremities

13 **In central cord syndrome what is the recommended mean arterial pressure goal?**

A. 60-65 mm Hg
B. 65-70 mm Hg
C. 75-80 mm Hg
D. 85-90 mm Hg

14 **Which vital sign findings are consistent with neurogenic shock?**

A. Bradycardia, hypotension
B. Bradypnea, hypotension
C. Tachycardia, hypotension
D. Tachypnea, hypotension

15 **Which patient should receive imaging of the neck per the Canadian cervical spine rule?**

A. 27-year-old man in a rear-end motor vehicle collision who has delayed neck pain and can rotate his neck
B. 35-year-old woman in a rear-end motor vehicle collision who has midline cervical spine tenderness
C. 45-year-old man in a rear-end motor vehicle collision who is sitting in triage and can rotate his neck
D. 64-year-old woman in a rear-end motor vehicle collision who is ambulatory and can rotate her neck

16 **Per ACEP's joint statement, which factor is not considered a reason to restrict neck mobility in blunt trauma?**

A. Age older than 55 years
B. Altered mental status or level of consciousness
C. Focal neurologic deficit
D. Midline tenderness

17 **What are possible complications of spinal board use?**

A. Increased pain
B. Pressure ulcers
C. Restriction of pulmonary expansion
D. All of these

18 **A 93-year-old woman with a past medical history of diabetes presents following a fall. She does not remember the fall. She denies numbness or weakness but on examination has midline tenderness to her cervical spine. What is the imaging modality of choice for this patient's cervical spine?**

A. Cervical spine x-rays
B. CT of the cervical spine
C. MRI of the cervical spine
D. No imaging required

19 **Which injury is not caused from a flexion injury?**

A. Atlantoaxial dislocation
B. Atlanto-occipital dislocation
C. Bilateral facet dislocation
D. C1 burst fracture

20 **What are the examination findings in anterior cord syndrome?**

A. Ipsilateral loss of motor function and contralateral loss of sensation
B. Motor paralysis and loss of pain and temperature sensation below the level of injury
C. Weakness in the upper extremities greater than the lower extremities
D. None of these

ANSWER KEY FOR FEBRUARY 2023, VOLUME 37, NUMBER 2

1	2	3	4	5	6	7	8	9	10	11	12	13	14	15	16	17	18	19	20
D	B	C	B	A	B	B	A	C	B	A	C	C	C	D	D	A	A	D	D

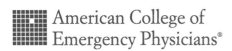

American College of
Emergency Physicians®

ADVANCING EMERGENCY CARE ___/_

Post Office Box 619911
Dallas, Texas 75261-9911

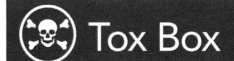

℞ Drug Box

Removal of X-Waiver Requirement

By Frank LoVecchio, DO, MPH, FACEP
Valleywise Health and ASU, Phoenix, Arizona

Objective
On completion of this column, you should be able to:
- Summarize how to prescribe buprenorphine for OUD.

Background
Previously, physicians in the United States had to apply for a federally required DATA 2000 waiver, or X-waiver, to prescribe buprenorphine for opioid use disorder (OUD). In January, the Consolidated Appropriations Act of 2023 removed this requirement. Now, physicians with a schedule III authority on their DEA registration can prescribe buprenorphine for OUD treatment if permitted by state law.

Dosing for Adults
Buprenorphine doses are adjusted depending on the condition being treated and patient response. Some institutions have instated a higher-dose buprenorphine induction protocol. Refer to www.samhsa.gov for more in-depth information.

Ensure the patient is in a state of mild to moderate opioid withdrawal by using the Clinical Opiate Withdrawal Scale (COWS). A COWS score ≥12 is indicative of mild to moderate withdrawal. Administer buprenorphine only when signs of withdrawal appear.

Day 1: Start transmucosal buprenorphine at a dose of 4 mg. Symptom relief can occur in minutes, but full effect takes 1 to 2 hours. Reassess in 1 to 2 hours. If withdrawal symptoms persist (COWS score ≥6), an additional dose of up to 4 mg can be administered. If symptoms are sufficiently relieved (COWS score <6) and there is no other reason for hospital admission, consider discharging. Have patients take home a second dose of buprenorphine to use if withdrawal symptoms or cravings worsen before the next morning. Federal guidelines recommend a maximum dose of 8 mg on the first day, but occasionally, a dose higher than 8 mg is needed. At discharge, transmucosal buprenorphine combined with naloxone is usually given to prevent diversion of the product.

Day 2: If patients return for a second day of treatment, administer a single dose equal to day 1's total dose and monitor for 1 to 2 hours. If the COWS score is ≥6, consider giving another 4 mg. Continue to monitor and give 4 mg every 2 hours if the COWS score remains ≥6. In general, a maximum total dose of 16 mg is recommended on day 2. If symptoms are sufficiently relieved, discharge with a prescription for a precise number of days specific to each patient and circumstance (eg, social supports, follow-up reliability). Follow-up for continuous or maintenance therapy should be established. Maintenance therapy aims to ensure that there is no withdrawal, craving, or illicit opioid use.

Warnings
Buprenorphine-related deaths have occurred in patients on maintenance therapy when used with substances like benzodiazepines or alcohol or when high doses of intravenous buprenorphine are misused. Death is caused by respiratory depression from oversedation. Dental problems, including dental caries and decay, are associated with dissolving buprenorphine formulations. Teeth and gums should be rinsed or brushed once the film has dissolved. Other adverse effects include headache, nausea, constipation, pain, and sweating.

REFERENCE
Removal of DATA waiver (X-waiver) requirement. Substance Abuse and Mental Health Services Administration. Last updated January 25, 2023. https://www.samhsa.gov/medications-substance-use-disorders/removal-data-waiver-requirement

☠ Tox Box

Vinyl Chloride Poisoning

By Christian A. Tomaszewski, MD, MS, MBA, FACEP
University of California San Diego Health

Objective
On completion of this column, you should be able to:
- Discuss how to identify and treat vinyl chloride exposure.

Introduction
Vinyl chloride monomer (VCM) is a colorless, sweet-smelling hydrocarbon widely used in the production of PVC, a substance ubiquitous in the construction of pipes and coatings. Exposure can happen at production sites and from releases during shipment as liquefied gas. VCM is highly flammable and can form explosive polymeric peroxides.

Toxicokinetics
- Exposure is primarily through inhalation.
  - OSHA-permissible exposure limit is 1 ppm.
  - 8,000 ppm for 5 minutes causes dizziness and CNS depression.
  - 120,000 ppm is potentially fatal.
- Metabolized by CYP2E1
- Renal excretion without accumulation of metabolites

Clinical Manifestations
Acute
- ***Neuro:*** headache, dizziness, CNS depression, and seizures
- ***Pulmonary:*** dyspnea, obstruction, and pneumonitis
- ***Cardiac:*** dysrhythmias from sensitization to catecholamines
- ***Mucous membranes:*** irritation
- ***Skin:*** frostbite if exposed to compressed gas

Chronic or Delayed
- ***Cancers***
  - Hepatic angiosarcoma (classic)
  - ***Others:*** hepatocellular, brain, lung, lymphoma, and leukemia
- ***Extremities***
  - Acro-osteolysis (lytic lesions of phalanges)
  - Skin thickening
- ***Axonal neuropathy***

Diagnostics
- No specific laboratory testing
- Chest x-ray for pulmonary symptoms

Treatment
- Removal of the individual from exposure source
- External decontamination
- Humidified oxygen and bronchodilator treatment for respiratory symptoms
- Benzodiazepines for seizures

Critical decisions
in emergency medicine

Volume 37 Number 4: **April 2023**

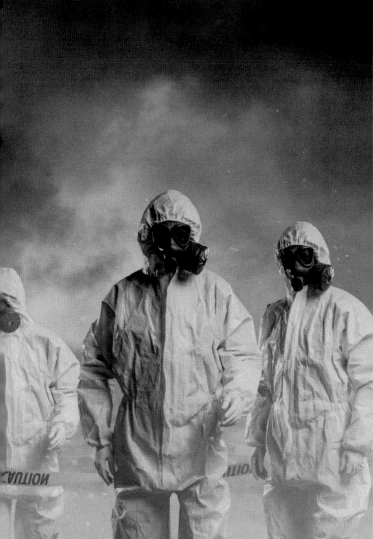

Bug Bombs

In an era of geopolitical unrest and interconnected populations, bioterrorism remains a genuine threat. Although the most dangerous biologic agents often present with nonspecific symptoms, emergency physicians must be able to recognize initial smaller outbreaks to prevent their spread and mitigate the fallout from a biologic attack.

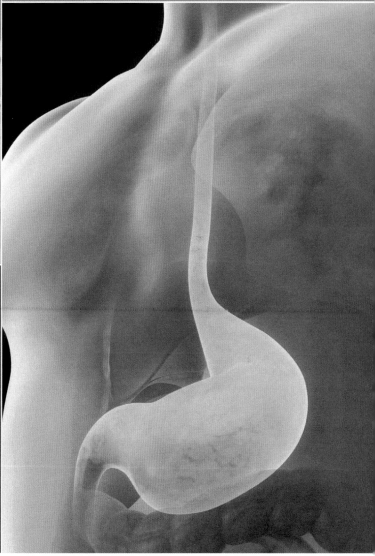

Seeing Red

Upper GI bleeding is a common condition encountered in the emergency department that has a variety of presentations and can lead to serious complications. Emergency physicians must differentiate between stable and unstable GI bleeds and act quickly to stabilize patients with unstable bleeds in preparation for more definitive management.

THE OFFICIAL CME PUBLICATION OF THE AMERICAN COLLEGE OF EMERGENCY PHYSICIANS

Individuals in Control of Content

1. Mariam Azim, MD – Faculty
2. Bethanne Bartscherer, MD – Faculty
3. Jeremy Berberian, MD – Faculty
4. William J. Brady, MD, FACEP – Faculty
5. Clare Charbonnet, MD – Faculty
6. Sullivan Hanback, MD – Faculty
7. Ashley Jackson, PharmD — Faculty
8. Adeola A. Kosoko, MD, FACEP, FAAP – Faculty
9. Brendan McGowan, DO – Faculty
10. Laura Welsh, MD – Faculty
11. Joshua S. Broder, MD, FACEP – Faculty/Planner
12. Andrew J. Eyre, MD, MS-HPEd – Faculty/Planner
13. John Kiel, DO, MPH, FACEP, CAQSM – Faculty/Planner
14. Danya Khoujah, MBBS, MEHP, FACEP – Faculty/Planner
15. Frank LoVecchio, DO, MPH, FACEP – Faculty/Planner
16. Sharon E. Mace, MD, FACEP – Faculty/Planner
17. Nathaniel Mann, MD – Faculty/Planner
18. Amal Mattu, MD, FACEP – Faculty/Planner
19. Christian A. Tomaszewski, MD, MS, MBA, FACEP – Faculty/Planner
20. Steven J. Warrington, MD, MEd, MS – Faculty/Planner
21. Tareq Al-Salamah, MBBS, MPH, FACEP – Planner
22. Michael S. Beeson, MD, MBA, FACEP – Planner
23. Wan-Tsu Chang, MD – Planner
24. Ann M. Dietrich, MD, FAAP, FACEP – Planner
25. Kelsey Drake, MD, MPH, FACEP – Planner
26. Walter L. Green, MD, FACEP – Planner
27. John C. Greenwood, MD – Planner
28. George Sternbach, MD, FACEP – Planner
29. Joy Carrico, JD – Planner/Reviewer

Contributor Disclosures. In accordance with the ACCME Standards for Integrity and Independence in Accredited Continuing Education, all relevant financial relationships, and the absence of relevant financial relationships, must be disclosed to learners for all individuals in control of content 1) before learners engage with the accredited education, and 2) in a format that can be verified at the time of accreditation. The following individuals have reported relationships with ineligible companies, as defined by the ACCME. These relationships, in the context of their involvement in the CME activity, could be perceived by some as a real or apparent conflict of interest. All relevant financial relationships have been mitigated to ensure that no commercial bias has been inserted into the educational content. Joshua S. Broder, MD, FACEP, is a founder and president of OmniSono Inc, an ultrasound technology company, and a consultant on the Bayer USA Cardiac Imaging Advisory Board. Sharon E. Mace, MD, FACEP, performs contracted research funded by Biofire Corporation, Genetesis, Quidel, and IBSA Pharma. Frank LoVecchio, DO, MPH, FACEP, receives speaking fees from ABBVIE for antibiotics. All remaining individuals with control over content have no relevant financial relationships to disclose.

This educational activity consists of two lessons, eight feature articles, a post-test, and evaluation questions; as designed, the activity should take approximately 5 hours to complete. The participant should, in order, review the learning objectives for the lesson or article, read the lesson or article as published in the print or online version until all have been reviewed, and then complete the online post-test (a minimum score of 75% is required) and evaluation questions. Release date: April 1, 2023. Expiration date: March 31, 2026.

Accreditation Statement. The American College of Emergency Physicians is accredited by the Accreditation Council for Continuing Medical Education to provide continuing medical education for physicians.

The American College of Emergency Physicians designates this enduring material for a maximum of 5 *AMA PRA Category 1 Credits™.* Physicians should claim only the credit commensurate with the extent of their participation in the activity.

Each issue of *Critical Decisions in Emergency Medicine* is approved by ACEP for 5 ACEP Category I credits. Approved by the AOA for 5 Category 2-B credits.

Commercial Support. There was no commercial support for this CME activity.

Target Audience. This educational activity has been developed for emergency physicians.

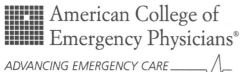

American College of Emergency Physicians®

ADVANCING EMERGENCY CARE

Critical decisions
in emergency medicine

Critical Decisions in Emergency Medicine is the official CME publication of the American College of Emergency Physicians. Additional volumes are available.

EDITOR-IN-CHIEF
Michael S. Beeson, MD, MBA, FACEP
Northeastern Ohio Universities, Rootstown, OH

SECTION EDITORS
Joshua S. Broder, MD, FACEP
Duke University, Durham, NC

Andrew J. Eyre, MD, MS-HPEd
Brigham and Women's Hospital/ Harvard Medical School, Boston, MA

John Kiel, DO, MPH, FACEP, CAQSM
University of Florida College of Medicine, Jacksonville, FL

Frank LoVecchio, DO, MPH, FACEP
Valleywise, Arizona State University, University of Arizona, and Creighton Colleges of Medicine, Phoenix, AZ

Sharon E. Mace, MD, FACEP
Cleveland Clinic Lerner College of Medicine/ Case Western Reserve University, Cleveland, OH

Amal Mattu, MD, FACEP
University of Maryland, Baltimore, MD

Christian A. Tomaszewski, MD, MS, MBA, FACEP
University of California Health Sciences, San Diego, CA

Steven J. Warrington, MD, MEd, MS
MercyOne Siouxland, Sioux City, IA

ASSOCIATE EDITORS
Tareq Al-Salamah, MBBS, MPH, FACEP
King Saud University, Riyadh, Saudi Arabia/ University of Maryland, Baltimore, MD

Wan-Tsu Chang, MD
University of Maryland, Baltimore, MD

Ann M. Dietrich, MD, FAAP, FACEP
University of South Carolina College of Medicine, Greenville, SC

Kelsey Drake, MD, MPH, FACEP
St. Anthony Hospital, Lakewood, CO

Walter L. Green, MD, FACEP
UT Southwestern Medical Center, Dallas, TX

John C. Greenwood, MD
University of Pennsylvania, Philadelphia, PA

Danya Khoujah, MBBS, MEHP, FACEP
University of Maryland, Baltimore, MD

Nathaniel Mann, MD
Greenville Health System, Greenville, SC

George Sternbach, MD, FACEP
Stanford University Medical Center, Stanford, CA

EDITORIAL STAFF
Suzannah Alexander, Editorial Director
salexander@acep.org

Joy Carrico, JD
Managing Editor

Alex Bass
Assistant Editor

Kyle Powell
Graphic Artist

ISSN2325-0186 (Print)   ISSN2325-8365 (Online)

Contents

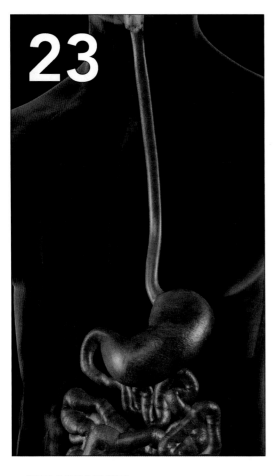

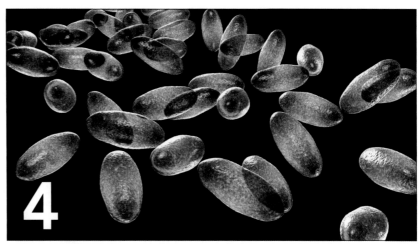

FEATURES

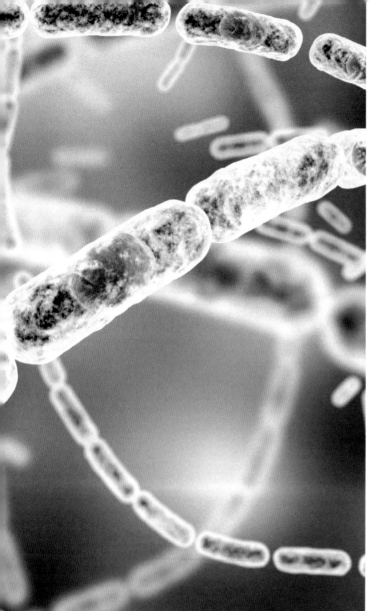

Bug Bombs

Identifying Illnesses of Bioterrorism

LESSON 7

By Clare Charbonnet, MD; and Sharon E. Mace, MD, FACEP
Dr. Charbonnet is an emergency medicine resident at MetroHealth Medical Center and the Cleveland Clinic Foundation in Ohio. Dr. Mace is a professor at Cleveland Clinic Lerner College of Medicine at Case Western Reserve University and the director of research at Cleveland Clinic's Emergency Services Institute.

Reviewed by Nathaniel Mann, MD

Objectives

On completion of this lesson, you should be able to:

1. Recall the history of biologic warfare in the United States.
2. Define the biologic agents that could be utilized in acts of terrorism.
3. List the CDC Category A biologic weapons.
4. Diagnose infections caused by the most dangerous of biologic warfare pathogens.
5. Use appropriate infection control measures.

From the EM Model

10.0 Systemic Infectious Disorders
    10.2 Biological Warfare Agents

▬ CRITICAL DECISIONS ▬

- ■ What makes a biologic agent a potential weapon?

- ■ What are the clinical presentation and treatment for anthrax?

- ■ What are the clinical presentation and treatment for plague?

- ■ What are the clinical presentation and treatment for tularemia?

- ■ What are the clinical presentation and treatment for the viral hemorrhagic fevers?

In an era of geopolitical unrest and interconnected populations, bioterrorism remains a genuine threat. The CDC categorizes possible bioweapons according to their potential for public health impact. Unfortunately, the most dangerous of these biologic agents often present with nonspecific symptoms. Emergency physicians must recognize initial smaller outbreaks to prevent their spread and mitigate the fallout from a biologic attack.

■ CASE ONE

A 42-year-old woman with a history of hypertension and type 2 diabetes mellitus presents with 2 days of severe fever, chills, headache, weakness, chest tightness, and dizziness. She opted to come to the emergency department when she became short of breath and coughed up blood-tinged sputum. Her vital signs are BP 105/93, P 101, R 24, and T 37.4°C (99.3°F); SpO_2 is 92% on room air. The examination reveals diminished breath sounds in the left upper lobe, and a chest x-ray demonstrates a corresponding segmental consolidation.

■ CASE TWO

An otherwise healthy 32-year-old man presented 3 days ago with 3 days of fever, chills, myalgia, chest pain, a nonproductive cough, and shortness of breath while at rest. He had also just developed abdominal pain and nonbloody emesis. His vital signs were BP 158/94, P 106, R 22, and T 38.1°C (100.6°F); SpO_2 was 97% on room air. The man was resuscitated with intravenous fluids and given symptomatic care. His vital signs and symptoms improved, so he was discharged from the emergency department. He has returned via EMS. His vital signs are now BP 92/48, P 126, R 32, and T 38.6°C (101.5°F); SpO_2 is 82% on room air. On examination, he is diaphoretic with marked diffuse lymphadenopathy. A chest x-ray shows a widened mediastinum.

■ CASE THREE

A 17-year-old boy with a history of asthma presents with 5 days of headache, sore throat, cough, chest pain, and myalgia, especially in his lower back. His chest pain is markedly exacerbated by inspiration. His vital signs are BP 112/68, P 76, R 22, and T 39.1°C (102.4°F); SpO_2 is 90% on room air. A chest x-ray shows pleural effusions and prominent hilar lymphadenopathy.

Introduction

From the contamination of local waterways with *Escherichia coli* after Hurricane Katrina in 2005 to the recurrence of cholera in Haiti following recent political instability, disease is a constant companion of disaster.[1] Traditional, nonbiologic weapons disrupt repositories of spores in warm soil. Refugee camps are notoriously plagued by illness. Livestock goes unvaccinated during times of tumult. Arthropod vectors are greeted by a new population of hosts previously unexposed to the diseases they transmit.

Authoritarian regimes, global energy shortages, and climate change may all contribute to both natural and man-made disasters and, therefore, an increased incidence of disaster-related diseases. In addition, the recent coronavirus pandemic demonstrates that disease itself can be the disaster. It also highlights the challenges of coordinating national and global responses to a zoonotic pathogen.

Biologic warfare is the deliberate release of microorganisms with the intention of causing mass casualties, severe economic disruption, or widespread public panic.[2] Examples of disease being used as a weapon of war far predate the German microbiologist Robert Koch's discovery of "Bacteridien" in the blood of sick rabbits in 1876.[3] For example, in the fourteenth century BCE, the Hittites drove their diseased livestock into the camps of their enemies. A millenium later, Scythian archers dipped their arrowheads into the rotting corpses of snakes.[4]

Naturally occurring zoonotic diseases pose significant danger as agents of biologic warfare. Germ warfare in North America dates back to the intentional distribution of blankets infested with smallpox to native populations during the French and Indian War. In 1943, the United States established a research center at Fort Detrick to weaponize *Yersinia pestis* and *Francisella tularensis*. A decade later, as concerns grew about epidemiologic risks, the program was terminated. The laboratories were repurposed to investigate medical countermeasures.[5]

This transition from production to detection and mitigation strategies was further formalized in 1972 with the ratification of the Biological and Toxin Weapons Convention (BWC) by the United States, the Soviet Union, and the United Kingdom. This accord is the first multilateral disarmament treaty banning an entire category of weapons of mass destruction and has since been ratified by over 140 nations.[5-7]

Signatories of the BWC in 1975 declared they would never "develop, produce, stockpile or otherwise acquire or retain microbiologic agents or toxins for hostile purposes or in armed conflict." However, research on this subject is known to have continued through the 1990s, and some national governments continue to interpret this statement loosely.[1]

Biologic attacks resurfaced in the collective American consciousness in 2001, when a perpetrator used the US Postal Service to mail *Bacillus anthracis* spores to members of Congress and the national press.[7] Although only 22 people became ill and 5 died, this event demonstrates the logistic and psychosocial complexities of bioterrorism on any scale. Several hundred facilities were tested for *B. anthracis* spores, and an estimated $320 million was needed for decontamination.[2] Approximately 32,000 people were started on antibiotic prophylaxis.[8] The word "anthrax" became a household name synonymous with biologic warfare.

CRITICAL DECISION

What makes a biologic agent a potential weapon?

Agents that could be utilized in biologic warfare include toxins, immune modulators, and pathogens. From the viewpoint of a terrorist, certain agents are more enticing for use in biologic warfare than others because they are readily available naturally, are environmentally stable, have long incubation periods, are inexpensive, and are difficult to detect.[5] The list of substances that could be used as dangerous bioweapons is overwhelmingly large.

The CDC prioritizes agents according to their potential for mass casualties and civil disruption. Agents are ranked into three categories depending on their delivery route, infectivity, latency period, mortality rate, and potential for public health impact, including the ramifications of national anxiety.[9,10] The

CDC designates pathogens of the highest priority as Category A agents. The six Category A agents are anthrax, botulism, plague, smallpox, tularemia, and the viral hemorrhagic fevers (ie, Ebola, Marburg, and Lassa viruses). Because smallpox is all but eradicated and most emergency physicians are familiar with the pathognomonic symptoms of botulism, this lesson focuses on the four remaining Category A agents.

Initial cases of Category A illnesses are often misdiagnosed in the emergency department because early symptoms are nonspecific and physicians, understandably, do not maintain a high index of suspicion for them. For example, during the anthrax scare, two postal workers were discharged from the emergency department only to later die. It is clear that in the context of a targeted attack, the health care system would become quickly overwhelmed by patients exhibiting the same nonspecific symptoms.[9]

Early detection of limited outbreaks from biologic warfare agents is essential so that testing and quarantine measures can be enacted as quickly as possible. During the early phases of the COVID-19 pandemic, the US health care system struggled to meet testing needs, and that event was free from the confusion created by the widespread panic of a public that feels under siege.[11]

CRITICAL DECISION

What are the clinical presentation and treatment for anthrax?

The gram-positive rod *B. anthracis* was the first bacterium to be identified in human history.[12] In the past, animals became ill from it by inhaling its spores in the soil, and outbreaks resulted from human contact with infected livestock. Natural outbreaks have become rare due to the vaccination of domestic animals, but heat-stable spores are still readily available around the world. Recent data extrapolation calculates that *B. anthracis* spores can survive over 600 years at room temperature and over a millennium in accommodating soil conditions.[13]

The symptoms of a *B. anthracis* infection depend on the route of entry into the body.[10] Cutaneous anthrax results from direct inoculation through a wound and causes a characteristic black eschar. The GI form of the illness occurs when a person consumes the undercooked meat of an infected animal. However, neither of these delivery routes are likely to be deployed as a biologic weapon given the low potential for widespread transmission.

Inhalation anthrax, a much more likely route of entry in biologic warfare, occurs when a person breathes in aerosolized spores. The disease course is biphasic. Early symptoms present in 1 to 4 days and include nonspecific symptoms such as fever, chills, myalgia, fatigue, chest pain, dyspnea, and a nonproductive cough. Several days later, untreated patients rapidly develop bacteremia, respiratory failure, and septic shock. The nearly pathognomonic hemorrhagic mediastinitis occurs because replicating bacteria are ingested by alveolar macrophages and carried to mediastinal lymph nodes, where they release toxins that cause hemorrhage and necrosis.[12] A chest x-ray can show lymphadenopathy or a widened mediastinum (*Figure 1*). Autopsies have failed to identify a bronchoalveolar pneumonic process, and physicians should not expect to see evidence of pulmonary hemorrhage on chest imaging.[1,5,14]

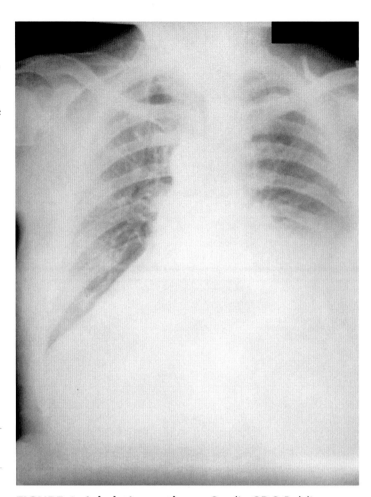

FIGURE 1. Inhalation anthrax. *Credit:* CDC Public Health Image Library, https://phil.cdc.gov/Details.aspx?pid=1795.

Unfortunately, latency periods can last up to 2 months. Untreated cases are almost universally fatal. Even with aggressive management, inhalation anthrax has a 45% mortality rate.[10] An index of suspicion for such a rare entity is likely to be piqued only if physicians recognize a pattern of multiple cases of a fulminant, toxic, and fatal influenza-like illness with a preponderance of hemorrhagic mediastinitis despite antibiotic treatment.[14,15]

Standard blood cultures can be used to identify *B. anthracis* and are likely to grow sufficiently large colonies within 24 to 48 hours.[14] Penicillins are the first-line antibiotic therapy for naturally occurring cases of anthrax. Patients with penicillin allergies can be treated with doxycycline. However, there are reports of *B. anthracis* strains that are engineered with resistance to both penicillins and tetracyclines. Therefore, if biologic warfare is suspected, patients of all ages should be treated empirically with a fluroquinolone (eg, ciprofloxacin) for 7 to 10 days until susceptibility can be determined (*Table 1*).[1,12] In addition to antimicrobial therapy, three antibody-based antitoxins have been approved by the FDA to treat anthrax. Two of the antitoxins are monoclonal antibodies, raxibacumab and obiltoxaximab. The third medication is an intravenous immune globulin solution derived from vaccinated donors called anthrax immune globulin.[16-19] These antitoxins should be administered only after consultation with the local department of public health and the CDC.[20]

First responders should wear a full-face respirator with high-efficiency particulate air (HEPA) filters or a self-contained breathing apparatus, or SCBA, in addition to gloves and splash-proof garments. Clothing should be removed and placed in airtight bags to prevent resuspension of anthrax molecules in the air. Exposed skin with gross contamination should be cleaned with bleach in a 1:10 dilution. Otherwise, exposed skin should be cleaned with soap and copious amounts of water. Quarantine is unnecessary because exposed patients are not contagious once decontaminated.[21] Following decontamination, these patients can be safely managed with standard infection control precautions.[5]

CRITICAL DECISION

What are the clinical presentation and treatment for plague?

Small rodents are the natural host for *Y. pestis*, the gram-negative coccobacillus that causes plague. Arthropods such as fleas serve as transmission vectors for bubonic plague between animals and humans. This illness presents with extreme lymph node edema until the node becomes hemorrhagic and necrotic.

About 5% to 15% of plague patients experience hematologic spread to the lungs and develop pneumonic plague. This disease presents with a very sudden onset of fever, chills, headache, generalized weakness, and pneumonia. This form of *Yersinia* is contagious and has a 2- to 6-day incubation period. Chest x-rays often show rapid progression from segmental to lobar to bilateral lung involvement (*Figure 2*). Untreated, pneumonic plague can progress to respiratory failure and septic shock within 2 days and is nearly universally fatal without the initiation of antibiotics within 1 day of symptom onset.[22,23]

Either bubonic or pneumonic plague can progress to septicemic plague, which includes abdominal pain, subcutaneous hemorrhage, and disseminated intravascular coagulation with quintessential digital necrosis. Unfortunately, although this late examination finding is helpful in raising clinical suspicion for plague, patients with this finding have a poor prognosis.[24]

Standard blood cultures will likely grow sufficiently large colonies within 24 to 48 hours in microbiology laboratories that use automated machines for bacterial identification; however, many of these machines may misdiagnose *Yersinia*, and manual identification can be difficult before 6 days. Immunoassays for rapid identification of plague are only available in special facilities.[25] Aminoglycosides such as streptomycin and gentamicin have classically been first-line antimicrobial therapies, but many different antibiotics have proven effective against this disease, including ciprofloxacin and doxycycline.[22] Penicillins are not an effective treatment for plague.[25]

Like anthrax, plague is most likely to be deployed as a biologic warfare agent in an aerosolized form. Unlike anthrax, plague is highly contagious through respiratory droplets, and most cases of transmission occur in the late stage when patients are coughing up purulent sputum.[1] Patients should be placed on strict droplet precautions until 48 hours after antibiotic initiation.[21,26] This means, in addition to standard precautions, health care professionals should wear surgical masks when working within 1 meter of a patient. Fitted N95 masks are only necessary during aerosolizing procedures, such as suctioning. Ideally, patients with plague should be placed in private rooms. Negative pressure rooms are unnecessary.

Agent	Antibiotic Regimen
Anthrax	Ciprofloxacin 400 mg IV twice daily *or* Doxycycline 200 mg IV one time then 100 mg twice daily *and* At least one additional antibiotic to which anthrax is susceptible including amoxicillin or clindamycin *and* Monoclonal antibodies raxibacumab or obiltoxaximab or polyclonal anthrax immune globulin IV
Plague	Streptomycin 1 g IM or IV twice daily for 10 to 14 days *or* Gentamicin 5 mg per kg IM or IV once daily for 10 to 14 days *or* Ciprofloxacin 400 mg IV twice daily until clinically improved, then 750 mg orally twice daily for 10 to 14 days *or* Doxycycline 200 mg IV one time, then 100 mg twice daily until clinically improved, then 100 mg orally twice daily for 10 to 14 days
Tularemia	Streptomycin 1 g IM or IV twice daily for 10 to 14 days *or* Gentamicin 5 mg per kg IM or IV once daily for 10 to 14 days *or* Doxycycline 100 mg twice daily *or* Ciprofloxacin 400 mg IV twice daily
Viral hemorrhagic fevers	Atoltivimab/maftivimab/odesivimab or ansuvimab for *Ebolavirus* Ribavirin for viral hemorrhagic fevers generally

TABLE 1. Possible regimens for inpatient treatment of patients infected with biologic warfare agents

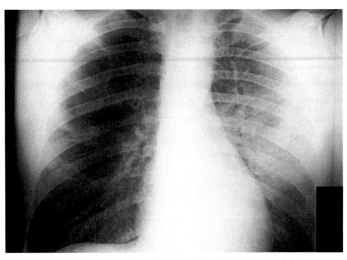

FIGURE 2. Pneumonic plague. *Credit:* CDC Public Health Image Library, https://phil.cdc.gov/Details.aspx?pid=1955.

Care should be taken to eliminate infected fleas and rodents. Although *Y. pestis* remains viable in most soil or grain for several weeks, air-dispersed bacteria are killed within a few hours of exposure to sunlight.[5]

CRITICAL DECISION

What are the clinical presentation and treatment for tularemia?

The bacterium *F. tularensis* is an aerobic, gram-negative coccobacillus that is commonly found in the northern hemisphere. The bacteria occur naturally in the United States in both rodents and rabbits. There are six different clinical manifestations of tularemia, depending on the route of inoculation: ulceroglandular, glandular, oculoglandular, oropharyngeal, typhoidal, and pneumonic. Most people contract tularemia by handling infected animals, but small outbreaks of inhalation tularemia have been traced to inhalation of contaminated lawn clippings or brush cuttings.[23,27]

As with anthrax and plague, tularemia is most effective as a bioweapon if aerosolized. In the 1960s, the US military developed and stockpiled devices that would disseminate aerosolized *F. tularensis*.[15] The bacteria are highly infective, meaning a very small number of organisms is needed to cause illness. The infective dose of tularemia is between 10 to 50 organisms, compared to 100 to 500 for plague and 2,500 to 50,000 spores for fatal inhalation anthrax.[1]

Once bacteria have penetrated skin or mucosal surfaces, they spread to regional lymph nodes, where replication leads to suppurative granulomatous lesions with central areas of necrosis. In most clinical presentations, pronounced afferent regional lymphadenopathy is present. If untreated, disease can rapidly disseminate.[15]

After an incubation period of 2 to 14 days, pneumonia progresses at highly variable rates. Patients complain of nonspecific symptoms such as headache, rigors, cough, sore throat, and myalgia, especially in the lower back. Some distinguishing features of this illness are pulse-temperature dissociation, severe pleuropneumonitis with pleural effusions, and prominent hilar lymphadenopathy (*Figure 3*). Up to 60% of patients infected with highly virulent strains die without antibiotics.[28]

Most hospital laboratories do not have the light microscopy equipment necessary for rapid identification of *F. tularensis*, and speciation through routine cultures can take several weeks. If physicians suspect an outbreak, they need to alert the laboratory to send samples to appropriate facilities. *Francisella* is rarely isolated from blood, and samples must include sputum, pharyngeal washings, and gastric aspirates. Antibiotic therapy for pneumonic tularemia is similar to regimens used to treat the plague. Aminoglycosides such as streptomycin and gentamicin are first line. Other possible options include ciprofloxacin and doxycycline. Treatment failure is common with beta-lactam and macrolide antibiotics.[15]

Despite the bacteria's infectivity, there are no documented cases of interpersonal transmission of pneumonic tularemia; therefore, standard barrier precautions are sufficient when caring for these patients.[21] Studies have shown that a 90% reduction of aerosolized *F. tularensis* particles occurs within 30 to 60 minutes of exposure to ambient air at common temperatures.[13]

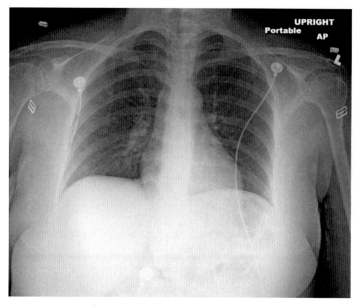

FIGURE 3. **Tularemia.** *Credit:* Copyright 2023 Jeffrey P. Kanne. Image courtesy of Jeffrey P. Kanne and Radiopaedia.org, rID: 98465. Used under license.

CRITICAL DECISION

What are the clinical presentation and treatment for the viral hemorrhagic fevers?

The viral hemorrhagic fevers (VHFs) that represent the greatest threat as bioweapons belong to four families of lipid-enveloped, single-stranded RNA viruses: Filoviridae, Arenaviridae, Bunyaviridae, and Flaviviridae.[5] Among the many pathogens in these families, only some have the infectivity, transmissibility, mortality, and availability necessary to pose a serious threat in biologic warfare.[29]

Although taxonomically distinct, the VHFs relevant to this discussion all cause vascular endothelial damage that results in flushing, edema, petechiae, ecchymosis, hemorrhage, and ultimately shock.[5] Owing to recent outbreaks, the most infamous of the VHFs is currently the filovirus Ebola. The epidemic in western African countries from 2013 to 2016 infected 30,000 people and resulted in 11,000 fatalities.[30]

Initial cases occur from exposure to animal carcasses or infected bats. Almost 99% of human cases are the result of direct person-to-person transmission. After an incubation period of up to 3 weeks, patients develop nonspecific symptoms such as fever and myalgia. The second phase of illness includes GI symptoms and resultant dehydration. The final stage is characterized by diffuse mucosal hemorrhage and multisystem organ failure.[30] Most laboratories in the United States are not equipped to rapidly diagnose any of the VHFs, and blood samples must be sent to either the CDC or the US Army Medical Research Institute of Infectious Diseases in Maryland.[29]

Therapy is primarily supportive, although the availability of pressors is limited in most endemic regions, and mortality can be as high as 90%.[5] A combination of three monoclonal antibodies, atoltivimab, maftivimab, and odesivimab, was the first FDA-approved treatment for *Ebolavirus*. The single antibody ansuvimab was approved in 2020.[31] The WHO recommends the antiviral medicine ribavirin for treatment of other VHFs, especially Crimean-Congo hemorrhagic fever and Lassa virus.[32] However, data remain inconclusive as to whether ribavirin imparts a mortality benefit.[33]

Most VHFs are transmitted either percutaneously or through mucosal contact, especially in the last stage of illness when patients hemorrhage from mucosal surfaces, including the mouth, eyes, and ears. Most transmission occurs through close contact with these bodily fluids, including indirectly from contaminated objects such as syringes and needles.[21] Even physical contact with corpses during burial practices is sufficient for inoculation.

Strict contact precautions are necessary for infection control.[29] Personal protective equipment (PPE) includes an inner layer of clothing (eg, scrubs), thin gloves, rubber boots or overshoes, a disposable gown with long sleeves and cuffs, a waterproof apron, a second pair of gloves, a HEPA filter, a head covering, and goggles.[34] Hand washing after removal of gloves is necessary. Items contaminated by patient excreta can be cleaned with household bleach. A 1:10 solution is used to disinfect bodies and excreta. A 1:100 bleach solution is used to disinfect surfaces, equipment, bedding, and reusable PPE.[34]

Summary

Biologic pathogens that are most likely to be utilized as weapons of terrorism are designated as Category A agents by the CDC. These agents are especially problematic for emergency physicians because they present with nonspecific symptoms, are nonresponsive to typical regimens of broad-spectrum antibiotics, and progress very rapidly with high mortality rates. Physicians should be cognizant of subtle examination and x-ray findings and advocate for testing for these microbes.

REFERENCES

1. Thomas D, Hawkins C. CBRNE preparedness. In: LaDou J, Harrison RJ, eds. *CURRENT Diagnosis & Treatment: Occupational & Environmental Medicine*. 6th ed. McGraw-Hill Education; 2021:722-739.

2. Rathjen NA, Shahbodaghi SD. Bioterrorism. *Am Fam Physician*. 2021 Oct 1;104(4):376-385.

3. Münch R. Robert Koch. *Microbes Infect*. 2003;5(1):69-74.

4. Barras V, Greub G. History of biological warfare and bioterrorism. *Clin Microbiol Infect*. 2014;20(6):497-502.

5. Dembek ZF, Cieslak TJ. Biological events. In: Koenig KL, Schultz CH, eds. *Koenig and Schultz's Disaster Medicine: Comprehensive Principles and Practices*. 2nd ed. Cambridge University Press; 2016:522-544.

6. United Nations Office for Disarmament Affairs. *The Biological Weapons Convention: An Introduction*. 2nd ed. 2022. https://www.un.org/disarmament/publications/the-biological-weapons-convention/

7. Joshi D, Kumar D, Maini AK, Sharma RC. Detection of biological warfare agents using ultra violet-laser induced fluorescence LIDAR. *Spectrochim Acta A Mol Biomol Spectrosc*. 2013 Aug;112:446-456.

8. Suchard JR. Biological weapons. In: Nelson LS, Howland MA, Lewin NA, Smith SW, Goldfrank LR, Hoffman RS, eds. *Goldfrank's Toxicologic Emergencies*. 11th ed. McGraw-Hill Education; 2019:1753-1762.

9. Suyama J. Bioterrorism. In: Tintinalli JE, Ma OJ, Yealy DM, et al, eds. *Tintinalli's Emergency Medicine: A Comprehensive Study Guide*. 9th ed. McGraw-Hill Education; 2020:41-47.

10. Bioterrorism agents/diseases. Centers for Disease Control and Prevention. Revised April 4, 2018. https://emergency.cdc.gov/agent/agentlist-category.asp

11. Lewis T. How the U.S. pandemic response went wrong – and what went right – during a year of COVID. *Scientific American*. 2021. March 11, 2021. https://www.scientificamerican.com/article/how-the-u-s-pandemic-response-went-wrong-and-what-went-right-during-a-year-of-covid/

12. Langston SM, Bales BD. Anthrax. In: Knoop KJ, Stack LB, Storrow AB, Thurman RJ, eds. *The Atlas of Emergency Medicine*. 5th ed. McGraw-Hill Education; 2021:724-726.

13. Sinclair R, Boone SA, Greenberg D, Keim P, Gerba CP. Persistence of category A select agents in the environment. *Appl Environ Microbiol*. 2008 Feb;74(3):555-563.

14. Inglesby TV, O'Toole T, Henderson DA, et al. Anthrax as a biological weapon, 2002: updated recommendations for management. *JAMA*. 2002 May 1;287(17):2236-2252.

15. Dennis DT, Inglesby TV, Henderson DA, et al. Tularemia as a biological weapon: medical and public health management. *JAMA*. 2001 Jun 6;285(21):2763-2773.

16. FDA approves raxibacumab to treat inhalational anthrax. United States Food & Drug Administration. Published December 14, 2012. https://wayback.archive-it.org/7993/20170111193902/http://www.fda.gov/NewsEvents/Newsroom/PressAnnouncements/ucm332341.htm

17. FDA approves new treatment for inhalation anthrax. United States Food & Drug Administration. Published March 21, 2016. https://www.fda.gov/news-events/press-announcements/fda-approves-new-treatment-inhalation-anthrax

18. FDA approves treatment for inhalation anthrax. United States Food & Drug Administration. Published March 25, 2015. https://web.archive.org/web/20180126014600/https://www.fda.gov/NewsEvents/Newsroom/PressAnnouncements/ucm439752.htm

19. Huang E, Pillai SK, Bower WA, et al. Antitoxin treatment of inhalation anthrax: a systematic review. *Health Secur*. 2015 Nov-Dec;13(6):365-377.

20. Datta KK, Singh J. Anthrax. *Indian J Pediatr*. 2002 Jan;69(1):49-56.

21. MacDonald RD. Infectious diseases and bioterrorism. In: Cooney DR, ed. *Cooney's EMS Medicine*. McGraw-Hill Education; 2016:325-344.

22. Prentice MB. Plague and other *Yersinia* infections. In: Loscalzo J, Fauci AS, Kasper DL, Hauser SL, Longo DL, Jameson JL, eds. *Harrison's Principles of Internal Medicine*. 21st ed. McGraw-Hill Education; 2022:1320-1328.

✔ Pearls

- The combination of lymphadenopathy and a widened mediastinum on chest x-ray of patients with fulminant respiratory failure is suspicious for inhalation anthrax.

- Digital necrosis in patients with bilateral pneumonia is suspicious for plague, although this is a late finding and portends a poor outcome.

- Pulse-temperature dissociation and severe pleuropneumonitis are features of inhalation tularemia.

- Although patients with inhalation anthrax and inhalation tularemia do not require more than standard precautions, patients with plague should be placed on droplet precautions, and patients with VHFs should be placed on contact precautions.

■ CASE ONE

The woman was started on ceftriaxone and azithromycin for presumed community-acquired pneumonia, and she was admitted to the regular nursing floor. She decompensated over the next several days and was transferred to the ICU; her antibiotics were changed to vancomycin and meropenem. Unfortunately, none of these common antibiotics were effective against engineered versions of plague, and the patient died on hospital day 4.

In the next week, six hospital employees developed symptoms of a respiratory illness, including hemoptysis. An astute intensivist noticed that several of them had petechial rashes and gangrenous digits in the later stages of disease. A report of a possible plague outbreak was made to the local department of public health, and special laboratory testing was sent out for confirmation. In the meantime, emergency physicians included either ciprofloxacin or doxycycline in broad-spectrum coverage for patients who presented with respiratory symptoms.

■ CASE TWO

The man was admitted to the hospital and started on vancomycin and cefepime. He rapidly developed acute respiratory distress syndrome, requiring intubation. On hospital day 2, blood cultures grew *Bacillus*. A physician reflected on the widened mediastinum on chest x-ray and the rapid progression of the disease. The laboratory was alerted to a possible case of anthrax, and additional speciation was performed. The patient improved on ciprofloxacin. Once the laboratory confirmed the presence of anthrax, the CDC was alerted. The patient's condition further improved with the administration of monoclonal antibodies.

■ CASE THREE

The emergency physician noticed the pulse-temperature dissociation and pleural effusions and recognized that the differential diagnosis for this case included pneumonic tularemia. In addition to traditional community-acquired pneumonia antibiotic coverage, the physician started the patient on streptomycin. Public health authorities were immediately alerted, and sputum and blood samples were transported to specially equipped laboratories for definitive identification. The patient slowly recovered during hospitalization and was successfully discharged. However, he continued to experience myalgia and generalized weakness for months.

23. Plague and other bacterial zoonotic diseases. In: Ryan KJ, ed. *Sherris & Ryan's Medical Microbiology*. 8th ed. McGraw-Hill Education; 2022:645-657.

24. Inglesby TV, Dennis DT, Henderson DA, et al. Plague as a biological weapon: medical and public health management. Working Group on Civilian Biodefense. *JAMA*. 2000 May 3;283(17):2281-2290.

25. Godfred-Cato S, Cooley KM, Fleck-Derderian S, et al. Treatment of human plague: a systematic review of published aggregate data on antimicrobial efficacy, 1939-2019. *Clin Infect Dis*. 2020 May 21;70(suppl 1):S11-S19.

26. Pacella CB. Occupational exposures, infection control, and standard precautions. In: Tintinalli JE, Ma OJ, Yealy DM, et al, eds. *Tintinalli's Emergency Medicine: A Comprehensive Study Guide*. 9th ed. McGraw-Hill Education; 2020:1092-1099.

27. Tularemia. Centers for Disease Control and Prevention. Reviewed December 18, 2018. https://www.cdc.gov/tularemia/index.html

28. Williams MS, Baker MR, Guina T, et al. Retrospective analysis of pneumonic tularemia in Operation Whitecoat human subjects: disease progression and tetracycline efficacy. *Front Med (Lausanne)*. 2019 Oct 22;6:229.

29. Borio L, Inglesby T, Peters CJ, et al. Hemorrhagic fever viruses as biological weapons: medical and public health management. *JAMA*. 2002 May 8;287(18):2391-2405.

30. Furuyama W, Marzi A. Ebola virus: pathogenesis and countermeasure development. *Annu Rev Virol*. 2019 Sep 29;6(1):435-458.

31. Sivanandy P, Jun PH, Man LW, et al. A systematic review of Ebola virus disease outbreaks and an analysis of the efficacy and safety of newer drugs approved for the treatment of Ebola virus disease by the US Food and Drug Administration from 2016 to 2020. *J Infect Public Health*. 2022 Mar;15(3):285-292.

32. World Health Organization Model List of Essential Medicines – 22nd List, 2021. World Health Organization. Published September 30, 2021. https://www.who.int/publications/i/item/WHO-MHP-HPS-EML-2021.02

33. Fillâtre P, Revest M, Tattevin P. Crimean-Congo hemorrhagic fever: an update. *Med Mal Infect*. 2019 Nov;49(8):574-585.

34. Lloyd E, Perry H. *Infection Control for Viral Haemorrhagic Fevers in the African Health Care Setting*. World Health Organization and Centers for Disease Control and Prevention; 1998.

✖ Pitfalls

- ■ Failing to recognize a pattern in similar presentations of rapidly progressing diseases in otherwise healthy individuals.

- ■ Neglecting to notify hospital laboratories when a Category A pathogen is suspected so that rapid definitive diagnostic testing can be achieved at specialized facilities.

- ■ Relying reflexively on classic combinations of antibiotics defined as broad spectrum in the setting of a possible outbreak from a biologic weapon.

- ■ Failing to perform proper decontamination and then maintain proper quarantine precautions for patients exposed to highly infectious biologic warfare agents.

Right Ventricular-Paced Myocardial Infarction

By Jeremy Berberian, MD; William J. Brady, MD, FACEP;
and Amal Mattu, MD, FACEP

Dr. Berberian is the associate director of emergency medicine residency education at ChristianaCare and assistant professor of emergency medicine at Sidney Kimmel Medical College, Thomas Jefferson University in Philadelphia, Pennsylvania. Dr. Brady is a professor of emergency medicine, medicine, and nursing, and vice chair for faculty affairs in the Department of Emergency Medicine at the University of Virginia School of Medicine in Charlottesville. Dr. Mattu is a professor, vice chair, and codirector of the Emergency Cardiology Fellowship in the Department of Emergency Medicine at the University of Maryland School of Medicine in Baltimore.

Objectives

On completion of this article, you should be able to:
- Describe the fundamentals of right ventricular pacing.
- Define the Sgarbossa criteria.
- Contrast the Sgarbossa criteria with the modified Sgarbossa criteria.
- Explain the role of the Sgarbossa criteria and modified Sgarbossa criteria in assessing for MI in the right ventricular-paced rhythm.

CASE PRESENTATION

An 87-year-old woman with a history of chronic atrial fibrillation status post AV node ablation and permanent implanted pacemaker presents with chest pain. An ECG is ordered (*Figure 1*).

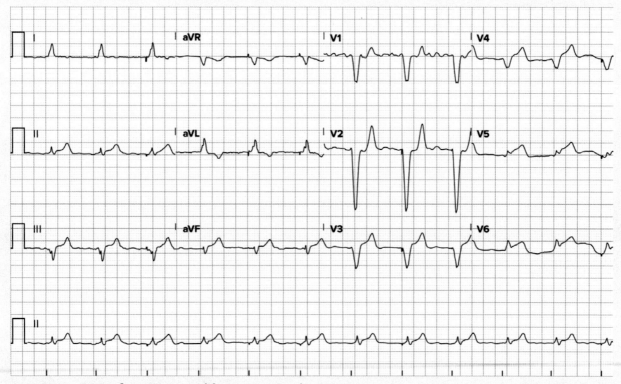

FIGURE 1. ECG of an 87-year-old woman. *Credit:* EMRA.

Discussion

This patient's ECG shows a ventricular-paced rhythm at 70 bpm, normal axis, prolonged QRS complex duration with a left bundle branch block–like (LBBB) morphology, and concordant ST-segment elevation (STE) in leads II, V_5, and V_6, suggesting acute myocardial infarction (AMI). The STE in either lead II, V_5, or V_6 meets Sgarbossa criteria, and the STE in leads V_5 and V_6 meets traditional ST-elevation myocardial infarction (STEMI) criteria.

The fundamentals of right ventricular pacing include the following:

- Depolarization is initiated in the apex of the right ventricle.
- An abnormal but predictable pattern is produced and mimics an intrinsic LBBB except for leads V_5 through V_6, which almost always have negatively oriented QRS complexes with a ventricular-paced rhythm.
- These repolarization abnormalities confound the ECG's ability to detect an AMI or other findings suggestive of acute coronary syndrome (ACS).

As with an intrinsic LBBB, the expected repolarization abnormalities in a paced rhythm follow the rule of

The patient was taken to the catheterization laboratory, where a 100% occlusion of the second obtuse marginal artery was successfully stented.

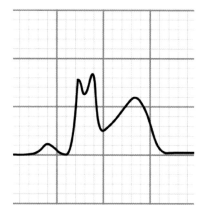

FIGURE 2. Sgarbossa criterion A: concordant STE of at least 1 mm in one or more leads (5 points is diagnostic of AMI). *Credit: EMRA.*

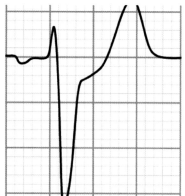

FIGURE 3. Sgarbossa criterion B: STD of at least 1 mm in V₁, V₂, or V₃ (3 points is diagnostic of AMI). *Credit: EMRA.*

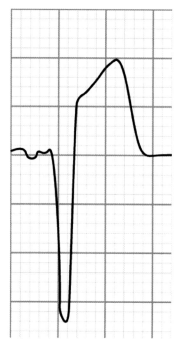

FIGURE 4. Sgarbossa criterion C: discordant STE of at least 5 mm in one or more leads (99% specific for AMI in the setting of a right ventricular–paced rhythm). *Credit: EMRA.*

appropriate discordance, which describes the relationship between the direction of the QRS complex and its ST segment (and usually the T wave). In other words, if the main vector of the QRS complex points up, there will be ST depression (STD) (and often T-wave inversion [TWI]), and if the QRS complex points down, there will be STE (and often upright T waves). Because these repolarization abnormalities confound the ECG's ability to detect an AMI and other ACS findings, an ECG suggestive of ACS requires using the Sgarbossa or modified Sgarbossa criteria to diagnose an AMI.[1] Notably, a significant number of patients with AMI and ventricular-paced rhythms do not have any abnormalities — Sgarbossa or otherwise — on their ECG.

The Sgarbossa criteria are based on the underlying principle that concordance and excessive discordance in an LBBB are abnormal. The criteria assign a point value for any concordant STE or excessively discordant STE (*Figures 2, 3,* and *4*). A score of three or greater is 98% specific for AMI, so the presence of criterion A or B is considered diagnostic of AMI. Criterion C is assigned only two points, so the presence of this criterion alone is not diagnostic of AMI.

The modified Sgarbossa criteria include Sgarbossa criteria A and B with a variation in criterion C. Instead of using a fixed cutoff of 5 mm for discordant STE, this modified version uses a ratio of the STE height to the S-wave depth (*Figure 5*). An STE:S ratio of at least 0.25 in one or more leads is considered diagnostic of AMI. This means that more than 5 mm of STE is permissible if there is a large S wave, and less than 5 mm of STE may be diagnostic if the accompanying S wave is small.

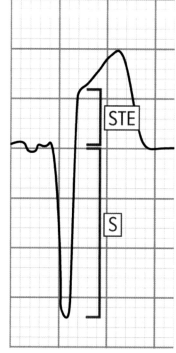

FIGURE 5. Modified Sgarbossa criterion C: STE/S ratio of at least 0.25 in one or more leads is diagnostic of AMI (but not mandated in current AHA/ACC STEMI guidelines).[2] *Credit: EMRA.*

REFERENCE

1. Writing Committee; Kontos MC, de Lemos JA, Deitelzweig SB, et al. 2022 ACC Expert Consensus Decision Pathway on the evaluation and disposition of acute chest pain in the emergency department: a report of the American College of Cardiology Solution Set Oversight Committee. *J Am Coll Cardiol.* 2022 Nov;80(20):1925-1960.

2. Dodd KW, Zvosec DL, Hart MA, et al. Electrocardiographic diagnosis of acute coronary occlusion myocardial infarction in ventricular paced rhythm using the modified Sgarbossa criteria. *Ann Emerg Med.* 2021 Oct;78(4):517-529.

— ACKNOWLEDGMENT —

This case is reprinted from *Emergency ECGs: Case-Based Review and Interpretations*, available at www.emra.org/amazon or by scanning the QR code.

The Broad Differential Diagnosis of a Posterior Auricular Mass

By Sullivan Hanback, MD; and
Adeola A. Kosoko, MD, FACEP, FAAP
McGovern Medical School, University of Texas
Health Sciences Center at Houston

Reviewed by Sharon E. Mace, MD, FACEP

Objective

On completion of this article, you should be able to:

- Discuss the differential diagnosis of a pediatric neck mass and how to differentiate between mass types.

CASE PRESENTATION

A previously healthy 6-year-old boy presents with his parents for swelling behind his left ear. The swelling was first noticed more than 1 week ago, shortly after he complained about pain behind his ear. His parents became concerned when the swelling worsened despite treatment with clindamycin and amoxicillin-clavulanate that was prescribed by urgent care clinics. The family denies that the boy had any trauma to the area, has a history of recurrent ear infections, or has any sick contacts. The patient's childhood immunizations are all up to date. In addition, he has no fever, chills, nausea, vomiting, headache, night sweats, or difficulty hearing. His behavior is normal, and he has normal intake and output.

His vital signs are BP 100/71, P 80, R 22, and T 37.1°C (98.8°F); SpO$_2$ is 99% on room air. The patient is well appearing, playful, and interactive. His tympanic membranes are normal bilaterally and so are his external ears. A left posterior auricular mass is noted; it is slightly larger than the diameter of a golf ball and is firm, fixed, and mildly tender to palpation. No lymphadenopathy is present. The patient also has left-sided facial weakness, including in his forehead, but no other cranial nerve or focal neurologic deficits. Basic laboratory results are unremarkable.

Discussion

Sarcoma is a broad term that refers to a tumor that originates from the bones or soft tissues, including fat, muscle, vessels, and lymphatics. These tumors are derived from mesenchymal cells that eventually develop into connective tissue. They make up less than 1% of adult malignancies and approximately 10% of pediatric cancers. Pediatric sarcomas can be classified as soft tissue sarcomas or osseous tumors. Soft tissue sarcomas are the sixth most common childhood malignancy, and half of them are rhabdomyosarcomas that usually occur in young children.[1] Nonrhabdomyosarcomas, by contrast, are most common in adolescents. The embryonal subtype of rhabdomyosarcomas is the most common in children; they generally occur when children are younger than 8 years and account for 60% of pediatric head and neck tumors.[1] Diagnosis is confirmed through biopsy with subsequent histopathologic analysis. Under the microscope, these rhabodmyosarcomas appear as primitive oval- to spindle-shaped cells with minimal cytoplasm and areas of small, round blue cells.[2] This malignancy has been associated with Li-Fraumeni syndrome as well as neurofibromatosis; it also appears to be associated with the *RAS* family of genes.[2]

Differential Diagnosis

Most head and neck masses in pediatric patients fall into one of three broad categories: inflammatory, congenital, or neoplastic. Although some masses are malignant, most are benign. Inflammatory lesions encompass a broad category, including common lymphadenitis. Lymphadenitis is often caused by an inflammatory response to an overgrowth of viruses or bacteria; viral upper respiratory pathogens are the most common cause, but other viral causes include HIV, cytomegalovirus, or mononucleosis, to name a few. Bacterial infections can lead to a suppurative adenitis, with *Staphylococcus aureus* as the leading cause. Tuberculosis is another important infectious cause of cervical adenitis, especially in children.[3] Other rarer causes of inflammatory pediatric head and neck masses include cat scratch disease (*Bartonella henslae*), tick-borne illnesses, and toxoplasmosis; these infections are suspected based on the history and can be confirmed by specialized testing.[4] Deep neck space infections can also lead to life-threatening neck masses like retropharyngeal abscessess.[3]

Congenital and developmental lesions span a large array of pathologies. Thyroglossal duct cysts appear as midline neck masses and are the second most common benign lesion after lymphadenopathy and lymphadenitis. A branchial cleft cyst typically occurs as a mass posterior to the sternocleidomastoid muscle. Other less common developmental lesions include epidermoid or dermoid cysts, vascular lesions, capillary malformations, lymphatic malformations, venous malformations, plunging ranulas, thymic cysts, torticollis, and hemangiomas.[3,4]

Of the head and neck neoplasms in children, teratomas are the most common but are rarely malignant. Benign lesions span from pilomatrixomas, which consist of hair follicle matrix cells, to lipomas, which are relatively rare in children. Malignant masses of the head and neck rarely occur in children. Nasopharyngeal carcinoma is more common in children of African or Asian descent and usually presents with epistaxis; it is one of the less common malignant masses and is highly

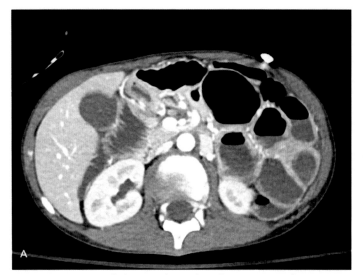
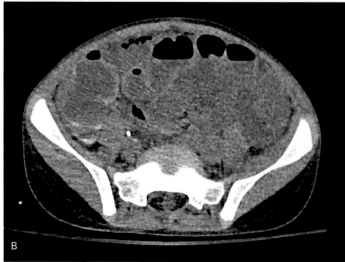

FIGURE 1. CT of the neck and soft tissue with intravenous contrast, axial view (A), coronal view (B)

associated with a previous Epstein-Barr virus infection. Lymphoma is the most common malignant pediatric neck mass and occurs predominantly in boys. In children younger than 5 years, neuroblastoma is the most common head and neck malignancy and is most often diagnosed in the first month after birth. The second most common malignant head or neck mass in the pediatric population is the highly aggressive rhabdomyosarcoma.[3,4]

Diagnosis

In the emergency department, advanced imaging is the test of choice to evaluate the composition of a head or neck mass. Emergency physicians should use imaging to determine if a mass is suppurative, if it is a hematoma, or if it is obstructive or invasive. Suppurative masses need to be evacuated or treated with antibiotics, and hematomas can indicate pathologic bleeding. CT and MRI are the most appropriate imaging modalities (*Figure 1*). Although ultrasound avoids ionizing radiation, it is more useful in detecting an abscess or vascular complication than in specifically delineating the composition of a mass.

Management

Before chemotherapy and radiation became available treatments in the late 1960s, the mainstay of treatment for pediatric sarcomas was surgery, which carried only a 10% to 15% survival rate.[2] The current standard of care includes a combination of surgical debulking, chemotherapy, and radiation to preserve the surrounding viable tissue. Outcomes have improved with these more modern approaches. However, the most promising factor for predicting outcomes is the timing of diagnosis. The 5-year survival rate for children diagnosed with a stage I sarcoma is 80%, while the survival rate for children diagnosed with a stage IV sarcoma is closer to 20%.[2]

CASE RESOLUTION

The working diagnosis based on the radiologist's imaging review and the pathologist's biopsy review was rhabdomyosarcoma of the embryonal subtype. The patient was admitted to pediatric acute care, with multiple specialties working to optimize his care, including neurosurgery, oncology, hematology, and otorhinolaryngology. An MRI of the brain and spinal cord was obtained to accurately stage the malignancy and evaluate for signs of obstruction, which would require more urgent surgical intervention. No intracranial or intraspinal extension was found, making outpatient management appropriate for the patient. He was discharged with recommendations for close follow-up with a specialized cancer center to obtain another biopsy and initiate multimodal therapy.

REFERENCES

1. Jackson DL. Evaluation and management of pediatric neck masses: an otolaryngology perspective. *Physician Assist Clin.* 2018 Apr;3(2):245-269.
2. Stuart A, Radhakrishnan J. Rhabdomyosarcoma. *Indian J Pediatr.* 2004 Apr;71(4):331-337.
3. Agaram NP. Evolving classification of rhabdomyosarcoma. *Histopathology.* 2022 Jan;80(1):98-108.
4. Gujar S, Gandhi D, Mukherji SK. Pediatric head and neck masses. *Top Magn Reson Imaging.* 2004 Apr;15(2):95-101.

Buprenorphine for Opioid Withdrawal in the Emergency Department

By Bethanne Bartscherer, MD; and Laura Welsh, MD
Boston Medical Center and Boston University
Chobanian & Avedisian School of Medicine,
Massachussetts

Reviewed by Andrew J. Eyre, MD, MS-HPEd

Objective

On completion of this article, you should be able to:

■ Explain when and how to initiate buprenorphine treatment of opioid withdrawal in the emergency department.

Herring AA, Perrone J, Nelson LS. Managing opioid withdrawal in the emergency department with buprenorphine. *Ann Emerg Med.* 2019 May;73(5):481-487.

KEY POINTS

■ Although opioid withdrawal itself is generally non–life-threatening, a subsequent opioid overdose from trying to counteract withdrawal symptoms carries a high mortality risk.

■ Emergency physicians who care for patients in opioid withdrawal can initiate medication-assisted therapy both as a withdrawal treatment and as a bridge to long-term treatment.

■ Buprenorphine should be considered for patients in opioid withdrawal who have abstained from short-acting opioids for over 12 hours, extended-release opioids for over 24 hours, and methadone for over 72 hours.

■ Approximately 30 to 60 minutes after an initial 8-mg dose of buprenorphine, an additional 8 to 24 mg can be given if withdrawal symptoms persist or are precipitated. After symptoms lessen, patients can be discharged with 16 mg buprenorphine-naloxone daily for 3 to 7 days until follow-up is established.

Emergency physicians play an integral role in addressing the public health crisis of opioid use disorder. Opioid withdrawal without medical therapy carries a high risk of mortality because it increases the chance of a subsequent fatal opioid overdose. Emergency physicians frequently care for patients in opioid withdrawal and can reduce its associated morbidity and mortality by initiating medication-assisted therapy.

To experience withdrawal, patients must be opioid dependent. Using short-acting opioids several times daily for as few as 2 weeks is enough to establish dependence. The intensity of dependence — and, thus, the severity of withdrawal — increases with higher doses that are consumed over longer periods of time. Withdrawing from opioids themselves (ie, without planning to take subsequent doses to self-treat withdrawal symptoms) is generally not life-threatening. Symptoms include restlessness, vomiting, diarrhea, piloerection, diaphoresis, yawning, mydriasis, and mild autonomic hyperactivity. Psychological symptoms such as pain, anxiety, irritability, and drug cravings can persist for weeks. Precipitated withdrawal that is caused by an opioid antagonist, partial agonist, or agonist-antagonist occurs abruptly and can be associated with vomiting, agitation, delirium, and autonomic instability. Most concerningly, precipitated withdrawal can cause massive catecholamine release that leads to pulmonary edema.

Opioid withdrawal is diagnosed clinically. The Clinical Opiate Withdrawal Scale (COWS) is a tool commonly used to assess withdrawal severity and can guide buprenorphine initiation. The Subjective Opiate Withdrawal Scale (SOWS) can guide unobserved buprenorphine inductions at home. Differences in personal practices and institutional cultures have led to wide differences in treatment approaches for opioid withdrawal. One approach involves mitigating withdrawal symptoms with nonopioid medications like α_2-adrenergic agonists and antiemetics. The evidence-based approach favors using an opioid agonist both as a treatment for withdrawal and as a bridge to long-term treatment. Although both buprenorphine and methadone are safe and effective opioid agonists that are used to treat withdrawal, buprenorphine is preferred in the emergency department.

Methadone is a full opioid agonist, and 10 to 20 mg orally can reduce opioid withdrawal symptoms without causing sedation or respiratory depression. Buprenorphine is a partial opioid agonist that does not cause euphoria, sedation, or respiratory depression. A definitive dosing approach in the emergency department is still lacking — the slow titration guidelines for the outpatient setting are impractical in the emergency department. Most patients require at least 8 mg SL buprenorphine to control withdrawal symptoms, and insufficient dosing can cause

Critical Decisions in Emergency Medicine's LLSA literature reviews feature articles from ABEM's 2023 Lifelong Learning and Self-Assessment Reading List. Available online at acep.org/moc/llsa and on the ABEM website.

Volume 37 Number 4: **April 2023**   15

withdrawal symptoms to return. Higher doses (a maximum daily dose is 32 mg) should be used cautiously in older adults and in those who use sedatives.

Buprenorphine precipitates withdrawal by displacing a full opioid agonist with a partial agonist. This displacement is also commonly seen with methadone, a full opioid agonist with low binding affinity, and will not occur when buprenorphine users receive full agonist opioids for analgesia. Larger initial doses of buprenorphine may be less likely to precipitate withdrawal symptoms because higher doses provide better partial agonist stimulation.

For patients in opioid withdrawal, buprenorphine initiation is appropriate when more than 12 hours have passed since using short-acting opioids, more than 24 hours since using extended-release formulations, and more than 72 hours since using methadone. For patients with COWS scores greater than 8, start with 4 to 8 mg SL buprenorphine based on withdrawal severity. If patients are still in withdrawal after 30 to 60 minutes, the initial dose is considered to have precipitated withdrawal, and additional buprenorphine (8-24 mg) should be administered.

After symptoms are under control, patients can be discharged from the emergency department with instructions to take 16 mg buprenorphine-naloxone daily for 3 to 7 days or until follow-up with a recovery physician is established. Emergency physicians may also want to consider providing patients with a take-home naloxone kit, screening for HIV and hepatitis C, and although pregnancy is not a contraindication to buprenorphine, providing reproductive health counseling.

Flexor Tenosynovitis of the Thumb

By Brendan McGowan, DO
University of Florida College of Medicine — Jacksonville

Reviewed by John Kiel, DO, MPH, FACEP, CAQSM

Objective

On completion of this article, you should be able to:
- State how to diagnose and manage FTS.

CASE PRESENTATION

A 49-year-old man presents for pain and swelling of the volar aspect of his right thumb. He states that he was cooking and cleaning with a wire brush when a bristle stabbed the area. Believing the bristle remained in his thumb, he attempted to remove it with a bobby pin. He complains of swelling, erythema, and tenderness of the right hand that is worse at the thumb and thenar eminence, with erythema tracking proximally to his wrist. The patient has one of four Kanavel signs of flexor sheath infection: tenderness to palpation along the flexor tendon sheath. He is admitted to the hospital for cellulitis versus FTS. Orthopedic consultation and MRI are pending.

Discussion

Flexor tenosynovitis (FTS) is a microbial infection within the flexor tendon sheath. It is the most common deep space infection of the hand, making up 2.9% to 9.4% of all hand infections.[1] FTS usually occurs secondary to trauma, although other causes include hematogenous spread, surgical manipulation, and open fractures.[1] In this patient's case, a puncture wound occurred on the volar aspect of the hand along the flexor tendon sheath.

Patients with FTS tend to present with complaints of finger and hand pain, swelling, redness, and warmth. On examination, the four classic Kanavel signs associated with flexor sheath infection may be present and include the following: the finger is passively held in flexion, pain occurs in the finger with passive extension, the finger demonstrates fusiform swelling, and tenderness to percussion occurs along the flexor tendon sheath. All four signs are unnecessary to diagnose FTS but the more signs, the higher the index of suspicion. The most common and typically first finding of FTS is pain with passive extension of the finger.

FTS is usually diagnosed based on the history, physical examination findings, and clinical gestalt. X-rays are insufficient for diagnosis but can be obtained to rule out a traumatic radiopaque foreign body (*Figure 1*). Ultrasound can be used to observe fluid within the tendon sheath and is 95% sensitive but only 74% specific, with a 95% negative predictive value (*Figures 2* and *3*).[2] MRI is the most sensitive imaging modality for clearly depicting all of the hand's anatomical structures (*Figure 4*).[3] Infectious and proinflammatory laboratory markers like WBCs, erythrocyte sedimentation rate, and C-reactive protein can be highly specific for FTS: All three have a 100% specificity and 100% positive predictive value in patients who need surgical management of FTS, but their sensitivity is low at 39%, 41%, and 76%, respectively, as is their negative predictive value at 4%, 3%, and 13%, respectively.[4] Also, the WBC count may not initially be elevated because only a low bacterial load is needed to infect the deep space of the hands. Overall, laboratory values are helpful in supporting the diagnosis but cannot reliably rule out infection; inflammatory markers can also be used to trend disease progression.

Gram-positive cocci, especially *Staphylococcus aureus* and *Streptococcus pyogenes*, are responsible for 30% to 80% of

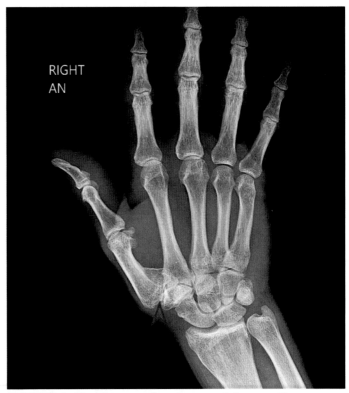

FIGURE 1. Hand x-ray showing post-traumatic osteoarthritis

infections.[4] Up to 75% of FTS wound cultures grow methicillin-sensitive *S. aureus* (MSSA), and 29% grow methicillin-resistant *S. aureus* (MRSA), with the latter continuing to increase in number.[1] Immunocompromised patients have mixed organisms, anaerobes, and gram-negative bacteria in their wound cultures.

Emergency physicians should strongly suspect FTS when corroborating history and signs are present. If there is concern for a deep space hand infection, intravenous access should be obtained; laboratory tests for inflammatory markers should be ordered; and intravenous antibiotics that cover MRSA, gram-negative bacteria, and anaerobes should be administered along with tetanus prophylaxis. An ultrasound or MRI should also

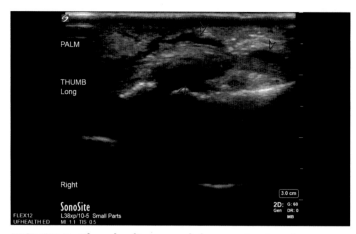

FIGURE 2. Thumb ultrasound, long axis showing peritendinous fluid

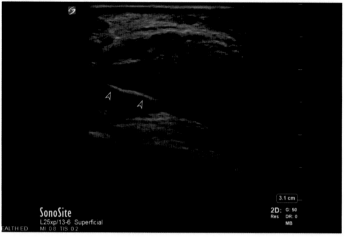

FIGURE 3. Wrist ultrasound showing arthrocentesis

be ordered. Early orthopedic consultation is also recommended because FTS complication rates can be as high as 38%, according to the literature, and surgery is necessary for irrigation and debridement of the infected space.[1] Even with successful eradication of the initial infection, a large portion of patients have complications, including chronic pain, contractures, stiffness, weakness, and recurrence of infection that requires amputation. If deep space hand infections are missed, complications can become limb- and life-threatening, highlighting the importance of keeping a high index of suspicion.

Patients with early presentation or fewer than two Kanavel signs within 48 hours of onset can be treated with antibiotics and re-evaluated in 24 hours.[1] If symptoms have improved at re-evaluation, antibiotic therapy can be continued, but if they have not improved, surgical intervention is indicated. Patients who are highly suspected of having FTS, including those with three to four Kanavel signs and moderate to severe symptoms, should be managed surgically.[1]

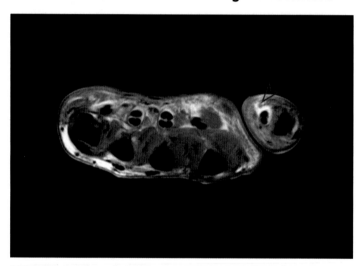

FIGURE 4. Thumb MRI puncture wound with peritendinous fluid

CASE RESOLUTION

The patient was seen and evaluated by orthopedic surgery for suspected FTS. Orthopedics recommended admission for intravenous antibiotics and serial examinations because the patient had only one of four Kanavel signs, and the orthopedic surgeon felt the patient's signs and symptoms were more consistent with cellulitis than FTS. The patient had soft tissue edema at the wrist; a wrist arthrocentesis with a culture of the aspirated fluid was completed in the emergency department. The patient also received a tetanus booster. The following day, MRI of the hand showed peritendinous fluid that extended proximal to and within the carpal tunnel and into the space of Parona; these findings were clinically significant for a horseshoe abscess (see *Figure 4*).

On day 2 of admission, the patient was taken to the operating room for debridement and irrigation of the thumb tendon sheath. During surgery, the patient had purulence from the first through fifth flexor tendons, with extension into the carpal tunnel. His cultures grew MSSA. The patient had been receiving vancomycin and ceftriaxone, so his antibiotics were adjusted according to his culture results. The infectious disease specialist recommended placement of a peripherally inserted central catheter for continued antibiotics. The patient returned to the operating room for reassessment on day 6 of admission. A repeat debridement and irrigation showed no evidence of purulence but did show extensive soft tissue cellulitis. The patient was discharged on day 7 of admission and advised to follow up with orthopedics. One month post procedure, his right hand's grip strength was significantly weak, and he had persistent neuropathy.

REFERENCES

1. Chapman T, Ilyas AM. Pyogenic flexor tenosynovitis: evaluation and treatment strategies. *J Hand Microsurg*. 2019 Dec;11(3):121-126.
2. Jardin E, Delord M, Aubry S, Loisel F, Obert L. Usefulness of ultrasound for the diagnosis of pyogenic flexor tenosynovitis: a prospective single-center study of 57 cases. *Hand Surg Rehabil*. 2018 Apr;37(2):95-98.
3. Malizos KN, Papadopoulou ZK, Ziogkou AN, et al. Infections of deep hand and wrist compartments. *Microorganisms*. 2020 Jun 3;8(6):838.
4. Bishop GB, Born T, Kakar S, Jawa A. The diagnostic accuracy of inflammatory blood markers for purulent flexor tenosynovitis. *J Hand Surg Am*. 2013 Nov;38(11):2208-2211.

The Critical Image

Chest Trauma in Older Patients

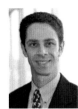

By Joshua S. Broder, MD, FACEP
Dr. Broder is a professor and the residency program director in the Department of Emergency Medicine at Duke University Medical Center in Durham, North Carolina.

Objectives

On completion of this article, you should be able to:

- Describe the morbidity and mortality associated with rib fractures in older patients.
- Identify patients who need a CT for a rib fracture diagnosis.
- Determine the disposition of patients 65 years and older with multiple rib fractures.

CASE PRESENTATION

An 80-year-old woman presents after falling from a ladder while changing a light bulb. She reports that she lost her balance and fell backward on her back. She denies striking her head or losing consciousness. After lying on the floor for a few minutes, she stood and walked to her bed, where she remained overnight. This morning, she called EMS because of ongoing pain. The patient complains of right-sided chest and back pain that is worse when she breathes in.

Her vital signs are BP 151/91, P 75, R 19, and T 37.1°C (98.8°F); SpO_2 is 95% on room air. She is stable and alert. Her lungs are clear, but her right anterior chest wall and right paraspinal thoracic region are tender to palpation. A deformity of the right clavicle is present. The patient states that this is chronic, and she has no tenderness in that location. A chest x-ray, followed by a CT, is performed (*Figures 1* and *2*).

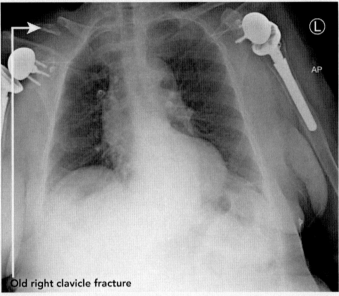

Old right clavicle fracture

FIGURE 1. Patient's initial chest x-ray showing no pneumothorax but an old right clavicle fracture. Rib fractures are present but may escape notice — none were reported in the radiology interpretation.

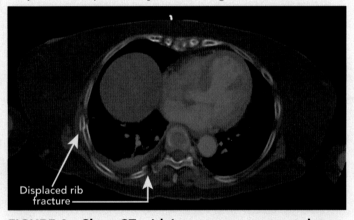

Displaced rib fracture

FIGURE 2. Chest CT with intravenous contrast, bone windows. Even in this single slice, multiple rib fractures are seen.

Discussion

Rib fractures are a common, painful, but often minor injury managed with supportive therapies such as analgesics and incentive spirometry. Often, imaging for confirmation of a rib fracture is unnecessary because the condition can be treated empirically. Imaging in patients with rib fractures is instead done to identify other serious traumatic injuries such as a pneumo- or hemothorax or an aortic injury. For minor blunt trauma, the American College of Radiology (ACR) finds chest x-rays "usually appropriate," rib x-rays "may be appropriate," and CT "usually not appropriate" for initial imaging.[1]

Rib fractures in patients aged 65 years or older take on a greater significance because an increasing number of rib fractures is associated with morbidity and mortality. A retrospective study found that mortality is 10% for older patients with one or two rib fractures, nearly 20% with three or four rib fractures, more than 20% with five or six rib fractures, and more than 30% with more than six rib fractures. By comparison, mortality rates in younger patients with six or fewer rib fractures are less than half of these values. Pneumonia, acute respiratory distress syndrome, ventilator days, and hospital length of stay are also strongly associated with an increasing number of rib fractures and occur at far greater rates in older patients than in patients younger than 65 years.[2] Delirium is another common complication (25% occurrence) in older patients with rib fractures.[3] Other injuries and comorbidities are important confounders — multiple rib fractures can be indicators of severe mechanisms of injury, and patients may die *with* rib fractures rather than *from* them. To reduce these confounders, some studies have focused on isolated rib fractures in older patients and have suggested lower morbidity and mortality rates.[4-6] However, even when older patients with other significant injuries are excluded, rates of pneumonia (15%-32%), mechanical ventilation (4%), and in-hospital mortality (4%) remain

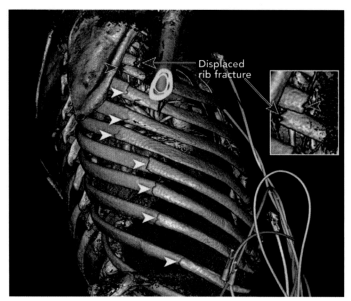

FIGURE 3. 3D CT reconstruction revealing eight consecutive rib fractures (ribs 4-11), including a displaced fracture of the fourth rib

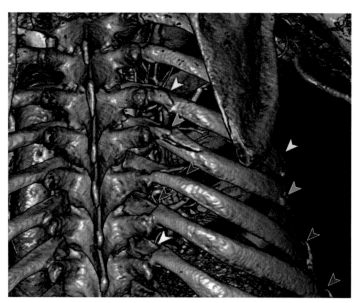

FIGURE 4. 3D CT reconstruction revealing posterior rib fractures. Colored pairs of arrows emphasize segmental rib fractures. Three or more segmentally fractured ribs can create a flail chest, which impairs respiratory mechanics. A free-floating segment of ribs can move inward during inspiration and create paradoxical chest wall motion that inhibits movement of air into the chest during inspiration.

high, despite relatively intensive monitoring and therapy, including ketamine or epidural pain control.[5] Care bundles that incorporate standardized analgesics, noninvasive positive-pressure ventilation, and incentive spirometry have shown mixed results. One study showed lower associated rates of unplanned ICU admission, unplanned intubation, and pneumonia.[7] Another study found that a care bundle improved pain control but increased ICU admission without reducing respiratory complications.[8]

Although CT is often performed to evaluate for other blunt traumatic injuries, its high sensitivity for rib fractures can also help identify older patients with an increased risk of morbidity and mortality (*Figures 3* and *4*). For hemodynamically stable patients with major blunt trauma, the ACR finds a chest CT with intravenous contrast to be "usually appropriate" for initial imaging. Contrast is not needed for detection of rib fractures or other bony

injuries but is required for vascular injury assessement.[9] In the National Emergency X-Radiography Utilization Study (NEXUS), 66% of patients with rib fractures were detected by CT only; chest x-rays were negative for rib fracture in these patients. Some previous investigators had suggested that rib fractures detected only by CT may be clinically insignificant. In the NEXUS study, however, the mortality of patients with rib fractures seen only on CT was not substantially different from patients with rib fractures also seen on x-ray, and the mortality rate of patients with rib fractures (5.6%) was higher than the mortality rate of patients without rib fractures (2.7%).[10]

CASE RESOLUTION

The patient was admitted for 1 week and then discharged to a rehabilitation facility. Two weeks later, she required readmission for worsened tachypnea; a chest tube was placed for interval development of a hemothorax, and she received a blood transfusion.

REFERENCES

1. Expert Panel on Thoracic Imaging; Henry TS, Donnelly EF, Boiselle PM, et al. ACR Appropriateness Criteria® Rib Fractures. *J Am Coll Radiol.* 2019 May;16(5S):S227-S234.
2. Bulger EM, Arneson MA, Mock CN, Jurkovich GJ. Rib fractures in the elderly. *J Trauma.* 2000 Jun;48(6):1040-1046; discussion 1046-1047.
3. Janssen TL, Hosseinzoi E, Vos DI, et al. The importance of increased awareness for delirium in elderly patients with rib fractures after blunt chest wall trauma: a retrospective cohort study on risk factors and outcomes. *BMC Emerg Med.* 2019 Jun 13;19(1):34.
4. Hoepelman RJ, Beeres FJP, Heng M, et al. Rib fractures in the elderly population: a systematic review. *Arch Orthop Trauma Surg.* 2023 Feb;143(2):887-893.
5. Cull JD, Ewing A, Metcalf A, Kitchens D, Manning B. Isolated rib fractures in elderly falls: not as deadly as we think. *J Trauma Nurs.* 2022 Mar-Apr;29(2):65-69.
6. Naar L, El Hechi MW, van Erp IA, et al. Isolated rib cage fractures in the elderly: do all patients belong to the intensive care unit? A retrospective nationwide analysis. *J Trauma Acute Care Surg.* 2020 Dec;89(6):1039-1045.
7. Kelley KM, Burgess J, Weireter L, et al. Early use of a chest trauma protocol in elderly patients with rib fractures improves pulmonary outcomes. *Am Surg.* 2019 Mar 1;85(3):288-291.
8. Carrie C, Stecken L, Cayrol E, et al. Bundle of care for blunt chest trauma patients improves analgesia but increases rates of intensive care unit admission: a retrospective case-control study. *Anaesth Crit Care Pain Med.* 2018 Jun;37(3):211-215.
9. Expert Panel on Major Trauma Imaging; Shyu JY, Khurana B, Soto JA, et al. ACR Appropriateness Criteria® Major Blunt Trauma. *J Am Coll Radiol.* 2020 May;17(5S):S160-S174.
10. Murphy CE, Raja AS, Baumann BM, et al. Rib fracture diagnosis in the panscan era. *Ann Emerg Med.* 2017 Dec;70(6):904-909.

Feature Editor: Joshua S. Broder, MD, FACEP. See also *Diagnostic Imaging for the Emergency Physician* (Winner of the 2011 Prose Award in Clinical Medicine, the American Publishers Award for Professional and Scholarly Excellence) and *Critical Images in Emergency Medicine* by Dr. Broder.

Dorsal Penile Nerve Block

By Steven J. Warrington, MD, MEd, MS
MercyOne Siouxland, Sioux City, Iowa

Objective

On completion of this article, you should be able to:
- Explain how to administer a dorsal penile nerve block.

Introduction

A dorsal penile nerve block is a regional anesthetic technique that can be used before procedures that involve the penis, such as laceration repairs or a paraphimosis reduction. It is low risk, quick, and useful in a number of uncommon situations.

Contraindications
- Infection overlying the injection site
- Concern for testicular torsion

Benefits and Risks

The primary benefit of this procedure is that it avoids or limits the use of systemic anesthesia or analgesia for patients with certain types of penile pathologies. Additionally, use of this regional anesthesia can prevent the distortion and distension of local tissues that could make certain procedures more difficult.

Potential risks of the procedure include an allergic reaction to a component of the anesthetic, hematoma formation, bleeding, urethral injuries, and infection (including osteomyelitis). Other potential risks are inadequately controlled pain, injection of the incorrect medication, or a foreign body from the needle tip breaking in the penis. In patients with suspected testicular torsion, the nerve block can prevent assessment for a successful manual detorsion.

Alternatives

Local anesthesia can be used in place of the dorsal penile nerve block. Procedural sedation or systemic anesthesia and analgesia are other alternatives to regional and local anesthetics.

Reducing Side Effects

Because the injection is given near the genitals, it can be anxiety inducing and perceived as painful. Adjunct medications such as oral or injectable anxiolytics and topical anesthetics that alleviate pain with needle insertion (eg, lidocaine and prilocaine cream or vapocoolants) can be beneficial. Even placing an ice pack over the injection site for a short time before administering the nerve block can reduce associated pain.

Special Considerations

Slowly injecting the anesthetic has been shown to reduce pain associated with the injection; an injection rate of 100 to 150 seconds is recommended. Using sodium bicarbonate to alkalinize lidocaine does not appear to be beneficial, and no studies have evaluated the technique of warming lidocaine prior to use.

The amount of anesthetic needed somewhat depends on the individual and type of anesthetic used. Suggestions for adults include 2 mL of 1% lidocaine, with 0.2 to 0.4 mL of anesthetic per side, up to a maximum of 4.5 mg/kg in younger populations.

TECHNIQUE

1. **Obtain** the patient's consent for the procedure and gather the necessary materials. Consider administering anxiolytics, analgesics, or local methods of pretreatment (eg, ice, vapocoolant, prilocaine and lidocaine cream).

2. **Clean** and prepare the area.

3. **Create** a topical wheal of anesthetic at the 2 o'clock and 10 o'clock positions as close to the base of the penis as possible.

4. **Insert** and advance the needle through the middle of the wheal, approximately 0.5 cm or until resistance is lost.

5. **Aspirate** to ensure the needle tip is not within a blood vessel; then, slowly inject the anesthetic at the suggested rate of 100 to 150 seconds per injection.

6. **Assess** for potential complications and the anesthesia's effectiveness, accounting for time to action.

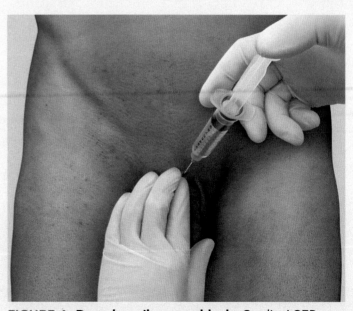

FIGURE 1. Dorsal penile nerve block. *Credit:* ACEP.

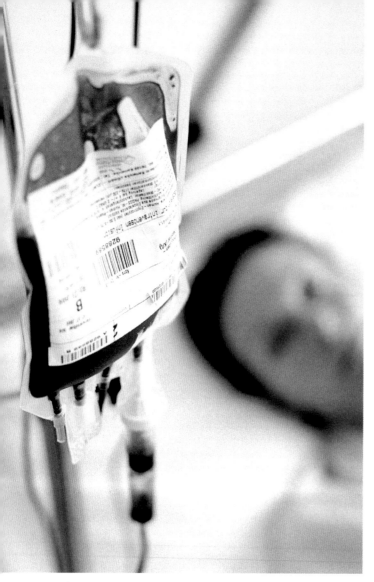

Seeing Red

Emergency Presentations of Upper GI Bleeds

LESSON 8

By Mariam Azim, MD

Dr. Azim is an emergency medicine resident at the University of Maryland in Baltimore.

Reviewed by Amal Mattu, MD, FACEP

Objectives

On completion of this lesson, you should be able to:

1. Recognize and manage critically ill patients with upper GI bleeds.
2. Apply the correct pharmacotherapies in upper GI bleeds.
3. Describe how to prepare and manage difficult airways.
4. Manage complications of massive blood transfusions.
5. Discuss steps for placing a balloon tamponade device.

From the EM Model

1.0   Signs, Symptoms, and Presentations
     1.3   General
          1.3.6   Bleeding
19.0 Procedures and Skills Integral to the Practice of Emergency Medicine
     19.4   Diagnostic and Therapeutic Procedures
          19.4.1   Abdominal and Gastrointestinal
               19.4.1.6 Mechanical Control of Upper Gastrointestinal Bleeding

▬ CRITICAL DECISIONS ▬

- How can unstable upper GI bleeds be identified and stabilized?

- What considerations help prepare for a difficult airway in patients with upper GI bleeds?

- How are upper GI bleeds managed?

- What are the treatment complications of upper GI bleeds?

- Do diagnostic and therapeutic management differ based on the etiology of bleeding?

Upper GI bleeding is a common condition encountered in the emergency department that has a variety of presentations and can lead to serious complications. Emergency physicians must differentiate between stable and unstable GI bleeds and act quickly to stabilize patients with unstable bleeds in preparation for more definitive management.

CASE ONE

A 45-year-old man presents via EMS with large volume hematemesis. EMS reports seeing multiple towels soaked with dark blood in his home. His vital signs include BP 85/50, P 112, and R 20; SpO_2 is 97% on room air. He appears lethargic and has a distended abdomen and scleral icterus. He is placed on a monitor while two large-bore intravenous lines are obtained. Emergency release of PRBCs from the blood bank are requested.

CASE TWO

A 40-year-old woman presents after three episodes of tarry stools in the past week. On examination, she is well appearing, and her abdomen is soft and nontender. Rectal examination demonstrates brown stool that is guaiac positive, and no hemorrhoids are seen. Vital signs include BP 140/83, P 70, and R 13; SpO_2 is 99% on room air. She denies any medication use and denies pain. Workup reveals a hemoglobin level of 13.9 g/dL, platelet count of 200,000 cells/μL, BUN level of 11 mg/dL, and creatinine level of 1.0 mg/dL.

CASE THREE

A 55-year-old man with a known history of esophageal varices presents with massive hematemesis. He is intubated and given a massive blood transfusion, but bleeding persists. The physician decides to place a Sengstaken-Blakemore tube down the oropharynx at roughly 50 cm until endoscopic and specialist care are available.

Introduction

Upper GI bleeding is commonly seen in the emergency department and is associated with high morbidity and mortality. Patients who are critically ill from an upper GI bleed must be quickly identified, prepared, and managed, with several key steps to guide the resuscitation. Like with all other kinds of shock, controlling the source of bleeding is the ultimate goal. Because treating hemorrhagic shock is time sensitive, knowing how to troubleshoot interventions can change outcomes. Physicians must also know their institutions' limitations so that the most appropriate dispositions and interventions are provided to patients.

CRITICAL DECISION

How can unstable upper GI bleeds be identified and stabilized?

Timely evaluation and diagnosis are crucial for differentiating stable and unstable upper GI bleeds. When unstable patients have an altered mental status and cannot provide their history, physicians should obtain information from EMS about the appearance of the scene, patient appearance, vital signs, surgical history, interventions or therapies administered, and medications suspected to have been taken, paying particular attention to NSAIDs, anticoagulants, or antiplatelets that raise suspicion for a bleeding ulcer or clotting issue. Physicians should quickly assess patients for more worrisome signs of GI bleeds, such as an elevated shock index (SI), signs of poor perfusion, a collapsed inferior vena cava on bedside ultrasound, and classic stigmata of liver disease. SI is calculated by dividing the heart rate by the systolic blood pressure; an SI greater than 0.8 is considered abnormal and is concerning for severe instability. Physicians should also search for the source of bleeding. Other signs such as severe abdominal pain with involuntary guarding are concerning for peritonitis or a perforated viscus.

For some patients, blood may be coming from the lungs instead of the GI tract. Blood from the lungs, or hemoptysis, can be frothy, small in volume, and associated with a cough. Blood from the upper GI tract can include melena or, if the upper GI bleeding is brisk enough, the brighter hematochezia (although the latter is normally associated with a lower GI bleed); upper GI bleeding can also appear as hematemesis, which is characteristically larger in volume, has the appearance of coffee grounds in vomit, and comes from proximal to the ligament of Treitz.[1] Hematemesis is more ominous than hematochezia because it is associated with a higher mortality rate.

The two most critical diagnoses to consider in patients with upper GI bleeds are variceal bleeding — usually in patients with known or suspected liver disease or heavy alcohol use — and peptic ulcer disease, which is most often caused by *Helicobacter pylori* infection and frequently associated with heavy NSAID use. Duodenal ulcers in particular are the most common cause of upper GI bleeding, even more so than gastric ulcers. Several other sources of upper GI bleeding include gastritis, malignancies, Dieulafoy lesions, and aortoenteric fistulae in patients with a history of aortic surgery or grafting.[2]

Regardless of the upper GI bleed's etiology, physicians should follow some basic universal first steps to stabilize patients; these steps include placing patients on a monitor, establishing two large-bore intravenous lines, and drawing blood for laboratory tests (CBC, blood chemistry panel, coagulation profile, fibrinogen test, type and screen, and viscoelastic testing, if available). After a rapid assessment of patients and their vital signs, their airway should be assessed to decide if intubation is necessary. The decision to intubate is multifactorial and takes into account patients' mental status, their risk of aspiration, the need for proper diagnostic evaluation, and the expected clinical course. However, prematurely performing rapid sequence intubation (RSI) on critically ill patients who are under-resuscitated can cause hemodynamic instability and rapid deterioration. As part of the airway plan, push-dose pressors or vasopressors should be ready to use in case postintubation hemodynamic decline occurs. Alternatively, because peri-intubation hypotension often occurs with hemorrhagic shock, starting these medications ahead of time may be beneficial. Norepinephrine infusion is recommended as the first-line vasopressor during peri-intubation fluid resuscitation and can be started peripherally.[3] Hemodynamically stable patients with upper GI bleeds still have a high risk of aspiration and may eventually need airway protection if they experience a delayed shock.

When treating hemorrhagic shock, blood transfusion is preferred over crystalloid fluids for volume expansion. For patients with unstable GI bleeding, volume resuscitation should target a mean arterial pressure (MAP) of 65 mm Hg. If time and resources allow, an arterial line can be used to assess the blood pressure response in real time. Appropriate selection of venous access is crucial in this time-sensitive condition (*Table 1*). Larger-gauge peripheral intravenous catheters (14 or 16 gauge) are faster than the standard 18- to 22-gauge catheters used in intravenous kits. For example, a 16-gauge intravenous catheter has a flow rate of 180 mL/min compared to an 18-gauge intravenous catheter that has a flow rate of 90 mL/min. If placement of two large-bore peripheral intravenous lines is delayed or cannot be obtained, central access should instead be obtained for rapid transfusion. Intravenous line length and diameter dictate the speed: Standard triple lumen central lines are long in length but have reduced flow rates that make them slower than the standard 18-gauge intravenous lines. Multilumen access catheters and hemodialysis catheters, especially, have larger diameters that allow for the fastest flow rates.

Access to blood products varies by facility and can be slow or limited. Generally speaking, hemodynamic instability, brisk bleeding, or an SI greater than 1.0 warrants more rapid transfusions. Importantly, physicians should remember that hemoglobin and hematocrit levels are slow to reflect blood loss. With stable GI bleeds, which are likely slower and more chronic, a restrictive transfusion strategy with a target hemoglobin level of 7 g/dL should be used. If access to blood products is delayed, a liter of crystalloid fluids and one or two units of uncrossmatched packed RBCs (PRBCs) should be administered immediately (in a warmer, if possible) while a massive transfusion protocol (MTP) is activated. Keep in mind that crystalloid fluids can dilute and impair the coagulation factors needed during fluid resuscitation. Consider starting vasopressors early during the active resuscitation if MAP goals are not met or if end-organ perfusion is compromised, signs of which can include changes in mental status or inadequate urine output. Administer blood products in a 1:1:1 ratio of PRBCs, fresh frozen plasma (FFP), and platelets. When available, viscoelastic testing can be used for more precise blood product administration. With each round of MTP (containing six units of PRBCs), administer intravenous calcium replacement. In certain cases, intravenous desmopressin can be an adjunct to blood products, especially for patients who have a known renal dysfunction, who are on antiplatelet medication, or who have thrombocytopenia. Additionally, some institutions include tranexamic acid (TXA) (at a loading dose of 1 gram IV) for cases of refractory bleeding, but the recent HALT-IT trial evaluated TXA for GI bleeding and found no mortality benefit and an increase in adverse events.[5]

CRITICAL DECISION

What considerations help prepare for a difficult airway in patients with upper GI bleeds?

When intubating critically ill bleeding patients, a plan for managing a difficult airway should be in place. At some institutions, emergency physicians may be the only physicians who provide critical care. When possible, however, other resources should be mobilized early on, such as notifying specialists from anesthesia, surgery, or dedicated airway teams, which can also include multiple surgical specialists. For more assistance, several checklists and cognitive aids are available for planning, preparation, setup, and postintubation care.

Many factors can lead to a difficult airway, including anatomy, obesity, neck mobility, mask ventilation abilities, airway contamination from blood or emesis, and previous intubation attempts. From an anatomic and physiologic standpoint, patients with unstable GI bleeds are usually considered to have difficult airways to manage. For one, these patients are at a higher risk of adverse outcomes; hypotension, acidosis, and an elevated SI are likely already present or impending when stabilizing patients with upper GI bleeds, and they are all risk factors that can lead to hemodynamic collapse or even cardiac arrest during the peri-intubation period. During setup for intubation, these patients should have reliable intravenous access and continuous monitoring, much like in the setup of an operating room where physicians have direct visual access to cardiac monitoring, frequent blood pressure checks (invasive or noninvasive), pulse oximetry, and capnography.

Size	Estimated Flow Rate (to Gravity)	Time to Administer 1 Liter
13F dialysis catheter	400 mL/min	2.5 min
14G	250 mL/min	4 min
16G	150 mL/min	7 min
8.5F sheath introducer	130 mL/min	8 min
18G	100 mL/min	10 min
16G distal port triple lumen	70 mL/min	15 min

TABLE 1. Vascular access flow rates[4]

In critically ill patients with unstable GI bleeds, preoxygenation should be started as early as possible because these patients can desaturate quickly. The goal of preoxygenation is to be efficient and create an adequate safe apnea time. Some methods include a nonrebreather face mask, which provides a 10- to 15-L/min flow of 80% to 95% FiO_2; a high-flow nasal cannula (HFNC), which provides humidified oxygen with a 40- to 70-L/min flow of up to 100% FiO_2; noninvasive positive-pressure ventilation (NPPV) (considering patients' aspiration risk and mental status); and bag-valve-mask (BVM) ventilation.[6] If a BVM is used for either preoxygenation or between intubation attempts, setting a positive end-expiratory pressure (PEEP) of 5 to 10 cm H_2O and using a PEEP valve can optimize oxygen saturation. Use caution with bagging. In a stressful situation, it can be easy to be overzealous with bagging, but this can cause gastric insufflation, which worsens vomiting and increases the risk of aspiration; some argue to avoid mask ventilation altogether because it can cause regurgitation. An oxygenation method involving the nares, such as a conventional nasal cannula (at flush rate) or HFNC, is recommended to maintain apneic oxygenation.[3] These methods can remain on patients after induction of chemical apnea and during laryngoscopy or insertion of the endotracheal tube without obscuring the view.

Before intubation, the necessary equipment, along with any backup equipment, should be set up. The setup should include different sizes of endotracheal tubes, end-tidal CO_2 capnography, proper suction, video or direct laryngoscopy, a bougie, and a naso- or oropharyngeal airway along with rescue supraglottic devices. The most experienced physician should make the first attempt at intubation. For a soiled airway, maintain two large-bore suction devices or use the suction-assisted laryngoscopy and airway decontamination (SALAD) technique to keep the airway decontaminated and prevent massive aspiration.[7] For active emesis, leave the tip of one suction device in the esophagus. Alternatively, intubate past the vocal cords with a large-bore suction catheter that can fit a bougie through it, withdraw the suction over the bougie, and then slide the endotracheal tube over the bougie. Importantly, in the event that intubation approaches fail, a surgical airway kit for a cricothyrotomy should be prepared and ready. The most challenging part of a cricothyrotomy is not the technique but deciding when to perform it — delaying it runs the risk of an anoxic brain injury. Material setup is crucial to this critically ill patient group because their safe apnea times are short.

Also while preparing for RSI, ensure patients are properly positioned and RSI medications are carefully selected. Etomidate and ketamine are less hemodynamically altering than propofol for the induction. During the induction, a lower or half dose of sedation medications can be used on persistently hypotensive patients. Sedation medications and analgesia post intubation are also vital for patient comfort; physicians must again consider the hemodynamic effects of medications administered during this time.

After intubation, ventilator settings should be adjusted according to each patient's needs and physiology. In the case of a "crashing" upper GI bleed, patients may become profoundly acidotic from hypoperfusion. Patients will physiologically compensate for severe metabolic acidosis through tachypnea and extremely high minute ventilation. Because anesthetic induction agents and neuromuscular blockers used in airway management decrease respiratory drive, the concentration of carbon dioxide (hypercarbia) will increase and the arterial pH will decrease. Consequently, intubation should proceed quickly and be performed by a physician with excellent intubation skills. Preoxygenation with NPPV is recommended in cases of severe metabolic acidosis except in patients with active hematemesis or altered mental status.[3] On the ventilator, the respiratory rate can initially be set higher and adjusted serially, keeping in mind how much the patient worked to breathe prior to intubation. If the patient has already aspirated and is having difficulty with oxygenation, PEEP and FiO_2 should be adjusted. Increased oxygen demand and pressure alarms on the ventilator should trigger suspicion for volume overload or acute respiratory distress syndrome (ARDS) from aspiration or rapid transfusion.

CRITICAL DECISION

How are upper GI bleeds managed?

Key medications for upper GI bleeds are intravenous proton pump inhibitors (PPIs) for acid suppression, somatostatin analogues for reducing blood flow, and prophylactic antibiotics for preventing infections. Intermittent dosing of PPIs (pantoprazole 40 mg twice daily) is now recommended rather than a bolus with the infusion. PPIs help increase pH in the stomach, and their use in peptic ulcer bleeding has been shown to reduce the likelihood of rebleeding and the need for surgical intervention.[8] After endoscopic therapy for hemostasis, high-dose PPI therapy should continue for 3 days, either as a bolus dose and intravenous infusion of 80 mg pantoprazole followed by 8 mg/hr or an intermittent dosing of 40 mg pantoprazole twice a day after an initial 80-mg bolus.[9] To reduce the risk of rebleeding in patients who are hospitalized for an unstable GI bleed and recent hemorrhage or who have high-risk findings on endoscopy, PPI therapy should be continued orally twice daily from day 4 until 2 weeks after endoscopic treatment, rather than the previously recommended once daily dosing.[9] Once patients are ready for discharge or their risk of rebleeding is low, they can typically be transitioned to oral PPI dosing.

For somatostatin analogues, octreotide is the analogue of choice. It is a splanchnic vasoconstrictor that decreases blood flow to the varices. Dosing starts with a 50-µg bolus followed by an infusion of 50 µg/hr. Although octreotide has not shown a mortality benefit, treatment with it can reduce the need for transfusions.

For patients with known or suspected cirrhosis, prophylactic antibiotics have been shown to decrease all-cause mortality and the incidence of bacterial infections. Ceftriaxone at a dosage of 1 g daily for 7 days is recommended to cover most infections, especially gram-negative bacterial infections; patients discharged prior to 7 days should transition to oral ciprofloxacin.[8]

Endoscopic therapy is the diagnostic and therapeutic modality of choice for variceal bleeding. Emergency physicians' role in this treatment is to initiate adjuncts. Varices develop in many patients with cirrhosis because as cirrhosis progresses, scarring and fibrous tissue that develop in the liver disrupt hepatic flow, which causes portal hypertension and collateral blood supplies to develop.[10] Gastric and esophageal varices continue to grow and are faced with increased blood pressure and flow, increasing their risk of rupture. A high percentage of patients with decompensated cirrhosis have variceal bleeding that is associated with high morbidity and mortality. A common laboratory abnormality seen in patients with liver failure is a decreased albumin level. Different treatments are classified as primary prophylaxis to prevent bleeding, therapies that control acute hemorrhages, and secondary prophylaxis for preventing future bleeding.

CRITICAL DECISION

What are the treatment complications of upper GI bleeds?

During stabilization, patients in shock can become acidotic, hypothermic, and coagulopathic. This has the potential to create a vicious cycle — for example, acidosis can impair the coagulation cascade. A dangerously low blood pH also affects intubation decisions, both during RSI and when managing the ventilator. In acidotic patients, any moment of apnea after RSI medications are given can cause rapid desaturation that leads to cardiac arrest. Therefore, ventilator settings should be optimized for blood pH. Temperature should also be monitored, and if low, warming should be started early on with fluid warmers or an external heat source. For patients who are coagulopathic at baseline or taking anticoagulants, reversal agents should be considered (*Table 2*).[11]

When administering blood products, patients' comorbidities should also be taken into consideration. Certain patients, such as those with congestive heart failure and end-stage renal disease, can deteriorate from rapid transfusion, even when their upper GI bleeds are stable. Transfusions in the stable GI bleed should be administered slowly to prevent volume overload and pulmonary edema, or the condition known as transfusion-associated circulatory overload (TACO). TACO can manifest as dyspnea, hypertension, and rales. TACO is difficult to distinguish from transfusion-related acute lung injury (TRALI) in the physical examination alone. TRALI is a noncardiogenic pulmonary edema that may require more invasive airway support.[12] Diuretics should be considered post transfusion in the appropriate patient

✔ Pearls

- MTP should be initiated early; blood should be replaced with blood products, and intravenous catheters with optimal flow rates should be selected.
- Physicians should start fluid resuscitation before intubation and have vasopressors and all intubation equipment set up for patients who may have difficult airways.
- Patients with known or suspected liver disease should be given PPIs as a bolus (rather than an infusion), octreotide, and ceftriaxone 1 g.
- Physicians should be familiar with the various balloon tamponade devices and their troubleshooting methods.

population. Massive amounts of fluid volume make certain patients more susceptible to ARDS.

Many potential complications must be considered during MTPs. Hypothermia can occur with each transfusion round administered.[13] Patients with cirrhosis who are already coagulopathic have difficulty clotting blood and so may need adjuncts of 10 mg IV vitamin K and cryoprecipitate (10 unit/kg) in addition to the 1:1:1 ratio for blood component replacement. Patients with chronic or end-stage renal disease can have hyperkalemia that is worsened by the potassium present in stored blood products. Rapid blood infusions can precipitate hypocalcemia and coagulopathy because of the citrate present in stored plasma that binds both calcium and magnesium. Eventually, citrate is metabolized into bicarbonate and helps improve low blood pH.[13,14] However, citrate is metabolized by the liver, so patients with liver disease can more quickly develop hypocalcemia and hypomagnesemia, which then increases their risk of cardiac dysrhythmias.

Blood products are given rapidly during MTP, so hemodynamic monitoring and clinical assessments, rather than laboratory studies, should be used to determine the end points of resuscitation. MTP should be stopped when patients become hemodynamically stable, after which laboratory tests can be run, including tests for coagulation factors, fibrinogen values, blood counts, and electrolyte levels that include ionized calcium. For patients with critical bleeding, the platelet level goal is at least 50,000 platelets/μL, especially before a procedure. In general, a restrictive transfusion strategy with a target hemoglobin level of 7 g/dL is used because overshooting the hemoglobin level can hasten bleeding, especially with variceal bleeds. If available, viscoelastic testing can provide useful information for more targeted transfusion end points. Patients should also be reassessed frequently to evaluate for improvement or decompensation, including examining body temperature, volume status, and signs of poor end-organ perfusion such as decreased mental status or decreased urinary output (these patients are at high risk of going into renal failure).

Anticoagulant	Reversal
Warfarin	Vitamin K 10 mg IV plus prothrombin complex concentrate (PCC) or FFP
Dabigatran	Idarucizumab 5 g
Argatroban, bivalirudin	PCC
Factor Xa inhibitors (rivaroxaban, apixaban, edoxaban)	4-factor PCC or andexanet alfa if available
Low-molecular-weight heparins (LMWH)	Protamine
Antiplatelet agents	Desmopressin acetate (DDAVP) and TXA (if needed)

TABLE 2. Approach to anticoagulant reversal[11]

CRITICAL DECISION

Do diagnostic and therapeutic management differ based on the etiology of bleeding?

Ideally, the ICU should manage patients with an unstable GI bleed. However, while patients are in the emergency department, disposition can be aided by emergency physicians mobilizing the correct consultants, such as interventional radiology, gastroenterology, and surgery. In the event of refractory bleeding, emergency physicians can place a balloon tamponade as a further temporizing measure until treatment from specialty services is available. Although not a definitive therapy, physicians should be familiar with each of the different balloon tamponade kits available (*Figure 1*). The Sengstaken-Blakemore tube has a 250-mL gastric balloon, an esophageal balloon, and one suction port; the Minnesota tube is similar to the Sengstaken-Blakemore but has an extra suction port; and the Linton-Nachlas tube has one 600-mL gastric balloon. Before using balloon tamponades, patients should be intubated, and their pain should be adequately controlled.

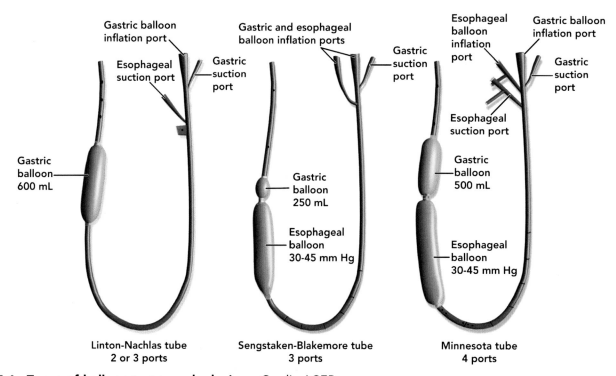

FIGURE 1. Types of balloon tamponade devices. *Credit: ACEP.*

After gathering supplies and inspecting the kit, place the tamponade tube next to a nasogastric (NG) or orogastric (OG) tube (if not already placed in the patient during intubation) and mark the NG or OG tube where the tip sits proximal to the gastric balloon of the tamponade tube. Mark the tamponade device around 50 cm and insert it so that the gastric balloon is in the stomach and not the esophagus to avoid perforation. Use a portable x-ray machine at bedside to verify the tamponade's location below the diaphragm before inflating and when beginning to inflate the gastric balloon with 50 mL of air; once the location is confirmed, fully inflate the gastric balloon (*Figure 2*). Clamp the port used for inflation and create a setup to maintain traction and prevent the balloon from pulling back against the gastric fundus — 250 to 500 grams of weight is usually enough to create tension.[1] Note the tube's measurement at the patient's teeth. The gastric port can then be placed for suction. If the NG or OG tube was marked before insertion, it can be positioned to localize esophageal bleeding. Place the NG or OG tube to the suction, and if ongoing bleeding is detected, the esophageal balloon needs to be inflated next by using a manometer attached to a three-way stopcock. Inflate the balloon to a goal pressure of 25 mm Hg and clamp the port. The balloon tamponade can be left in place for 24 to 48 hours until the appropriate medical teams are mobilized or the patient is transferred to a facility with the required specialty services.

Getting consultants involved in managing an upper GI bleed as soon as possible can influence patient outcomes. Endoscopy is typically the first step toward determining the etiology of the upper GI bleed. The American College of Gastroenterology (ACG) no longer follows the 2012 recommendation of considering endoscopy within 12 hours after presentation; it now recommends endoscopy within 24 hours after presentation and an administration of erythromycin infusion immediately prior to the procedure. Erythromycin is a prokinetic agent that can improve the diagnostic yield of endoscopy by improving visualization and decreasing the need for repeat endoscopies.[9]

Treatments for upper GI bleeds differ depending on whether the etiology is variceal or nonvariceal. Procedures for variceal bleeding include ligation, sclerotherapy, and obturation. Endoscopic ligation is typically the preferred first step in management. In certain cases of refractory bleeding, esophageal stents have also been used.[15] Although treating bleeding gastric varices can be more difficult than treating esophageal varices, both types of patients are at a high risk of rebleeding. Variceal size and appearance as well as the extent of liver disease are all factors that affect the severity of bleeding. A transjugular intrahepatic portosystemic shunt (TIPS) is often the next step if

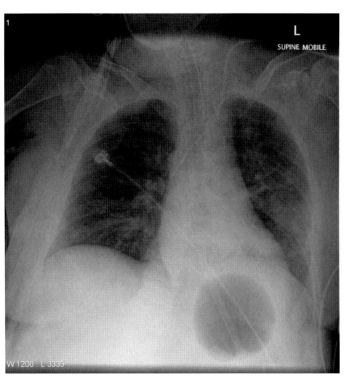

FIGURE 2. Chest x-ray demonstrating a Sengstaken-Blakemore tube in situ. *Credit:* Copyright 2023 Frank Gaillard. Image courtesy of Frank Gaillard and Radiopaedia.org, rID: 12118. Used under license.

ligation fails. TIPS is meant to reverse portal hypertension by shunting the portal system to the systemic circulation; however, diverting the portal system sometimes requires surgical shunting.

Guidelines have also expanded for nonvariceal upper GI bleeds. Endoscopic therapy fails when bleeding persists. Indicators of potential recurrent bleeds include, but are not limited to, the following: new melena or hematochezia after stool color returned to normal, large drops in hemoglobin levels, hemodynamic instability without a better explanation, or new or recurrent hematemesis several hours after the first endoscopy.[16] If initial endoscopic therapy appears to have failed, a subsequent endoscopy can be performed unless there is an urgent indication for surgery.[9] Another option after failed endoscopy is transcatheter arterial embolization (TAE), if appropriate and if resources allow. TAE is associated with fewer complications and shorter hospital stays compared to surgical treatment.[9]

CT angiography (CTA) also carries a diagnostic and therapeutic role and may be more appropriate than endoscopy, depending on the etiology of the bleed and whether interventional radiology or surgery will be needed for treatment. In the event of catastrophic or rapid bleeding, CTA can visualize an area of active extravasation. Surgical interventions also still play a role in some cases of upper GI bleeding, especially if endoscopy is unavailable, if less invasive therapies have failed, or if concomitant issues like surgical abdomen are occurring. Surgery specialists should be involved early as part of the team approach for cases of massive bleeding and persistent hemodynamic instability.

By contrast, a subset of patients with upper GI bleeds can present with less severe symptoms. Their presentation may include an isolated episode of hematemesis or melena or small volumes of blood produced. The physical examination is crucial for distinguishing stable from unstable patients. Signs indicative of more severe, life-threatening bleeds include vital signs that worsen or are already consistent with hemorrhagic shock, lethargy, and declining mental status. Some patients who are deemed low risk are discharged and managed as

✖ Pitfalls

- Failing to facilitate a multidisciplinary approach. Specialists should be contacted as early as possible, so the source of upper GI bleeding can be identified and treated.
- Providing overly aggressive crystalloid fluid resuscitation instead of resuscitation with blood products early on.
- Inadequately managing complications such as electrolyte abnormalities or hypothermia, which can hasten coagulopathy in critically ill patients.
- Failing to correct hypoxemia, hypotension, and acidosis as best as possible prior to intubation.

CASE ONE

This unstable patient was found to have an upper GI bleed. He had the classic stigmata of cirrhosis, including scleral icterus and a distended abdomen secondary to ascites. Hemodynamic instability and altered mental status suggested hemorrhagic shock. Initial assessment focused on the airway, breathing, and circulation. He was placed on a monitor, and two 18-gauge intravenous catheters were secured. Intubation was successfully performed while the first two units of PRBCs were transfused; this transfusion only briefly augmented his blood pressure, so a norepinephrine infusion was started to maintain an adequate MAP while awaiting further blood products. After intubation, he was given a pantoprazole bolus, an octreotide bolus followed by the infusion, and ceftriaxone. Gastroenterology was consulted to facilitate definitive management, and the patient was admitted to the ICU.

CASE TWO

This patient had developed an upper GI bleed. Her GBS was 0, which suggested she could be safely discharged. After the physician discussed her results with her, they agreed on discharge plans. The patient had a caretaker for assistance and no barriers to outpatient medical care. She agreed to close follow-up with a gastroenterologist.

CASE THREE

After placement of the balloon tamponade, the patient's blood pressure and heart rate stabilized. He was continuously monitored and transferred to the ICU shortly thereafter, where he awaited an emergent GI evaluation and further steps for definitive management.

outpatients. The Glasgow-Blatchford bleeding score (GBS) is one of the clinical decision-making tools used to risk stratify patients with upper GI bleeds. It is calculated using variables that include serum BUN levels, hemoglobin levels, systolic blood pressure, heart rate, physical examination findings, and comorbidities.[17,18] A score of 0 places patients in a low-risk category that makes outpatient treatment more appropriate; higher scores (up to 23) can detect patients who need further intervention such as transfusions, endoscopy, or other procedures.[19] Other important factors to consider when making discharge plans include patients' perspectives on being discharged, their ability to access prompt outpatient GI follow-up and take a daily PPI in the interim, the stability of their vital signs, and any significant comorbidities that may be a barrier to discharge.

Summary

Emergency department presentations of upper GI bleeding can range from stable to catastrophic. Early preparation, setup, and aggressive fluid resuscitation are the most important steps to begin managing upper GI bleeds. Emergency physicians play an important role in initiating adequate intravenous access, protecting the airway, and detecting and managing hemorrhagic shock with adequate volume resuscitation and vasopressor support, as needed, in these patients. Controlling the source of bleeding is imperative, and ACG guidelines now recommend an endoscopy within 24 hours of patient presentation. From diagnostics and orchestrating a multidisciplinary team approach to therapeutics and disposition, emergency physicians must be adept at identifying and managing upper GI bleeds.

REFERENCES

1. Mihata RGK, Bonk JA, Keville MP. Resuscitation of the patient with massive upper gastrointestinal bleeding. *EM Critical Care.* 2013;3(2):1-12.
2. Nguyen T. Upper GI bleeding. In: Mattu A, Swadron S, eds. *CorePendium.* Updated January 18, 2022. https://www.emrap.org/corependium/chapter/recBREJHrprcRlvRg/Upper-GI-Bleeding
3. Butler K, Winters M. The physiologically difficult intubation. *Emerg Med Clin North Am.* 2022 Aug;40(3):615-627.
4. Reddick AD, Ronald J, Morrison WG. Intravenous fluid resuscitation: was Poiseuille right? *Emerg Med J.* 2011 Mar;28(3):201-202.
5. HALT-IT Trial Collaborators. Effects of a high-dose 24-h infusion of tranexamic acid on death and thromboembolic events in patients with acute gastrointestinal bleeding (HALT-IT): an international randomised, double-blind, placebo-controlled trial. *Lancet.* 2020 Jun 20;395(10241):1927-1936.
6. Parker BK, Manning S, Winters ME. The crashing obese patient. *West J Emerg Med.* 2019 Mar;20(2):323-330.
7. DuCanto J, Serrano KD, Thompson RJ. Novel airway training tool that simulates vomiting: suction-assisted laryngoscopy assisted decontamination (SALAD) system. *West J Emerg Med.* 2017 Jan;18(1):117-120.
8. Chavez-Tapia NC, Barrientos-Gutierrez T, Tellez-Avila F, et al. Meta-analysis: antibiotic prophylaxis for cirrhotic patients with upper gastrointestinal bleeding – an updated Cochrane review. *Aliment Pharmacol Ther.* 2011 Sep;34(5):509-518.
9. Loren L, Barkun AN, Saltzman JR, Martel M, Leontiadis GI. ACG clinical guideline: upper gastrointestinal and ulcer bleeding. *Am J Gastroenterol.* 2021 May 1;116(5):899-917.
10. Garcia-Tsao G, Bosch J. Management of varices and variceal hemorrhage in cirrhosis. *NEJM.* 2010 Mar 4;362(9):823-832.
11. Farkas J. Anticoagulant reversal. The Internet Book of Critical Care. Published September 25, 2021. https://emcrit.org/ibcc/reverse
12. Moskoff J. Transfusion reactions and complications. In: Wolfson A, Cloutier RL, Hendey GW, et al, eds. *Harwood-Nuss' Clinical Practice of Emergency Medicine.* 7th ed. Wolters Kluwer; 2021:1015-1019.
13. Davis JE, Isserman J. Anemia and transfusion. In: Mattu A, Swadron S, eds. *CorePendium.* Updated October 14, 2022. https://www.emrap.org/corependium/chapter/rec5IV3F4iDi4fk5f/Anemia-and-Transfusion
14. Flint AWJ, McQuilten ZK, Wood EM. Massive transfusions for critical bleeding: is everything old new again? *Transfus Med.* 2018 Apr;28(2):140-149.
15. Gralnek IM, Duboc MC, Garcia-Pagan JC, et al. Endoscopic diagnosis and management of esophagogastric variceal hemorrhage: European Society of Gastrointestinal Endoscopy (ESGE) Guideline. *Endoscopy.* 2022 Nov;54(11):1094-1120.
16. Laine L, Spiegel B, Rostom A, et al. Methodology for randomized trials of patients with nonvariceal upper gastrointestinal bleeding: recommendations from an international consensus conference. *Am J Gastroenterol.* 2010 Mar;105(3):540-550.
17. Simon TG, Travis AC, Saltzman JR. Initial assessment and resuscitation in nonvariceal upper gastrointestinal bleeding. *Gastrointest Endosc Clin N Am.* 2015 Jul;25(3):429-442.
18. Chen I-C, Hung M-S, Chiu T-F, Chen J-C, Hsiao C-T. Risk scoring systems to predict need for clinical intervention for patients with nonvariceal upper gastrointestinal tract bleeding. *Am J Emerg Med.* 2007 Sep;25(7):774-779.
19. Stanley AJ, Ashley D, Dalton HR, et al. Outpatient management of patients with low-risk upper-gastrointestinal haemorrhage: multicentre validation and prospective evaluation. *Lancet.* 2009 Jan 3;373(9657):42-47.

MDCALC REFERENCE

Glasgow-Blatchford bleeding score. MDCalc. https://www.mdcalc.com/calc/518/glasgow-blatchford-bleeding-score-gbs

CME Questions

Reviewed by Nathaniel Mann, MD; and Amal Mattu, MD, FACEP

Qualified, paid subscribers to *Critical Decisions in Emergency Medicine* may receive CME certificates for up to 5 ACEP Category I credits, 5 *AMA PRA Category 1 Credits*™, and 5 AOA Category 2-B credits for completing this activity in its entirety. Submit your answers online at acep.org/cdem; a score of 75% or better is required. You may receive credit for completing the CME activity any time within 3 years of its publication date. Answers to this month's questions will be published in next month's issue.

1 Following an initial phase of disease that is characterized by nonspecific respiratory symptoms, which biologic weapon rapidly progresses to a second phase of disease that is characterized by respiratory failure?
   A. *Bacillus anthracis*
   B. *Francisella tularensis*
   C. Viral hemorrhagic fevers
   D. *Yersinia pestis*

2 Antibody-based antitoxins are approved by the FDA for treatment of which pathogen?
   A. *Bacillus anthracis*
   B. *Francisella tularensis*
   C. *Lassa mammarenavirus*
   D. *Yersinia pestis*

3 Which biologic warfare agent requires contact precautions?
   A. *Bacillus anthracis*
   B. *Francisella tularensis*
   C. *Yersinia pestis*
   D. *Zaire ebolavirus*

4 A 28-year-old man presents for the second time in a week. He was initially discharged with a presumed diagnosis of a viral syndrome. He returns with a widened mediastinum on chest x-ray and requires intubation. In the setting of a possible biologic warfare attack, what antibiotic regimen is most likely to treat the responsible pathogen?
   A. Ciprofloxacin
   B. Streptomycin
   C. Vancomycin and cefepime
   D. Vancomycin and piperacillin-tazobactam

5 Which biologic warfare agent rapidly replicates in regional lymph nodes and causes suppurative necrotic granulomas?
   A. *Bacillus anthracis*
   B. *Francisella tularensis*
   C. Viral hemorrhagic fevers
   D. *Yersinia pestis*

6 A landscaper presents with gradual-onset respiratory symptoms and pleuritic chest pain. His vital signs are BP 142/86, P 64, R 28, and T 40.2°C (104.3°F); SpO$_2$ is 90% on room air. What finding on his chest x-ray is to be expected?
   A. Diffuse ground-glass opacifications
   B. Lobar opacification
   C. Pleural effusions and perihilar lymphadenopathy
   D. Widened mediastinum

7 Which pathogen can reliably be identified within 48 hours by standard blood cultures performed in most microbiology laboratories in the United States?
   A. *Bacillus anthracis*
   B. *Francisella tularensis*
   C. Viral hemorrhagic fevers
   D. *Yersinia pestis*

8 Which specimen is least likely to grow colonies of *Francisella tularensis*?
   A. Blood
   B. Gastric aspirates
   C. Pharyngeal washings
   D. Sputum

9 A 23-year-old female nurse presents with a petechial rash, scattered ecchymoses, diffuse myalgia, and severe diarrhea. She recently returned from a medical mission trip to Sierra Leone. Her vital signs are BP 84/46, P 118, R 28, and T 38.4°C (101.1°F); SpO$_2$ is 94% on room air. In addition to supportive therapy, which medication is strongly recommended by the WHO for treatment of this patient's illness?
   A. Nirmatrelvir
   B. Oseltamivir phosphate
   C. Ribavirin
   D. Sofosbuvir

10 A 62-year-old man is intubated in the emergency department for acute respiratory distress syndrome. The following day, his blood cultures grow gram-negative coccobacilli, and the patient receives broad-spectrum antibiotics. Unfortunately, laboratory values are consistent with disseminated intravascular coagulation, and the patient develops digital necrosis and diffuse ecchymoses. What type of isolation precautions are appropriate?
   A. Airborne
   B. Contact
   C. Droplet
   D. Standard

11 What is the most common cause of upper GI bleeding?
   A. Aortoenteric fistula
   B. Duodenal ulcers
   C. Gastritis
   D. Varices

12 **Which access method is the most rapid for administering blood products (to gravity without pressure)?**
    A. 16-gauge intravenous catheter
    B. Intraosseous catheter
    C. Single lumen sheath introducer
    D. Triple lumen central venous catheter

13 **Which is most commonly associated with peptic ulcer disease?**
    A. Alcohol use
    B. Dieulafoy lesions
    C. Gastric cancer
    D. NSAID use

14 **What electrolyte abnormality can occur in critically ill patients during rapid, massive blood transfusions?**
    A. Hypercalcemia
    B. Hyperkalemia
    C. Hypocalcemia
    D. Hypokalemia

15 **Which clinical scenario raises suspicion for a perforated viscus?**
    A. 32-year-old woman with sudden onset abdominal pain that is associated with unrelenting nausea and intermittent vomiting
    B. 39-year-old woman with 4 days of right lower quadrant abdominal pain, vomiting, and fevers
    C. 45-year-old woman with 3 days of severe gnawing abdominal pain, vomit that is dark in color, and abdominal guarding
    D. 65-year-old woman with 3 days of diffuse abdominal pain that she noticed after eating and that is out of proportion to her physical examination

16 **A 56-year-old man with a history of progressive nonischemic cardiomyopathy that required a left ventricular assist device 1 year ago is awaiting cardiac transplantation. He takes warfarin and hydralazine. He presents after four large bowel movements today that he describes as black, tarry, and sometimes maroon; a low-flow alarm prompted him to call 911. On examination, he is diaphoretic, and a manual mean arterial pressure is difficult to obtain. A mechanical hum is heard over the precordium. His respiratory rate is 20, and his SpO$_2$ is 98% on room air. A large-volume GI bleed is suspected. What is the best next step in managing his condition?**
    A. Administer a 4-factor prothrombin complex concentrate
    B. Place an arterial line
    C. Start a norepinephrine infusion
    D. Transfuse 2 units of uncrossmatched packed RBCs

17 **What intervention in upper GI bleeding has been shown to have a mortality benefit for patients with cirrhosis?**
    A. Ceftriaxone
    B. Octreotide
    C. Pantoprazole
    D. Platelets

18 **A patient with an unstable GI bleed has ongoing hematemesis. The emergency physician decides to secure the patient's airway because they anticipate a decline in the patient's clinical course and mental status. After a nasogastric tube is placed to decompress the patient's stomach, 300 mL of output that has the appearance of coffee grounds is collected. About 30 minutes later, the patient remains hypoxemic, with an SpO$_2$ of 82% despite maximal FiO$_2$, and has equal breath sounds on auscultation. What is the best next step?**
    A. Disconnect from the ventilator and use bag-valve-mask ventilation
    B. Increase the positive end-expiratory pressure (PEEP)
    C. Increase the tidal volume
    D. Withdraw the endotracheal tube by 2 cm

19 **A 49-year-old woman presents after having a "black and sticky" bowel movement. Her vital signs include BP 148/77, P 82, and R 13; SpO$_2$ is 98% on room air. She has been previously diagnosed with progressive liver disease secondary to alcohol use disorder. Which laboratory abnormality is most likely?**
    A. Decreased albumin level
    B. Decreased prothrombin time
    C. Elevated ALT that is greater than AST
    D. Low mean corpuscular volume

20 **A 55-year-old man with a history of alcohol use disorder presents with multiple episodes of "coffee-ground" emesis. On examination, he has scleral icterus, gynecomastia, and a distended abdomen. Vital signs include BP 91/68, P 107, and R 15; SpO$_2$ is 98% on room air. Laboratory results are notable for a hemoglobin level of 8 g/dL, a platelet level of 34,000 cells/µL, an INR of 1.0, a PT of 16 sec, an ALT of 84 IU/L, an AST of 75 IU/L, and an alkaline phosphatase level of 82 IU/L. In addition to volume resuscitation, what would be most beneficial for the patient at this time?**
    A. Ciprofloxacin
    B. Nasogastric tube
    C. Octreotide
    D. Pantoprazole

ANSWER KEY FOR MARCH 2023, VOLUME 37, NUMBER 3

1	2	3	4	5	6	7	8	9	10	11	12	13	14	15	16	17	18	19	20
D	B	C	A	D	A	B	B	A	C	C	C	D	A	B	A	D	B	D	B

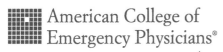

American College of Emergency Physicians®

ADVANCING EMERGENCY CARE

Post Office Box 619911
Dallas, Texas 75261-9911

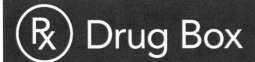

Fomepizole in APAP-Induced Liver Injury

By Ashley Jackson, PharmD; and
Frank LoVecchio, DO, MPH, FACEP
Valleywise Health Medical Center and ASU, Phoenix, Arizona

Objective
On completion of this column, you should be able to:
■ Describe the indications for fomepizole in APAP overdose.

Background
Acetaminophen (APAP) is a readily available, nonopioid analgesic and antipyretic that is considered safe at therapeutic levels. Accidental and intentional overdoses are a significant concern because of APAP-induced hepatoxicity.

At therapeutic levels, APAP is metabolized in the liver by glucuronidation, sulfation, or the cytochrome P450 enzyme CYP2E1. Only a small portion of APAP is metabolized through CYP2E1 (<10%) to form the reactive metabolite N-acetyl-p-benzoquinone imine (NAPQI). With therapeutic dosing, NAPQI toxicity is avoided because it readily conjugates with glutathione (GSH) to create mercapturic acid.

When toxicity occurs, the GSH pathway becomes saturated, depleting GSH and leaving extensive amounts of NAPQI. NAPQI then binds to the cytosol and mitochondria, which ultimately leads to the phosphorylation of c-Jun N-terminal kinase (JNK). The phosphorylated JNK amplifies the formation of mitochondrial superoxides that will react with nitric oxide and generate peroxynitrite, the final oxidant responsible for APAP toxicity.

N-acetylcysteine (NAC) is the only FDA-approved treatment for APAP toxicity and is most effective when used within 8 hours of ingestion. NAC serves as a glutathione substitute that binds to NAPQI to create the nontoxic mercapturic acid that is excreted from the body.

NAC's efficacy is reduced in patients who present later for treatment, but fomepizole has been shown to be of use in these patients or patients who have ingested more than 30 to 40 g of APAP. Fomepizole acts as a CYP2E1 inhibitor and prevents the formation of all oxidative metabolites. It also inhibits the activation of JNK in the mitochondria. Based on these mechanistic findings, fomepizole decreases the amount of peroxynitrite and prevents severe or acute liver failure. Animal studies and case studies in humans suggest fomepizole is a beneficial adjunct antidote for APAP overdose, but controlled clinical trials are needed to support its efficacy.

Uses
■ Acetaminophen overdose, adjunct
■ Ethylene glycol or methanol toxicity

Dosing
15 mg/kg, followed by 10 mg/kg every 12 hours as needed

REFERENCES

Akakpo JY, Ramachandran A, Curry SC, Rumack BH, Jaeschke H. Comparing N-acetylcysteine and 4-methylpyrazole as antidotes for acetaminophen overdose. *Arch Toxicol.* 2022 Feb;96(2):453-465.

Jaeschke H, Akakpo JY, Umbaugh DS, Ramachandran A. Novel therapeutic approaches against acetaminophen-induced liver injury and acute liver failure. *Toxicol Sci.* 2020 Apr 1;174(2):159-167.

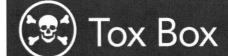

Hydrogen Peroxide Ingestion

By Christian A. Tomaszewski, MD, MS, MBA, FACEP
University of California San Diego Health

Objective
On completion of this column, you should be able to:
■ State how to treat hydrogen peroxide ingestions.

Introduction
Hydrogen peroxide is available in a diluted (3%-5%) solution for medicinal and household use and in a concentrated (10%-35%) solution for bleaching and sterilizing (ie, food grade). Although typically innocuous, ingestions of concentrated or massive amounts of dilute solution can lead to serious GI and neurologic complications.

Mechanism of Action
■ Local tissue injury (oxidizer), irritant or caustic (depending on the concentration)
■ Liberation of oxygen with embolization (10 mL of 35% can liberate approximately 1 L of gas)

Toxicity
■ Sips of household grade products (<3%) are usually nontoxic.
■ Massive ingestions of dilute (<10%) or any concentrated products (>10%) can lead to caustic injury and gas embolism.

Clinical Manifestations
■ ***GI:*** vomiting, irritation, erosions, gas embolism
■ ***Cardiac:*** hypotension, infarction
■ ***Pulmonary:*** lung injury with massive ingestions
■ ***Metabolic:*** acidosis
■ ***CNS:*** seizures, strokes

Diagnostics
■ Chest x-ray and kidney-bladder-ureter x-ray may reveal GI gas if symptomatic
■ Endoscopy for symptomatic cases after high-volume or high-concentration ingestions
■ Brain CT or MRI for neurologic abnormalities
■ Abdominal CT or ultrasound for pain (can diagnose portal venous emboli)

Treatment
■ Maintain the patient flat or in Trendelenburg position if portal gas is suspected
■ Intubate for upper airway obstruction
■ Nasogastric tube for gastric decompression
■ Endoscopy for signs of GI injury
■ IV benzodiazepines for seizures
■ Hyperbaric oxygen for arterial gas embolism, if neurologic findings

Disposition
■ At-home observation for asymptomatic ingestions of dilute products
■ Further observation and diagnostic workup for symptomatic ingestions, especially of concentrated products

Critical decisions
in emergency medicine

Volume 37 Number 5: **May 2023**

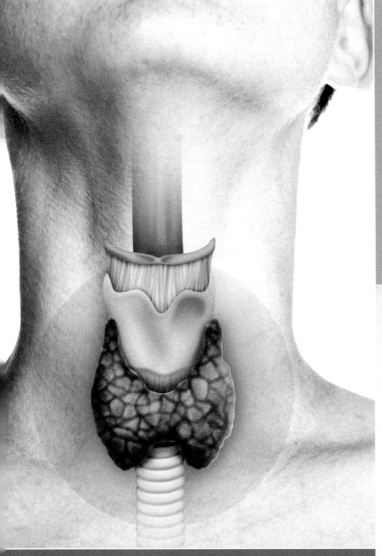

Under the Weather

Thyroid storm is a rare but deadly form of hyperthyroidism that can be easily overlooked by even the most experienced physician. Diagnosing the condition can be extremely difficult because its symptoms are nonspecific and can mimic many other pathologies. Emergency physicians must be aware of thyroid storm's presentation and initial management steps to avoid potential multiorgan failure.

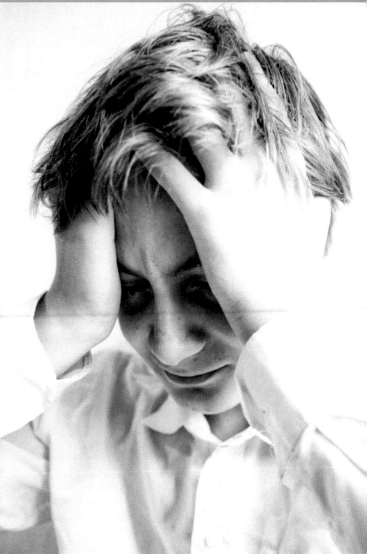

Head Scratcher

More than half of children and adolescents experience a headache at some point in their lifetime. Although most pediatric headaches are benign, some are indicators of a potentially fatal illness. Emergency physicians must recognize the red flags that can point to life-threatening causes of headaches, such as brain tumors and meningitis.

THE OFFICIAL CME PUBLICATION OF THE AMERICAN COLLEGE OF EMERGENCY PHYSICIANS

Individuals in Control of Content

1. Muhammad Ramdhan Abd Aziz, MD, MMed – Faculty
2. Jeremy Berberian, MD – Faculty
3. William J. Brady, MD, FACEP — Faculty
4. Alan Chan, MD – Faculty
5. Avery Elifritz, DO – Faculty
6. Rosemary Mallonée, MD — Faculty
7. Chang Woo Park, MD – Faculty
8. Jeremiah Duane Smith, MD, FAAP – Faculty
9. Allen Williams, MD – Faculty
10. Michael Platzer, DO, LT, MC, USN – Faculty
11. Daphne Morrison Ponce, MD, CDR, MC, USN – Faculty
12. Joshua S. Broder, MD, FACEP – Faculty/Planner
13. Ann M. Dietrich, MD, FAAP, FACEP – Faculty/Planner
14. Kelsey Drake, MD, MPH, FACEP – Faculty/Planner
15. Andrew J. Eyre, MD, MS-HPEd – Faculty/Planner
16. John Kiel, DO, MPH, FACEP, CAQSM – Faculty/Planner
17. Frank LoVecchio, DO, MPH, FACEP – Faculty/Planner
18. Sharon E. Mace, MD, FACEP – Faculty/Planner
19. Nathaniel Mann, MD – Faculty/Planner
20. Amal Mattu, MD, FACEP – Faculty/Planner
21. Christian A. Tomaszewski, MD, MS, MBA, FACEP – Faculty/Planner
22. Steven J. Warrington, MD, MEd, MS – Faculty/Planner
23. Tareq Al-Salamah, MBBS, MPH, FACEP – Planner
24. Michael S. Beeson, MD, MBA, FACEP – Planner
25. Wan-Tsu Chang, MD – Planner
26. Walter L. Green, MD, FACEP – Planner
27. John C. Greenwood, MD – Planner
28. Danya Khoujah, MBBS, MEHP, FACEP – Planner
29. George Sternbach, MD, FACEP – Planner
30. Joy Carrico, JD – Planner/Reviewer

Contributor Disclosures. In accordance with the ACCME Standards for Integrity and Independence in Accredited Continuing Education, all relevant financial relationships, and the absence of relevant financial relationships, must be disclosed to learners for all individuals in control of content 1) before learners engage with the accredited education, and 2) in a format that can be verified at the time of accreditation. The following individuals have reported relationships with ineligible companies, as defined by the ACCME. These relationships, in the context of their involvement in the CME activity, could be perceived by some as a real or apparent conflict of interest. All relevant financial relationships have been mitigated to ensure that no commercial bias has been inserted into the educational content. Joshua S. Broder, MD, FACEP, is a founder and president of OmniSono Inc, an ultrasound technology company, and a consultant on the Bayer USA Cardiac Imaging Advisory Board. Sharon E. Mace, MD, FACEP, performs contracted research funded by Biofire Corporation, Genetesis, Quidel, and IBSA Pharma. Frank LoVecchio, DO, MPH, FACEP, receives speaking fees from ABBVIE for antibiotics. Christian A. Tomaszewski, MD, MS, MBA, FACEP does contracted research (Roche, Pfizer, AstraZeneca — Site PI with financial support provided to institution). All remaining individuals with control over content have no relevant financial relationships to disclose.

This educational activity consists of two lessons, eight feature articles, a post-test, and evaluation questions; as designed, the activity should take approximately 5 hours to complete. The participant should, in order, review the learning objectives for the lesson or article, read the lesson or article as published in the print or online version until all have been reviewed, and then complete the online post-test (a minimum score of 75% is required) and evaluation questions. Release date: May 1, 2023. Expiration date: April 30, 2026.

Accreditation Statement. The American College of Emergency Physicians is accredited by the Accreditation Council for Continuing Medical Education to provide continuing medical education for physicians.

The American College of Emergency Physicians designates this enduring material for a maximum of 5 *AMA PRA Category 1 Credits™*. Physicians should claim only the credit commensurate with the extent of their participation in the activity.

Each issue of *Critical Decisions in Emergency Medicine* is approved by ACEP for 5 ACEP Category I credits. Approved by the AOA for 5 Category 2-B credits.

Commercial Support. There was no commercial support for this CME activity.

Target Audience. This educational activity has been developed for emergency physicians.

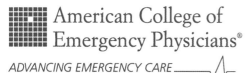

American College of Emergency Physicians®

ADVANCING EMERGENCY CARE

Critical decisions
in emergency medicine

Critical Decisions in Emergency Medicine is the official CME publication of the American College of Emergency Physicians. Additional volumes are available.

EDITOR-IN-CHIEF

Michael S. Beeson, MD, MBA, FACEP
Northeastern Ohio Universities, Rootstown, OH

SECTION EDITORS

Joshua S. Broder, MD, FACEP
Duke University, Durham, NC

Andrew J. Eyre, MD, MS-HPEd
Brigham and Women's Hospital/Harvard Medical School, Boston, MA

John Kiel, DO, MPH, FACEP, CAQSM
University of Florida College of Medicine, Jacksonville, FL

Frank LoVecchio, DO, MPH, FACEP
Valleywise, Arizona State University, University of Arizona, and Creighton Colleges of Medicine, Phoenix, AZ

Sharon E. Mace, MD, FACEP
Cleveland Clinic Lerner College of Medicine/Case Western Reserve University, Cleveland, OH

Amal Mattu, MD, FACEP
University of Maryland, Baltimore, MD

Christian A. Tomaszewski, MD, MS, MBA, FACEP
University of California Health Sciences, San Diego, CA

Steven J. Warrington, MD, MEd, MS
MercyOne Siouxland, Sioux City, IA

ASSOCIATE EDITORS

Tareq Al-Salamah, MBBS, MPH, FACEP
King Saud University, Riyadh, Saudi Arabia/University of Maryland, Baltimore, MD

Wan-Tsu Chang, MD
University of Maryland, Baltimore, MD

Ann M. Dietrich, MD, FAAP, FACEP
University of South Carolina College of Medicine, Greenville, SC

Kelsey Drake, MD, MPH, FACEP
St. Anthony Hospital, Lakewood, CO

Walter L. Green, MD, FACEP
UT Southwestern Medical Center, Dallas, TX

John C. Greenwood, MD
University of Pennsylvania, Philadelphia, PA

Danya Khoujah, MBBS, MEHP, FACEP
University of Maryland, Baltimore, MD

Nathaniel Mann, MD
Greenville Health System, Greenville, SC

George Sternbach, MD, FACEP
Stanford University Medical Center, Stanford, CA

EDITORIAL STAFF

Suzannah Alexander, Editorial Director
salexander@acep.org

Joy Carrico, JD
Managing Editor

Alex Bass
Assistant Editor

Kyle Powell
Graphic Artist

ISSN2325-0186 (Print)   ISSN2325-8365 (Online)

Contents

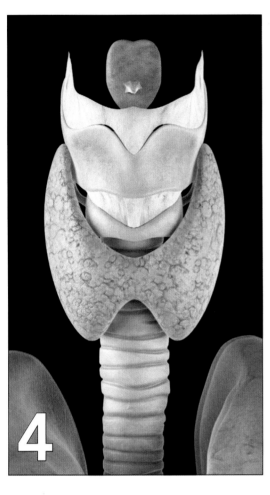

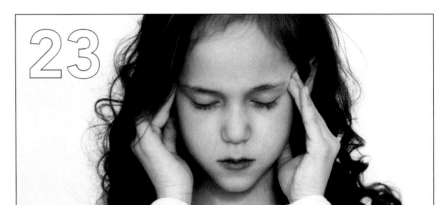

FEATURES

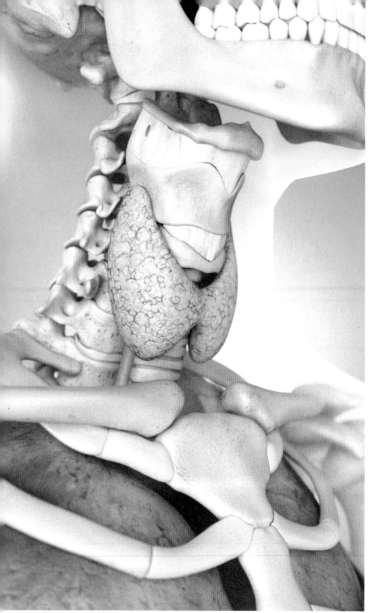

Under the Weather

Thyroid Storm in the Emergency Department

LESSON 9

By Avery Elifritz, DO; Chang Woo Park, MD; and Allen Williams, MD

Dr. Elifritz and Dr. Park are emergency medicine residents at The University of Toledo in Ohio. Dr. Williams is an assistant professor of emergency medicine at The University of Toledo.

Reviewed by Kelsey Drake, MD, MPH, FACEP

Objectives

On completion of this lesson, you should be able to:

1. Distinguish between the symptoms of hyperthyroidism and thyroid storm.
2. Identify patients who are at a high risk of clinical deterioration from thyroid storm.
3. Use the BWPS to predict thyroid storm.
4. Name the causative pathologies and appropriate treatments for thyroid storm.
5. Describe complications of thyroid storm.
6. State the evidence-based guidelines for effectively managing thyroid storm.

From the EM Model

5.0 Endocrine, Metabolic, and Nutritional Disorders
    5.8 Thyroid Disorders
        5.8.4 Thyroid Storm

▬ CRITICAL DECISIONS ▬

- What is the pathophysiology of thyroid storm?

- How is thyroid storm recognized and diagnosed?

- What factors can lead to thyroid storm?

- What comorbidities can develop during emergency care of thyroid storm?

- What blood work and imaging should be obtained in patients with thyroid storm?

- What is the initial management of thyroid storm in the emergency department?

Thyroid storm is a rare but deadly form of hyperthyroidism that can be easily overlooked by even the most experienced physician. Diagnosing the condition can be extremely difficult because its symptoms are nonspecific and can mimic many other pathologies. Emergency physicians must be aware of thyroid storm's presentation and initial management steps to avoid potential multiorgan failure.

■ CASE ONE

A 22-year-old woman presents with left lower quadrant abdominal pain. On examination, she is severely agitated, so her husband supplies her history. She has been in pain for around 12 hours and has never experienced anything like this before. She is also approximately 6 weeks pregnant and is having vaginal bleeding, causing them to worry about a miscarriage. Prenatal care has not yet started. She recently stopped taking her thyroid medication after reading online that it can harm babies.

Her vital signs are BP 84/52, P 163, R 26, and T 39.1°C (102.3°F); SpO$_2$ is 99% on room air. Her physical examination is remarkable for diaphoresis and agitation. She is oriented to name and place but not to month. She has significant tenderness in the left lower and right upper quadrants as well as a mild amount of vaginal bleeding.

■ CASE TWO

An 83-year-old man presents with altered mental status, generalized weakness, fatigue, and respiratory distress over the past 24 hours. He is accompanied by his two children who say that he is not himself and seems off. Based on prior infections and symptoms, they think he may have a urinary tract infection or pneumonia again. They also state that he has lost a significant amount of weight in the last 3 months. The patient could not supply any further history due to his acute mental status changes.

His vital signs are BP 102/72, P 136, R 28, and T 38.4°C (101.1°F); SpO$_2$ is 92% on 2 L of oxygen via nasal cannula. Physical examination reveals a disheveled man who minimally participates in the examination. He is awake and alert but does not follow commands. His neck examination is notable for a goiter, and he is jaundiced and has a fine tremor. Cardiopulmonary auscultation is remarkable for tachycardia, an irregularly irregular rhythm, tachypnea, and bibasilar rales. His work of breathing is slightly increased, but he does not appear to be in respiratory distress. He also has bipedal edema.

■ CASE THREE

A 23-year-old man presents as a level II trauma activation patient 30 minutes after a motor vehicle collision in which he was the restrained passenger. On arrival, the patient's primary survey is largely negative. His Glasgow Coma Scale score is 14; his one-point deduction is for slight confusion and repetitive questions. His secondary survey is significant for a seatbelt sign across his right anterior neck and left anterior chest as well as minor abrasions to his face. Chest and pelvis x-rays are both negative, as is a focused assessment with sonography in trauma examination. Noncontrast CT of the head, CT angiogram of the neck, and CT with contrast of the chest, abdomen, and pelvis are all also negative. While his scans are being read, the patient becomes progressively more agitated, confused, and combative despite treatment with several doses of lorazepam and haloperidol. He also becomes progressively tachycardic, hypertensive, and develops a low-grade fever. He is intubated and chemically sedated for airway protection and control.

Introduction

Thyroid storm is a severe, life-threatening form of thyrotoxicosis that comes with a high mortality rate, between 8% to 25%, despite aggressive management.[1] It is a multisystem disease that must be recognized quickly to reduce the risk of multiorgan failure and death. Thankfully, it is quite rare, accounting for only a small portion of all hyperthyroidism admissions. Risk factors include a history of poorly managed hyperthyroidism and stressors such as infection, trauma, pregnancy, surgical manipulation to the thyroid, abrupt cessation of thyroid medication, stroke, and myocardial infarction, among others.[2]

CRITICAL DECISION

What is the pathophysiology of thyroid storm?

Thyroid storm is a hyperadrenergic state caused by excess thyroid hormones in the periphery. Hyperthyroidism is relatively common in the United States, with studies estimating decreased thyroid-stimulating hormone (TSH) levels in 1.2% to 2.2% of the population and signs and symptoms of overt hyperthyroidism in 0.5% of the population.[3,4] In a normal physiologic state, the hypothalamus releases thyrotropin-releasing hormone (TRH), which stimulates the anterior pituitary gland to release TSH. TSH, in turn, stimulates the thyroid follicular cells to release both triiodothyronine (T3) and thyroxine (T4) into the bloodstream, both of which are bound to thyroxine-binding globulin. T4 is considered metabolically inactive and is converted in the periphery to the more metabolically active T3. Both T3 and T4 provide feedback to the hypothalamus and anterior pituitary gland to reduce or stimulate the release of more thyroid hormone

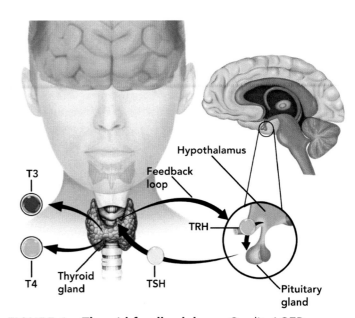

FIGURE 1. **Thyroid feedback loop.** *Credit:* ACEP.

(*Figure 1*).[5] Thyroid storm and thyroid disease in general represent an aberrancy in this feedback loop.

During a thyroid storm, patients have an excess amount of and increased sensitivity to T3 along with an increased amount of catecholamines in the bloodstream; this combination leads to a severe hypermetabolic state. Emergency management of thyroid storm targets several different steps in the synthesis of T3. Additionally, long-standing hyperthyroidism is associated with a depleted adrenocortical reserve, which can also complicate diagnosis and care.[6]

CRITICAL DECISION

How is thyroid storm recognized and diagnosed?

Thyroid storm is largely a clinical diagnosis, and can be difficult because the condition can mimic many other pathologies. The most common presenting signs and symptoms include derangements in the nervous, cardiopulmonary, GI, and hepatic systems.

CNS symptoms are among the most common and include fever and altered mental status, which can appear as agitation, depression, psychosis, or even coma. Hyperreflexia, tremor, and diplopia can also occur.[7]

Cardiopulmonary symptoms most often include tachycardia that is out of proportion to any associated fever; sinus tachycardia is the most common, but new-onset atrial fibrillation occurs as well. In severe cases, tachycardia can progress to high-output cardiac failure, which manifests as bipedal edema, rales, or pulmonary edema. High-output cardiac failure can progress to low-output cardiac failure with progressive cardiac myocyte fatigue. Patients often present with hypertension but can experience hypotension and subsequent shock if multisystem organ failure occurs. A widened pulse pressure is often found.[8]

GI and hepatic symptoms include abdominal pain, nausea, vomiting, diarrhea, hepatic dysfunction, and jaundice. Additionally, patients can present with the stigmata of undiagnosed hyperthyroidism: goiter and exophthalmos (*Figures 2* and *3*).[9]

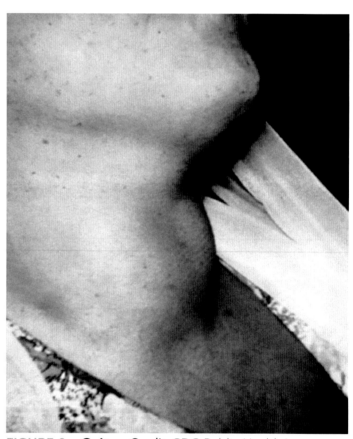

FIGURE 2. **Goiter.** *Credit:* CDC Public Health Image Library (Public Domain; https://phil.cdc.gov/Details.aspx?pid=1700).

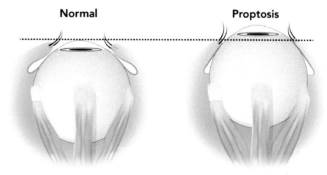

FIGURE 3. **Exophthalmos.** *Credit:* ttsz/iStock/Getty Images Plus.

Category	Range	Score
Temperature	37.2°C-37.7°C (99°F-99.9°F)	5
	37.8°C-38.2°C (100°F-100.9°F)	10
	38.3°C-38.8°C (101°F-101.9°F)	15
	38.9°C-39.3°C (102°F-102.9°F)	20
	39.4°C-39.9°C (103°F-103.9°F)	25
	≥40.0°C (104°F)	30
Central nervous system effects	Absent	0
	Mild (agitation)	10
	Moderate (delirium, psychosis, or extreme lethargy)	20
	Severe (seizure or coma)	30
GI-hepatic dysfunction	Moderate (diarrhea, nausea or vomiting, or abdominal pain)	10
	Severe (unexplained jaundice)	20
Cardiovascular dysfunction	Tachycardia 99-109 bpm	5
	110-119 bpm	10
	120-129 bpm	15
	130-139 bpm	20
	≥140 bpm	25
	Atrial fibrillation	10
Heart failure	Mild (pedal edema)	5
	Moderate (bibasilar rales)	10
	Severe (pulmonary edema)	15
Precipitant history	Positive	0
	Negative	10

Total: <25, thyroid storm is unlikely; 25-45, impending thyroid storm; >45, thyroid storm

TABLE 1. **The Burch-Wartofsky Point Scale (BWPS) for thyrotoxicosis**

The Burch-Wartofsky Point Scale (BWPS) can be used to predict the likelihood of thyroid storm when patients present with a biochemical thyrotoxicosis (*Table 1*). The American Thyroid Association (ATA) endorses the scale, and it has been both internally and externally validated.[10] Points are assigned to patients based on CNS, cardiopulmonary, and GI symptoms. Scores less than 25 are unlikely to represent thyroid storm. With scores greater than 45, thyroid storm is likely, and scores in between may indicate an impending thyroid storm.[11]

The scoring tool developed by the Japanese Thyroid Association (JTA) has also been shown to be a good diagnostic tool for thyroid storm. It includes similar criteria to the BWPS and classifies thyroid storm into two levels based on a combination of various symptoms.[12] Multiple studies, however, have shown an increased sensitivity with the BWPS, without a difference in specificity between the two scoring tools.[2]

Notably, older patients may not present with the common symptoms of thyroid storm but rather can present with a constellation of predominantly psychiatric symptoms, referred to as apathetic thyroid storm. Apathetic thyroid storm includes complaints of generalized weakness, fatigue, apathy, and depression.[13] Generalized weakness and altered mental status are among the most common presenting complaints in the emergency department in general, so remembering that these symptoms can present in older adults with thyroid storm is especially important for narrowing down the diagnosis.

CRITICAL DECISION

What factors can lead to thyroid storm?

The most common thyroid condition that can lead to thyroid storm is Graves disease, followed by toxic multinodular goiter and toxic adenoma.[4] Other associated conditions include thyroiditis, struma ovarii tumor, and a TSH-secreting pituitary tumor.[2] Thyroid storm almost never occurs independently; it most often occurs secondary to another condition like diabetic ketoacidosis, pregnancy, a postpartum state, ectopic pregnancy, gestational trophoblastic disease, sepsis, trauma, toxidrome, surgery, discontinuation of antithyroid medications, or exogenous thyroid hormone abuse.[14,15] Even an excess amount of iodine, such as an iodine load from amiodarone administration or iodinated contrast, can result in thyroid storm by causing too much thyroid hormone to be released, a condition known as the Jod-Basedow phenomenon.[16] On presentation, patients with thyroid storm may report a history of Graves disease or symptoms such as weight loss, heat intolerance, goiter, thinning hair, and exophthalmos.

The underlying cause of thyroid storm needs to be investigated for proper diagnosis and management. However, diagnosing its cause can be particularly difficult because of its many confounding symptoms. For example, a trauma patient's symptoms of hypotension and tachycardia from thyroid storm would most likely be attributed to hemorrhagic shock. The same can be said for patients with diabetic ketoacidosis who are experiencing thyroid storm; their tachycardia and acidosis would likely be attributed to ketosis and hypovolemia rather than

thyroid storm. Symptoms of thyroid storm in patients with sepsis — such as fever, leukocytosis, acidosis, tachycardia, hypotension, and multisystem organ failure — are also easily misattributed because they overlap with symptoms of sepsis. In some cases, thyroid storm can appear like a toxidrome or be precipitated by one.[17] Physicians should keep all of the potential diagnoses in mind based on the patient's history to avoid missing a diagnosis of thyroid storm.

CRITICAL DECISION

What comorbidities can develop during emergency care of thyroid storm?

Multisystem organ failure due to global hypoperfusion is the most common cause of death in thyroid storm.[12] Organs affected include the heart, liver, kidneys, and pancreas. Other comorbidities that can arise during emergency care of thyroid storm include coagulopathy from disseminated intravascular coagulation (DIC), adrenocortical insufficiency, and seizures.

Although rare, thyrotoxic periodic paralysis can occur as a complication as well. It is a gradual paralysis that primarily affects the extremities and occurs because of a rapid intracellular potassium shift. It often resolves spontaneously and can be mistaken for familial periodic paralysis. Fortunately, thyrotoxic periodic paralysis rarely affects the respiratory muscles, but intubation has been required in some cases.[18]

CRITICAL DECISION

What blood work and imaging should be obtained in patients with thyroid storm?

Laboratory analysis for thyroid storm includes a thyroid panel. However, physicians must be wary of laboratory results because they do not always reflect the severity of the illness; thyroid storm is a clinical diagnosis. Thyroid levels may appear similar to levels in patients with compensated hyperthyroidism.[11] However, thyroid laboratory tests should still be used to aid in diagnosis. TSH levels will typically be low, while T3 and T4 levels will be high. Occasionally, TSH

—— ✔ **Pearls** ——

- Early recognition of thyroid storm is difficult, so emergency physicians must remember to include it on the differential diagnosis.

- The order in which thyroid medications are given is important for successful management of thyroid storm.

- Physicians must remember to investigate for and treat concomitant organ failure.

- Fever associated with thyroid storm should never be treated with NSAIDs or salicylates because they can worsen symptoms. Instead, treat fever with acetaminophen and external cooling.

levels will be normal or even elevated if thyroid storm is caused by a TSH-secreting pituitary tumor. If suspicion for thyroid storm is high, physicians should not delay initiating treatment pending laboratory results.[1,19]

Additional blood work should be broad and include a workup to rule out common pathologies that can mimic thyrotoxicosis and thyroid storm. Many complications that arise from thyroid storm can also be recognized in the blood work. Laboratory tests should include a bedside glucose test, CBC, basic metabolic panel (BMP), liver panel, troponin test, coagulation studies, lactate level, arterial blood gas (ABG) or venous blood gas (VBG) analysis, urinalysis, pregnancy test, and blood cultures.[1]

Patients can have reactive leukocytosis or leukopenia, elevated lactate levels, and severe acidosis (from elevated lactate or β-hydroxybutyrate). The BMP may show acute renal failure and a variety of electrolyte derangements, including hypercalcemia due to enhanced bone resorption and hyperglycemia due to catecholaminergic surge. Hepatic function panels may show transaminitis and elevated lipase levels. Coagulopathy from DIC or liver failure is not uncommon. Troponin levels may be elevated, and an ECG will most likely show sinus tachycardia or atrial fibrillation; atrial fibrillation occurs in 10% to 22% of patients with hyperthyroidism, more often in patients with underlying structural heart disease.[20]

Imaging is aimed at diagnosing the underlying cause of thyroid storm. However, iodinated contrast studies can worsen symptoms if an inappropriate iodine load is administered. A chest x-ray is always indicated to evaluate for infection and vascular congestion, as is a head CT to evaluate for alternative causes of altered mental status.[1] Bedside or formal echocardiography can help distinguish between high- and low-output cardiac failure. Thoracic ultrasound can also reveal B-lines that correspond to pulmonary edema.

CRITICAL DECISION

What is the initial management of thyroid storm in the emergency department?

Thyroid storm treatment is performed sequentially to properly address the physiologic derangement. The ATA describes five main treatment strategies for thyroid storm: "(i) therapy directed against thyroid hormone secretion and synthesis; (ii) measures directed against the peripheral action of thyroid hormone at the tissue level; (iii) reversal of systemic decompensation; (iv) treatment of the precipitating event or intercurrent illness; and (v) definitive therapy."[2] Treatment reduces the severity of symptoms and helps manage unstable vital signs. A β-blocker, such as propranolol or esmolol, should be given as a first-line medication immediately after recognizing thyroid storm and should immediately be followed by a thionamide, such as propylthiouracil or methimazole. One hour later, iodine and steroids should be administered. Some experts also recommend administering bile acid sequestrants, such as cholestyramine. Patients eventually need definitive thyroid management from an endocrinologist, which can include surgical resection, radioactive iodine ablation, or ongoing use of thionamide medications (*Table 2*).

β-blockers for thyroid storm can be given either orally or intravenously. They decrease sympathetic hyperactivity and reduce heart rate, which increase cardiac filling times and improve cardiac output. β-blockers also help to reduce blood pressure. Nitrates, by contrast, are contraindicated for treating hypertension because they rapidly reduce heart preload, which worsens cardiac failure in patients with thyroid storm.[1,21] Although all β-blockers prevent T4 from converting to T3 in the periphery, propranolol is the most effective at this and, therefore, the preferred agent. Preexisting comorbidities should also be considered when administering β-blockers because β-blockers can worsen some conditions such as systolic heart failure and can precipitate severe hypotension. In these cases, esmolol is preferred because of its short half-life and ability to easily be discontinued if significant side effects occur. β-blockers are also relatively contraindicated in asthma and chronic obstructive pulmonary disease. Cardioselective medications, like metoprolol, or calcium channel blockers, like diltiazem, can be used instead to control heart rate in these patients; keep in mind, however, that calcium channel blockers are ineffective at preventing the conversion of T4 to T3.[22] Calcium channel blockers for thyroid storm can also be used as adjuncts to β-blockers when blood pressure is not adequately controlled by β-blockers alone.

In addition to β-blockers, thionamides should also be immediately administered. Both propylthiouracil and methimazole decrease the synthesis of new thyroid hormone and decrease peripheral conversion of T4 to T3. They are oral medications that can be given through a nasogastric tube if needed. Propylthiouracil is the preferred treatment in critically ill patients because it blocks T4 to T3 conversion more effectively and has a faster onset — propylthiouracil leads to a 45% drop in T3 conversion in the first 24 hours of treatment compared to methimazole's 10% to 15% drop.[23] However, propylthiouracil has a shorter half-life and needs to be readministered more often. Thionamides do not block the release of stored hormones from the thyroid gland. Their known side effects include agranulocytosis, hepatotoxicity, and pruritic rash. If patients have a previous intolerance to one or both thionamides, urgent thyroidectomy should be considered. For critically ill patients, however, one thionamide can be substituted for the other if patients have a history of poor tolerance of either one (eg, use methimazole if propylthiouracil was not previously tolerated).[24,25] Methimazole is contraindicated in the first trimester of pregnancy because it is highly teratogenic.[2]

Approximately 1 hour after β-blocker and thionamide administration, iodine should be given orally. The iodine load is therapeutic because it induces the Wolff-Chaikoff effect in which the thyroid gland is prevented from releasing T3 and T4. The 1-hour delay between thionamide and iodine administration, however, is important to prevent the Jod-Basedow phenomenon, wherein more thyroid hormone is synthesized and released and the symptoms of thyroid storm are worsened in patients with toxic adenoma or toxic multinodular goiter.[16]

For severe or refractory cases of thyroid storm, steroids can be used. Hydrocortisone is the first-line steroid, and dexamethasone is the second. Steroids also block the peripheral conversion of T4 to T3 and have the added benefit of treating

Medication	Uses	Mechanism	PO Dosing	IV Dosing	Special Information	Contraindications
Propranolol	Control of hyperadrenergic state, reduction in heart rate, cardiac contractility, and blood pressure	Nonselective ß2 blockage, decreases peripheral T4 to T3 conversion	60-80 mg every 4-6 hr based on hemodynamics	0.5-1 mg given over 10 min. Can repeat every few hours until PO therapy begins to work.	First-line ß-blocker	Avoid in low-output cardiac failure. Be careful in asthma and COPD patients.
Esmolol	Control of hyperadrenergic state, reduction in heart rate, cardiac contractility, and blood pressure	Nonselective ß1 blockage, decreases peripheral T4 to T3 conversion	N/A	Loading dose of 250-500 µg/kg, followed by a continuous infusion of 50-100 µg/kg/min. Adjust dose based on heart rate and blood pressure.	Use when unsure if the patient's hemodynamics will remain stable when given ß-blockers. Esmolol is short acting and can be easily discontinued.	Avoid in low-output cardiac failure.
Propylthiouracil	Reduction of circulating thyroid hormone	Blocks thyroid peroxidase synthase, decreases synthesis of new thyroid hormone, and decreases peripheral conversion of T4 to T3	Loading dose of 500-1,000 mg, followed by 200-250 mg every 4 hr	N/A	Can be given via nasogastric tube or rectally, if needed. Preferred over methimazole in the acute setting.	Use methimazole if allergic to propylthiouracil.
Methimazole	Reduction of circulating thyroid hormone	Blocks thyroid peroxidase synthesis of new thyroid hormone and decreases peripheral conversion of T4 to T3	20 mg every 4-6 hr	N/A	Can be given via nasogastric tube or rectally, if needed.	Teratogenic, avoid in first trimester of pregnancy. Use propylthiouracil if allergic to methimazole.
Iodine	Reduction of circulating thyroid hormone	Prevents T3 and T4 release from the thyroid via the Wolff-Chaikoff effect	Can be given in two forms: SSKI (5 drops, 50 mg iodide/drop [0.05 mL]) orally every 6 hr or Lugol's solution (10 drops, 6.25 mg iodide/drop [0.05 mL]) orally three times per day. Can be given rectally.	10 drops of Lugol's solution can be given in IV fluids	Discontinue after clinical improvement is noted. Watch for rare esophageal injury.	N/A
Hydrocortisone	Reduction of circulating thyroid hormone	Short-acting corticosteroid, blocks conversion of T4 to T3, and treats adrenal insufficiency.[25] May also address underlying autoimmune disorders (eg, Graves).	N/A	Loading dose of 300 mg followed by 100 mg every 8 hr	Preferred over dexamethasone. Has not been shown to decrease mortality.[26] Duration of therapy remains unknown.	N/A
Cholestyramine	Reduction of circulating thyroid hormone	Prevents reabsorption of intestinal thyroid hormone, which instead is excreted in the feces	4 g four times per day until thyroid storm resolves	N/A	N/A	N/A

TABLE 2. **Medications used to treat thyroid storm**

underlying autoimmune effects that may have precipitated thyroid storm (as in Graves disease) and underlying adrenal insufficiency from shock and cortisol depletion (secondary to overstimulation).[2,6]

Recently, the bile acid sequestrant cholestyramine has been used to reduce intestinal reabsorption and enterohepatic circulation of thyroid hormone. Thyroid hormone is normally metabolized by the liver, released in bile in a conjugated form, and later reabsorbed in the intestines. Cholestyramine binds to bile to remove thyroid hormone from the small intestine, aids in fecal excretion, and prevents reabsorption. Physicians should be cautious when administering medications alongside bile acid sequestrants because they reduce the absorption of other medications.[26]

Plasmapheresis can be used as a final effort before considering an emergent thyroidectomy.[27,28] Lithium has also been used to treat thyroid storm for its ability to gather in thyroid follicular cells and prevent iodine absorption, but its use is limited by its neurologic and renal side effects.[29]

When treating symptoms and managing comorbidities in critically ill patients, airway, breathing, and circulation must be considered, and the airway must be secured if needed.[30] Hemodynamic instability should be managed with fluid resuscitation and β-blockers. Expect patients with thyroid storm to be volume depleted from fever, agitation, and hyperpnea. Fever can be treated with acetaminophen. Passive external cooling techniques, such as removing clothes and lowering the room temperature can also be used. The use of cooling blankets and ice packs has been recommended by the ATA and JTA. Salicylates and NSAIDs should never be used in patients with thyroid storm; they can worsen thyroid storm by displacing bound thyroid hormone from thyroxine-binding globulin.[31] Agitation can be managed with benzodiazepines and antipsychotics as needed, and seizures can be managed with benzodiazepines and antiepileptics. Physicians, however,

must remain cognizant of how these medications affect patients' ability to maintain their airway.[32] Electrolyte abnormalities and any underlying conditions should also be treated.[2,28] Patients with thyroid storm should always be admitted to the ICU. Definitive treatment varies by etiology but can include thyroidectomy or radioactive iodine ablation.

Summary

Although thyroid storm can be difficult to diagnose, emergency physicians must be able to recognize and treat it. Patients' history and physical examinations are important in clinically identifying thyroid storm. Calculators such as the BWPS and the JTA's scoring tool for thyroid storm can aid in diagnosis. Physicians must also examine patients for any precipitating causes and developing complications. Treating thyroid storm involves following multiple steps in a specific order for successful outcomes.

REFERENCES

1. Idrose AM. Acute and emergency care for thyrotoxicosis and thyroid storm. *Acute Med Surg.* 2015 May 12;2(3):147-157.

2. Ross DS, Burch HB, Cooper DS, et al. 2016 American Thyroid Association guidelines for diagnosis and management of hyperthyroidism and other causes of thyrotoxicosis. *Thyroid.* 2016 Oct;26(10):1343-1421.

3. Canaris GJ, Manowitz NR, Mayor G, Ridgway EC. The Colorado thyroid disease prevalence study. *Arch Intern Med.* 2000 Feb 28;160(4):526-534.

4. Singer PA, Cooper DS, Levy EG, et al. Treatment guidelines for patients with hyperthyroidism and hypothyroidism. Standards of Care Committee, American Thyroid Association. *JAMA.* 1995 Mar 8;273(10):808-812.

5. Costanzo LS. *BRS Physiology.* 8th ed. Wolters Kluwer; 2022.

6. Tsatsoulis A, Johnson EO, Kalogera CH, Seferiadis K, Tsolas O. The effect of thyrotoxicosis on adrenocortical reserve. *Eur J Endocrinol.* 2000 Mar;142(3):231-235.

7. Kudrjavcev T. Neurologic complications of thyroid dysfunction. *Adv Neurol.* 1978;19:619-636.

8. Biondi B, Palmieri EA, Lombardi G, Fazio S. Effects of thyroid hormone on cardiac function: the relative importance of heart rate, loading conditions, and myocardial contractility in the regulation of cardiac performance in human hyperthyroidism. *J Clin Endocrinol Metab.* 2002 Mar;87(3):968-974.

9. Devereaux D, Tewelde SZ. Hyperthyroidism and thyrotoxicosis. *Emerg Med Clin North Am.* 2014 May;32(2):277-292.

10. Nayak B, Burman K. Thyrotoxicosis and thyroid storm. *Endocrinol Metab Clin North Am.* 2006 Dec;35(4):663-686.

11. Burch HB, Wartofsky L. Life-threatening thyrotoxicosis. Thyroid storm. *Endocrinol Metab Clin North Am.* 1993 Jun;22(2):263-277.

12. Satoh T, Isozaki O, Suzuki A, et al. 2016 guidelines for the management of thyroid storm from the Japan Thyroid Association and Japan Endocrine Society (first edition). *Endocr J.* 2016 Dec 30;63(12):1025-1064.

13. Boelaert K, Torlinska B, Holder RL, Franklyn JA. Older subjects with hyperthyroidism present with a paucity of symptoms and signs: a large cross-sectional study. *J Clin Endocrinol Metab.* 2010 Jun;95(6):2715-2726.

14. Hamidi OP, Barbour LA. Endocrine emergencies during pregnancy: diabetic ketoacidosis and thyroid storm. *Obstet Gynecol Clin North Am.* 2022 Sep;49(3):473-489.

15. Liang C-M, Ho M-H, Wu X-Y, Hong Z-J, Hsu S-D, Chen C-J. Thyroid storm following trauma: a pitfall in the emergency department. *Injury.* 2015 Jan;46(1):169-171.

✖ Pitfalls

- Waiting on laboratory test results before initiating treatment for suspected thyroid storm. Thyroid storm is primarily a clinical diagnosis, and laboratory test results may not accurately reflect the severity of the condition.

- Overlooking the diagnosis of apathetic thyroid storm in older adults, who often present with unique symptoms.

- Failing to investigate comorbidities of or precipitating factors for thyroid storm to aid in more effective treatment.

- Forgetting to wait 1 hour between treatment with thionamides and treatment with an iodine load. Administering an iodine load too soon after thionamide administration can worsen thyroid storm symptoms.

CASE ONE

The emergency physician noticed a history of Graves disease when reviewing the patient's chart. The patient's ECG revealed sinus tachycardia. Laboratory results were significant for acute blood loss anemia, acute renal failure, hyperkalemia, transaminitis, and low β-human chorionic gonadotropin levels for her gestational age. Her TSH level was low, while her T3 and T4 levels were high. Transvaginal ultrasound confirmed an ectopic pregnancy. The patient was subsequently treated for thyroid storm and admitted to the ICU with orders for an emergent obstetrics evaluation for a ruptured ectopic pregnancy.

CASE TWO

Laboratory analysis was significant for leukocytosis and transaminitis with elevated total bilirubin. Urinalysis had positive leukocyte esterase and nitrates. CT of the head was negative, but his chest x-ray revealed pulmonary vascular congestion and pulmonary edema without pneumonia. The patient was treated for urosepsis with ceftriaxone and supportive care. He became increasingly tachycardic with worsening hypotension and was started on peripheral vasopressors. His respiratory status worsened, necessitating intubation. The patient died 3 days later in the ICU. Postmortem studies revealed a toxic multinodular goiter.

CASE THREE

A fourth-year medical student noticed the patient's history of Graves disease during chart review. The patient's last refill for his 30-day supply of methimazole was filled 90 days ago. Thyroid laboratory studies were added to his trauma workup; his TSH level was low, while his T3 and T4 levels were significantly elevated. The patient was diagnosed with thyroid storm and then admitted to the ICU. It is unknown whether his thyroid storm was caused by neck trauma from his seat belt or by the iodine load during imaging, but the patient recovered well and was eventually discharged from the hospital.

16. Rose HR, Zulfiqar H, Anastasopoulou C. Jod Basedow syndrome. *StatPearls [Internet]*; 2022. Updated March 2, 2023. https://www.ncbi.nlm.nih.gov/books/NBK544277/

17. Viswanath O, Menapace DC, Headley DB. Methamphetamine use with subsequent thyrotoxicosis/thyroid storm, agranulocytosis, and modified total thyroidectomy: a case report. *Clin Med Insights Ear Nose Throat.* 2017 Nov 17;10:1179550617741293.

18. Lam L, Nair RJ, Tingle L. Thyrotoxic periodic paralysis. *Proc (Bayl Univ Med Cent).* 2006 Apr;19(2):126-129.

19. Cimino-Fiallos N. Thyroid storm and hyperthyroidism. CorePendium. Updated October 20, 2021. https://www.emrap.org/corependium/chapter/rec1SP9oNI2GZgKKF/Thyroid-Storm-and-Hyperthyroidism

20. Wald DA. ECG manifestations of selected metabolic and endocrine disorders. *Emerg Med Clin North Am.* 2006 Feb;24(1):145-157.

21. Ikram H. The nature and prognosis of thyrotoxic heart disease. *Q J Med.* 1985 Jan;54(213):19-28.

22. Milner MR, Gelman KM, Phillips RA, Fuster V, Davies TF, Goldman ME. Double-blind crossover trial of diltiazem versus propranolol in the management of thyrotoxic symptoms. *Pharmacotherapy.* 1990;10(2):100-106.

23. Abuid J, Larsen PR. Triiodothyronine and thyroxine in hyperthyroidism. Comparison of the acute changes during therapy with antithyroid agents. *J Clin Invest.* 1974 Jul;54(1):201-208.

24. Sundaresh V, Brito JP, Wang Z, et al. Comparative effectiveness of therapies for Graves' hyperthyroidism: a systematic review and network meta-analysis. *J Clin Endocrinol Metab.* 2013 Sep;98(9):3671-3677.

25. Otsuka F, Noh JY, Chino T, et al. Hepatotoxicity and cutaneous reactions after antithyroid drug administration. *Clin Endocrinol (Oxf).* 2012 Aug;77(2):310-315.

26. Solomon BL, Wartofsky L, Burman KD. Adjunctive cholestyramine therapy for thyrotoxicosis. *Clin Endocrinol (Oxf).* 1993 Jan;38(1):39-43.

27. Muller C, Perrin P, Faller B, Richter S, Chantrel F. Role of plasma exchange in the thyroid storm. *Ther Apher Dial.* 2011 Dec;15(6):522-531.

28. Scholz GH, Hagemann E, Arkenau C, et al. Is there a place for thyroidectomy in older patients with thyrotoxic storm and cardiorespiratory failure? *Thyroid.* 2003 Oct;13(10):933-940.

29. Prakash I, Nylen ES, Sen S. Lithium as an alternative option in Graves thyrotoxicosis. *Case Rep Endocrinol.* 2015;2015:869343.

30. Nai Q, Ansari M, Pak S, et al. Cardiorespiratory failure in thyroid storm: case report and literature review. *J Clin Med Res.* 2018 Apr;10(4):351-357.

31. Samuels MH, Pillote K, Asher D, Nelson JC. Variable effects of nonsteroidal antiinflammatory agents on thyroid test results. *J Clin Endocrinol Metab.* 2003 Dec;88(12):5710-5716.

32. Carroll R, Matfin G. Endocrine and metabolic emergencies: thyroid storm. *Ther Adv Endocrinol Metab.* 2010 Jun;1(3):139-145.

MDCALC REFERENCE

Burch-Wartofsky Point Scale (BWPS) for Thyrotoxicosis. MDCalc. https://www.mdcalc.com/calc/3816/burch-wartofsky-point-scale-bwps-thyrotoxicosis

The Critical ECG

Ectopic Atrial Rhythm

By Jeremy Berberian, MD; William J. Brady, MD, FACEP; and Amal Mattu, MD, FACEP

Dr. Berberian is the associate director of emergency medicine residency education at ChristianaCare and assistant professor of emergency medicine at Sidney Kimmel Medical College, Thomas Jefferson University in Philadelphia, Pennsylvania. Dr. Brady is a professor of emergency medicine, medicine, and nursing, and vice chair for faculty affairs in the Department of Emergency Medicine at the University of Virginia School of Medicine in Charlottesville. Dr. Mattu is a professor, vice chair, and codirector of the Emergency Cardiology Fellowship in the Department of Emergency Medicine at the University of Maryland School of Medicine in Baltimore.

Objectives

On completion of this article, you should be able to:

- Describe the morphologies for normal P waves in adults in normal sinus rhythm.
- Identify the morphologies for normal T waves in adults in normal sinus rhythm.
- Formulate a differential diagnosis for inverted P waves in a narrow complex rhythm with normal ventricular rates.

CASE PRESENTATION

An 84-year-old man presents after an abnormal preoperative ECG. He has no complaints. His ECG shows an ectopic atrial rhythm with a ventricular rate of 82 bpm; normal axis; normal intervals; negative P waves in leads I, II, III, aVF, and V_4 through V_6; and positive P waves in lead aVR.

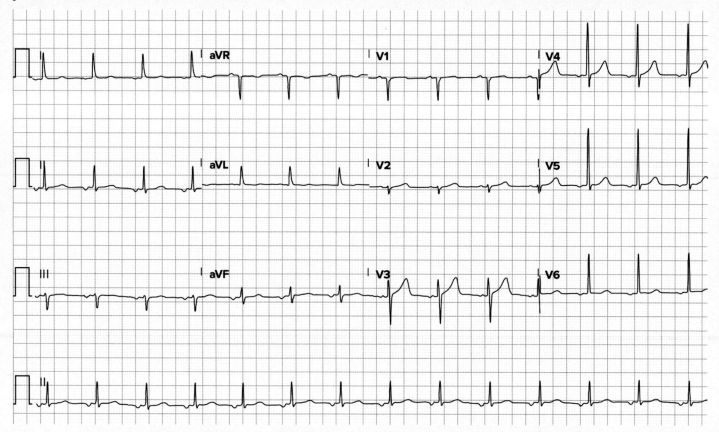

FIGURE 1. ECG of an 84-year-old man. *Credit:* EMRA.

The key to interpreting this ECG is to identify the abnormal P waves, in particular the negative P wave in lead II, which is never present in a normal sinus rhythm (*Figure 2*). The characteristics of normal P waves include:

- Leads I and II: always upright and monophasic
- Lead III: upright, inverted, or biphasic (positive-negative)
- Lead aVR: always inverted and monophasic
- Lead aVL: upright, inverted, or biphasic (negative-positive)
- Lead aVF: usually upright but can be flat or biphasic
- Lead V_1: usually biphasic (positive-negative) but can be entirely upright or inverted
- Lead V_2: usually biphasic (positive-negative) but can be entirely upright (entirely inverted is rare)
- Leads V_3 through V_6: always upright and monophasic
- The PR interval, which includes the time for atrial depolarization and conduction through the atrioventricular (AV) node, is 120 to 200 msec for adults and 70 to 180 msec for pediatric patients.

CASE RESOLUTION

Ectopic atrial rhythms occur when the ectopic atrial rate exceeds the SA node rate or when the SA node rate slows to below the ectopic atrial rate. In this patient's ECG, the normal PR interval suggests an ectopic atrial rhythm. This patient had an unremarkable workup and was discharged.

ACKNOWLEDGMENT

This case is reprinted from *Emergency ECGs: Case-Based Review and Interpretations,* available at www.emra.org/amazon or by scanning the QR code.

The differential diagnosis for inverted P waves in a regular narrow complex rhythm with normal ventricular rates includes:
- Ectopic atrial rhythm
- Junctional rhythm with retrograde P waves that precede the QRS complex

An ectopic atrial rhythm originates from a site in the atria other than the sinoatrial (SA) node and has a rate of 60 to 100 bpm. Ectopic P waves will differ from sinus P waves in their morphology (ie, shape), axis (ie, positive or negative), or both. The PR interval is typically 120 to 200 msec but can be less than 120 msec when the ectopic atrial focus is located near the AV node.

A junctional rhythm originates from the AV node or proximal Purkinje system and has a rate of 40 to 60 bpm. It is called an

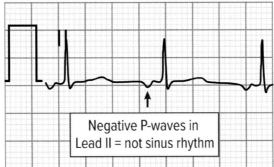

Negative P-waves in Lead II = not sinus rhythm

FIGURE 2. The P wave in lead II should be upright in sinus rhythm. *Credit:* EMRA.

accelerated junctional rhythm when the rate is 61 to 100 bpm. In junctional rhythms, the depolarization of the cardiac conduction system starts in the middle, so there is anterograde conduction to the ventricles and retrograde conduction to the atria. This retrograde conduction creates P waves that are typically inverted compared to the sinus P waves. If the junctional focus initiates conduction in the AV node, the retrograde P waves can appear before the QRS complex with a short PR interval. If the junctional focus is farther down the conduction system, the retrograde P waves can appear after the QRS complex, can be buried in the QRS complex, or can be hidden in the QRS complex and not appear at all.

NORMAL P WAVE AND T WAVE LEARNING POINTS

- Normal P wave and T wave morphologies in adults in normal sinus rhythm in the absence of conduction abnormalities, ischemia, structural abnormalities, etc, include[1,2]:

I	aVR	V$_1$	V$_4$
P: always upright	P: always inverted	P: usually biphasic (+/–) but can be entirely upright or inverted	P: upright
T: always upright	T: always inverted	T: upright or inverted	T: almost always upright
II	aVL	V$_2$	V$_5$
P: always upright	P: upright, inverted, or biphasic (–/+)	P: usually biphasic (+/–) but can be entirely upright (entirely inverted is rare)	P: upright
T: always upright	T: upright or inverted	T: usually upright	T: always upright
III	aVF	V$_3$	V$_6$
P: upright, inverted, or biphasic (+/–)	P: usually upright but can be flat or biphasic	P: upright	P: upright
T: upright or inverted	T: usually upright	T: usually upright	T: always upright

- Inverted, flat, or positive-negative biphasic T waves in lead V$_1$ (less so in leads V$_2$-V$_3$) can be normal.
- Positive-negative biphasic T waves in leads V$_1$ through V$_3$ can be abnormal or a normal variant.
- T-wave amplitude is typically <6 mm in limb leads and <10 mm in precordial leads.

ECTOPIC ATRIAL RHYTHM LEARNING POINTS

- Ectopic focus from the atria other than the SA node
- ECG shows ventricular rate of 60 to 100 bpm with normal QRS complex duration unless there is a concurrent conduction abnormality (eg, bundle branch block).
- P waves will have different morphology or axis than sinus P waves.
- PR interval is typically normal at 120 to 200 msec but can be <120 msec if the focus is near the AV node.

REFERENCES

1. Knilans T, Surawicz B. *Chou's Electrocardiography in Clinical Practice.* 6th ed. Elsevier; 2020.
2. Berberian, JG. Normal P-waves and T-waves. In: Berberian JG, Brady WJ, Mattu A. *EMRA EKG Guide.* 2nd ed. EMRA; 2022.

Clinical Pediatrics

Pediatric Stroke in a Patient With Congenital Nephrotic Syndrome

By Alan Chan, MD; and Nathaniel Mann, MD
University of South Carolina School of Medicine
and Prisma Health Children's Hospital,
Greenville, South Carolina
Reviewed by Sharon E. Mace, MD, FACEP

Objective

On completion of this article, you should be able to:

- Recognize the risk factors for pediatric AIS for faster diagnosis of this rare condition.

CASE PRESENTATION

A 4-year-old boy presents with right arm weakness. He has a medical history of hypothyroidism and hyperlipidemia but is not on medications for these conditions at presentation. He recently completed a kidney biopsy and is awaiting confirmation for a diagnosis of nephrotic syndrome. The patient's parents noticed that he has been unable to move his right arm since noon yesterday, has diminished right hand strength, and has been dragging his feet while walking. They also noticed right facial drooping but attributed it to facial swelling from nephrotic syndrome. No other symptoms, such as fever, chills, nausea, vomiting, abdominal discomfort, hematuria, or diarrhea are reported. The parents deny any trauma in the child's past or a history of familial neuromuscular dysfunction.

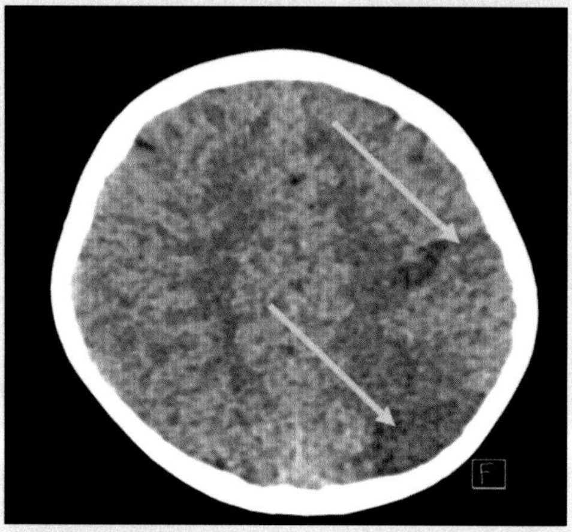

FIGURE 1. Head CT showing hypodensities in the left parietal and left posterior frontal lobes that suggest ischemic changes.
Credit: Nathaniel Mann, MD.

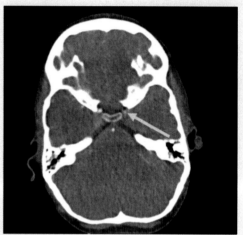

FIGURE 2. CTA of the head and neck showing an occlusion of the paraophthalmic segment of the left internal carotid artery. The left carotid segment has a lack of contrast compared to the analogous right carotid segment.
Credit: Nathaniel Mann, MD.

The patient's physical examination shows vital signs of BP 115/87, P 106, R 21, and T 36.7°C (98.1°F); SpO$_2$ is 98% on room air. He has mild facial asymmetry, with drooping of his right face; nearly complete right arm paralysis; and mild weakness in his right lower extremity. Given the patient's presentation, the emergency physician activates the stroke alert protocol.

Before the patient gets a CT, intravenous access is established, and laboratory tests are obtained. A point-of-care glucose level is 110 mg/dL. His other laboratory results reveal a WBC count of 9.2 K/μL, a hemoglobin level of 15.3 g/dL with a hematocrit level of 41.6%, and a platelet count of 431 K/μL. His basic metabolic panel is unremarkable except for a creatinine level of 0.29 mg/dL. Results from a PT/INR and PTT are both within normal limits. His lipid panel shows an elevated triglyceride level of 1,222 mg/dL and a total cholesterol level of 480 mg/dL. A noncontrast head CT captures left posterior frontal lobe and left parietal lobe hypodensities that are concerning for ischemic changes (*Figure 1*). A CT angiogram (CTA) of the head and neck shows an occlusion of the paraophthalmic segment of the left internal carotid artery (*Figure 2*).

Discussion

Acute ischemic stroke (AIS) accounts for approximately half of all cerebrovascular accidents.[1] However, AIS is a rare event in children — the overall estimated incidence of childhood stroke is 1.3 to 13/100,000 per year, with 25 to 40 strokes/100,000 births in neonates.[2] Childhood strokes can be further categorized by age. Perinatal strokes take place between the prenatal period and the end of the newborn period; childhood strokes occur between the 28th postnatal day to 18 years old.[3,4] The presentation of AIS varies, so emergency physicians must consider it among the differential

diagnosis when evaluating patients with concerning signs and symptoms (*Table 1*).[3]

The primary risk factors for strokes in adults are hypertension, diabetes, and atherosclerosis. In children, however, the risk factors are more varied. Between 15% and 30% of pediatric AIS cases are associated with an underlying cardiac disease, including endocarditis, rheumatic heart disease, prosthetic valves, or a patent foramen ovale.[1,5] Approximately 20% to 50% of strokes occur in children who have thrombotic disorders, either hereditary or acquired.[5] Prothrombotic hematologic disorders such as sickle cell disease, polycythemia,

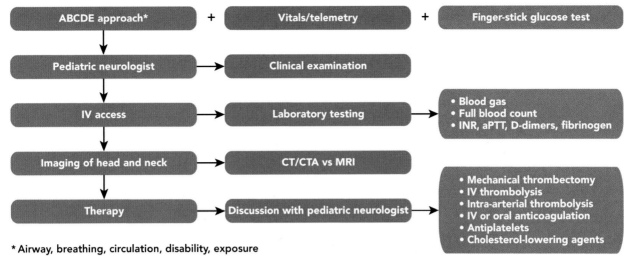

FIGURE 3 Initial approach to a pediatric patient with suspected AIS. *Credit:* ACEP.

and protein C and S deficiencies (associated with nephrotic syndrome) can also increase the risk of AIS.[1] In pediatric patients with sickle cell disease, the risk of AIS is nearly 200 times that of the general pediatric population.[6] Infections, vasculitis, arteriovenous malformations, malignancy, trauma, and drugs can also increase the risk of pediatric AIS.[1]

The imaging workup begins with CT, which may include a noncontrast head CT or CTA. MR angiography can also be considered. Treatment of pediatric AIS varies. There are no concrete guidelines for using thrombolytics or invasive interventions like thrombectomy in the pediatric population. Initiation of anticoagulation is critical but should be done in conjunction with a pediatric neurologist, if available (*Figure 3*).[7] Although younger patients are said to have more neuroplasticity, AIS at a younger age is associated with worse cognitive and neuropsychologic outcomes.[8] The mortality rate of AIS in the pediatric population is 6% to 30%.[9] AIS has a recurrence rate of approximately 1.2% in the perinatal stroke population compared to 19% in the childhood

stroke population.[6] Even though the incidence of pediatric stroke is rising, comprehensive treatment and prevention guidelines are still lacking.[10] More scientific research is needed to determine the best treatment course for this vulnerable population.

Perinatal AIS	Childhood AIS	Potential Stroke Mimics
• Seizure (focal and unilateral) • Cardiovascular symptoms • Altered consciousness • Failure to thrive • Feeding intolerance	• Hemiparesis • Facial unilateral weakness • Speech disorder • Vision abnormalities • Altered consciousness	• Migraine • Headache • Confusion • Syncope • Nausea and vomiting • Seizures with Todd paralysis • Bell palsy • Altered consciousness

TABLE 1. Possible AIS presentations

CASE RESOLUTION

After the CT was obtained and a pediatric neurologist was consulted, the emergency physician decided to place the patient on a heparin drip for anticoagulation. The patient was not a good candidate for thrombolysis and mechanical thrombectomy because his time since symptom onset was greater than 24 hours. He was admitted to the pediatric ICU and started on fenofibrate, lisinopril, and levothyroxine before a hypercoagulable workup was initiated. An MRI of his brain that was obtained 4 days after his initial presentation showed stability of his lesions. He transitioned to oral aspirin and was discharged 13 days later with physical and occupational therapy. Since discharge, the patient has had mild improvement in the function of his right upper extremity.

REFERENCES

1. Earley CJ, Kittner SJ, Feeser BR, et al. Stroke in children and sickle-cell disease: Baltimore-Washington Cooperative Young Stroke Study. *Neurology*. 1998 Jul;51(1):169-176.
2. Mallick AA, O'Callaghan FJK. The epidemiology of childhood stroke. *Eur J Paediatr Neurol*. 2010 May;14(3):197-205.
3. Ferriero DM, Fullerton HJ, Bernard TJ, et al. Management of stroke in neonates and children: a scientific statement from the American Heart Association/American Stroke Association. *Stroke*. 2019 Mar;50(3):e51-e96.
4. Nelson KB, Lynch JK. Stroke in newborn infants. *Lancet Neurol*. 2004 Mar;3(3):150-158.
5. Ohene-Frempong K, Weiner SJ, Sleeper LA, et al. Cerebrovascular accidents in sickle cell disease: rates and risk factors. *Blood*. 1998 Jan 1;91(1):288-294.
6. Ciceri EF, Cuccarini V, Chiapparini L, Saletti V, Valvassori L. Paediatric stroke: review of the literature and possible treatment options, including endovascular approach. *Stroke Res Treat*. 2011;2011:781612.
7. Klučka J, Klabusayová E, Musilová T, et al. Pediatric patient with ischemic stroke: initial approach and early management. *Children (Basel)*. 2021 Jul 28;8(8):649.
8. Paediatric Stroke Working Group. *Stroke in Childhood: Clinical Guidelines for Diagnosis, Management and Rehabilitation*. Royal College of Physicians of London; 2004. https://cdn.shopify.com/s/files/1/0924/4392/files/stroke-in-childhood-guideline.pdf
9. Irazuzta J, Sullivan KJ. Hyperacute therapies for childhood stroke: a case report and review of the literature. *Neurol Res Int*. 2010;2010:497326.
10. Hollist M, Au K, Morgan L, et al. Pediatric stroke: overview and recent updates. *Aging Dis*. 2021 Jul;12(4):1043-1055.

The Importance of Lactate

By Michael Platzer, DO, LT, MC, USN; and
Daphne Morrison Ponce, MD, CDR, MC, USN
Navy Medical Center in Portsmouth, Virginia

Reviewed by Andrew J. Eyre, MD, MS-HPEd

Objective

On completion of this article, you should be able to:

- State the diseases associated with elevated lactate levels and the importance of lactate in guiding treatment in the emergency department.

Wardi G, Brice J, Correia M, Liu D, Self M, Tainter C. Demystifying lactate in the emergency department. *Ann Emerg Med.* 2020 Feb;75(2):287-298.

KEY POINTS

- Elevated lactate levels can be caused by overproduction, decreased clearance, or a combination of both; they are associated with acute and chronic disease states and with an increased mortality rate.

- Increased tissue perfusion and circulation or treatment of underlying disease improves outcomes of patients with elevated lactate levels in most instances.

- Elevated lactate levels should be trended and used as a continuous measure to guide treatment and fluid resuscitation efforts.

In their review article, Wardi et al discuss the biochemistry and pathophysiology of elevated lactate levels and address both the previously accepted and emerging explanations for hyperlactatemia. The authors also review treatments for hyperlactatemia and the condition's impact on mortality.

Lactic acid is a naturally occurring organic acid that converts to the lactate ion. In humans, lactate is used at both rest and during exercise for two functions: to maintain blood glucose levels through its role in gluconeogenesis and to support oxidative phosphorylation through its role as an oxidizable agent. The heart and brain increase lactate metabolism during metabolic stress; each uses lactate for its energy demand (up to 60% for the heart and 25% for the brain). Lactate was traditionally believed to be a waste product of skeletal muscle metabolism, mostly from anaerobic metabolism, based on the "oxygen debt model." Contemporary understanding is that lactate is important for both energy use and oxidation-reduction reactions, even in aerobic conditions. Lactate levels can also rise in response to an increased metabolic state caused by proinflammatory cytokine cascades during physiologic stress, such as in cases of sepsis.

Approximately 70% to 75% of lactate is metabolized by the liver, while the remaining 25% to 30% is metabolized by the kidneys. Lactic acidosis refers to elevated serum lactate levels and a pH of less than or equal to 7.35. Type A lactic acidosis occurs from poor tissue perfusion when oxygen supply and demand are mismatched. Type B lactic acidosis occurs due to medications or other disease states that do not result in cellular hypoxia.

Measurements and Monitoring

Lactate measurements are accurate and repeatable when done correctly. Lactate is generated by drawing serum samples in a gray-top tube or by cooling samples to inhibit RBC metabolism. Processing fresh serum samples within 15 minutes of collection does not significantly distort values. Whole blood and finger-stick samples are both accurate methods for point-of-care lactate measurements. Venous tourniquet use has not been shown to significantly affect the accuracy of readings. Although arterial samples most accurately indicate the level of centrally circulating lactate, venous samples are still appropriate for trending — trending of the sample should be done from the same sample type. According to published studies, patients who receive infusions of lactated Ringer solution, which contains sodium lactate, do not show significant lactate elevations in their blood samples as long as samples are not collected in the immediate vicinity of the infusion.

Lactate in Sepsis

In patients with sepsis, the majority of lactate is thought to be generated in the lungs and skeletal muscle. Lactate elevation in sepsis is a result of leukocyte glycolysis: These inflammatory cells undergo accelerated aerobic glycolysis and produce markedly increased lactate. Increasing evidence shows that hyperlactatemia does not directly correlate with tissue hypoperfusion in patients with sepsis and, therefore, may not be a direct symptom of tissue hypoxia. Cryptic shock or occult hypoperfusion are terms that describe the presence of hyperlactatemia with a normal blood pressure. Patients with this finding (with lactate levels >4 mmol/L) have a relatively high mortality rate.

Lactate in Other Disease Processes

Increased lactate levels in trauma patients are also associated with an increased mortality rate. In general, failure to clear lactate is a strong independent predictor of mortality and can indicate infectious complications, organ dysfunction, mortality, or inadequate resuscitation. Elevated lactate levels in these instances are defined as greater than 2 mmol/L and may outperform base excess as a treatment goal for fluid resuscitation. Seizures, convulsions, and extreme exertion increase lactate levels, but

Critical Decisions in Emergency Medicine's LLSA literature reviews feature articles from ABEM's 2023 Lifelong Learning and Self-Assessment Reading List. Available online at acep.org/moc/llsa and on the ABEM website.

lactate levels do not correlate with patient outcomes in these cases. Thiamine deficiency, which can occur in patients with chronic alcoholism or poor nutritional status, causes hyperlactatemia because pyruvate undergoes anaerobic metabolism. Acetaminophen toxicity can cause lactic acidosis by directly inhibiting the mitochondrial electron transport chain, and lactate elevation in cases of acute liver failure portends a poor prognosis. β-adrenergic agonists (eg, albuterol) accelerate glycolysis and cause transient hyperlactatemia, although hyperlactatemia from these medications does not predict mortality. Cyanide toxicity impairs oxidative phosphorylation and is associated with lactate levels greater than 10 mmol/L. Ethanol intoxication, along with other comorbidities present in patients with this condition, can also increase lactate levels. Metformin overdose can cause a profound hyperlactatemia, but levels do not predict a poor prognosis.

Prognostic Value and Lactate Clearance

For many disease processes, elevated lactate levels and an inability to clear lactate are associated with a worse prognosis. Lactate levels greater than 4 mmol/L are associated with a 28% increased rate of inhospital mortality, independent of shock rate. Even mildly elevated lactate levels can be associated with mortality and a poor prognosis (depending on the cause), and levels should be used as a continuous variable to guide treatment. In the emergency department, an elevated lactate level should prompt investigation into its cause and should guide fluid resuscitation. Lactate levels must be interpreted in the context of the patient's medical history and presentation because they are not an exclusive indicator of disease severity, and physicians should not be falsely assured by low levels.

Disclosures

The views expressed in this article are those of the authors and do not necessarily reflect the official policy or position of the Department of the Navy, Department of Defense, or the United States Government.

This work was prepared as part of our official duties as military service members. Title 17 USC § 105 provides that "copyright protection under this title is not available for any work of the United States Government." A United States Government work is defined in 17 USC § 101 as a work prepared by a military service member or employee of the United States Government as part of that person's official duties.

Traumatic Hemipelvectomy

By Rosemary Mallonée, MD
University of Florida College of Medicine – Jacksonville

Reviewed by John Kiel, DO, MPH, FACEP, CAQSM

Objective

On completion of this article, you should be able to:

- Describe how to manage the uncommon presentation of THP in the emergency department.

CASE PRESENTATION

A 27-year-old man with a history of schizophrenia presents to the trauma bay after a pedestrian versus motor vehicle collision. EMS reports that the patient was walking when a vehicle struck him at highway speeds. He arrives on a backboard with an obvious deformity of the left hemipelvis. Although he is confused, he can protect his airway and, therefore, does not require immediate intubation. His physical examination reveals trauma to the left hip and leg, with a visible anterior superior iliac spine (ASIS) of the left hemipelvis, visible vasculature, and a visible quadricep muscle (*Figure 1*). He is unable to move his left lower extremity beneath the level of the hip. He also has an open left tibia-fibula fracture, a disrupted pubic symphysis, and an insensate left lower extremity without palpable pulses. He is in hemorrhagic shock, but his blood pressure improves after he receives two units of whole blood through a rapid infuser. X-rays and a CT are obtained and detect a traumatic hemipelvis disarticulation, an abrupt occlusion or thrombosis of the external iliac artery at the level of the left sacroiliac joint, a left common femoral artery transection, and a right both-column acetabular fracture (*Figures 2* and *3*). After consulting the trauma surgery team, the patient is taken directly to the operating room.

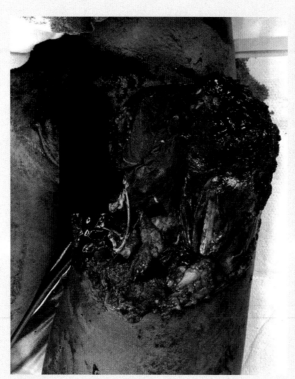

FIGURE 1. Gross appearance of the patient's left hip after a pedestrian versus motor vehicle collision, with gauze packing for hemostasis. *Credit:* Rosemary Mallonée, MD.

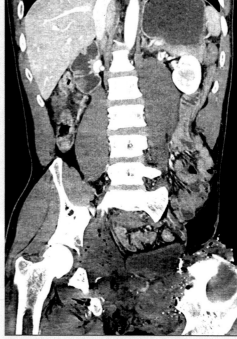

FIGURE 2. Initial CT showing complete disarticulation of the left hemipelvis, multiple comminuted pelvic fractures, a right acetabular fracture with intra-articular air, and a large pelvic hematoma. *Credit:* Rosemary Mallonée, MD.

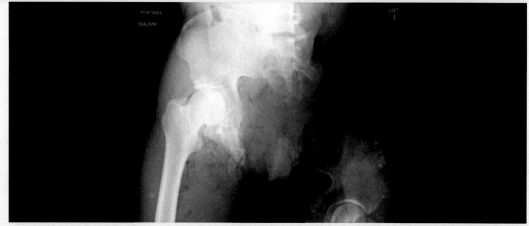

FIGURE 3. Pelvis x-ray on initial presentation showing an amputation injury of the left lower extremity with involvement of the left sacrum through pubic symphysis. *Credit:* Rosemary Mallonée, MD.

Discussion

Despite advances in prehospital resuscitation, traumatic hemipelvectomy (THP) remains a devastating and often fatal injury. Although classified in several ways, the most common classifications for THP are complete or partial. Complete THP is a complete dislocation of the hemipelvis, with disruption of the pubic symphysis and sacroiliac joint from trauma to the iliac vessels.[1] In complete THP, the hindquarter is dissociated from the axial skeleton. In partial THP, the soft tissue is intact, and the lower extremity is still attached to the trunk. Partial THP injuries can be further classified as closed or open, while all complete THP injuries are open by definition. Although documented cases of THP are rare (THP accounts for only 0.6% to 1.8% of all pelvic trauma), its true incidence is unknown because a large percentage of these patients die before arriving at the hospital.[2]

On arrival, patients with THP should undergo a standard Advanced Trauma Life Support (ATLS) protocol, which includes a primary survey, aggressive resuscitation, and hemorrhage control, if needed. Broad-spectrum antibiotics and tetanus prophylaxis should be administered to patients with open fractures or suspected partial or complete THP. Physical examination should include assessment of the typically obvious deformity, skin and soft tissue evaluation, and evaluation for hard or soft signs of vascular injury. Neurologic examination is indicated in alert patients. Assessment for neurovascular injury and hard or soft vascular signs can help distinguish closed partial THP from reconstructible pelvic trauma.

CT angiography (CTA) is the gold standard for diagnosing THP; however, patient stability and delays in care will affect the decision to obtain advanced imaging.

Once THP is suspected or diagnosed, the patient should be transferred to the nearest trauma center for definitive care. Operative treatment of THP has historically favored early hemipelvectomy without other operative intervention because it allows for complete hemorrhage control and is associated with reduced complication rates. However, abdominal aorta balloon occlusion, laparotomy, and packing prior to hemipelvectomy yield superior results according to small case studies of partial THP.[3] Revascularization is unfavored for closed THP cases because it can lead to rhabdomyolysis, renal failure, and compartment syndrome. In most cases, limb salvage and pelvic fixation are not recommended.

THP is also associated with damage to the anorectum (in 60% of cases) and genitourinary tract (in 85% of cases).[4] For anorectal damage, a diverting colostomy or ileostomy is indicated. Some sources recommend a colostomy even in THC patients without anorectal injury to avoid contaminating the pelvic wound.[5] Initial management of urethral injuries focuses on diverting urine to prevent contamination. Urethral reconstruction can occur immediately or later — secondary repair at a later date is associated with lower rates of urinary fistulas.[6] Patients with THP have complicated hospital courses and typically return to the operating room multiple times for debridement or placement of wound vacuum systems.

CASE RESOLUTION

The patient underwent CTA, which showed no evidence of perfusion distal to the left common iliac artery at the level of the proximal sacroiliac joint. Vascular surgery and orthopedics were consulted. After an interdisciplinary discussion with trauma surgery, vascular surgery, and orthopedics, the left limb was deemed unsalvageable, and a left hemipelvectomy was performed. The prostatic urethra appeared transected, so a suprapubic catheter was placed. Because of concern for a bleeding left internal iliac artery, the patient was taken to interventional radiology. The left internal iliac artery was found to be spastic, so embolization of the hypogastric artery was performed.

During the patient's initial stabilization, his right lower extremity was placed in traction for managing his right both-column acetabular fracture. Once clinically stable, he returned to the operating room for an open reduction and fixation (ORIF) of his right acetabular fracture by the orthopedics team and for a colostomy by the trauma surgery team. He had a prolonged hospital course of more than 2 months. Approximately 1 month after admission, he reported ongoing hip pain; pelvis x-rays were repeated to rule out hardware failure (*Figure 4*). During his hospital course, he returned to the operating room for a sphincterotomy, multiple debridements and drain placements, and placement of a wound vacuum system. He was discharged to inpatient rehab and eventually transitioned to full weight-bearing on the right leg. He attended regular postoperative appointments without issues.

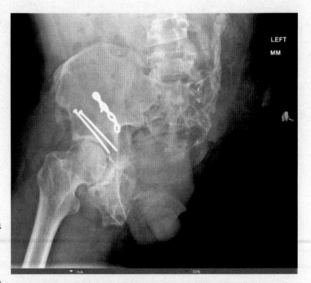

FIGURE 4. X-ray 1 month post operation showing plate-screw fixation without hardware migration or dislocation.
Credit: Rosemary Mallonée, MD.

REFERENCES

1. Labler L, Trentz O, Keel M. Traumatic hemipelvectomy. *Eur J Trauma.* 2005 Nov;31(6):543-550.
2. Patch DA, Hess MC, Spitler CA, Johnson JP. Diagnosis and management of traumatic hemipelvectomy. *J Am Acad Orthop Surg.* 2022 Sep 15;30(18):888-895.
3. Wang G, Zhou D, Shen W-J, et al. Management of partial traumatic hemipelvectomy. *Orthopedics.* 2013 Nov;36(11):e1340-e1345.
4. Schoderbek RJ, Battaglia TC, Dorf ER, Kahler DM. Traumatic hemipelvectomy: case report and literature review. *Arch Orthop Trauma Surg.* 2005 Jun;125(5):358-362.
5. Moore WM, Brown JJ, Haynes JL, Viamontes L. Traumatic hemipelvectomy. *J Trauma.* 1987 May;27(5):570-572.
6. Rieger H, Dietl KH. Traumatic hemipelvectomy: an update. *J Trauma.* 1998 Aug;45(2):422-426.

The Critical Image

Foreign Body Ingestions

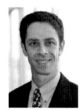

By Joshua S. Broder, MD, FACEP
Dr. Broder is a professor and the residency program director in the Department of Emergency Medicine at Duke University Medical Center in Durham, North Carolina.

Objectives

On completion of this article, you should be able to:

- Describe the complications of foreign body ingestions.
- Explain the risk of magnet ingestions.
- Apply a standard imaging approach for suspected recent GI foreign body ingestions.

CASE PRESENTATION

A 10-year-old girl presents after ingesting a foreign body approximately 1 hour ago. She accidentally swallowed a small toy that she was playing with and now has mild abdominal pain but no vomiting and no respiratory symptoms. Her vital signs are BP 107/72, P 82, R 18, and T 36.5°C (97.7°F); SpO₂ is 100% on room air. The patient is not distressed, and her abdominal examination shows normal bowel sounds and no tenderness. An abdominal x-ray is obtained (*Figure 1*).

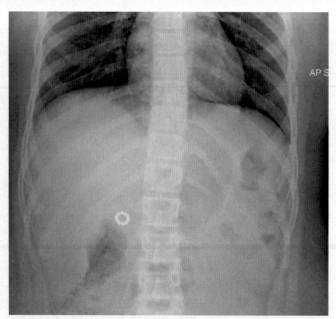

FIGURE 1. An anteroposterior supine x-ray demonstrating a radiopaque foreign body overlying the right upper quadrant. An object outside of the patient (anterior or posterior) would have a similar appearance; a lateral view could help confirm that the object is within the patient. The size of the object can be magnified slightly by x-ray if it lies closer to the x-ray source and farther from the detector.

Feature Editor: Joshua S. Broder, MD, FACEP. See also *Diagnostic Imaging for the Emergency Physician* (Winner of the 2011 Prose Award in Clinical Medicine, the American Publishers Award for Professional and Scholarly Excellence) and *Critical Images in Emergency Medicine* by Dr. Broder.

Discussion

Foreign body ingestion requires no intervention in 80% to 90% of cases. However, 10% to 20% require endoscopic removal, and 1% necessitate a surgical procedure to remove the foreign body.[1] Intentional ingestions are associated with much higher rates of intervention, with surgery required in as many as 28% of cases. Death from foreign body ingestions occurs in approximately 1,500 cases annually in the United States, although this often-cited number is based on older data.[2] Foreign bodies can enter the GI or respiratory tracts. Signs and symptoms can indicate which system is involved, but imaging or endoscopy may be required for uncertain cases. Foreign bodies in the GI tract can cause morbidity and mortality from bowel obstruction, perforation, pharmacologic effects (as with ingested packages of illicit or prescription drugs), and chemical or even radiologic toxicity (as with heavy metals or ingested radioactive material). Rare catastrophic effects such as aortoenteric fistula have been reported.

Important clinical information that helps determine the need for intervention includes the size (affecting the likelihood of spontaneous passage), shape or sharpness (affecting the perforation risk), number (affecting the passage and obstruction risk), and composition (affecting toxicity, perforation, and obstruction risks) of ingested foreign bodies. The timing of ingestion and the current location of the object also affect the urgency, feasibility, and manner of retrieval.[1,3]

Diagnostic imaging can assist with defining the characteristics of size, shape, and number as well as provide clues to location and composition. However, imaging has several important limits. Foreign bodies are not typically visible with plain x-rays when they have the same density as adjacent anatomic structures. For this reason, plastics, wood, small bones, and other organic materials are not reliably identified. Metal and glass (except for thin aluminum and small glass fragments) and gas-filled objects are usually visible on x-rays. Contrast agents can outline foreign bodies in the bowel lumen, and air is an intrinsic contrast agent that can make otherwise radiolucent objects visible.[1,3] Oral contrast agents are controversial because they can be aspirated, can impair subsequent endoscopic visualization, and can potentially obscure any foreign bodies of a similar density. If perforation is suspected, only water-soluble contrast agents should be used.[3]

Plain x-rays magnify objects that are closer to the x-ray source and farther from the detector, similar to how the shadow of a hand gets larger the closer the hand travels to the light source in a game of shadow puppets. The size of foreign bodies is relevant to potential endoscopic removal, which can be necessary for gastric

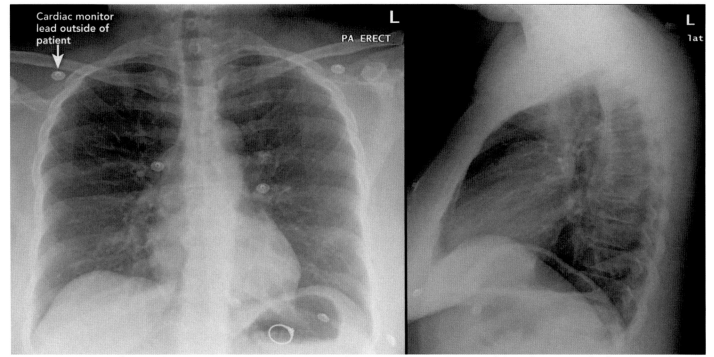

FIGURE 2. In another patient, a posteroanterior image demonstrating a ring overlying the stomach that is not seen on the lateral image. The ring was later discovered outside of the patient. Multiple cardiac leads on the patient's skin surface are also visible in both views and have a similar appearance, potentially leading to confusion in image interpretation.

foreign bodies greater than 2.5 cm in smallest dimension, which may not pass the pylorus spontaneously.

Although the magnetic fields from ingested magnets are not in themselves dangerous, magnets pose the risks of pressure necrosis and consequent perforation, fistula, and obstruction if they adhere to one another across adjacent bowel walls.[1,3] To avoid these complications, magnets within reach of an endoscope should be urgently removed. Multiple adherent magnets can simulate a single object on x-ray. Gaps between foreign bodies can suggest entrapped tissue, particularly if the gaps do not change on serial imaging.[3]

The following are recommendations for management of patients who present within hours of suspected GI foreign body ingestions:

- Use x-ray as the initial imaging modality for most cases, unless the ingested material is believed to be radiolucent, in which case CT may be needed. CT may also be warranted for delayed presentations with suspected complications such as obstruction or perforation or when x-rays are negative but suspicion persists. Ultrasound for ingested foreign bodies is not as well studied, but case reports describe its use.[4]
- Image as soon as possible. The opportunity to endoscopically retrieve a foreign body can be lost as the object progresses through the GI tract, which can leave surgical intervention as the only option if the object fails to progress or poses substantial perforation or other risk. Complications such as perforation can also be time dependent.
- Remove external objects that create confusion in image interpretation, such as jewelry, clothing, and unnecessary medical equipment.
- Obtain orthogonal views (eg, frontal and lateral) to confirm the foreign body's location within the patient (*Figure 2*).
- Image liberally (eg, x-rays of the neck, chest, abdomen, and pelvis) to avoid missing an ingested object if its location is uncertain.

REFERENCES

1. Kramer RE, Lerner DG, Lin T, et al. Management of ingested foreign bodies in children: a clinical report of the NASPGHAN Endoscopy Committee. *J Pediatr Gastroenterol Nutr.* 2015 Apr;60(4):562-574.
2. Schwartz GF, Polsky HS. Ingested foreign bodies of the gastrointestinal tract. *Am Surg.* 1976 Apr;42(4):236-238.
3. Guelfguat M, Kaplinskiy V, Reddy SH, DiPoce J. Clinical guidelines for imaging and reporting ingested foreign bodies. *AJR Am J Roentgenol.* 2014 Jul;203(1):37-53.
4. Pak SM, Lee YJ, Hwang JY. Diagnosis of nonmigrating metallic foreign bodies in the abdomen using ultrasound: an alternative approach using a traditional method. *Pediatr Gastroenterol Hepatol Nutr.* 2022 Jan;25(1):87-91.

CASE RESOLUTION

On further questioning, the patient revealed the ingested objects were magnets. These foreign bodies were quickly removed using endoscopy (*Figure 3*).

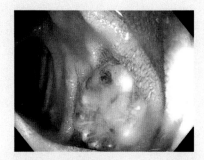

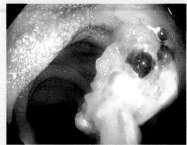

FIGURE 3. Endoscopic images of the ingested objects in the distal duodenum. The objects were ensnared in a net and removed.

The Critical Procedure

Cold Gastric Lavage

By Steven J. Warrington, MD, MEd, MS
MercyOne Siouxland, Sioux City, Iowa

Objective

On completion of this article, you should be able to:

■ Describe how to perform a cold gastric lavage for hyperthermia.

Introduction

There are multiple techniques for cooling patients who have hyperthermia. Evaporative cooling is an often-recommended route for external cooling. Certain situations, however, may necessitate the use of adjunct techniques for core cooling, such as cold gastric lavage.

Contraindications

■ An unprotected airway
■ A symptom or condition that would make placement of an oro- or nasogastric tube inadvisable

Benefits and Risks

A cold gastric lavage as an adjunct therapy can increase how quickly the body is cooled. Although invasive, it is less invasive relative to other cooling measures like thoracic or peritoneal lavage.

In addition to the risks associated with the required oro- or nasogastric tube placement, the cold gastric lavage carries other risks. Aspiration is one of them, so recommendations are to intubate patients with a cuffed endotracheal tube prior to the procedure. Electrolyte derangement is another risk, especially for patients at age extremes; this risk is variable based on the fluid selected for lavage. Dysrhythmias are a theoretical risk because of the proximity of the heart during rapid cooling, but no cases of dysrhythmia during cold gastric lavage have been reported. Patients who undergo rapid cooling also have a risk of developing hypothermia from overcorrection of their hyperthermic state.

Alternatives

External cooling techniques, such as evaporative cooling, ice packing (specific or general), and cold water immersion, are generally considered first-line cooling methods. Alternative approaches to core cooling include peritoneal, intrathoracic, or bladder lavage; infusion of chilled intravenous fluids; and respiratory therapy with cool air.

The cold gastric lavage technique described below uses instillation and suction, but an alternative technique can be used for a faster rate of lavage. In the alternative technique, a lavage with a large-bore gastric tube is placed. The bag for the lavage is opened and hung above the height of the patient, and ice and saline are added as needed. The bag and suction are connected to the gastric tube by a Y connector, which allows for faster instillation and withdrawal of chilled fluids.

Reducing Side Effects

Ensuring the patient's airway is protected can reduce the risk of aspiration and allow for sedation, which helps the procedure succeed. Additionally, a protected airway allows for paralysis to prevent shivering. Using normal saline instead of tap water or other solutions can help limit electrolyte abnormalities from developing.

Special Considerations

Cooling strategies used in the emergency department depend on multiple factors related to each patient, location, and the resources available. Using multiple cooling approaches can be beneficial, but close temperature monitoring is necessary to prevent hypothermia from developing.

TECHNIQUE

1. **Consider** a noninvasive, external method of cooling and initiate it if appropriate.
2. **Consider** if any contraindications to an orogastric tube exist.
3. **Ensure** the patient's airway is protected, such as with a cuffed endotracheal tube.
4. **Obtain** materials, including an orogastric tube, container for saline and ice, and a large-volume syringe for instillation and aspiration. Chill the saline bags, then open a bag and place it in the container with ice to lower its temperature more rapidly. Routinely monitor the bag's temperature, such as with a temperature-sensing Foley catheter.
5. **Instill** up to 10 mL/kg of iced saline through the orogastric tube.
6. **Wait** approximately 1 minute.
7. **Suction** contents through the orogastric tube.
8. **Repeat** the process until the cold gastric lavage is no longer a necessary part of therapy.

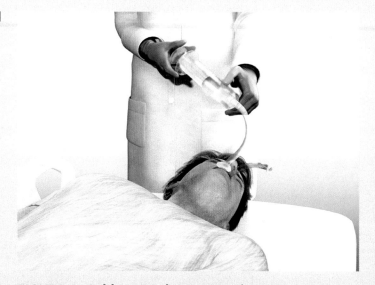

FIGURE 1. Cold gastric lavage. *Credit:* ACEP.

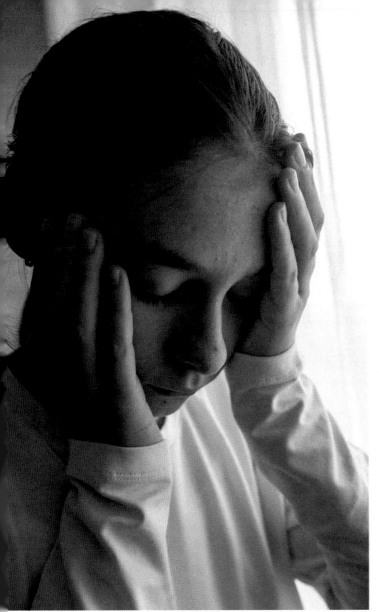

Head Scratcher

Pediatric Headache

LESSON 10

By Muhammad Ramdhan Abd Aziz, MD, MMed; and Jeremiah Duane Smith, MD, FAAP

Dr. Aziz is an emergency physician and pediatric emergency medicine fellow, and Dr. Smith is a pediatric emergency physician and clinical assistant professor at Prisma Health Greenville Memorial Hospital in Greenville, South Carolina.

Reviewed by Ann M. Dietrich, MD, FAAP, FACEP

Objectives

On completion of this lesson, you should be able to:

1. Obtain a complete history and physical examination of children with a headache.
2. Recognize the red flags of headache in children.
3. Differentiate between primary and secondary headache.
4. Apply relevant diagnostic investigations of pediatric headache based on history and physical examination findings.

From the EM Model

1.0 Signs, Symptoms, and Presentations
    1.2 Pain
        1.2.2 Headache
12.0 Nervous System Disorders
    12.3 Headache

■ CRITICAL DECISIONS

- How can primary and secondary pediatric headaches be distinguished?
- What are the most important aspects of the history and physical examination of children with a headache?
- Which red flags in pediatric headache patients warrant a CT of the brain?
- What laboratory studies should be ordered to investigate a pediatric headache?
- Which pediatric headache cases require urgent referral and hospitalization?
- How safe is it to discharge children with a headache?

Headache is a common complaint of children who present to the emergency department. More than half of children and adolescents experience a headache at some point in their lifetime. Although most pediatric headaches are benign, some are indicators of a potentially fatal illness. Emergency physicians must recognize the red flags that can point to life-threatening causes of headaches, such as brain tumors and meningitis.

CASE ONE

A 14-year-old girl presents with a throbbing headache on the right side of her head. It has been constant throughout the day, aggravated by physical activity, and reduced by sleep. She has no history of illness and states that this is her first time to have a headache. On examination, she is afebrile and holds her head while keeping her eyes closed. The findings of her neurologic examination are otherwise normal.

CASE TWO

A 9-year-old boy presents with a history of headaches that started 2 months ago. The headaches are increasing in frequency and severity. His father reports that the child had two episodes of vomiting this morning and now has a "wobbly" walk. He is worried and frustrated because he has visited several physicians who have told him to give the boy ibuprofen, but the headaches keep worsening. The child is awake and alert with a Glasgow Coma Scale score of 15 and no focal neurologic deficits. He refuses to lie flat on the bed because he fears the headache will worsen. He declines to walk and says he is afraid he will fall.

CASE THREE

A family medicine physician sends an 11-year-old boy to the emergency department with a concern for meningitis. The boy has a 2-day history of headache, neck pain, and nausea but no vomiting. His mother reports that the child's urine was dark brown this morning. On examination, he is febrile. Vital signs include P 105 and T 38.0°C (100.4°F); SpO$_2$ is 99% on room air. The neurologic examination reveals no abnormalities. There is mild left costophrenic tenderness to palpation and no stiffness of the neck. Kernig and Brudzinski signs are negative.

Introduction

The majority of children experience a headache at some point before reaching adulthood.[1] Fortunately, most headaches in children are benign.[2] However, children are frequently brought into the acute care setting for severe headaches or headaches that persist or do not respond to acetaminophen or ibuprofen. Parents may also be concerned about a brain tumor or more serious life-threatening etiology for the headache. In addition to providing pain control, physicians must determine whether the headache is a primary headache (usually a migraine or tension headache) or a secondary headache from a potentially life-threatening cause (eg, meningitis, an intracranial bleed, or a brain tumor). Determining the etiology of a headache relies heavily on the history and physical examination — laboratory and imaging tests are rarely needed. However, given the innate challenges of obtaining a thorough history and physical examination in young children, emergency physicians should be on the alert for red flags, which can be subtle, that indicate a serious underlying pathology.[3]

CRITICAL DECISION

How can primary and secondary pediatric headaches be distinguished?

The third edition of the International Classification of Headache Disorders (ICHD-3), published by the International Headache Society, provides detailed criteria for headache disorders, including primary and secondary headaches and facial pain.[4] Primary headache disorders include migraines, tension-type headaches, and trigeminal autonomic cephalgias, such as cluster headaches. Primary headaches are painful and may be disabling, but they are not a sign of underlying disease. By contrast, secondary headaches have an underlying etiology that may be life-threatening. Examples of underlying causes include brain tumors, idiopathic intracranial hypertension (IIH), or infections of the CNS.[5,6]

The two most common primary headache disorders are tension-type headache and migraine, which both present with normal physical examination findings (*Table 1*). Although tension-type headache has the greatest prevalence in the general population, the most common cause of primary headache seen in the emergency department is migraine. The occurrence of migraine is 1% to 3% in children 3 to 7 years and 3% to 8% in adolescents. Boys tend to have more migraines in early childhood, and girls tend to have more frequent headaches after puberty.[7] Migraine is typically characterized by intermittent headaches lasting for 2 to 72 hours, which is classified as with or without aura. An aura is typically visual but may also include numbness, weakness, dysarthria, coordination difficulties, or confusion. The headache onset is gradual, with moderate to severe intensity. The pain is often described as pulsing or throbbing. Unlike in adults, pediatric migraine is more often bilateral and may be frontal or temporal. The adult migraine is usually a unilateral temporal throbbing. Migraine is aggravated by physical activity, and patients prefer to be in a dark, quiet

Characteristic	Tension-Type	Migraine
Location	Diffuse	Bilateral or unilateral
Onset and duration	Minutes to days	Hours to days; gradual onset; develops in stages
Pain type	Pressure, tightness	Pulsing, throbbing
Physical activity	Does not worsen	Worsens
Photophobia, phonophobia	One may be present, but not both	Both are common
Nausea or vomiting	No	Yes
Cranial autonomic symptoms	No	Yes
Aura	No	May be present

TABLE 1. **Comparing pediatric tension-type headache (most common overall) and pediatric migraine (most common in the emergency department)[4]**

room. When present, aura can occur before or during the headache phase. Phonophobia, photophobia, nausea, vomiting, and cranial autonomic symptoms are also frequently present.[8]

The ICHD-3 criteria for the diagnosis of migraine without aura are:
A. At least five headache attacks that fulfill criteria B through D.
B. Two to 72 hours of an untreated or unsuccessfully treated headache for children younger than 18 years.
C. The headache has at least two of the following characteristics:
   1. Unilateral or bilateral location (and often frontal) in children younger than 18 years;
   2. A pulsating quality;
   3. Moderate or severe pain intensity; and
   4. The headache is either aggravated by or causes avoidance of normal physical activity.
D. During a headache, at least one of the following occurs:
   1. Nausea or vomiting; and
   2. Photophobia and phonophobia.
E. Another ICHD-3 diagnosis fails to account for the symptoms.

The ICHD-3 criteria for the diagnosis of migraine with aura are:
A. At least two headache attacks that fulfill criteria B and C.
B. One or more of the following fully reversible aura disturbances: visual, sensory, speech or language, motor, brainstem, or retinal.
C. At least three of the following characteristics:
   1. At least one aura symptom spreading gradually over 5 minutes or more;
   2. Two or more symptoms occurring in succession;
   3. Each individual aura symptom lasting 5 to 60 minutes;
   4. At least one aura symptom that is unilateral;
   5. At least one aura symptom that is positive; and
   6. The headache accompanies the aura or follows it within 60 minutes.
D. Another ICHD-3 diagnosis fails to account for the symptoms.

A family history of migraine contributes to the likelihood that a child's headache is primary, but there are no diagnostic laboratory tests or imaging studies specific to migraine.

Management of migraine in children is a multidisciplinary approach that consists of lifestyle modifications, abortive agents, and preventive agents. In addition to basic lifestyle modifications, including rest and hydration, most patients respond to the use of an over-the-counter medication (eg, NSAID or acetaminophen), which has been found to be effective in children with migraine.[9] Triptan therapy or a combination of NSAID, antiemetic, and oral fluids may be used as an abortive agent. Nasal sumatriptan and nasal zolmitriptan have the best efficacy in pediatrics.

Other primary headaches include tension-type and cluster headaches. Although it may be difficult to distinguish primary headaches in children too young to describe their pain, tension-type headache is far more common than cluster headache and other trigeminal autonomic cephalgias. Tension-type headache is characterized by a diffuse, nonthrobbing pain that lasts minutes to days. It is often described as a pressing or tightening sensation over the head. The pain does not worsen with routine physical activity and is not associated with nausea or vomiting, but photophobia or phonophobia may be present. Relief can usually be achieved with acetaminophen or ibuprofen.[3]

The ICHD-3 diagnostic criteria for infrequent episodic tension-type headache are:
A. At least 10 episodes of headache at a frequency of less than 1 day per month on average (<12 days per year) and that fulfill criteria B through D.
B. The headache lasts from 30 minutes to 7 days.
C. At least two of the following characteristics:
   1. Bilateral location;
   2. Pressing or tightening (nonpulsating) quality;
   3. Mild or moderate intensity; and
   4. Unaffected by routine physical activity such as walking or climbing stairs.
D. No nausea or vomiting and either photophobia or phonophobia may be present, but not both.
E. Another ICHD-3 diagnosis fails to account for the symptoms.

Cluster headaches are rare in children younger than 10 years. Classically, they are characterized by attacks of severe pain in a unilateral distribution, that typically affects the orbital and temporal areas of the head; ipsilateral cranial parasympathetic autonomic signs include nasal congestion, rhinorrhea, lacrimation, facial sweating, miosis, and ptosis or eyelid edema.[10]

Secondary headaches are caused by an underlying condition and may resolve with proper management of the causal disease. Some etiologies of secondary headache in children include acute febrile illness (eg, recurrent rhinosinusitis or influenza), medications (eg, overuse of analgesics), acute or chronic meningitis, hydrocephalus, brain tumors, IIH, and intracranial hemorrhage.[4] One helpful way to differentiate between primary and secondary headaches is by using the SNOOP mnemonic (Table 2):
- **S**ystemic signs and symptoms: Fever; weight loss; history of cancer; and abnormal blood test results that could point to meningitis, cancer, or other illness causing the headache.
- **N**eurologic examination: If the findings (eg, speech, gait, mental status) are abnormal, then a secondary headache should be suspected.
- **O**nset: If the onset is sudden, a secondary headache, such as from an aneurysm or bleed, should be suspected. An onset of shorter than 2 weeks could indicate meningitis; an onset of longer than 6 months usually points to a benign primary headache condition.
- **O**nset age: If the patient is younger than 3 years, a secondary headache should always be considered. It is uncommon for younger children to suffer from primary headaches.
- **P**rogressive: A headache pattern that progressively worsens and is associated with other progressive symptoms, such as weight loss or neurologic changes, is suggestive of a secondary headache.

Differentiating Between Primary and Secondary Headaches
Systemic signs and symptoms
Neurologic examination
Onset
Onset age
Progressive

TABLE 2. **SNOOP mnemonic**

What are the most important aspects of the history and physical examination of children with a headache?

A good history will provide important information for the assessment of children with a headache. It is also critical to complete a careful physical examination, particularly the neurologic assessment, to avoid unnecessary investigations and neuroimaging. The history should be obtained from both the child and caregivers. Some important components of a headache history for children include:

- Age of onset: Headaches are unusual in children younger than 3 years. Migraines frequently begin in the first decade of life.
- Mode of onset: Abrupt onset (a "thunderclap headache" or "the worst headache of my life") may indicate intracranial hemorrhage.
- Frequency and duration: Headaches that become progressively more frequent or increase in intensity should raise suspicion for a more serious underlying condition.
- Time of occurrence: Headaches that wake a child from sleep or occur on waking may indicate elevated intracranial pressure.
- Aggravating and relieving factors: Migraine usually responds to analgesic, and routine physical activities may aggravate the pain.
- Associated symptoms: Altered mental status, ataxia, and diplopia may indicate a space-occupying lesion. A stiff neck may occur in meningitis or intracranial hemorrhage. Vomiting associated with morning headaches may indicate increased intracranial pressure. Growth curves can also be helpful. An escalating head circumference (usually measured until 3 years of age), split sutures, or an enlarging fontanelle is suspicious for an intracranial process. Weight loss or a drop in percentile on the growth curve that is accompanied by a headache and vomiting is concerning for an intracranial process. Developmental regression and headaches are also concerning for an intracranial process. Neurologic deficits, including ataxia, associated with headaches are highly suggestive of an intracranial tumor.

A child's history of headache can be unreliable, especially in younger children. In infants, episodes of colic or intermittent torticollis may be early signs of a headache. Toddlers may appear pale and become less active than usual. They may also vomit, rock in place, or hide. Sometimes, they may act as though they are afraid to walk due to acute intermittent vertigo. School-age children are usually better at describing the headache and its associated feelings.[11]

Medication overuse headache (MOH) describes a headache that occurs on 15 or more days per month in a patient with a preexisting primary headache.[4] It is a consequence of over 3 months of overuse of one or more drugs that are used for acute or symptomatic treatment of a headache. The headache is temporarily relieved by medications, leading to more medication usage. It is essential to recognize if medication overuse is contributing to a patient's headache because management through the elimination of acute abortive agent overuse may reduce the patient's symptoms.

A child who appears ill may have a more serious underlying condition, such as meningitis or an intracranial hemorrhage. Meningitis may initially present with subtle signs, especially in younger children, so a high degree of suspicion is necessary. Following the Pediatric Emergency Care Applied Research Network or American College of Emergency Physicians/American Academy of Pediatrics guidelines for fever in well-appearing children younger than 60 days can help prevent missing a more serious illness in the youngest patients. An older child may complain of fever, headache, photophobia, nausea, and vomiting and exhibit the classic signs of meningism. The onset may present as a rapidly progressive illness that is characterized by shock, coma, or status epilepticus. An infectious etiology of headache, including meningitis, is possible even in the absence of fever. One systematic review found that the presence of meningeal signs (eg, nuchal rigidity, photophobia, and a positive Kernig or Brudzinski sign) increased the likelihood of the diagnosis of meningitis, and conversely, their absence decreased the probability (*Figure 1*).[12] However, other studies have shown that the presence of classic signs and symptoms of meningitis cannot accurately distinguish between children with and without meningitis. Thus, they should be interpreted with caution.[13]

Intracranial hemorrhage can be associated with aneurysm, vascular malformation, coagulopathy, and hemoglobinopathy (intracranial hemorrhage accounts for one-third of cerebrovascular events in patients with sickle cell disease).[14]

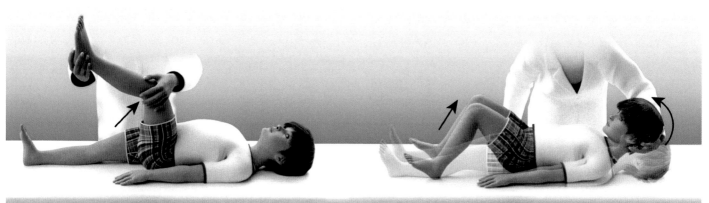

Kernig sign:
Resistance to extension of the leg while the hip is flexed

Brudzinski sign:
Flexion of the hips and knees in response to neck flexion

FIGURE 1. Kernig and Brudzinski signs. *Credit:* ACEP.

The symptoms include abrupt onset of headache, nausea, and vomiting. Signs frequently include hemiparesis and seizures.

Under normal circumstances, opting to forgo a blood pressure reading in the pediatric population is acceptable; however, when children present with a headache, a blood pressure reading must be taken. Hypertension in pediatric patients can be an indicator of undiagnosed renal disease or an undiagnosed narrowing of the aorta, both of which are potentially dangerous causes of headaches. Measuring the head circumference provides valuable information: Hydrocephalus or a brain tumor can cause macrocephaly. The neurologic examination should focus on mental status, speech, strength, sensation, gait, coordination, and cranial nerve function; a fundoscopic assessment should also be made. Look for signs of trauma and examine the skin for evidence of a neurocutaneous disease. For example, multiple café-au-lait lesions suggest neurofibromatosis and a possible intracranial tumor.[15] Neurofibromatosis (usually type I) is an autosomal dominant disorder of the NF1 gene that encodes the protein neurofibromin. A child with neurofibromatosis has visible hyperpigmented macules (ie, café-au-lait lesions) and soft papules and nodules on the skin (ie, neurofibromata). Neurofibromatosis increases the risk of having CNS gliomas and other malignant tumors.[3]

Three or more hypopigmented lesions, ash leaf spots, can be associated with tuberous sclerosis, which can also be associated with intracranial tumors.

CRITICAL DECISION

Which red flags in pediatric headache patients warrant a CT of the brain?

Red flags are historical and physical examination findings that increase suspicion of a secondary headache and warrant further evaluation, including urgent neuroimaging and potential subspecialty referral. Common red flag symptoms include:
- Headache in a child younger than 3 years[16];
- Recent onset (<6 months) with a steadily worsening pattern (frequency or intensity)[16];
- Early-morning awakening with a headache or vomiting[16];
- Double vision[17,18];
- Worsening of the headache while straining;
- Presence of seizures;
- Associated mood, mental status, or school performance change[16,19]; and
- Neurocutaneous stigmata (café-au-lait macules, hypopigmented macules).[16]

Children who present with red flag symptoms require evaluation for a brain tumor or space-occupying lesion.[19] CNS imaging may be accomplished with CT or MRI, depending on the facility's resources. An urgent head CT scan may be a better choice to evaluate a patient with the potential for intracranial hemorrhage, head trauma, cerebral edema, hydrocephalus, or herniation syndrome because CT is faster and more readily available than MRI and typically does not require sedation. A noncontrast CT scan is superior to MRI, especially in detecting acute subarachnoid hemorrhage (SAH) from a ruptured aneurysm or arteriovenous malformation (AVM). If SAH is detected, further evaluation for any aneurysm or AVM should be performed. CT is sometimes performed before a lumbar puncture (LP) in cases of suspected intracranial infection

and elevated intracranial pressure; it helps to determine if the procedure is safe by excluding any mass lesion or cerebral edema that produces midline shift or herniation.[19] Patients with evidence of an intracranial process such as a bleed or a mass need emergent intervention by the neurosurgical team. MRI with urgent follow-up with a primary care physician or neurologist is appropriate for a patient with chronic progressive headaches and normal physical examination findings. MRI provides much more detailed information and spares the patient from radiation exposure.[3,20]

CRITICAL DECISION

What laboratory studies should be ordered to investigate a pediatric headache?

According to the American Academy of Neurology, there is inadequate documentation in the literature to support any recommendations of routine laboratory studies or LPs for children presenting with a headache. Recurrent headaches are common in children and are diagnosed on a clinical basis. Diagnostic studies are not indicated when physical examination results are normal and there are no associated risk factors from the clinical history.[21]

When laboratory tests are used, they should be tailored to the circumstance based on clinical suspicion from the history and clinical examination. For example, when children present with a possibly severe infection that causes a headache, they may require numerous laboratory investigations, including a CBC, blood cultures, and an LP. Serum electrolytes, BUN, creatinine levels, and a urinalysis should be obtained to rule out nephritic syndrome and nephropathy if children with a headache have unexplained elevated blood pressure. Serum or urine toxicology screenings should be ordered for cases of suspected acute or chronic intoxication, especially in teenagers who present with severe headache, vomiting, or delirium.

CRITICAL DECISION

Which pediatric headache cases require urgent referral and hospitalization?

Emergency physicians generally see patients who have been referred to the emergency department because of onsets of worsening headaches, therapy failures, concerning neurologic examination findings, or other red flags. In the emergency

✔ Pearls

- The history and physical examination are critical to recognizing red flags for more serious causes of pediatric headaches.

- Migraines are diagnosed clinically. There are no diagnostic laboratory tests or imaging studies specific to migraine.

- A noncontrast CT may be indicated in the emergency department to rule out any space-occupying lesions or an acute hemorrhage.

department, these patients are evaluated to identify red flags suggestive of life-threatening disease. Urgent consultation with a pediatric neurologist is indicated in cases with neurologic signs and symptoms, such as hemiparesis or other stroke-like symptoms that may require stroke team activation and evaluation. An urgent referral to the pediatric neurology team should be made if there are concerns about specific headache patterns, treatment failures, or patients with complex migraines with atypical presentations. Patients with headache and papilledema can require ophthalmology confirmation of papilledema, especially in the younger age groups; visual testing must also be performed to identify any vision loss. Children who present with visual complaints should receive ophthalmologic evaluation. Imaging is required prior to checking CSF pressure and may require inpatient admission for an MRI with sedation.[3]

The ICHD-3 criteria for a headache attributed to IIH includes[22]:
A. A new or significantly worsened headache or one that has significantly worsened, fulfilling criterion C.
B. Both:
1. IIH has been diagnosed; and
2. CSF pressure exceeds 250 mm CSF (or 280 mm CSF in obese children).
C. Either or both:
1. The headache has developed or significantly worsened in temporal relation to IIH, or led to its discovery; or
2. The headache is accompanied by either or both:
a. Pulsatile tinnitus; or
b. papilledema.
D. Another ICHD-3 diagnosis fails to account for the symptoms.[22]

If imaging reveals no obstruction or structural lesions, an LP needs to be performed to determine the opening pressure. If a secondary etiology for the headache is identified, including hydrocephalus or an intracranial mass, the appropriate pediatric subspecialists should be contacted and an appropriate admission arranged (most likely to a pediatric tertiary care center).

Although most pediatric patients with headaches can be safely discharged with appropriate follow-up, some require admission for further evaluation and treatment. Hospitalization is generally indicated for patients with concerning neurologic examination findings (eg, papilledema, acute behavior changes, or seizure), abnormal vital signs, and concerning imaging results. For example, a hypertensive child with a headache should be admitted for blood pressure control and to find the underlying cause. Patients with intractable headaches warrant admission for more effective pain control.

CRITICAL DECISION

How safe is it to discharge children with a headache?

Some pediatric patients experience a recurrence of headache symptoms after discharge and return to the emergency department. The return rate in patients with headaches has been reported to range from 3% to 12%.[23,24] There has been limited investigation into the frequency of missed serious neurologic and non-neurologic diagnoses (SNNDs) among children discharged from the emergency department. A multicenter retrospective cohort study found that 0.5% of patients had an SNND identified within 30 days. According to the study, benign intracranial hypertension, cerebral edema and compression, and seizures were the most common SNNDs identified. The most common SNND (essential hypertension) carried lower morbidity and mortality. Other more serious SNNDs that require acute interventions, such as ventricular shunt malformation and malignant neoplasm, occurred at low rates.[25] Despite the low incidence rate of SNNDs, it is wise to establish safeguards for discharged patients, such as close outpatient follow-up.

Summary

Headache is a common complaint in the emergency department, especially in children. Physicians must be able to distinguish benign headaches from more ominous cases. Differentiating various headaches is usually achievable through a complete history and physical examination and, when warranted, laboratory tests and imaging. Proper referrals to the neurology or neurosurgery team are also key to properly managing children with headaches, whether for urgent intervention or appropriate follow-up.

✖ Pitfalls

- Failing to recognize the signs that may point to a headache in small children, such as crying, rocking, hiding, or decreased activity levels.

- Ignoring the patient's history of recurrent visits for headaches or parental concerns, which may point to inadequate treatment or an unresolved underlying illness.

- Neglecting to take a blood pressure reading during the physical examination in pediatric patients who present with a headache.

REFERENCES

1. Abu-Arafeh I, Razek S, Sivaraman B, Graham C. Prevalence of headache and migraine in children and adolescents: a systematic review of population-based studies. *Dev Med Child Neurol.* 2010 Dec;52(12):1088-1097.

2. Kang BS, Lee J, Choi JH, Kwon HH, Kang JW. Clinical manifestations of headache in children younger than 7 years. *Korean J Pediatr.* 2018 Nov;61(11):355-361.

3. Pauzé DR, Malabanan C. Pain: headache. In: Shaw KN, Bachur EG, Chamberlain JM, Lavelle J, Nagler J, Shook JE, eds. *Fleisher & Ludwig's Textbook of Pediatric Emergency Medicine.* 8th ed. Wolters Kluwer; 2021:394-401.

4. Headache Classification Committee of the International Headache Society (IHS). The international classification of headache disorders, 3rd ed. *Cephalalgia.* 2018 Jan;38(1):1-211.

5. Susy J. Children and headache: red flags, triggers, and rescue treatments. Contemporary Pediatrics. Published May 11, 2021. https://www.contemporarypediatrics.com/view/children-and-headaches-red-flags-triggers-and-rescue-treatments

CASE RESOLUTIONS

■ CASE ONE
Based on this patient's history and physical examination, she most likely had a primary headache syndrome. Her throbbing unilateral headache lasted for days, occured with photophobia, and was aggravated by physical activity, suggesting a migraine. The patient was assessed for signs of an infection, including meningitis, and she was found to have no fever, no meningeal signs, and no signs of sinusitis. Following an oral analgesic dose in the emergency department, her headache pain went from 5 to 1. She was discharged home with an oral analgesic, counseling on avoidance of possible migraine triggers, and a referral to a neurologist for follow-up.

■ CASE TWO
Patients with repeat visits for a chief complaint, such as this patient's persistent headache, warrant a thorough history and physical examination. The father's concern about worsening headaches was justified. This child had several warning signs, including morning emesis, a "wobbly" walk (possible cerebellar sign), and refusal to lie down (possible increased intracranial pressure). Because of these red flags, the child needed neuroimaging. His refusal to lie down was determined to be most likely secondary to pain from increased intracranial pressure. The pain was addressed with a nonsedating agent to facilitate the imaging test. He was placed on a cardiac monitor with the head of the bed elevated, and intravenous access was initiated. The physician in charge ordered a noncontrast head CT, which showed a mass in the posterior fossa with hydrocephalus. The child required urgent transfer to a tertiary center for definitive intervention by neurosurgery.

■ CASE THREE
This patient's symptoms were vague and nonspecific. There were clues in the systemic findings, including tachycardia, dark urine, and costophrenic tenderness. Additional questions about the character, timing, intensity, and associated symptoms were important to delineate an appropriate differential. Blood pressure was not obtained, which is typical in actual practice, especially in younger children. This patient had a blood pressure of 160/100 mm Hg, which was severely hypertensive for an 11 year old and placed her at risk of seizures and intracranial bleeding. A urinalysis showed microscopic hematuria and proteinuria, but no pyuria. Based on the history, clinical findings, and urinalysis, the child was suspected to have acute glomerulonephritis. An antihypertensive was started, and the nephrology unit was consulted urgently. Because headache can be a sign of systemic illness, a thorough history and clinical examination are always required, including a complete set of vital signs.

6. Bonthius DJ, Hershey AD. Headache in children: Approach to evaluation and general management strategies. UpToDate. Updated September 19, 2022. https://www.uptodate.com/contents/headache-in-children-approach-to-evaluation-and-general-management-strategies

7. Hershey AD. Current approaches to the diagnosis and management of paediatric migraine. *Lancet Neurol.* 2010;9(2):190-204.

8. Gelfand AA. Pathophysiology, clinical features, and diagnosis of migraine in children. UpToDate. Updated January 31, 2023. https://www.uptodate.com/contents/pathophysiology-clinical-features-and-diagnosis-of-migraine-in-children

9. Richer L, Billinghurst L, Linsdell MA, et al. Drugs for the acute treatment of migraine in children and adolescents. *Cochrane Database Syst Rev.* 2016 Apr 19;4(4):CD005220.

10. Lampl C. Childhood-onset cluster headache. *Pediatr Neurol.* 2002 Aug;27(2):138-140.

11. Rothner AD. The evaluation of headaches in children and adolescents. *Semin Pediatr Neurol.* 1995 Jun;2(2):109-118.

12. Curtis S, Stobart K, Vandermeer B, Simel DL, Klassen T. Clinical features suggestive of meningitis in children: a systematic review of prospective data. *Pediatrics.* 2010 Nov;126(5):952-960.

13. Amarilyo G, Alper A, Ben-Tov A, Grisaru-Soen G. Diagnostic accuracy of clinical symptoms and signs in children with meningitis. *Pediatr Emerg Care.* 2011 Mar;27(3):196-199.

14. Ohene-Frempong K, Weiner SJ, Sleeper LA, et al. Cerebrovascular accidents in sickle cell disease: rates and risk factors. *Blood.* 1998 Jan 1;91(1):288-294.

15. Honig PJ, Charney EB. Children with brain tumor headaches. Distinguishing features. *Am J Dis Child.* 1982 Feb;136(2):121-124.

16. Lewis DW, Koch T. Headache evaluation in children and adolescents: when to worry? When to scan? *Pediatr Ann.* 2010 Jul;39(7):399-406.

17. Tsze DS, Ochs JB, Gonzalez AE, Dayan PS. Red flag findings in children with headaches: prevalence and association with emergency department neuroimaging. *Cephalalgia.* 2019 Feb;39(2):185-196.

18. Manoyana A, Angkurawaranon S, Katib S, Wiwattanadittakul N, Sirikul W, Angkurawaranon C. Diagnostic values of red flags and a clinical prediction score for emergent intracranial lesions in non-traumatic pediatric headaches. *Children (Basel).* 2022 Jun 10;9(6):863.

19. Lewis DW, Koch T. Headache evaluation in children and adolescents: when to worry? When to scan? *Pediatric Ann.* 2010 Jul;39(7):399-406.

20. Hayes LL, Palasis S, Bartel TB, et al; Expert Panel on Pediatric Imaging. ACR Appropriateness Criteria® Headache — Child. *J Am Coll Radiol.* 2018 May;15(5)(suppl):S78-S90.

21. Lewis DW, Ashwal S, Dahl G, et al. Practice parameter: evaluation of children and adolescents with recurrent headaches: report of the Quality Standards Subcommittee of the American Academy of Neurology and the Practice Committee of the Child Neurology Society. *Neurology.* 2002 Aug 27;59(4):490-498.

22. Moavero R, Sforza G, Papetti L, et al. Clinical features of pediatric idiopathic intracranial hypertension and applicability of new ICHD-3 criteria. *Front Neurol.* 2018 Sep 28;9:819.

23. Cobb-Pitstick KM, Hershey AD, O'Brien HL, et al. Factors influencing migraine recurrence after infusion and inpatient migraine treatment in children and adolescents. *Headache.* 2015 Nov-Dec;55(10):1397-1403.

24. Hong A, Shah Y, Singh K, Karkare S, Kothare S. Characteristics and predictors of 7- and 30-day hospital readmissions to pediatric neurology. *Neurology.* 2019 Apr 16;92(16):e1926-e1932.

25. Zhou AZ, Marin JR, Hickey RW, Ramgopal S. Serious diagnoses for headaches after ED discharge. *Pediatrics.* 2020 Nov;146(5):e20201647.

CME Questions

Reviewed by **Kelsey Drake, MD, MPH, FACEP**; and Ann M. Dietrich, MD, FAAP, FACEP

Qualified, paid subscribers to *Critical Decisions in Emergency Medicine* may receive CME certificates for up to 5 ACEP Category I credits, 5 *AMA PRA Category 1 Credits™*, and 5 AOA Category 2-B credits for completing this activity in its entirety. Submit your answers online at acep.org/cdem; a score of 75% or better is required. You may receive credit for completing the CME activity any time within 3 years of its publication date. Answers to this month's questions will be published in next month's issue.

1 Which patient has the highest risk of thyroid storm?

A. 28-year-old woman with a history of multiple drug use who presents with agitation. She is not answering questions but has a family history of "thyroid issues" in her chart. Her vital signs include BP 172/87, P 132, R 32, and T 40.1°C (104.2°F). On examination, she is febrile, agitated, and vomiting.

B. 42-year-old woman with a recent thyroidectomy who presents with muscle spasms. Her vital signs include BP 98/65, P 92, and T 39.1°C (102.4°F). Laboratory tests are remarkable for a thyroid-stimulating hormone level of 0.2 µu/mL (normal 0.5-5 µu/mL), a free T4 level of 64 µg/dL (normal 5-12 µg/dL), and an ionized calcium level of 2.0 mg/dL (normal 4.5-5.6 mg/dL).

C. 56-year-old man with a history of hyperthyroidism, heart failure, and hypertension who presents with fever and cough. He has not been compliant with his medications. A chest x-ray shows right lower lobe pneumonia. His examination is remarkable for grade +2 pitting edema in the lower extremities and bilateral crackles in the lower lung lobes that are worse in the right lung than the left. He is otherwise alert and oriented. His vital signs include BP 157/79, P 88, R 22, and T 38.2°C (100.8°F).

D. 74-year-old man with a history of atrial fibrillation who presents with an afebrile urinary tract infection. He is currently in atrial fibrillation with a heart rate of 101 bpm and takes amiodarone.

2 A 42-year-old woman with a history of Graves disease and asthma presents with dyspnea, tachycardia, and chest pain. She has an elevated Wells score for pulmonary embolism. Diffuse wheezing is noted on examination. Laboratory tests, imaging, and nebulized breathing treatments are ordered. After finishing her workup, the patient becomes belligerent and tachycardic, and her dyspnea worsens. What most likely resulted in these changes to her clinical status?

A. CT angiography of the chest
B. Flash pulmonary edema
C. Intravenous fluids
D. Medication side effect

3 In the emergency department, a patient is diagnosed with thyroid storm. What is the initial therapeutic sequence in managing this condition?

A. Hydrocortisone, propylthiouracil, propranolol, iodine
B. Propranolol, propylthiouracil, iodine, hydrocortisone
C. Propylthiouracil, propranolol, hydrocortisone, iodine
D. Propylthiouracil, propranolol, iodine, hydrocortisone

4 Which medication is most likely to exacerbate hyperthyroidism and increase the risk of thyroid storm?

A. Amiodarone
B. Ciprofloxacin
C. Glipizide
D. Lisinopril

5 A patient is being treated for suspected thyroid storm and also undergoing a workup to rule out infection as the cause. The patient has a fever of 40.2°C (104.4°F). What medication would be best for treating the fever?

A. Acetaminophen
B. Ibuprofen
C. Ketorolac
D. Meperidine

6 What is the mechanism of action of thionamides in treating thyroid storm?

A. Blocking the synthesis of thyroid hormone
B. Decreasing sympathetic hyperactivity
C. Inhibiting release of stored thyroid hormone
D. Targeting the autoimmune process behind hyperthyroidism

7 A 22-year-old woman presents with palpitations. She appears anxious and complains of worsening anxiety, a fast heart rate, and bloating that have occurred over the past 2 months. Her periods have been irregular, and she experiences nausea and vomiting every morning. She has no prior medical history. Her vital signs include BP 98/67, P 153, R 22, and T 38.1°C (100.6°C). Which laboratory test(s) will most likely reveal the cause of her symptoms?

A. Antithyroid antibody test
B. Bedside glucose and A1C tests
C. β-human chorionic gonadotropin test
D. Comprehensive metabolic panel

8 A patient presents with altered mental status, fever, and tachycardia. Thyroid storm is suspected. What is the best next step for aggressive management of this patient?

A. Administer iodine
B. Administer metoprolol
C. Discharge the patient home with supportive care, reassurance, and strict return precautions
D. Order laboratory tests and wait for results to confirm the diagnosis

9 A 47-year-old man with a history of Graves disease and depression presents with altered mental status. He has been increasingly agitated and confused for the past 2 days and has had intermittent fevers and rhinorrhea, which he thought were symptoms of a viral illness. His vital signs are BP 190/86, P 143, R 24, and T 39.1°C (102.4°F); SpO₂ is 97% on room air. On examination, he is agitated, tremulous, tachycardic, and diaphoretic, and he has grade +2 pitting edema. An ECG shows sinus tachycardia, and a chest x-ray shows bilateral pleural effusions. What is the most appropriate next step?

A. Furosemide
B. Iodine
C. Nicardipine
D. Propranolol

10 A 31-year-old woman presents with a 1-week history of worsening dyspnea, palpitations, and excessive sweating. She reports that she recently started using a holistic medication she found online to try to lose weight but cannot remember its name. She has a history of depression and anxiety and is now increasingly anxious and unable to sleep. Her vital signs include BP 162/95, P 156, R 22, and T 38.9°C (102°F). An ECG shows an irregularly irregular rhythm with tachycardia. She also has crackles bilaterally in her lower lung lobes and a grade +2 pitting edema in her lower extremities. Which medication should be avoided?

A. Dexamethasone
B. Ketorolac
C. Nicardipine
D. Propranolol

11 **What is a sign of raised intracranial pressure when coexisting with a headache?**

   A. Aura
   B. Fever
   C. Photophobia
   D. Waking from sleep due to pain

12 **What is the most appropriate investigation for headaches with clinical neurologic signs in the emergency department?**

   A. Electroencephalogram
   B. Lumbar puncture
   C. Noncontrast CT of the brain
   D. Toxicology screen

13 **What most likely represents a primary headache illness?**

   A. Headache associated with changes in behavior
   B. Headache following recent trauma
   C. Headache with a known case of diabetes type 1
   D. Unilateral throbbing headache that lasts 24 hours with photophobia

14 **Which condition warrants urgent imaging in the emergency department?**

   A. 3 year old with morning headaches that have increased in intensity over the last month
   B. Gradual onset of a severe headache
   C. Headache that lasts more than 24 hours
   D. Persistent headache after concussion

15 **What is least likely to suggest a headache associated with a brain tumor?**

   A. Behavioral changes
   B. Headache that occurs later in the day
   C. Multiple hyperpigmented spots all over the body
   D. Polydipsia or polyuria

16 **A 6-year-old boy is brought in by his mother for a headache. She reports that pain has been waking him up at night for the past week. Sometimes, he vomits on awakening. His vital signs are normal, but on examination, some ataxia is noted. What is the next step in management?**

   A. Admit and obtain a sedated MRI in the morning
   B. Discharge home and recommend the patient see an optometrist for glasses
   C. Obtain an urgent head CT
   D. Provide ibuprofen and discharge home

17 **A 16-year-old girl comes in complaining of a frontal headache. The headache does not occur daily, but she does complain of headaches multiple times during the week. The headache never wakes her up, and she has no vomiting. She has had no changes in vision or other complaints. She takes ibuprofen daily. She has normal physical examination results and reassuring vital signs. What is the best recommendation?**

   A. Discontinue daily ibuprofen use
   B. Obtain a lumbar puncture and opening pressure
   C. Obtain an urgent head CT
   D. Obtain a psychiatric consultation for somatic symptom disorder

18 **A 6-month-old boy is brought in by his mother because he has been very fussy for the last week. The mother has tried giving him acetaminophen, which seems to help for a few hours but then wears off. He is still eating but seems to be spitting up more than usual. His mother also feels he is not sitting up as well as he had been. What physical examination or vital sign finding would be most worrisome for a secondary cause of the patient's fussiness?**

   A. Blood pressure of 80/40 mm Hg
   B. Head circumference greater than the 99th percentile
   C. No sign of a hair tourniquet
   D. Soft abdomen

19 **A mother brings in her 14-year-old son for a headache. It is primarily a frontal headache. It resolves with ibuprofen. He only complains about it once or twice a week, and it has not impacted school or home life. He sleeps well, and he enjoys school. He recently had normal eye examination results. What is the most likely diagnosis?**

   A. Depression
   B. Myopia
   C. Primary headache
   D. Secondary headache

20 **An 8-year-old girl is brought in by her father for a fever and headache. The patient's fever has been up to 39.4°C (103°F) at home. The headache has been primarily occipital. She is not drinking well, and her father notes a rash on her feet that has just started. The patient refuses to move her head during the examination. When the patient's history is obtained, her father states that she is unvaccinated. What is the best management plan?**

   A. Discharge home with antibiotics
   B. Lumbar puncture, admission, and intravenous antibiotics for presumed meningitis
   C. MRI with contrast
   D. Social work consultation

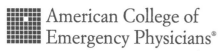

American College of
Emergency Physicians®

ADVANCING EMERGENCY CARE

Post Office Box 619911
Dallas, Texas 75261-9911

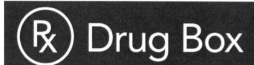

Zavegepant

Frank LoVecchio, DO, MPH, FACEP
Valleywise Health Medical Center and ASU, Phoenix, Arizona

Objective
On completion of this column, you should be able to:
- Describe zavegepant usage and benefits.

Zavegepant is an antimigraine medication with a newer mechanism of action: calcitonin gene-related peptide (CGRP) receptor antagonism. To date, it is the only CGRP receptor antagonist formulated as a nasal spray.

Mechanism of Action and Evidence
Zavegepant blocks the effects of the calcitonin peptide, a neuropeptide and vasodilator produced by neurons in the central and peripheral nervous systems. CGRP release in trigeminal neurons is associated with the release of vasoactive neuropeptides and vasodilation of the cerebral vasculature, and exogenous CGRP triggers migraine headaches. Elevated blood and salivary CGRP levels occur in patients with migraines, cluster headaches, neuralgias such as trigeminal neuralgia, and even rhinosinusitis.

CGRP receptor antagonists are unassociated with medication abuse, overuse, or rebound headaches. The nasal formulation is helpful in patients with nausea and vomiting. In a recent study, zavegepant had an advantage over placebo in 13 of 17 additional outcome measures, including time-based endpoints such as pain relief at 15 and 30 minutes, return to normal function within 30 minutes, sustained pain relief for 2 to 24 hours, and pain freedom for 2 to 48 hours. Statistically, zavegepant was not significantly different from placebo in restoring normal function 15 minutes post dosage. Zavegepant's onset of action is ~15 minutes, its half-life is ~6.5 hours, and its time-to-peak effect is ~30 minutes. Zavegepant is an alternative if triptans are ineffective or contraindicated (eg, cardiovascular risk factors).

Similar Medications
FDA-approved CGRP signal-blocking drugs used in migraine treatment or prophylaxis include monoclonal antibodies that act against the CGRP receptor — erenumab, eptinezumab, galcanezumab, and fremanezumab — and CGRP receptor antagonists — rimegepant and ubrogepant. Oral rimegepant and ubrogepant are used for the acute treatment of migraine with or without aura. Additionally, atogepant and vazegepant are other CGRP receptor antagonists undergoing clinical trials, but they are not yet approved by the FDA.

Side Effects
Hypersensitivity reactions can occur with zavegepant. The medication has not been studied in patients with hepatic or renal impairment (creatinine clearance value <30 mL/min) or in children or pregnant patients. The most common adverse reactions for zavegepant (occurring in ≥2% of patients treated with zavegepant and >placebo) were taste disorders including dysgeusia and ageusia (18% treatment group vs 4% placebo group), nausea (4% vs 1%), nasal discomfort (3% vs 1%), and vomiting (2% vs 1%).

Dosing
A single intranasal dose is one spray (10 mg/spray) in one nostril. Maximum dose is one spray per 24 hr.

REFERENCE
Lipton RB, Croop R, Stock DA, et al. Safety, tolerability, and efficacy of zavegepant 10 mg nasal spray for the acute treatment of migraine in the USA: a phase 3, double-blind, randomised, placebo-controlled multicentre trial. *Lancet Neurol.* 2023 Mar;22(3):209-217.

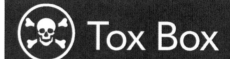

Buspirone Toxicity

By Christian Tomaszewski, MD, MS, MBA, FACEP
University of California San Diego Health

Objective
On completion of this column, you should be able to:
- Discuss the effects and treatment of buspirone toxicity.

Introduction
Buspirone is an anxiolytic of the azapirone class that has more recently been used to treat depression. Because it does not affect gamma-aminobutyric acid (GABA) levels, it tends to be safer than benzodiazepines. Doses up to 375 mg are tolerated with minimal side effects.

Mechanism of Action
- Partial serotonin 5-HT1A receptor agonist (can lead to serotonin syndrome)
- Some antagonism at the D2 dopamine receptor (akathisia)

Toxicokinetics
- Absorption
  - Low oral bioavailability <5%
  - Peak level at 0.9-1.5 hr post ingestion
- Metabolism
  - Half-life of 2-3 hr
  - Metabolized by CYP3A4 (interactions possible)

Clinical Manifestations
- ***Ocular:*** miosis
- ***GI:*** nausea and vomiting
- ***CNS:*** dizziness, sedation, hyperreflexia, and seizures
- ***Neuro:*** dyskinesia, akathisia, parkinsonism, and dystonia
- ***Cardiac:*** bradycardia and hypotension

Diagnostics
- Routine screening of glucose and acetaminophen levels
- ECG if symptoms are severe

Treatment
- Can give activated charcoal orally if <1 hr post ingestion (avoid in patients with altered mental status)
- IV fluid bolus for hypotension or norepinephrine for fluid-unresponsive hypotension
- Benzodiazepines or levetiracetam for seizures
- Benzodiazepines (or cyproheptadine if oral intake is possible) for serotonin syndrome

Disposition
- If asymptomatic, monitor for up to 4-6 hr after an oral overdose.
- If symptomatic or ECG changes are present, observe or admit.

Critical decisions
in emergency medicine

Volume 37 Number 6: **June 2023**

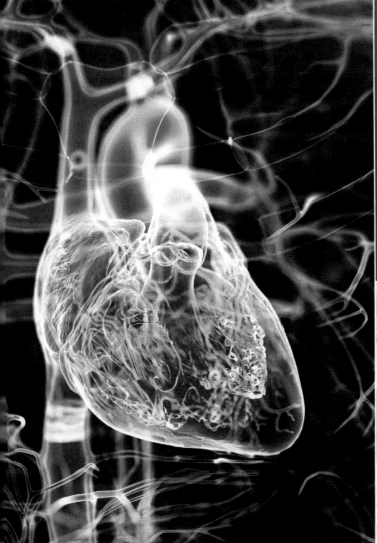

Under the Weather

Thyroid storm is a rare but deadly form of hyperthyroidism that can be easily overlooked by even the most experienced physician. Diagnosing the condition can be extremely difficult because its symptoms are nonspecific and can mimic many other pathologies. Emergency physicians must be aware of thyroid storm's presentation and initial management steps to avoid potential multiorgan failure.

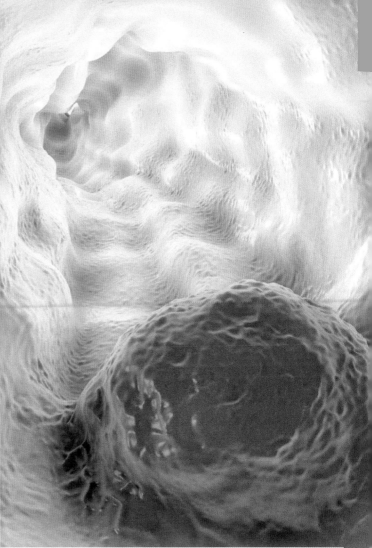

Head Scratcher

More than half of children and adolescents experience a headache at some point in their lifetime. Although most pediatric headaches are benign, some are indicators of a potentially fatal illness. Emergency physicians must recognize the red flags that can point to life-threatening causes of headaches, such as brain tumors and meningitis.

THE OFFICIAL CME PUBLICATION OF THE AMERICAN COLLEGE OF EMERGENCY PHYSICIANS

Contributor Disclosures. In accordance with the ACCME Standards for Integrity and Independence in Accredited Continuing Education, all relevant financial relationships, and the absence of relevant financial relationships, must be disclosed to learners for all individuals in control of content 1) before learners engage with the accredited education, and 2) in a format that can be verified at the time of accreditation. The following individuals have reported relationships with ineligible companies, as defined by the ACCME. These relationships, in the context of their involvement in the CME activity, could be perceived by some as a real or apparent conflict of interest. All relevant financial relationships have been mitigated to ensure that no commercial bias has been inserted into the educational content. Joshua S. Broder, MD, FACEP, is a founder and president of OmniSono Inc, an ultrasound technology company, and a consultant on the Bayer USA Cardiac Imaging Advisory Board. Sharon E. Mace, MD, FACEP, performs contracted research funded by Biofire Corporation, Genetesis, Quidel, and IBSA Pharma. Frank LoVecchio, DO, MPH, FACEP, receives speaking fees from ABBVIE for antibiotics. Christian A. Tomaszewski, MD, MS, MBA, FACEP does contracted research (Roche, Pfizer, AstraZeneca — Site PI with financial support provided to institution). All remaining individuals with control over content have no relevant financial relationships to disclose.

This educational activity consists of two lessons, eight feature articles, a post-test, and evaluation questions; as designed, the activity should take approximately 5 hours to complete. The participant should, in order, review the learning objectives for the lesson or article, read the lesson or article as published in the print or online version until all have been reviewed, and then complete the online post-test (a minimum score of 75% is required) and evaluation questions. Release date: June 1, 2023. Expiration date: May 31, 2026.

Accreditation Statement. The American College of Emergency Physicians is accredited by the Accreditation Council for Continuing Medical Education to provide continuing medical education for physicians.

The American College of Emergency Physicians designates this enduring material for a maximum of 5 *AMA PRA Category 1 Credits™*. Physicians should claim only the credit commensurate with the extent of their participation in the activity.

Each issue of *Critical Decisions in Emergency Medicine* is approved by ACEP for 5 ACEP Category I credits. Approved by the AOA for 5 Category 2-B credits.

Commercial Support. There was no commercial support for this CME activity.

Target Audience. This educational activity has been developed for emergency physicians.

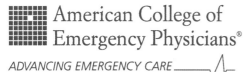

American College of Emergency Physicians®

ADVANCING EMERGENCY CARE

Critical decisions
in emergency medicine

Critical Decisions in Emergency Medicine is the official CME publication of the American College of Emergency Physicians. Additional volumes are available.

EDITOR-IN-CHIEF

Michael S. Beeson, MD, MBA, FACEP
Northeastern Ohio Universities,
Rootstown, OH

SECTION EDITORS

Joshua S. Broder, MD, FACEP
Duke University, Durham, NC

Andrew J. Eyre, MD, MS-HPEd
Brigham and Women's Hospital/
Harvard Medical School, Boston, MA

John Kiel, DO, MPH, FACEP, CAQSM
University of Florida College of Medicine,
Jacksonville, FL

Frank LoVecchio, DO, MPH, FACEP
Valleywise, Arizona State University, University of Arizona,
and Creighton Colleges of Medicine, Phoenix, AZ

Sharon E. Mace, MD, FACEP
Cleveland Clinic Lerner College of Medicine/
Case Western Reserve University, Cleveland, OH

Amal Mattu, MD, FACEP
University of Maryland, Baltimore, MD

Christian A. Tomaszewski, MD, MS, MBA, FACEP
University of California Health Sciences,
San Diego, CA

Steven J. Warrington, MD, MEd, MS
MercyOne Siouxland, Sioux City, IA

ASSOCIATE EDITORS

Tareq Al-Salamah, MBBS, MPH, FACEP
King Saud University, Riyadh, Saudi Arabia/
University of Maryland, Baltimore, MD

Wan-Tsu Chang, MD
University of Maryland, Baltimore, MD

Ann M. Dietrich, MD, FAAP, FACEP
University of South Carolina College of Medicine,
Greenville, SC

Kelsey Drake, MD, MPH, FACEP
St. Anthony Hospital, Lakewood, CO

Walter L. Green, MD, FACEP
UT Southwestern Medical Center, Dallas, TX

John C. Greenwood, MD
University of Pennsylvania, Philadelphia, PA

Danya Khoujah, MBBS, MEHP, FACEP
University of Maryland, Baltimore, MD

Nathaniel Mann, MD
Greenville Health System, Greenville, SC

George Sternbach, MD, FACEP
Stanford University Medical Center, Stanford, CA

EDITORIAL STAFF

Suzannah Alexander, Editorial Director
salexander@acep.org

Joy Carrico, JD
Managing Editor

Alex Bass
Assistant Editor

Kyle Powell
Graphic Artist

ISSN2325-0186 (Print)   ISSN2325-8365 (Online)

Contents

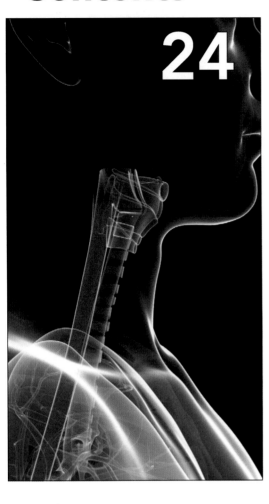

24

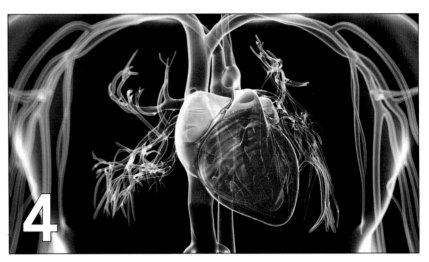

4

FEATURES

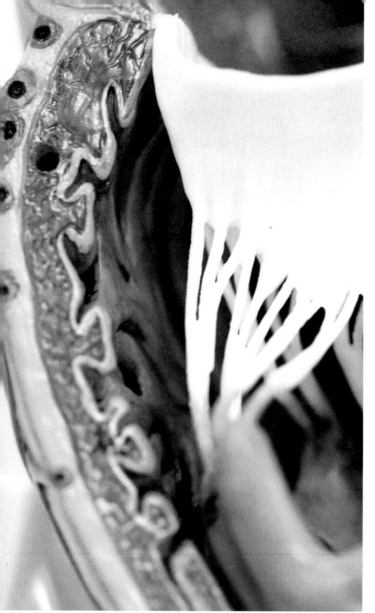

Tight Squeeze

Pericarditis Presentations in the Emergency Department

LESSON 11

By Connie Wu Klasek, MD, MPH; and
Leen Alblaihed, MBBS, MHA, FACEP
Dr. Klasek is a resident at the University of Maryland Medical
Center, and Dr. Alblaihed is an assistant professor in the
Department of Emergency Medicine at the University of Maryland
School of Medicine in Baltimore.

Reviewed by Amal Mattu, MD, FACEP

Objectives

On completion of this lesson, you should be able to:

1. Define pericarditis and describe its pathophysiology.
2. State what guidelines and workup findings are used to diagnose pericarditis.
3. Recognize the complications of pericarditis and their treatment strategies.
4. Differentiate between the signs and symptoms of infectious, uremic, and post-MI pericarditis.
5. List the recommended treatment strategies for the different types of pericarditis.

From the EM Model

3.0 Cardiovascular Disorders
    3.6   Diseases of the Pericardium
          3.6.2   Pericarditis

▬ CRITICAL DECISIONS ▬

- What are the pathophysiology and presentation of pericarditis?

- What does the workup for pericarditis include?

- How is pericarditis treated, and what are its treatment complications?

- How do viral, tuberculous, bacterial, and parasitic pericarditis differ in their presentations and treatments?

- How does uremic pericarditis differ in its pathophysiology, presentation, and treatment?

- How does post-MI pericarditis differ from other causes in its pathophysiology, presentation, and treatment?

Pericarditis is diagnosed in 5% of patients who present with acute chest pain and can be an elusive diagnosis because of its various presentations. It has many different causes, so treatment varies as well. Emergency physicians must astutely recognize and differentiate pericarditis from other causes of chest pain to ensure patients receive the most direct and appropriate therapy.

CASE PRESENTATIONS

■ CASE ONE

A 21-year-old man presents with chest pain that began 1 week ago. The pain is worse when he lies down and when he takes a deep breath. He and his roommates were sick with a sore throat and cough 3 weeks ago. His vital signs are BP 127/72, P 97, R 17, and T 37.3°C (99.1°F); SpO$_2$ is 96% on room air. Overall, he is well appearing. An ECG is obtained and shows diffuse ST elevations and PR downsloping but no ST depressions.

■ CASE TWO

A 62-year-old man presents with a cough and new, sharp chest pain that radiates to his shoulders. He has a history of a recent myocardial infarction and had a percutaneous coronary intervention with stent placement to the circumflex artery 10 days ago. His vital signs include BP 89/63, P 119, and T 38.7°C (101.7°F);

SpO$_2$ is 92% on room air. He appears ill and uncomfortable. On examination, his heart sounds are difficult to hear. His ECG shows diminished QRS amplitude, Q waves in the inferior leads, and diffuse ST elevations throughout all 12 leads.

■ CASE THREE

A 69-year-old woman with a history of hypertension and end-stage renal disease presents with chest pain and a fever. She reports that she missed a dialysis session this week due to illness. In triage, her vital signs are BP 172/56, P 109, R 21, and T 38.2°C (100.8°F); SpO$_2$ is 93% on room air. During examination, she appears uncomfortable and has mild crackles and a friction rub on lung auscultation. Her ECG shows nonspecific T-wave changes in the lateral leads that are consistent with a prior ECG from 3 months ago. Laboratory tests are ordered, including CBC, BMP, ESR, CRP, and troponin tests.

Introduction

Pericarditis is inflammation of the pericardial sac from many potential etiologies, including infection, uremia, and myocardial infarction (MI). Clinical diagnosis of pericarditis can be difficult because of its many presenting symptoms, and a combination of diagnostic criteria, laboratory evaluation, and imaging is often necessary.

Infectious causes differ significantly based on geographic location. Tuberculosis is the most common cause of infectious pericarditis in endemic areas. In developed parts of the world, postviral infectious pericarditis is the most common presumed etiology; in these cases, empiric treatment of pericarditis outweighs determining the specific infectious agent. Uremic pericarditis occurs either pre or post dialysis. Pericarditis following an MI is generally divided into early and late types, with the latter primarily driven by an inappropriate immune response.

General treatments of pericarditis exist, but treatment strategies can be tailored to the underlying cause. Additional options are available for refractory cases. Complications from treatment can arise, and emergency physicians must be able to recognize and treat them as well.

CRITICAL DECISION

What are the pathophysiology and presentation of pericarditis?

The pericardium is a sac-like structure that encases the heart to protect it and facilitate smooth contraction. It is composed of two contiguous layers: an inner visceral layer that consists of serous tissue and adheres to the underlying myocardium and an outer parietal layer that consists of fibroserous tissue that anchors the heart to nearby mediastinal structures. A small amount of pericardial fluid (generally ≤50 mL) separates and decreases friction between the two layers. In physiologic conditions, the pericardium also creates a functional pressure-volume relationship between the right and left sides of the heart. By contrast, in pathologic conditions that alter cardiac pressure and volume, the pericardium can have significant clinical consequences. The pericardium transmits afferent signals through the phrenic nerve and receives efferent signals primarily from the vagus nerve and sympathetic trunk.

Pericarditis is inflammation of the pericardium. It has many potential causes that can be broadly divided into infectious and noninfectious categories. Occasionally, this inflammation extends to and injures the myocardium, which leads to elevated troponin levels in laboratory tests. Concomitant myocarditis occurs in roughly one-third of patients with acute pericarditis of the same etiology.[1] Although

myocarditis and pericarditis are distinguished by an elevated troponin level and can also occur separately, the two clinical entities are sometimes placed on a spectrum of myopericardial disease.

The presenting symptoms of pericarditis can vary widely, and the condition can be acute or chronic and isolated or recurrent. Acute pericarditis is generally defined as a new and acute presentation of pericarditis symptoms, while chronic pericarditis is the occurrence of symptoms that last longer than 3 months. Diagnosing pericarditis can be challenging, as can estimating its incidence and prevalence — around 5% of non-MI chest pain in the emergency department is thought to be from pericarditis.[2] A recent article examined more than 2,000 patients with chest pain at a Swedish emergency department. A pericarditis diagnosis was made in 1.9% of patients, and the researchers estimated its incidence rate to be 6/100,000 people in the overall population. Approximately 50% of the patients diagnosed with pericarditis in this study were admitted to the hospital.[3] In general, men are more likely than women to be diagnosed with pericarditis, and the incidence appears to decrease with age.[3,4]

Determining the specific etiology of pericarditis is often clinically unimportant because most cases resolve; therefore, the burden of further testing often outweighs its clinical significance. The European Society of Cardiology (ESC) recommends a workup for determining the etiology of pericarditis in patients who are at risk of developing complications and whose presentation suggests an underlying systemic cause. For all other patients, the ESC recommends empiric treatment and outpatient follow-up.

Findings in Pericarditis

Pericardial chest pain is classically described as pleuritic; it is worse when lying flat and improved by sitting up or leaning forward. Because of the pericardium's innervation, the pain associated with it can be difficult to describe and can mimic ischemic chest precordial pain or the substernal pain that is associated with radiation to the arms or jaw. A pericardial friction rub over the left sternal border can be heard on auscultation in approximately one-third of cases.[5] The finding of a pericardial friction rub is highly specific for pericarditis — nearly 100% — but its sensitivity is much lower. Also, a friction rub may be present only intermittently, and several emergency department factors like the difficulty of frequently reassessing patients and a noisy environment can make auscultation less practical. When a rub is detected, it is usually described as a triphasic rasping or scratching sound. Auscultating during end expiration while patients are leaning forward may increase the likelihood of hearing a friction rub.

To promote standardization, the ESC published diagnosis guidelines for pericarditis in 2004 and updated them in 2015. According to these guidelines, acute pericarditis can be diagnosed when at least two of the following are present: chest pain (classic pericardial chest pain that tends to be sharp, positional, and pleuritic), a pericardial friction rub, ECG changes suggestive of pericarditis, or new or worsening pericardial effusion. Findings that suggest acute pericarditis include elevated inflammatory markers and imaging evidence of an inflamed pericardium (*Table 1*).[6]

CRITICAL DECISION

What does the workup for pericarditis include?

A workup for chest pain generally encompasses the workup for pericarditis. A basic metabolic panel (BMP), CBC, ECG, and chest x-ray are usually indicated. An additional laboratory workup can include tests for the erythrocyte sedimentation rate (ESR) and levels of C-reactive protein (CRP); elevations in these inflammatory markers and accompanying leukocytosis can assist with diagnosing pericarditis and are included in the ESC guidelines. Classic ECG findings in pericarditis include widespread ST-segment elevation and associated downsloping PR segments (*Figures 1* and *2*); however, these findings are not sensitive, and pericarditis can present with a normal or nonspecific ECG.[5] When classic ECG findings do occur, they are more often seen in young men with pericarditis. The presence of ST elevation on ECG can make distinguishing between pericarditis and ST-elevation MI (STEMI) challenging, especially when pericarditis patients present with ischemic-like chest pain. Other ECG patterns, however, can help with this distinction. The presence of ST depression in any leads other than aVR and V_1, greater ST elevation in lead III than in lead II, and the absence of PR depression increase the likelihood of STEMI over pericarditis. Although they may also occur with STEMI, the Spodick sign — or a downsloping TP segment indicative of an overall downsloping ECG baseline — and PR depression increase the likelihood of pericarditis.[7] If the ECG shows low voltage (R-wave amplitude <5 mV in all limb leads or <10 mV in all precordial leads) or electrical alternans, large pericardial effusion should be suspected.

Imaging Modalities in the Workup of Pericarditis

Guidelines based on expert opinion have proposed incorporating multimodal imaging to assist in the diagnosis of pericarditis, starting with chest x-ray and echocardiography. An initial chest x-ray can be unremarkable unless a significant amount of pericardial fluid

Criterion	
Two of these	• Pericardial chest pain (sharp, pleuritic, improved with leaning forward and worsened when supine) • Friction rub • ECG findings of widespread ST elevation and PR depression • New or worsening pericardial effusion
Supportive findings	• Elevated inflammatory markers • Imaging findings that are consistent with pericardial inflammation

TABLE 1. Criteria for diagnosing acute pericarditis[6]

(generally >250 mL) has accumulated.[7] If significant pericardial effusion occurs, the cardiac silhouette may be enlarged or have the classic water bottle shape. Echocardiography can show increased echogenicity of the pericardium — a nonspecific finding that is consistent with acute inflammation — and the presence of pericardial effusion; it is the imaging modality of choice for unstable patients with pericarditis because it can be used at bedside and can identify any hemodynamically significant pericardial effusion or tamponade physiology. Findings suggestive of cardiac tamponade are right ventricular collapse during diastole and right atrial collapse during systole; suspicion for a tamponade should be further raised by the finding of a distended inferior vena cava (*Figure 3*). Echocardiography is also recommended as an evaluation modality for constrictive pericarditis. Specific findings of constrictive pericarditis on echocardiography include septal motion variation that correlates with respiration and specific measures of flow velocity at the mitral valve, tricuspid valve, and hepatic veins.[8]

CT of the chest can also be used. Although motion artifact is likely to interfere with image interpretation, it can be minimized by ECG-synchronized imaging. The pericardium has a normal thickness of ≤2 mm and is best visualized along the right ventricular wall, where there is less epicardial fat. CT findings of acute pericarditis show thickening and contrast enhancement of the pericardium; the degree of attenuation can differentiate between simple and purulent disease.[9]

MRI is the preferred imaging modality because it can show a range of cardiac states in real time. Its use is limited by a patient's ability to tolerate and cooperate with the examination and by the contraindications of pregnancy, incompatible implanted devices, and hemodynamic instability (as with cardiac tamponade). A fully comprehensive cardiac MRI assesses cardiac morphology, biventricular function, ventricular interdependence, cardiac tissue, and pericardial mobility. Gadolinium-enhanced MRI can visualize inflammation of the pericardium, and further specialized sequences can reveal edema

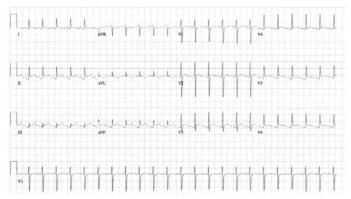

FIGURE 1. ECG consistent with pericarditis, example 1. Diffuse ST elevations with concave upward morphology and PR depressions are shown. ST depressions in leads other than aVR and V_1 are absent, and ST elevation in lead II is greater than in lead III. *Credit:* Image courtesy of Amal Mattu, MD, FACEP.

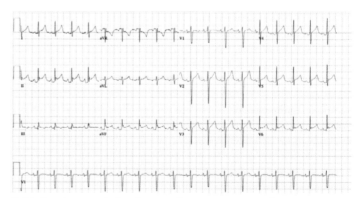

FIGURE 2. ECG findings of acute pericarditis, example 2. Diffuse ST elevations and prominent PR depressions are shown. *Credit:* Image courtesy of Amal Mattu, MD, FACEP.

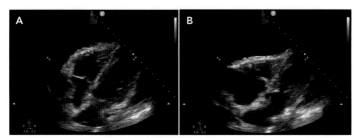

FIGURE 3. Cardiac tamponade on echocardiography.
A. Pericardial effusion seen surrounding the heart with right atrial collapse during systole. **B.** Right ventricular collapse seen during diastole. *Credit:* Images courtesy of the University of Maryland School of Medicine, Department of Emergency Medicine.

within the pericardial layers. Perhaps one of the most useful benefits of MRI is its ability to detect constrictive pericarditis. An MRI of constrictive pericarditis will show diffuse pericardial thickening, most notably over the right ventricle, and may show concomitant ventricular chamber flattening. Previously, pericardial thickening greater than 4 mm was believed to suggest constrictive pericarditis, and thickening greater than 5 to 6 mm was specific for the disease; however, more recent evidence has shown that constrictive pericarditis is associated with a wide range of pericardial thicknesses. Pericardial calcifications, a common sign of constrictive pericarditis, can also be seen on MRI but are better detected by CT. The hemodynamic effects of constrictive pericarditis can be visualized on MRI as enhanced early filling and decreased late filling that are secondary to high filling pressures from a noncompliant pericardium. Furthermore, real-time MRI visualization of enhanced filling-pattern changes through the respiratory cycle can also identify constrictive pericarditis. Other MRI findings of constrictive pericarditis include septal flattening and S-shaped motion due to increased ventricular coupling.

Selection of Patients for Admission

Not all patients with suspected pericarditis require hospital admission and further workup. Many can be started empirically on medical therapy and instructed to follow up for outpatient medical care. Several risk factors, however, warrant consideration for admission: fever (>38°C [100.4°F]), leukocytosis, large pericardial effusion (echo-free space >20 mm), subacute onset, cardiac tamponade, concurrent anticoagulation, and refractory symptoms after a trial of medical therapy.[2,10] Additional factors also warrant admission, including preceding trauma, an immunocompromised state, and concurrent myocardial involvement as indicated by elevated troponin levels. One proposed stepwise approach to triaging patients with acute pericarditis includes using clinical features and epidemiology to see if a specific etiology is highly suspected and then identifying any high-risk features. Patients should be admitted and a workup pursued if both an etiology is suspected and high-risk features are present.[10]

CRITICAL DECISION

How is pericarditis treated, and what are its treatment complications?

Despite a lack of high-quality evidence, NSAIDs are the main treatment for the most common cause of pericarditis (ie, idiopathic or a presumed viral cause), and some other etiologies have additional treatment recommendations. For idiopathic pericarditis, the 2015 ESC guidelines recommend using either high-dose aspirin, 750 to 1,000 mg every 8 hours, or ibuprofen, 600 mg every 8 hours, for 1 to 2 weeks followed by a taper. Additionally, colchicine can be given for 3 months as either 0.5 mg once daily for patients weighing less than 70 kg (154 lb)

	Dosage	Duration
Aspirin	750-1,000 mg every 8 hr	1-2 wk
Ibuprofen	600 mg every 8 hr	1-2 wk
Colchicine	<70 kg: 0.5 mg once per day ≥70 kg: 0.5 mg twice per day	3 mo
Prednisone	0.25-0.5 mg/kg/day, followed by taper	2-4 wk

TABLE 2. Potential medical treatment regimens for pericarditis

or 0.5 mg twice daily with or without a taper (*Table 2*). Colchicine is a broad anti-inflammatory medication that disrupts microtubule assembly in proinflammatory leukocytes, enhances the likelihood of early pericarditis resolution, and appears to decrease the likelihood of recurrent pericarditis. However, colchicine carries a higher risk of adverse side effects, predominantly diarrhea and other GI manifestations.

For patients with contraindications to NSAIDs (eg, a history of GI bleeds or ongoing anticoagulation therapy), a low to moderate dose of steroids, such as prednisone 0.25 to 0.5 mg/kg/day, should be considered. Treatment should be tailored primarily to symptom resolution, although serum markers of inflammation such as CRP can also be trended. If patients do not respond to first- and second-line treatments, other treatment options include azathioprine and other disease-modifying antirheumatic drugs as well as intravenous immune globulin. Rare case reports exist of pericardiectomy as a final treatment for refractory pericarditis.[5]

Complications

By far, the most common complication of acute pericarditis is its recurrence. Acute pericarditis recurs in approximately one-third of diagnosed patients. If symptoms reappear after 4 to 6 weeks, the syndrome is termed recurrent or relapsing pericarditis; if no symptom-free interval of at least 4 to 5 weeks occurs, the clinical entity is termed incessant pericarditis. The term chronic pericarditis is used if symptoms persist for longer than 3 months.

One of the most feared complications of pericarditis is cardiac tamponade. It should be suspected in patients with pericarditis who develop hemodynamic instability, particularly with concurrent quiet heart sounds and jugular venous distention. Cardiac tamponade can occur in patients with large pericardial effusions that equalize intracardiac pressures or in patients with small pericardial effusions that accumulate rapidly. It can be a presenting symptom of pericarditis or develop along the clinical course. When associated with a cardiac tamponade, pericarditis is more likely to be secondary to bacterial or uremic rather than viral or idiopathic etiologies. Echocardiography should be obtained for suspected cardiac tamponade, and pericardiocentesis or a pericardial window should be performed once the diagnosis is confirmed.

Constrictive pericarditis is a long-term complication that can develop secondary to scarring of the pericardium. In this condition, pericardial elasticity is lost; diastolic filling also becomes impaired, but systolic function is generally preserved. Although it is most common in individuals with pericarditis from bacterial or purulent causes, it can develop in any pericarditis patient.

CRITICAL DECISION

How do viral, tuberculous, bacterial, and parasitic pericarditis differ in their presentations and treatments?

Idiopathic or Viral Pericarditis

The etiology of infectious pericarditis varies significantly by geographic location. In Europe and the United States, pericarditis is most often labeled idiopathic, with a presumed viral etiology 80% to

90% of the time.[5] However, because most pericarditis cases resolve after empiric treatment, a definitive workup to investigate the etiology is not commonly done, so these statistics are only estimates; for instance, collecting a pericardial fluid sample is generally uncommon in patients who are not critically ill. Common viruses implicated in idiopathic or viral pericarditis are enteroviruses, especially coxsackieviruses, herpes viruses, and adenoviruses. The classic presentation is a patient with pericarditis-like chest pain that started after a viral prodrome of fever and myalgia.

Pericarditis and the SARS-CoV-2 Vaccine

As the COVID-19 pandemic progressed in 2020, the world responded by rapidly developing vaccines. In the Western Hemisphere, the predominant initial vaccines produced and distributed were BNT162b2 and mRNA-1273 vaccines. Although the vaccines demonstrated effectiveness against severe disease with early strains, pericarditis and myocarditis quickly became recognizable vaccine side effects in countries like Israel that adopted it early, which prompted a wave of attention as the vaccines were rolled out globally.

In an analysis of open data from a vaccine adverse event surveillance network in the United Kingdom, the incidence of myocarditis and pericarditis was approximately 48/1,000,000 recipients of at least one dose of the BNT162b2 vaccine and 203/1,000,000 recipients of at least one dose of the mRNA-1273 vaccine. A European Union surveillance network, whose data relied on self-reports, showed a pericarditis incidence of 17/1,000,000 recipients of at least one dose of the BNT162b2 vaccine and 32/1,000,000 recipients of at least one dose of the mRNA-1273 vaccine. Data from an equivalent surveillance network in the United States showed a pericarditis incidence of approximately 9/1,000,000 fully vaccinated recipients (two doses) of BNT162b2 or mRNA-1273 vaccines.[11] In the United States and the United Kingdom, cases were reported more frequently in younger recipients (ages 18 to 39 years), but this finding was not seen in data from the European Union surveillance network. Overall, vaccine-induced pericarditis is exceedingly rare, and symptoms are generally mild, with most patients making a full recovery.

In the United States, a review of cases of pericarditis or myocarditis from four large claims databases that included over 100 million beneficiaries aged 18 to 64 years reported similarly low incidence rates for men between 18 and 25 years: 0.88/100,000 people after any dose of the BNT162b2 vaccine and 1.27/100,000 people after any dose of the mRNA-1273 vaccine. The incidence rate of these conditions increased for all recipients after subsequent doses. In young men, the observed rate of cases was higher than the expected rate in the first week after vaccination compared to pre vaccination. Overall, the adjusted incidence rate was higher in young recipients (18-25 years) and in men. The incidence did not appear to be affected by the type of vaccine received.[12] By contrast, a study from Canada showed an increased risk of myocarditis, pericarditis, or both with the mRNA-1273 vaccine compared to the BNT162b2 vaccine, especially after the second dose.[13]

Tuberculous Pericarditis

Tuberculosis is the most common cause of pericarditis in endemic parts of the world, and most patients who develop tuberculous pericarditis are coinfected with HIV. The incidence of tuberculous pericarditis is estimated to be as high as 70% in Africa and less than 5% in Europe.[5] The predominant theory on its pathogenesis is that the mycobacteria enter the pericardial space

through lymphatic spread or hematogenous dissemination and then initiate a strong, delayed hypersensitivity reaction (hematogenous dissemination may be more common in patients coinfected with HIV).[14] Pericardial disease then develops in four pathologic stages.

- Stage 1 is characterized by the presence of acid-fast bacilli, polymorphonuclear leukocytes, and predominantly fibrinous exudate.
- Stage 2 is characterized by lymphocytic exudate with serosanguinous effusion.
- Stage 3 is characterized by pericardial thickening, granuloma formation, and fibrosis development.
- Stage 4 shows constrictive scarring of the visceral and parietal pericardium.

Clinical symptoms of pericarditis are usually seen in the first stage. Patients in the second stage generally have symptoms of heart failure or cardiac tamponade, while patients in the third and fourth stages have constrictive pericarditis.[14] Patients most frequently present in the second stage with heart failure.

Diagnosing tuberculous pericarditis is done either directly through pericardiocentesis — if resources allow and the effusion is large enough to sample — or indirectly through clinical judgment and empiric concern. If pericardiocentesis is performed, the presence of adenosine deaminase (ADA) in pericardial fluid is the biggest indicator of tuberculous pericarditis, although the presence of acid-fast bacilli also suggests the diagnosis. Culturing the pericardial fluid is the most sensitive method, but results can take several weeks.[14,15] Many diagnoses are made indirectly, particularly in endemic countries where pericarditis is generally considered tuberculous unless an alternative etiology is obvious. Tuberculous pericarditis is likely in patients with signs of pericarditis and tuberculosis, with lymphocytic exudative pericardial fluid and ADA activity, or with good response to tuberculosis treatment.[14]

Tuberculous pericarditis is primarily treated by treating the underlying systemic tuberculosis with the four-drug regimen of rifampin, isoniazid, ethambutol, and pyrazinamide and by treating any cardiac symptoms. Patients generally remain on the four-drug regimen for 2 months, after which isoniazid and rifampin are taken for an additional 4 months. Adjunctive treatment with steroids may be beneficial — the ESC currently states that a course of steroids with a taper may be reasonable for patients without HIV coinfection based on trials that associated steroid use with improved mortality and fewer complications.[14] It is unclear what role NSAIDs such as colchicine may play in tuberculous pericarditis.

✔ Pearls

- Pericarditis should be suspected in patients with two of these: sharp pleuritic or positional chest pain, a friction rub, diffuse ST elevations and PR depressions on ECG, and new or worsening pericardial effusion.
- ECG findings of ST depression (aside from in leads aVR or V₁) and ST elevation in lead III greater than in lead II should raise suspicion for STEMI instead of pericarditis.
- Hospital admission should be considered for patients with fever, leukocytosis, subacute onset, large pericardial effusion, and failure of outpatient treatment.
- High-dose aspirin is the first-line treatment for post-MI pericarditis.
- Uremic pericarditis is treated by initiating or increasing the intensity of dialysis.

Nontuberculous Bacterial, Fungal, and Parasitic Pericarditis

Nontuberculous forms of bacterial pericarditis are much less common, especially in the era of antibiotics, and were previously identified mostly on postmortem evaluation. The incidence of bacterial pericarditis is likely less than 1% in Western Europe and North America, and when seen, the condition tends to indicate a worse prognosis.[5] The most common nonmycobacterial organisms identified in these cases of pericarditis are *Coxiella burnetii* and *Borrelia burgdorferi*; less frequently, streptococcal, meningococcal, and staphylococcal species are implicated. Overall, epidemiologic data is sparse and often limited to case reports in the literature. Generally, patients with bacterial pericarditis are ill and toxic appearing, with high fevers and systemic symptoms of infection. Bacterial pericarditis is thought to develop after direct spread of infections from other areas such as adjacent thoracic infection (eg, pulmonary empyema) or myocardial infection (eg, from a ruptured paravalvular abscess secondary to endocarditis), hematogenous spread, or direct seeding through trauma or medical procedures.[16]

Because of their fulminant presentation, most patients with bacterial pericarditis undergo pericardiocentesis. Pericardial fluid is often frankly purulent; culturing the fluid can identify the causative organism to tailor the antibiotic treatment. Even before culture results return, however, patients should be placed on empiric systemic antibiotics that cover both gram-negative and gram-positive bacteria. Possible regimens include a carbapenem or intravenous vancomycin with a third-generation cephalosporin or aminoglycoside. Drainage of purulent pericardial fluid is often necessary, and irrigation of the pericardium with catheter-directed fibrinolytic agents can be considered. If these procedures do not remove enough fluid or the fluid is too fibrotic, the next treatment option would be a pericardial window with accompanying manual lysis of loculations and adhesions. A pericardiectomy can be considered in refractory cases, but this procedure carries significant risks.

Fungal and parasitic causes of pericarditis are exceedingly rare. In immunocompetent patients, *Histoplasma capsulatum* is the most common causative fungus, while *Candida* and *Aspergillus* are more common culprits in immunocompromised patients.[17] Patients with fungal pericarditis tend to present with toxic systemic signs and may have an associated mediastinitis. Fungal pericarditis should generally be considered in patients with a predisposing factor such as parenteral nutrition, prolonged antibiotic or steroid use, or malignancy. Pericardial fluid analysis in these cases should always include a fungal stain in addition to a bacterial workup. Intravenous antifungals such as fluconazole and amphotericin B should be administered in at-risk patients with suspected fungal pericarditis. The most common causes of parasitic pericarditis are *Echinococcus* and *Toxoplasma* species, although *Trypanosoma cruzi*, the parasite that causes Chagas disease, is a significant cause in endemic regions. Occasionally, *Entamoeba histolytica* infection can also lead to pericardial involvement. Patients with parasitic pericarditis will generally be systemically ill and have other manifestations of the underlying disease. Treatment is targeted to the parasite (eg, albendazole for *Echinococcus*, pyrimethamine and sulfadiazine for *Toxoplasma*, and benznidazole for *Trypanosoma cruzi*).

CRITICAL DECISION

How does uremic pericarditis differ in its pathophysiology, presentation, and treatment?

Uremia is a clinical entity that is seen in patients with decreased kidney function, most often in end-stage renal disease once creatinine clearance is less than 10 mL/min (or <15 mL/min in patients with diabetes). The condition is characterized by fluid, electrolyte, hormone, and metabolic derangements. Pericarditis that occurs in patients with uremia is classified by whether it occurs before or after initiation of dialysis, but it is uncertain if the two types are distinct entities or exist on a spectrum. Pericarditis that occurs before or within 8 weeks of dialysis initiation is considered uremic pericarditis, while pericarditis that develops 8 weeks after dialysis initiation is considered dialysis-associated pericarditis. Why patients on long-standing dialysis develop pericarditis remains unknown, but this type of pericarditis generally improves with more frequent sessions.[18]

The incidence of uremic pericarditis is difficult to estimate for many of the same reasons that the general incidence of pericarditis is difficult to estimate. The earliest epidemiologic data on uremic pericarditis came from autopsy data of patients with uremia. Current estimates of uremic and dialysis-associated pericarditis range widely, with a reported incidence anywhere from 2% to 21% based on clinical criteria. Their incidence is believed to be decreasing, perhaps because of improvement in dialysis techniques that allow for better toxin clearance and volume control.[18,19]

Uremic pericarditis is thought to be caused by uremic toxins that accumulate and inflame the pericardium's layers.[20] Uremic toxins are not specific toxins themselves but rather are a combination of toxic metabolites and nitrogenous waste products; even baseline shifts in fluid and electrolyte balances can trigger pericarditis. Furthermore, patients with end-stage renal disease may have concomitant underlying cardiac problems that contribute to the overall clinical picture, and uremia can lead to cardiomyopathy, which worsens cardiac function and fluid balance. Notably, BUN levels do not correspond with the symptoms of uremic pericarditis.[19]

The presentation of uremic pericarditis is largely the same as the presentation of other types of pericarditis, except that symptoms of uremic pericarditis can take longer to develop.[21] Pleuritic chest pain continues to be a key feature, and the presence of a pericardial friction rub remains the most specific clinical sign. Occasionally, patients have associated symptoms of fever, malaise, and dyspnea. ECGs of patients with uremic pericarditis may fail to show diffuse ST elevations as frequently as in patients with nonuremic pericarditis. Laboratory evaluation for uremic pericarditis may reveal leukocytosis along with elevated ESR and CRP levels; troponin levels may also be elevated but can be difficult to interpret when renal clearance is decreased at baseline. Hyperkalemia, hypocalcemia, and tachycardia are said to be highly specific for pericardial effusion in patients with end-stage renal disease; patients with these findings should undergo a prompt imaging evaluation.[18]

Uremic pericarditis is treated with hemodialysis. Most patients with the condition who are not yet on dialysis respond well and rapidly to the treatment, often within the first 2 weeks of initiation. Dialysis should be frequent, but specific recommendations vary. Some sources recommend daily sessions for 5 to 7 days or 10 to 14 days, while others recommend continuing with treatment until cessation of the pericardial friction rub. Dialysis-associated pericarditis is treated by increasing the intensity of dialysis, but evidence does not clearly state if more frequent sessions or longer sessions are more beneficial. Because anticoagulants are used during dialysis, the intensity of treatment should be carefully considered in patients at a higher risk of hemorrhagic tamponade.

NSAIDs (eg, indomethacin) and corticosteroids are considered adjuncts for treating uremic pericarditis and are usually used for refractory cases. Systemic NSAIDs should be used cautiously because patients in renal failure are already at a higher risk of bleeding complications. Current guidelines recommend considering an intrapericardial infusion of NSAIDs. Corticosteroids can be trialed at a low dose (0.25-0.5 mg/kg/day) and can be administered as an intrapericardial infusion as well. Colchicine is contraindicated in uremic pericarditis patients. If these patients develop cardiac tamponade, an immediate pericardiocentesis or pericardial window should be performed. Pericardiectomy is reserved for those who progress to constrictive physiology despite maximal hemodialysis and medical management.

CRITICAL DECISION

How does post-MI pericarditis differ from other causes in its pathophysiology, presentation, and treatment?

Pericarditis that occurs after an acute MI (AMI) can be divided into early and late categories. Early post-MI pericarditis occurs within the first few days after an AMI and usually is benign and self-resolving; late post-MI pericarditis generally occurs weeks to months after an AMI and is associated with a greater burden of symptoms.[22] The term Dressler syndrome is occasionally used to refer to late post-MI pericarditis but can also refer to the entire spectrum of post-MI disease. Although this temporal division is the easiest one to apply clinically, the underlying pathology of post-MI pericarditis may offer a clearer distinction between early and late forms. Early post-MI pericarditis involves localized inflammation in the cardiac tissue that was damaged by the AMI; any subsequent pericarditis is thought to persist because of an ongoing, aberrant immune response that continues to damage the pericardium after recovery from the AMI.[23] Often, the AMI's time of occurrence is unknown, so the onset of pericarditis symptoms relative to the AMI can be unclear. In the emergency department, the precise differentiation between early and late forms is less important than the clinical presentation.

Some argue that post-MI pericarditis should be part of the broader post–cardiac injury syndrome spectrum, which includes cases of pericarditis seen after cardiac interventions such as percutaneous coronary intervention and cardiac surgery.[24] This push is driven partly by the changing epidemiology of post-MI pericarditis now that cardiac interventions occur much more frequently. The incidence of early post-MI pericarditis dropped from an estimated range of 10% to 20% to an estimated range of 1% to 6% after thrombolysis and percutaneous intervention became available.[24,25] The incidence of late post-MI pericarditis has also decreased from an estimated range of 3% to 4% to less than 1%.[24] Both early and late post-MI pericarditis are more common in patients with larger infarct sizes, failed percutaneous intervention, or delayed presentation for definitive treatment.

The development of post-MI pericarditis is largely thought to be from an immune response to antigens that are released by an injured myocardium. Some proposed antigens include antiheart and antimyosin antigens, which activate various immune mechanisms like complement activation and micro-RNA

expression when released.[25] Post-MI pericarditis is diagnosed based on the same signs and symptoms and ECG and laboratory findings as other forms of pericarditis but with the additional history of an AMI. Patients with post-MI pericarditis can also present with concomitant pleural effusion or pulmonary infiltrates. Later presentations of post-MI pericarditis tend to have more frequent effusion, tamponade, and other complications.[23]

Although post-MI pericarditis is diagnosed the same way as other types of pericarditis, some factors can make the diagnosis more difficult, especially when symptoms present close to the time of the original infarct. If troponin levels are still elevated after a recent AMI, distinguishing between persistently elevated AMI biochemical markers and post-MI pericarditis complications like myopericarditis can be difficult. Similarly, because AMI is generally a proinflammatory state, other inflammatory markers like ESR and CRP can also be elevated. Persistent ischemic and reperfusion changes from an AMI can also make it difficult to detect ECG patterns associated with pericarditis.[26] Imaging may aid in diagnosing post-MI pericarditis in these instances. Transthoracic echocardiography is a method that requires relatively few resources and can rapidly visualize pericardial effusion and tamponade physiology. Cardiac MRI can visualize pericardial thickness, edema, and delayed clearance of contrast that is consistent with pericarditis. It can also give further information on the time of infarct and the presence of any additional AMI complications such as ventricular scar, ventricular aneurysm, or cardiomyopathy.[25] When contraindications to cardiac MRI are encountered, CT can be used to estimate pericardial thickness and evaluate any pericardial effusion.

Post-MI pericarditis has nearly the same treatment as idiopathic pericarditis. NSAIDs and colchicine are the mainstays of treatment, but aspirin is the preferred NSAID because of its antiplatelet and anti-inflammatory properties. Aspirin is dosed higher for post-MI pericarditis than for post-MI therapy. Some regimens suggest oral dosages as high as 800 mg every 6 to 8 hours for 7 to 10 days, while others suggest 650 mg every 6 to 8 hours until symptomatic relief is achieved. Dosing is then tapered to and maintained at the usual post-MI dosage. If symptoms are refractory to aspirin alone, colchicine is added. Indomethacin for post-MI pericarditis is not recommended because it can decrease coronary blood flow.[25] The role of steroids for post-MI pericarditis is controversial. Although a second-line treatment in idiopathic pericarditis, steroids in post-MI pericarditis may weaken the myocardium affected by the infarct and increase the risk of aneurysm and rupture. Oral prednisone at a low dose (0.25-0.5 mg/kg/day) followed by a taper can be cautiously considered.

Overall, the prognosis of post-MI pericarditis is affected by the MI prognosis and any sequelae, unless complications of pericarditis develop. Such complications are mostly the same as those in other types of pericarditis, including cardiac tamponade and constrictive pericarditis. Recurrent post-MI pericarditis occurs approximately 10% to 15% of the time and should be carefully distinguished from recurrent ischemia.[23,24] Refractory cases can be treated with the same third-line agents used in idiopathic pericarditis, with close follow-up with rheumatology and cardiology given their side effects. Although cardiac tamponade develops infrequently, prompt echocardiography should be performed when the complication is suspected, along with pericardiocentesis or a pericardial window if necessary. Patients with constrictive pericarditis can still undergo medical therapy because sometimes the condition is transient. Any prior MI-directed interventions must be considered before any surgical intervention for post-MI pericarditis.

✖ Pitfalls

- Assuming a diagnosis of pericarditis purely based on ECG findings of ST elevations and PR depressions.
- Overlooking pericarditis as a cause of chest pain.
- Ruling out pericarditis because no friction rub is present.
- Failing to use echocardiography in patients with suspected cardiac tamponade.

CASE RESOLUTIONS

CASE ONE

The patient's chest x-ray was unremarkable. CBC, BMP, ESR, and CRP revealed mildly elevated CRP and ESR values. He appeared comfortable and had stable vital signs during his visit. On reassessment and auscultation, a faint friction rub was heard. His symptoms improved after he was given 600 mg of ibuprofen. He was discharged in stable condition, with instructions to continue ibuprofen three times per day and follow up with his primary care physician.

CASE TWO

A bedside echocardiogram was immediately performed; it detected moderate pericardial effusion and right ventricular collapse during diastole. The patient's systolic blood pressure decreased into the 70s.

The patient underwent bedside pericardiocentesis and placement of a pericardial drainage catheter, which improved his systolic blood pressure into the 100s. He was admitted to the cardiac ICU for further monitoring and was diagnosed with post-MI pericarditis that was complicated by cardiac tamponade.

CASE THREE

The patient's laboratory results revealed a mildly elevated creatinine level from baseline, elevated CRP and ESR values, and mild leukocytosis. Her first troponin test was mildly elevated, but repeat troponin tests did not show any further increase. Her ECG did not show any evolutions. She was admitted for daily dialysis sessions and experienced rapid improvement of her chest pain by day 3.

Summary

Pericarditis is associated with a variety of presentations but classically presents with some combination of pleuritic chest pain, a pericardial friction rub, specific ECG changes, pericardial effusion, an inflamed pericardium on imaging, and elevated inflammatory markers. Causes can be infectious, most commonly from tuberculosis and viruses, or noninfectious, as from uremia or MI. The most useful imaging modalities for pericarditis are an initial chest x-ray and echocardiogram. CT and MRI can also help with the diagnosis by identifying pericardial thickening and inflammation. Recurrent pericarditis is the most common complication of acute pericarditis. Other complications include cardiac tamponade and constrictive pericarditis. Most pericarditis cases can be empirically treated, without hospital admission. However, hospital admission is warranted in patients with fever, leukocytosis, large pericardial effusions, a subacute course, and failure to respond to initial medical therapy. Medical treatment varies by cause, but NSAIDs and colchicine are first-line treatments for the most common type, idiopathic or presumed viral pericarditis. Pericardiectomy is reserved for refractory cases.

REFERENCES

1. Imazio M, Gaita F. Diagnosis and treatment of pericarditis. *Heart.* 2015 Jul;101(14):1159-1168.
2. Khandaker MH, Espinosa RE, Nishimura RA, et al. Pericardial disease: diagnosis and management. *Mayo Clin Proc.* 2010 Jun;85(6):572-593.
3. Prepoudis A, Koechlin L, Nestelberger T, et al; APACE investigators. Incidence, clinical presentation, management, and outcome of acute pericarditis and myopericarditis. *Eur Heart J Acute Cardiovasc Care.* 2022 Feb 8;11(2):137-147.
4. Kytö V, Sipilä J, Rautava P. Clinical profile and influences on outcomes in patients hospitalized for acute pericarditis. *Circulation.* 2014 Oct 28;130(18):1601-1606.
5. Imazio M, Gaita F, LeWinter M. Evaluation and treatment of pericarditis: a systematic review. *JAMA.* 2015 Oct 13;314(14):1498-1506.
6. Adler Y, Charron P, Imazio M, et al; ESC Scientific Document Group. 2015 ESC guidelines for the diagnosis and management of pericardial diseases: The Task Force for the Diagnosis and Management of Pericardial Diseases of the European Society of Cardiology (ESC) endorsed by: The European Association for Cardio-Thoracic Surgery (EACTS). *Eur Heart J.* 2015 Nov 7;36(42):2921-2964.
7. Witting MD, Hu KM, Westreich AA, Tewelde S, Farzad A, Mattu A. Evaluation of Spodick's sign and other electrocardiographic findings as indicators of STEMI and pericarditis. *J Emerg Med.* 2020 Apr;58(4):562-569.
8. Rammos A, Meladinis V, Vovas G, Patsouras D. Restrictive cardiomyopathies: the importance of noninvasive cardiac imaging modalities in diagnosis and treatment — a systematic review. *Radiol Res Pract.* 2017;2017:2874902.
9. Bogaert J, Francone M. Pericardial disease: value of CT and MR imaging. *Radiology.* 2013 May;267(2):340-356.
10. Imazio M, Trinchero R. Triage and management of acute pericarditis. *Int J Cardiol.* 2007 Jun 12;118(3):286-294.
11. Lane S, Yeomans A, Shakir S. Reports of myocarditis and pericarditis following mRNA COVID-19 vaccination: a systematic review of spontaneously reported data from the UK, Europe and the USA and of the scientific literature. *BMJ Open.* 2022 May 25;12(5):e059223.
12. Wong HL, Hu M, Zhou CK, et al. Risk of myocarditis and pericarditis after the COVID-19 mRNA vaccination in the USA: a cohort study in claims databases. *Lancet.* 2022 Jun 11;399(10342):2191-2199.
13. Abraham N, Spruin S, Rossi T, et al. Myocarditis and/or pericarditis risk after mRNA COVID-19 vaccination: a Canadian head to head comparison of BNT162b2 and mRNA-1273 vaccines. *Vaccine.* 2022 Jul 30;40(32):4663-4671.
14. Isiguzo G, Du Bruyn E, Howlett P, Ntsekhe M. Diagnosis and management of tuberculous pericarditis: what is new? *Curr Cardiol Rep.* 2020 Jan 15;22(1):2.
15. Mayosi BM, Burgess LJ, Doubell AF. Tuberculous pericarditis. *Circulation.* 2005 Dec 6;112(23):3608-3616.
16. Pankuweit S, Ristić AD, Seferović PM, Maisch B. Bacterial pericarditis: diagnosis and management. *Am J Cardiovasc Drugs.* 2005;5(2):103-112.
17. Imazio M, Brucato A, Derosa FG, et al. Aetiological diagnosis in acute and recurrent pericarditis: when and how. *J Cardiovasc Med (Hagerstown).* 2009 Mar;10(3):217-230.
18. Chugh S, Singh J, Kichloo A, Gupta S, Katchi T, Solanki S. Uremic- and dialysis-associated pericarditis. *Cardiol Rev.* 2021 Nov-Dec 01;29(6):310-313.
19. Rehman KA, Betancor J, Xu B, et al. Uremic pericarditis, pericardial effusion, and constrictive pericarditis in end-stage renal disease: insights and pathophysiology. *Clin Cardiol.* 2017 Oct;40(10):839-846.
20. Greenberg KI, Choi MJ. Hemodialysis emergencies: core curriculum 2021. *Am J Kidney Dis.* 2021 May;77(5):796-809.
21. Sadjadi SA, Mashahdian A. Uremic pericarditis: a report of 30 cases and review of the literature. *Am J Case Rep.* 2015 Mar 22;16:169-173.
22. Spodick DH. Decreased recognition of the post-myocardial infarction (Dressler) syndrome in the postinfarct setting: does it masquerade as "idiopathic pericarditis" following silent infarcts? *Chest.* 2004 Nov;126(5):1410-1411.
23. Mehrzad R, Spodick DH. Pericardial involvement in diseases of the heart and other contiguous structures: part I: pericardial involvement in infarct pericarditis and pericardial involvement following myocardial infarction. *Cardiology.* 2012;121(3):164-176.
24. Montrief T, Davis WT, Koyfman A, Long B. Mechanical, inflammatory, and embolic complications of myocardial infarction: an emergency medicine review. *Am J Emerg Med.* 2019 Jun;37(6):1175-1183.
25. Verma BR, Montane B, Chetrit M, et al. Pericarditis and post-cardiac injury syndrome as a sequelae of acute myocardial infarction. *Curr Cardiol Rep.* 2020 Aug 27;22(10):127.
26. Imazio M, Negro A, Belli R, et al. Frequency and prognostic significance of pericarditis following acute myocardial infarction treated by primary percutaneous coronary intervention. *Am J Cardiol.* 2009 Jun 1;103(11):1525-1529.

The Critical ECG

Lead Reversals

By Jeremy Berberian, MD; William J. Brady, MD, FACEP;
and Amal Mattu, MD, FACEP

Dr. Berberian is the associate director of emergency medicine residency education at ChristianaCare and assistant professor of emergency medicine at Sidney Kimmel Medical College, Thomas Jefferson University in Philadelphia, Pennsylvania. Dr. Brady is a professor of emergency medicine, medicine, and nursing, and vice chair for faculty affairs in the Department of Emergency Medicine at the University of Virginia School of Medicine in Charlottesville. Dr. Mattu is a professor, vice chair, and codirector of the Emergency Cardiology Fellowship in the Department of Emergency Medicine at the University of Maryland School of Medicine in Baltimore.

Objectives

On completion of this article, you should be able to:

- Identify the ECG abnormalities that suggest a lead reversal.

- Describe the ECG findings seen with LA-LL and RA-RL lead reversal.

CASE PRESENTATION

A 74-year-old man is being admitted for a hip fracture and completes a preoperative ECG (*Figure 1*).

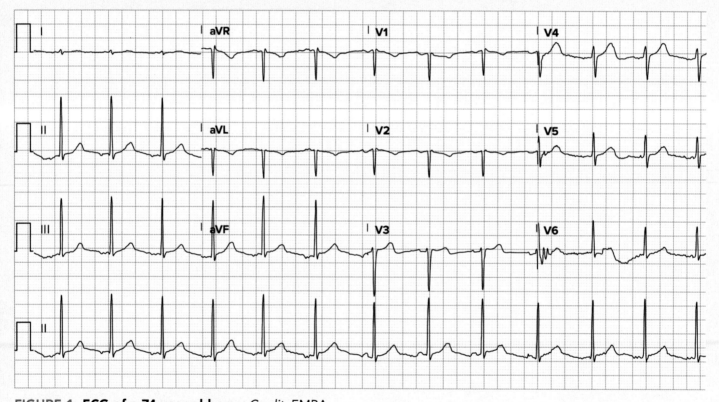

FIGURE 1. ECG of a 74-year-old man. *Credit:* EMRA.

ECG Findings

His ECG shows left arm-left leg (LA-LL) and right arm-right leg (RA-RL) lead reversal. The most easily recognizable abnormality in this ECG that should prompt concern for lead reversal is that lead I is almost flatline, with barely discernible P-QRS-T complexes. This finding is often referred to as pseudo asystole.

ECG findings seen with LA-LL and RA-RL lead reversal include (*Figure 2* and *Table 1*):

- Lead I is almost a straight line, with barely discernible P-QRS-T complexes.
- Leads aVR and aVL are identical.
- Lead III is inverted, meaning the P-QRS-T complexes are all oriented in the opposite direction from the normal P-QRS-T complexes (ie, normal sinus rhythm with normal lead placement).
- Leads II, III, and aVF are identical.

A repeat ECG with correct lead placement was obtained and was unremarkable.

ACKNOWLEDGMENT

This case is reprinted from *Emergency ECGs: Case-Based Review and Interpretations*, available at www.emra.org/amazon or by scanning the QR code.

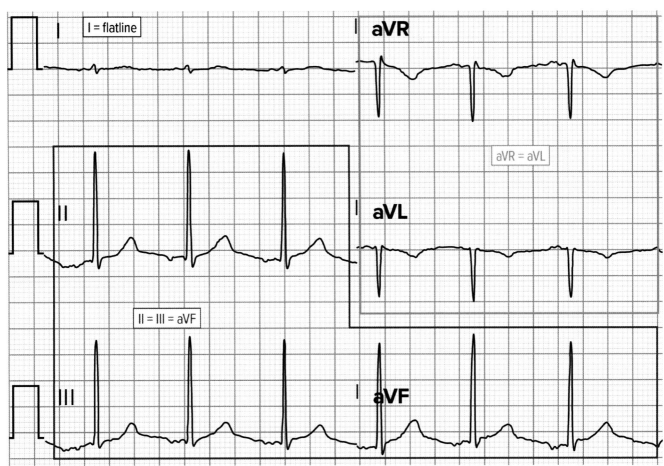

FIGURE 2. Examples of lead reversal on ECG. *Credit:* EMRA.

	I	II	III	aVR	aVL	aVF	V1-V6
LA-RA	Inverted	Switches with III	Switches with II	Switches with aVL	Switches with aVR	No change	No change
LA-LL	Switches with II	Switches with I	Inverted	No change	Switches with aVF	Switches with aVL	No change
LA-RL	Looks like II	Unchanged	Flatline	Looks like inverted II	Looks identical to aVF	Looks identical to aVL	No change
RA-LL	Switches with inverted III	Inverted	Switches with inverted I	Switches with aVF	No change	Switches with aVR	No change
RA-RL	Looks like inverted III	Flatline	Unchanged	Looks identical to aVF	Looks like inverted III	Looks identical to aVR	No change
LA-LL + RA-RL	Flatline	Looks like inverted III	Inverted	Looks identical to aVL	Looks identical to aVR	Looks like inverted III	No change
Dextrocardia	Inverted	Switches with III	Switches with II	Switches with aVL	Switches with aVR	No change	Dominant S wave and poor R-wave progression

Note: RL is a ground lead, so RL-LL reversal does not result in any significant changes

TABLE 1. Characteristics of lead reversals

Clinical Pediatrics

Defying the Rule of Twos: Meckel Diverticulum

By Valerie McLure, MD; and Erika Crawford, MD, FAAP, FACEP
Prisma Health Greenville Memorial Hospital in
South Carolina

Reviewed by Sharon E. Mace, MD, FACEP

Objective

On completion of this article, you should be able to:

- Describe the common presentation of Meckel diverticulum and when to consider it in the differential diagnosis.

CASE PRESENTATION

A 12-year-old girl presents after an episode of profuse bloody diarrhea. She has a history of iron deficiency anemia that was treated with iron supplementation. The patient states that she awoke with slight abdominal discomfort. When she went to the bathroom, she had profuse diarrhea that was dark red in color and appeared to consist of mainly blood clots. Afterward, she felt like she was going to faint, but this feeling resolved quickly. Since her arrival, she has had no further symptoms or episodes of bloody diarrhea. She is pale and tachycardic but otherwise hemodynamically stable; she also has a soft, benign abdomen. A rectovaginal examination does not reveal any vaginal bleeding, but a stool sample from a digital rectal examination is positive for occult blood. Laboratory evaluation is significant for normocytic anemia with a hemoglobin level of 8.7 g/dL, and an ECG shows sinus tachycardia. She is given a normal saline bolus, and her tachycardia improves. After consultation with pediatric gastroenterology, the emergency physician gives the patient a dose of intravenous pantoprazole, and EMS transfers her to a pediatric emergency department for further management.

At the pediatric emergency department, further laboratory evaluation is performed to narrow the differential diagnosis for hematochezia, and the results reveal a slightly elevated erythrocyte sedimentation rate of 31 mm/hr, stable hemoglobin and hematocrit levels, and a normal urinalysis and C-reactive protein level. A Meckel scan, or a ^{99m}Tc sodium pertechnetate scan, is performed based on high clinical suspicion but is read as negative for Meckel diverticulum.

Discussion

Meckel diverticulum is the most common congenital GI tract malformation, occurring in 0.3% to 3% of the population. It is a true diverticulum because its outpouching contains all three layers of the intestinal wall; it also has its own mesentery and blood supply.[1-5] It forms after the omphalomesenteric duct fails to completely obliterate at 7 weeks' gestation. The omphalomesenteric duct, also called the vitelline duct, is an embryonic structure that connects the yolk sac to the forming intestinal tract.[1,4] Because cells in the omphalomesenteric duct are pluripotent, Meckel diverticulum can contain ectopic gastric, pancreatic, duodenal, colonic, Brunner gland, hepatobiliary, or endometrial mucosa. Ectopic gastric mucosa is the most common, and it can cause ulcerations near the ileal mucosa that lead to painless GI bleeding. Other symptomatic presentations of Meckel diverticulum include GI obstruction, inflammation, perforation, tumor, herniation, and abdominal discomfort. Between 4% and 9% of people with Meckel diverticulum become symptomatic. Of those who are symptomatic, 20% to 25% present with GI bleeding.[1,3-6] Hematochezia from Meckel diverticulum can be brick or currant jelly colored and can lead to anemia that requires blood transfusions, but many episodes are self-limited because the vasculature contracts in response to acute blood loss. A large proportion of patients are symptomatic before 2 years of age, and the majority are symptomatic by 10 years, but the risk of complications decreases with age.[1-5,7] For patients with symptoms that are concerning for Meckel diverticulum, a ^{99m}Tc sodium pertechnetate scintigram (ie, Meckel scan) is the standard for diagnosis: It is the most accurate noninvasive test and can identify ectopic gastric tissue associated with the condition. It has a sensitivity of 81% to 85% and a specificity of 95% to 97%; however, false negatives are common and can be caused by insufficient gastric tissue, quick dilution of the ^{99m}Tc marker due to the rate of bleeding, a reduced vascular supply, or anemia. Medications like cimetidine, ranitidine, glucagon, and pentagastrin can be used to enhance uptake and increase sensitivity.[1,2,4-7] If clinical suspicion remains high after a negative Meckel scan, other tests can be performed. When a symptomatic Meckel diverticulum is found, surgical resection is the definitive treatment. Discussions about the need for treatment and the type of treatment for asymptomatic Meckel diverticulum are ongoing.[3]

The Rule of Twos can help recall the characteristics of Meckel diverticulum: It occurs in 2% of the population, in a 2:1 male to female ratio, and within 2 feet of the ileocecal valve; it is 2 cm in length, symptomatic in patients younger than 2 years, and usually associated with two common types of ectopic tissue.[1,2,4] Even when patients do not fit the exact criteria but have some of these characteristics, Meckel diverticulum should be included in the differential diagnosis. The patient in the case presentation, for instance, fulfills the criteria of having ectopic tissue that is 2 feet from the ileocecal valve and 2 inches in length but would seem less likely to have the condition based on her age and sex. Her differential diagnosis is broad and should include Meckel diverticulum among other conditions like gynecological bleeding, ulcers, polyps, coagulopathy, hemolytic uremic syndrome, hemorrhoids, inflammatory bowel disease, and infectious colitis.

Even though the Meckel scan was read as negative, the patient was admitted by the pediatric hospitalist team for monitoring and to complete further workup. A CT scan was obtained and showed Meckel diverticulum without evidence of an acute GI bleed (*Figure 1*). The radiologist then reviewed the Meckel scan and noted an area of uptake in the right lower quadrant that was similar to findings on CT (*Figure 2*). The patient was transferred to the pediatric surgery service for a surgical resection. While waiting for definitive management, her hemoglobin level continued to drop, with a nadir of 6.8 g/dL, so she was given one unit of packed RBCs prior to surgery and responded well. During laparoscopic examination, the Meckel diverticulum was 2 feet proximal to the ileocecal valve. She underwent a small bowel resection with primary anastomosis without complications. She completed a 2-day course of cefazolin, was able to tolerate oral intake, and had well-controlled pain before she was discharged home. Pathology later confirmed a 3.5-cm diverticulum at its greatest dimension that was consistent with Meckel diverticulum of the gastric-type epithelium.

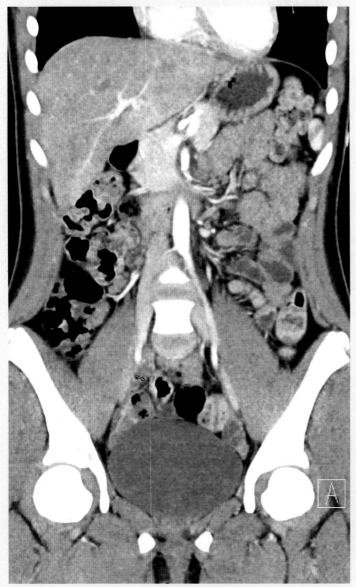

FIGURE 1. CT scan revealing a Meckel diverticulum

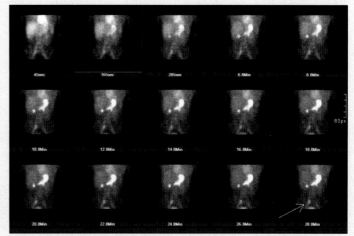

FIGURE 2. On reevaluation, Meckel scan (initially read as negative) showing some uptake in the same configuration as the CT scan

REFERENCES

1. Sagar J, Kumar V, Shah DK. Meckel's diverticulum: a systematic review. *J R Soc Med*. 2006 Oct;99(10):501-505.

2. Takei R, Guttadauria B. Meckel diverticulum. In: Ferri FF, ed. *Ferri's Clinical Advisor 2023*. Elsevier; 2022:950.

3. Hansen, CC, Søreide, K. Systematic review of epidemiology, presentation, and management of Meckel's diverticulum in the 21st century. *Medicine (Baltimore)*. 2018 Aug;97(35):e12154.

4. Kennedy M, Liacouras CA. Intestinal duplications, Meckel diverticulum, and other remnants of the omphalomesenteric duct. In: Kliegman RM, Stanton BF, Schor NF, St Geme JW III, Behrman RE, eds. *Nelson Textbook of Pediatrics*. Vol 2. 20th ed. Elsevier; 2016:1804-1805.

5. McDonald JS, Horst KK, Thacker PG, Thomas KB, Klinkner DB, Kolbe AB. Meckel diverticulum in the pediatric population: patient presentation and performance of imaging in prospective diagnosis. *Clin Imaging*. 2022 Nov;91:37-44.

6. Malek M, Mollen K, Richardson W. Surgery. In: Zitelli B, McIntire S, Nowalk AJ, Garrison J, eds. *Atlas of Pediatric Physical Diagnosis*. 8th ed. Elsevier; 2023:615-64557.

7. Kong MS, Chen CY, Tzen KY, Huang MJ, Wang KL, Lin JN. Technetium-99m pertechnetate scan for ectopic gastric mucosa in children with gastrointestinal bleeding. *J Formos Med Assoc*. 1993 Aug;92(8):717-720.

Treating Patients With Recurrent, Low-Risk Chest Pain

By Adam Howell, MD, LT, MC, USN; and
Daphne Morrison Ponce, MD, CDR, MC, USN
Navy Medical Center in Portsmouth, Virginia

Reviewed by Andrew J. Eyre, MD, MS-HPEd

Objective

On completion of this article, you should be able to:

■ Explain the recommended guidelines for managing patients with recurrent, low-risk chest pain who present to the emergency department.

Musey PI, Bellolio F, Upadhye S, et al. Guidelines for reasonable and appropriate care in the emergency department (GRACE): recurrent, low-risk chest pain in the emergency department. *Acad Emerg Med.* 2021 Jul;28(7):718-744.

KEY POINTS

■ The guidelines from the article represent standards for reasonable and appropriate care, and emergency physicians should always use clinical judgment when applying them.

■ Shared decision-making and dissemination of relevant, patient-accessible information should be considered alongside these care guidelines to accommodate for variations in patients' values, preferences, and understanding of medical processes.

■ Further prospective investigation into how to manage patients with recurrent, low-risk chest pain is warranted — there is still a paucity of direct evidence to address priority questions.

The Society for Academic Emergency Medicine sponsored the Guidelines for Reasonable and Appropriate Care in the Emergency Department (GRACE) for recurrent, low-risk chest pain. A multidisciplinary panel developed eight questions to assess the certainty of evidence and the strength of the published recommendations on caring for adults with recurrent, low-risk chest pain. The multidisciplinary panel consisted of emergency personnel, a cardiologist, a patient representative, and three methodologists. Their clinical questions emphasized patient-focused outcomes, namely 30-day major adverse cardiac events (MACE). Forty-one studies were included to address the specified questions; however, no direct evidence was available for several of the questions. The expert panelists reached a consensus on all recommendations. The certainty of evidence was assessed using the Grading of Recommendations Assessment Development and Evaluation approach, and each recommendation's strength was labeled as either strong or conditional to indicate the panel's confidence that the management strategy's desirable effects would outweigh its undesirable efffects. The final guidelines were analyzed by the Agency for Healthcare Research and Quality's National Guideline Clearinghouse Extent of Adherence to Trustworthy Standards instrument to ensure the best possible adherence to the Institute of Medicine's 2011 standards for trustworthy guidelines. The panel's questions used consensus definitions for targeted key terms.

Recurrent chest pain was defined as chest pain that prompted a previous visit to the emergency department, including two or more visits in a 12-month period, and prompted an evaluation that used a diagnostic protocol but did not demonstrate acute coronary syndrome (ACS) or flow-limiting coronary stenosis. *Low risk* refers to a low risk of ACS or MACE in emergency department patients with recurrent chest pain and was determined by a HEART score (**H**istory, **E**CG, **A**ge, **R**isk factors, and **T**roponin) of less than 4 or an equivalent score from another validated measure that is used in the emergency department. The term *expedited* refers to a follow-up that occurs within 3 to 5 days.

The Eight Priority Questions and Recommendations

In adult patients with recurrent, low-risk chest pain:

1. **Are serial troponin measurements or a single troponin measurement needed to determine ACS outcomes within 30 days?**
Recommendation: Adult patients with recurrent, low-risk chest pain that lasts longer than 3 hours should have a single high-sensitivity troponin measurement that is below a validated threshold to reasonably exclude ACS within 30 days (low level of evidence; for [conditional]).

2. **If they also have normal or nondiagnostic stress testing within the last 12 months, does repeat stress testing affect MACE within 30 days?**
Recommendation: In patients who also had a normal stress test within the previous 12 months, repeat routine stress testing is not recommended to decrease rates of MACE at 30 days (low level of evidence; against [conditional]).

Critical Decisions in Emergency Medicine's LLSA literature reviews feature articles from ABEM's 2023 Lifelong Learning and Self-Assessment Reading List. Available online at acep.org/moc/llsa and on the ABEM website.

3. **Is admission to the hospital, a stay in the emergency department's observation unit, or outpatient follow-up recommended for ACS outcomes within 30 days?**

Recommendation: Evidence is insufficient to recommend hospitalization (either standard inpatient admission or an observation stay) over discharge as a strategy to mitigate MACE within 30 days (no evidence; either).

4. **For patients who also have negative cardiac catheterization results (defined as <50% stenosis), what is their risk of subsequent ACS and the time to ACS?**

Recommendation: For patients with nonobstructive coronary artery disease (CAD) (<50% stenosis) on prior angiography within 5 years, referral for expedited outpatient testing as warranted rather than admission for inpatient evaluation is recommended (low level of evidence; for [conditional]).

5. **For patients who also have negative cardiac catheterization results (defined as no CAD, or 0% stenosis), what is their risk of subsequent ACS and the time to ACS?**

Recommendation: In adult patients with recurrent, low-risk chest pain and no occlusive CAD (0% stenosis) on prior angiography within 5 years, the recommendation is a referral for expedited outpatient testing as warranted rather than admission for inpatient evaluation (low level of evidence; for [conditional]).

6. **In patients who also have a negative coronary CT angiogram (CTA), what is their risk of subsequent ACS and the time to ACS?**

Recommendation: If patients have a coronary CTA within the past 2 years that showed no coronary stenosis, no further diagnostic testing is warranted other than a single high-sensitivity troponin measurement below a validated threshold to exclude ACS within that 2-year time frame (moderate level of evidence; for [conditional]).

7. **What is the effect of depression and anxiety screening tools on patients' health care use and return visits to the emergency department?**

Recommendation: Depression and anxiety screening tools should be used because they may affect health care use and returns to the emergency department (very low level of evidence; either [conditional]).

8. **What is the impact of anxiety and depression referrals on patients' health care use and emergency department return visits?**

Recommendation: Referrals should be made for anxiety or depression management because these conditions may affect health care use and returns to the emergency department (low level of evidence; either [conditional]).

Disclosures

The views expressed in this article are those of the authors and do not necessarily reflect the official policy or position of the Department of the Navy, Department of Defense, or the United States Government.

This work was prepared as part of our official duties as military service members. Title 17 USC §105 provides that "copyright protection under this title is not available for any work of the United States Government." A United States Government work is defined in 17 USC §101 as a work prepared by a military service member or employee of the United States Government as part of that person's official duties.

Trans-Scaphoid Perilunate and Complete Radiocarpal Dislocations

By Ian Benjamin, MD, MS
University of Washington in Seattle

Reviewed by John Kiel, DO, MPH, FACEP, CAQSM

Objective

On completion of this article, you should be able to:

■ Identify and manage trans-scaphoid perilunate and complete radiocarpal dislocations in the emergency department.

CASE PRESENTATION

A 32-year-old man arrives via ambulance after an 80-mph, helmeted motorcycle collision. His chief complaint is pain in his left arm and shoulder. On evaluation, a left wrist deformity with exposed bone is noted. His sensorimotor examination reveals reduced sensation along the left fifth digit. Subsequent x-rays identify a trans-scaphoid perilunate dislocation and a complete radiocarpal dislocation (*Figure 1*). In the operating room, the patient is found to have a transected ulnar nerve and artery as well as complete disruption of the radioscaphocapitate ligament. No other injuries are identified.

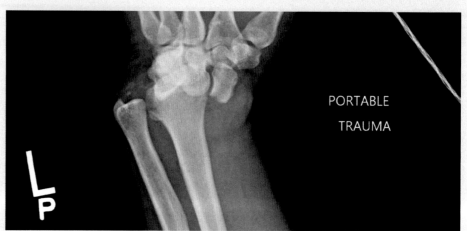

FIGURE 1. A perilunate dislocation and complete radiocarpal dislocation

Discussion

Perilunate dislocations and trans-scaphoid fracture dislocations are rare orthopedic traumatic injuries that are mainly seen in children after high-energy trauma. Perilunate dislocations occur when the lunate remains located in its fossa, but the remainder of the carpus is dorsally dislocated. In trans-scaphoid injury patterns, the proximal pole of the scaphoid travels with the lunate and may also be dislocated into the carpal tunnel, which would cause median nerve dysfunction.[1] The mechanism of injury involves hyperextension of the wrist that leads to intercarpal supination and a cascade of transmitted forces. The initial force is sent through the scaphoid or the scapholunate interval, which can cause scapholunate and radioscaphocapitate ligament tears. Thereafter, the capitolunate articulation is disrupted, followed by the lunotriquetral joint.[2,3]

Although these injuries are rare overall, perilunate dislocations are the most common type of carpal dislocation and account for roughly 10% of all carpal injuries.[4] Approximately 25% of these dislocations are missed and so are not managed surgically, which is problematic because trans-scaphoid perilunate injuries that are managed nonsurgically have universally poor outcomes.[5] These injuries, however, are associated with classic x-ray signs including the disruption of Gilula arcs, "slice of pie" (on anteroposterior x-rays) and "spilled teacup" signs (on lateral x-rays), and

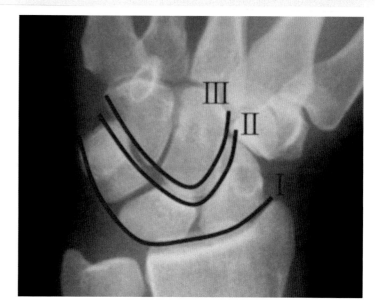

FIGURE 2. Gilula lines — three arcs that are evaluated on an anteroposterior x-ray of the wrist to assess the carpal bones' alignment. A disrupted arc can indicate a ligamentous injury or a fracture where the lines are disrupted.[2] The first arc runs along the proximal convexity of the scaphoid, lunate, and triquetrum. The second arc runs along the distal concavities of the scaphoid, lunate, and triquetrum. The third arc runs along the proximal curvatures of the capitate and hamate.

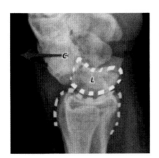

FIGURE 3. The piece of pie sign showing the abnormal triangular appearance of the lunate on the posterior-anterior x-ray of the wrist. It represents either lunate or perilunate dislocation.

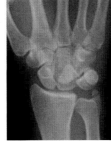

FIGURE 4. The spilled teacup sign showing the abnormal volar displacement and tilt of a dislocated lunate on lateral x-rays of the wrist

overlapping of the carpal bones (*Figures 2, 3,* and *4*). Recognizing these signs can prevent these dislocations from being overlooked.

All perilunate dislocations must be reduced in the emergency department as soon as possible to reverse median nerve compression at the carpal tunnel and to decompress the vasculature that supplies the displaced carpal bones.[6] After appropriate analgesia and anesthesia, the physician should apply uninterrupted finger trap traction while the patient's elbow is flexed at 90° for 10 to 15 minutes. Once the hand muscles are fatigued, a closed reduction can be performed with the following method:

1. While maintaining longitudinal traction during the entire procedure, extend the patient's wrist with one hand and use the thumb of the other hand to stabilize the lunate by pushing dorsally on the palmar surface of the wrist. Gradual wrist flexion allows the capitate to relocate into the concavity of the lunate.
2. Once the lunocapitate joint is reduced, gradually re-extend the wrist while applying dorsal pressure on the lunate.[1,4] If the patient also has a complete radiocarpal dissociation, as with the patient in the case presentation, a radially directed force should be applied to the distal ulna, and an ulnar-directed force should be applied to the carpals.
3. Immediately splint the wrist with a sugar tong splint.

CASE RESOLUTION

The patient underwent a successful closed reduction of the radiocarpal dislocation in the emergency department after procedural sedation; he was admitted to orthopedic surgery for surgical exploration the next day. In the operating room, the patient had an ulnar nerve and artery repair, a proximal row carpectomy (secondary to a denuded lunate), a carpal tunnel release, and a radioscapholunate ligament repair after debridement and irrigation of the wound. He was seen as an outpatient in the orthopedic surgery clinic, adhered well to hand therapy, and continued to make excellent progress with range of motion and returning to activities of daily living (*Figures 5* and *6*).

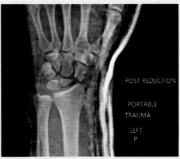

FIGURE 5. Status post reduction

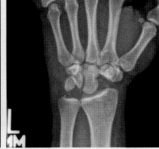

FIGURE 6. Two months post operation

REFERENCES

1. Budoff JE. Treatment of acute lunate and perilunate dislocations. *J Hand Surg Am.* 2008 Oct;33(8):1424-1432.
2. Muppavarapu RC, Capo JT. Perilunate dislocations and fracture dislocations. *Hand Clin.* 2015 Aug;31(3):399-408.
3. Obert L, Loisel F, Jardin E, Gasse N, Lepage D. High-energy injuries of the wrist. *Orthop Traumatol Surg Res.* 2016 Feb;102(1)(suppl):S81-S93.
4. Blazar PE, Murray P. Treatment of perilunate dislocations by combined dorsal and palmar approaches. *Tech Hand Up Extrem Surg.* 2001 Mar;5(1):2-7.
5. Herzberg G, Comtet JJ, Linscheid RL, Amadio PC, Cooney WP, Stalder J. Perilunate dislocations and fracture-dislocations: a multicenter study. *J Hand Surg Am.* 1993 Sep;18(5):768-779.
6. Stanbury SJ, Elfar JC. Perilunate dislocation and perilunate fracture-dislocation. *J Am Acad Orthop Surg.* 2011 Sep;19(9):554-562.

The Critical Image

An Elbow Injury in a Child

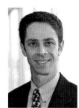

By Joshua S. Broder, MD, FACEP
Dr. Broder is a professor and the residency program director in the Department of Emergency Medicine at Duke University Medical Center in Durham, North Carolina.

Objectives

On completion of this article, you should be able to:

■ Describe the recommended initial imaging and normal and abnormal findings for pediatric elbow injuries.

■ Identify pitfalls and complications of occult elbow injuries.

■ Select the next steps when imaging is negative but elbow injury is still suspected.

CASE PRESENTATION

A 12-year-old boy presents after falling from a tree the previous evening. The patient reports that a branch broke and he fell onto his outstretched left arm, causing immediate pain in his left elbow. He was evaluated at that time in another emergency department, informed that no fracture was present, and discharged with his arm in a sling. This second visit is prompted by the patient's increased pain, swelling, and ecchymosis of the left elbow. He denies other injuries or neurologic complaints. His vital signs are BP 118/73, P 78, R 17, and T 36.9°C (98.4°F); SpO$_2$ is 98% on room air.

The patient is awake and alert and has a normal physical examination except for the findings in his left arm: His elbow is held in 90° of flexion and has edema and patchy ecchymosis. The patient is unable to flex and extend the elbow because of pain, and he also complains of pain with attempted pronation and supination. The proximal and distal examinations are normal, including neurovascular examinations. X-rays from the initial visit are reviewed, and additional x-rays are obtained (*Figures 1* and *2*).

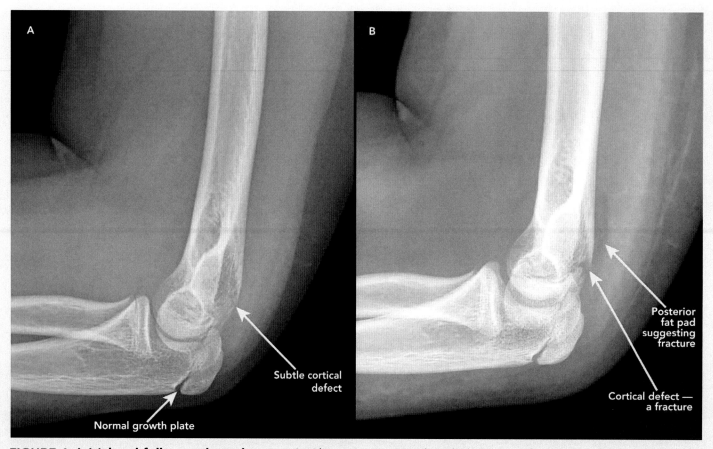

FIGURE 1. Initial and follow-up lateral x-rays. A. Alignment is normal, including normal anterior humeral and radiocapitellar lines. No significant effusion is seen. A subtle cortical defect is present along the distal posterior humerus. **B.** The cortical defect now shows displacement and a posterior fat pad, another indication of fracture.

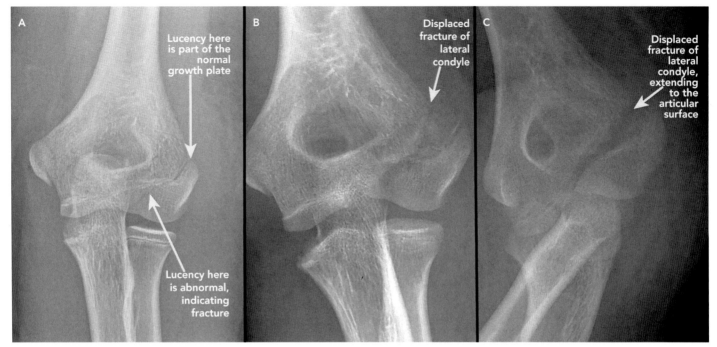

FIGURE 2. Initial and follow-up images. A. The initial x-ray shows a lucency from the lateral condyle to the articular surface, which can be mistaken for a growth plate. **B.** A displaced fracture is now evident — a Salter-Harris type IV injury because it crosses the growth plate. **C.** An oblique image from the second visit reveals the severity of the fracture displacement.

Discussion

Standard images of the elbow include anterior-posterior (performed with the elbow in extension and the forearm supinated) and lateral (performed with the elbow flexed to 90° and the forearm supinated) views.[1] In addition to obvious dislocations and fractures, images should be reviewed for other common surrogate findings (*Figure 3*). On the lateral x-ray, the anterior humeral line should normally intersect the center of the capitellum. In supracondylar humeral fractures, the distal humerus is often displaced posteriorly, which causes the anterior humeral line to intersect the capitellum anterior to its center. Anterior and posterior fat pads can become visible because blood or effusion from fractures displaces fat from its normally hidden position within fossae. A posterior fat pad has a high positive predictive value for fractures, hence the phrase "posterior is pathological." One prospective study found that fractures of the elbow were present in 76% of children with a posterior fat pad and no other evidence of fracture on anterior-posterior, lateral, and oblique x-rays.[2] The normal finding on lateral and anterior-posterior images of a radiocapitellar line that intersects the center of the capitellum is absent when radial head dislocation occurs.

When fracture is suspected but not visualized on standard anterior-posterior and lateral images, several approaches can be applied:
- Additional imaging with oblique views of the elbow may demonstrate fractures.[1]
- Comparison views of the unaffected side can reveal asymmetry and also clarify bone ossification centers and growth plates, distinguishing these from fractures in some cases.[1]
- Ultrasound may demonstrate fractures not seen on x-ray.[3,4]

- CT is considered highly sensitive but is often avoided in children because of radiation exposure concerns and expense.[5]
- MRI is sensitive for fracture and soft tissue injuries but is usually avoided because of expense and limited availability in the emergency department.[1,6]
- Empiric splinting or casting rather than additional imaging in the emergency department may be indicated. Follow-up x-rays are then obtained approximately 4 to 7 days later.[1,7]

In children, lateral condyle fractures of the distal humerus are the second most common elbow fracture after supracondylar fractures, accounting for 12% to 17% of distal humerus fractures.[7] In contrast to supracondylar fractures, which also occur after a fall on an outstretched arm, lateral condylar fractures are rarely complicated by nerve or vascular injuries. Salter-Harris fracture patterns are common because the ossification centers of the distal humerus remain unfused in children during the peak years of incidence for lateral condyle fractures. Nondisplaced fractures and fracture lines through physes *may be occult on x-rays*; these fractures often extend to the articular surface of the elbow and can render the elbow unstable. Surgical fixation is then required to stabilize the articular surface, preserving smooth joint motion and limiting further injury to growth plates.

Missed injury can lead to displacement of fracture fragments, which can convert an injury that can be treated with casting alone to one that requires surgery. Fractures with 2 mm or more of displacement require operative fixation. Other complications of the injury include nonunion (failure to heal by 12 weeks), spur formation, cubitus varus or valgus deformities (in which the forearm is directed toward or away from the midline, respectively), and avascular necrosis (the blood supply to the lateral condyle along with the lateral collateral ligament and extensor muscles of the elbow may be disrupted).[7]

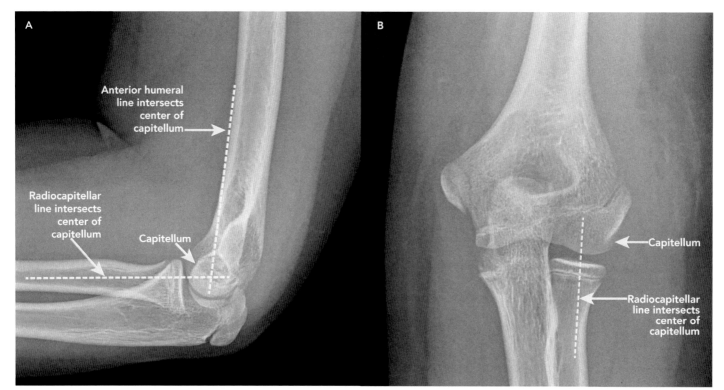

FIGURE 3. The anterior humeral and radiocapitellar lines can assist with identifying occult fractures and dislocations. The anterior humeral line is drawn on the lateral x-ray and normally intersects the center of the capitellum. A posteriorly displaced supracondylar humerus fracture should be suspected when the line intersects the anterior half of the capitellum. On both the anterior-posterior and lateral views, the radiocapitellar line should intersect the center of the capitellum; if this is not the case, the radial head is likely dislocated or the capitellum is not in its usual position.

CASE RESOLUTION

Orthopedics was consulted and placed a long arm cast. Outpatient surgery was recommended with closed or open reduction of the fracture and percutaneous pinning of the lateral condyle fracture with Kirschner wires (K-wires).

REFERENCES

1. Iyer RS, Thapa MM, Khanna PC, Chew FS. Pediatric bone imaging: imaging elbow trauma in children — a review of acute and chronic injuries. *AJR Am J Roentgenol.* 2012 May;198(5):1053-1068.
2. Skaggs DL, Mirzayan R. The posterior fat pad sign in association with occult fracture of the elbow in children. *J Bone Joint Surg Am.* 1999 Oct;81(10):1429-1433.
3. Vocke-Hell AK, Schmid A. Sonographic differentiation of stable and unstable lateral condyle fractures of the humerus in children. *J Pediatr Orthop B.* 2001 Apr;10(2):138-141.
4. Wu X, Li X, Yang S, et al. Determining the stability of minimally displaced lateral humeral condyle fractures in children: ultrasound is better than arthrography. *J Orthop Surg Res.* 2021 Jan 9;16(1):32.
5. Chapman VM, Kalra M, Halpern E, Grottkau B, Albright M, Jaramillo D. 16-MDCT of the posttraumatic pediatric elbow: optimum parameters and associated radiation dose. *AJR Am J Roentgenol.* 2005 Aug;185(2):516-521.
6. Kamegaya M, Shinohara Y, Kurokawa M, Ogata S. Assessment of stability in children's minimally displaced lateral humeral condyle fracture by magnetic resonance imaging. *J Pediatr Orthop.* 1999 Sep-Oct;19(5):570-572.
7. Shaerf DA, Vanhegan IS, Dattani R. Diagnosis, management and complications of distal humerus lateral condyle fractures in children. *Shoulder Elbow.* 2018 Apr;10(2):114-120.

Feature Editor: Joshua S. Broder, MD, FACEP. See also *Diagnostic Imaging for the Emergency Physician* (Winner of the 2011 Prose Award in Clinical Medicine, the American Publishers Award for Professional and Scholarly Excellence) and *Critical Images in Emergency Medicine* by Dr. Broder.

The Critical Procedure

Drainage of an Acute Paronychial Abscess

By Steven J. Warrington, MD, MEd, MS
MercyOne Siouxland, Sioux City, Iowa

Objective

On completion of this article, you should be able to:

■ List the steps for a successful drainage of an acute paronychial abscess in the emergency department.

Introduction

Nail infections can form at the edge or base of the nail, lead to an abscess, and spread underneath the nail. Swelling at the base of the nail without fluctuance or signs of an abscess generally requires only antibiotics and supplemental soaks. Any accompanying drainage, however, can indicate an abscess. These cases can be treated with adjunctive procedures like trephination of the nail, removal of the nail, or reflection of the proximal nail fold, with follow-up for reevaluation and treatment.

Contraindications

■ The presence of herpetic whitlow

Benefits and Risks

Draining a paronychial abscess prevents the infection from progressing. Most cases are successfully treated with incision and drainage, but adjunct antibiotic therapy may be needed depending on the surrounding infection.

Risks of the procedure include failure to heal the infection, injury to the nail or nail matrix, and spreading of the infection to healthy tissue. Cases of herpetic whitlow may also be misdiagnosed as acute paronychia and, therefore, treated incorrectly.

Alternatives

Anesthetization with a digital nerve block is often performed before drainage, but alternatives exist for superficial paronychia. One alternative is to use a warm soak to soften skin. Another is to use a vapocoolant or ice to help decrease sensation.

The approach to incision is dictated by the presence, location, and chronicity of the abscess. For individuals with no definitive abscess, a pre-incision trial of antibiotics and warm soaks is appropriate. If an abscess is excessive, packing with a single strip of gauze for 24 to 48 hours allows for ongoing drainage. If the abscess appears to have spread beneath the nail, then trephination can be an alternative to removing or lifting the nail to allow for drainage. If the infection appears severe at the base of the nail or involves each nail fold, reflection of the proximal nail fold skin, also known as the Swiss roll technique, can be used. For more chronic paronychia, eponychial marsupialization may be necessary.

Reducing Side Effects

Although some physicians believe adjunctive antibiotics should be used less often for acute paronychia, the literature seems to recommend antibiotic therapy. It suggests that increased antibiotic use decreases therapy failure and prevents infections from spreading. Oral antibiotics are formally recommended in the literature, but topical antibiotics can be adequate in some cases. After the incision and drainage, additional care includes daily soaks and early range of motion exercises.

TECHNIQUE

1. **Obtain** the patient's consent.
2. **Arrange** equipment for the procedure at the bedside.
3. **Anesthetize** the affected digit with a digital block.
4. **Assess** for appropriate anesthesia of the affected area.
5. **Place** a digital tourniquet, if desired.
6. **Use** a number 11 scalpel parallel to the nail to incise under the eponychium.
7. **Assess** for potential residual infection. If present, consider trephination of the nail, removal of a portion of the nail, or lifting of the nail.
8. **Consider** placing a single strip of packing material if excessive purulence is present.
9. **Dress** the wound if indicated.
10. **Discuss** appropriate home care, antibiotics, pain control, and follow-up with the patient.

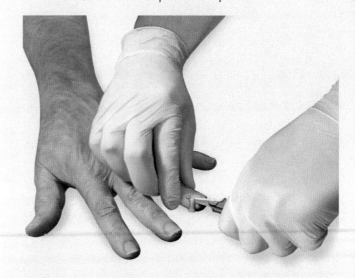

FIGURE 1. Draining an acute paronychial abscess.
Credit: ACEP.

Special Considerations

Physicians must determine if each case of paronychia is acute, acute on chronic, or chronic because chronic paronychia is treated differently from acute paronychia and may require additional workup. Any residual infection underneath the nail or within the finger pulp must also be adequately drained. Although many cases do not require it, a digital tourniquet may be of benefit prior to incision and drainage, especially for patients with large abscesses or those who are anticoagulated.

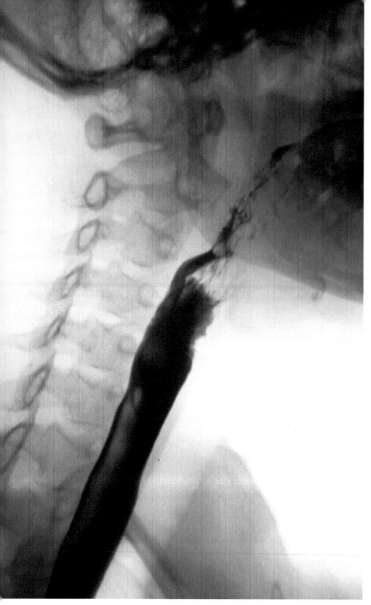

All Choked Up

Esophageal Emergencies

LESSON 12

By Zachary Hagen, MD; and Jerrah Pickle, MD

Dr. Hagen is an emergency physician at Carroll Hospital and Northwest Hospital in Baltimore, and Dr. Pickle is an otolaryngology resident at the University of Maryland in Baltimore.

Reviewed by Amal Mattu, MD, FACEP

Objectives

On completion of this lesson, you should be able to:

1. Describe how to evaluate patients with esophageal pathology.
2. Identify emergent and urgent esophageal pathology.
3. Explain the different types of esophageal foreign bodies.
4. Describe how to manage esophageal food impactions.
5. List the indications, contraindications, and risks associated with NG tubes.

From the EM Model

1.0 Signs, Symptoms, and Presentations
   1.3 General
      1.3.15 Dysphagia
2.0 Abdominal and Gastrointestinal Disorders
   2.2 Esophagus
      2.2.2 Inflammatory Disorders
         2.2.2.1 Esophagitis

▬ CRITICAL DECISIONS ▬

- What types of dysphagia are emergency physicians likely to encounter?
- What are the key historical elements for patients with dysphagia?
- When should esophagitis be considered as a cause of chest pain?
- How does esophageal anatomy affect the location of esophageal pathologies?
- What are common causes of esophageal perforation?
- How should esophageal food impactions be managed?
- What are the common complications of NG tube placement?

Problems with the esophagus are often diagnosed as gastroesophageal reflux disease (GERD), but the esophagus can harbor many often-disregarded emergent pathologies. Emergency physicians encounter serious esophageal conditions, ranging from perforation to impaction. They must be able to distinguish emergent from nonemergent conditions and avoid treatment complications.

CASE PRESENTATIONS

■ CASE ONE

A 2-year-old boy presents with poor oral intake for 2 weeks. His mother reports that the patient seems to be in pain any time he eats thick or solid food. He had been tolerating liquids but, over the past week, has also begun vomiting immediately after drinking. He seems to be averse to any oral intake at this point. The patient has a history of esophageal atresia and had an associated tracheoesophageal fistula repaired when he was an infant. He is up to date on all his vaccines.

On physical examination, the boy is awake and seated upright in bed but appears tired and dehydrated. The boy drools more than is expected for his age. Cardiopulmonary examination reveals a heart rate of 130 bpm, clear lungs, and no stridor or respiratory distress. The patient's abdomen is soft and nontender but slightly scaphoid; he appears underweight for his age.

■ CASE TWO

A 57-year-old man presents after dining at a local steak house. He states that he was eating a large piece of steak that he now feels is trapped in his chest. He tried to drink both water and soda but immediately vomited both. He denies respiratory symptoms but states he has been spitting his saliva into a basin because he cannot swallow it. He takes amlodipine for hypertension. During his physical examination, the patient must stand because sitting or lying down is uncomfortable. His lungs are clear, and he spits into the basin every few minutes. His abdominal examination is unremarkable.

■ CASE THREE

An HIV-positive 23-year-old woman presents with chest pain that has worsened over the past 2 weeks and is exacerbated by eating and drinking. The pain is constant, nonexertional, and unassociated with shortness of breath. The patient reports no fevers or chills at home. She has questionable compliance with her antiretroviral therapy based on outpatient notes from her infectious disease specialist. On physical examination, she is thin, her lungs are clear, and she has a regular rate and rhythm. Her oropharyngeal examination shows no intraoral lesions or plaques.

Introduction

Esophageal pathology is an often-overlooked area in emergency medicine despite its inclusion on the differential diagnosis for many conditions. Usually, the esophagus is deemed the nonemergent culprit in chest pain that is attributed to GERD — a frequently incorrect diagnosis for patients with chest pain. This dichotomy can lead to a missed or late diagnosis in esophageal emergencies.

Another equally challenging aspect to managing esophageal emergencies is the lack of a clear understanding of which specialties should be involved. Gastroenterology, general surgery, and sometimes thoracic surgery all have a role in managing these conditions, but policies for which specialties to include vary by institution. Clear communication between multiple consultants is helpful for appropriately triaging esophageal emergencies.

Iatrogenic etiologies are the leading cause of many esophageal complications. Although esophageal endoscopy is not within the scope of emergency medicine, naso- and orogastric tube placement is, as is managing any associated complications. Emergency physicians must be well prepared to diagnose and begin the treatment process for esophageal emergencies.

CRITICAL DECISION

What types of dysphagia are emergency physicians likely to encounter?

Patients with esophageal pathology can present in a variety of ways. Dysphagia, odynophagia, chest pain, and foreign body sensation are all common presenting symptoms of esophageal emergencies. Intrinsic etiologies of esophageal dysphagia are classified as either motility or structural (ie, obstructive) disorders.

The most common esophageal motility disorder that causes dysphagia is achalasia. Although the exact cause of achalasia is unknown, theories suggest that a loss of the Auerbach plexus impairs esophageal peristalsis and prevents relaxation of the lower esophageal sphincter (LES). Esophagram in patients with achalasia classically shows a bird beak appearance, with dilation of the proximal esophagus and narrowing at the LES.[1] The American College of Gastroenterology published a detailed and evidence-based approach to the workup, management, and follow-up of achalasia that can facilitate testing and treatment for this difficult diagnosis.[2]

Diffuse esophageal spasm is another motility disorder; it can cause sudden, severe chest pain and is commonly mistaken for myocardial infarction. Patients with esophageal spasm are unable to swallow solids or liquids during these episodes, but the spasms are usually short-lived. The etiology is overactivity of the excitatory innervation of the esophagus or overreaction of the esophageal smooth muscle to these excitatory nerves. Diagnosis is confirmed by esophageal manometry in an outpatient setting, and the condition has the classic finding of a corkscrew esophagus on esophagram (*Figure 1*). Treatment for the condition includes treating the associated GERD symptoms and prescribing calcium channel blockers if GERD treatment alone is ineffective.[3] Systemic connective tissue disorders — most notably cutaneous scleroderma, or CREST syndrome — are another cause of esophageal dysmotility; scleroderma can also lead to acute kidney injury and elevated liver enzymes, along with dysfunctions in other organ systems.

Structural, or obstructive, dysphagia occurs when a structural change to the esophagus affects its function. Esophageal webs are thin extensions of the mucosal and submucosal layers of the esophagus that cause structural dysphagia. They are usually found in the proximal or middle esophagus and are commonly associated with Plummer-Vinson syndrome and iron deficiency anemia.[4] A Schatzki ring, a fibrous structure that develops at or near the gastroesophageal (GE) junction, can also cause food impaction or structural dysphagia.[5]

Esophagitis, which is covered more in a later section, is another structural condition that causes dysphagia and chest pain. The differential diagnosis for esophagitis is broad, and it is rarely diagnosed in the emergency department.

A less common cause of dysphagia is functional esophageal dysphagia. Functional dysphagia is often not initially considered because it is a diagnosis of exclusion. To qualify for this diagnosis, patients must have experienced symptoms once a week or more for the last 3 months, with symptom onset at least 6 months ago. These stringent criteria and the fact that a workup is required to rule out most other causes of dysphagia make functional dysphagia difficult to diagnose in the emergency department. The Rome IV diagnostic criteria for functional dysphagia can be used if all prior workup has been completed.[6]

An emergent diagnosis that can masquerade as esophageal in origin is an acute stroke. Although rarely the only sign or symptom, esophageal dysmotility can be one of the main symptoms of a stroke. Swallowing is a neurologically complex event that involves cranial nerves V, VII, IX, X, and XII. Thus, evaluating a patient's swallowing ability during the physical examination can quickly assess multiple nerves. Prior to evaluating swallow function, however, emergency physicians must first assess the patient's airway and mentation because deficits with either one can further increase the risk of aspiration, which is a common complication of strokes that affect these nerves. A detailed neurologic examination can help reveal possible central causes of upper esophageal dysmotility.[7]

CRITICAL DECISION

What are the key historical elements for patients with dysphagia?

A thorough history of patients with swallowing disorders should include multiple key elements to narrow down the likely causes and locations of the pathology. The time course and chronicity of the dysphagia should be ascertained to determine if the onset was sudden or indolent and progressive. Progressive worsening or a transition from difficulty swallowing solids to difficulty with liquids can also indicate the source of the swallowing pathology. Odynophagia, in particular, is associated with acute processes like foreign body impaction and pharyngitis. Knowing whether food is digested or undigested when regurgitated and whether the patient has a history of GERD can trace the source of the pathology to either above or below the GE junction.

A recent or recurrent history of aspiration, frequent pneumonia, or even simply coughing after swallowing can indicate that patients are not safely swallowing their diet. Recent pneumonias tend to increase the risk of poor outcomes from swallowing disorders. Signs of reduced ability to masticate and salivate decrease a patient's ability to properly form a food bolus before swallowing. A history of drooling is important to obtain for any patient suspected of having a foreign body or other airway obstruction. Patients with a slowly progressive dysphagia should be asked about risk factors that can increase their risk of esophageal carcinomas and head and neck cancers, like smoking and heavy alcohol use.[7]

CRITICAL DECISION

When should esophagitis be considered as a cause of chest pain?

Esophagitis is divided into two broad categories: infectious and noninfectious. Infectious causes of esophagitis include fungi, viruses, and least commonly, bacteria (*Table 1*). Risk factors for these infections are HIV, systemic or inhaled steroids, and antibiotic use (for *Candida* esophagitis in particular). Esophageal candidiasis is the most common cause of infectious esophagitis, can occur in healthy individuals, and most often presents as pain and dysphagia. Intraoral lesions (ie, thrush) may or may not be present with *Candida* esophagitis, and treatment is with oral antifungals such as fluconazole. Less commonly, esophagitis is caused by a virus. A variety of viruses can cause esophagitis, but the most common culprits include herpes simplex virus, cytomegalovirus, and HIV. Viral esophagitis is characterized by shallow-based ulcerations in the mucosa, and its diagnosis is confirmed by biopsy. Concurrent viral and fungal esophagitis can occur, so viral esophagitis should be suspected in immunocompromised patients who do not respond to outpatient fluconazole treatment.

Common causes of noninfectious esophagitis include pill-induced esophagitis, eosinophilic esophagitis, and GERD-related esophagitis. Multiple medications can cause esophageal inflammation and injury that lead to pill-induced esophagitis. Smooth muscle relaxers like alcohol and nicotine increase the risk of medication reflux and, thus, pill-induced esophagitis. In addition to esophageal damage from reflux, pills can also directly injure the esophagus if they become lodged in it. Medications that are classically known to cause pill-

induced esophagitis include doxycycline, clindamycin, NSAIDs, bisphosphonates, and iron pills.[7] Eosinophilic esophagitis is a common cause of dysphagia and food intolerance, especially in atopic patients, and can cause stricture formation.[8] It is an IgE-mediated chronic inflammatory pathology that is definitively diagnosed on endoscopy. Endoscopy will show concentric rings within the esophagus, often termed trachealization of the esophagus. Endoscopic biopsy will reveal diffuse eosinophils within the superficial epithelium. Even with endoscopy, however, eosinophilic esophagitis can be difficult to differentiate from simple GERD. One study attempted to

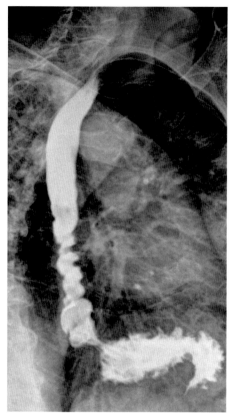

FIGURE 1. Corkscrew esophagus. *Credit:* Copyright 2023 Mohammadtaghi Niknejad. Image courtesy of Mohammadtaghi Niknejad and Radiopaedia.org, rID: 94889. Used under license.

determine predictive features on history and endoscopy to differentiate the two. Its predictive model found that younger age; male sex; the presence of dysphagia and food allergies; the presence of esophageal rings, furrows, and plaques; and the lack of a hiatal hernia were all predictive of eosinophilic esophagitis over GERD.[9] GERD-related esophagitis is the most common noninfectious type of esophagitis and is associated with decreased tone in the LES. Hormonal changes and increased intra-abdominal pressure from the uterus during pregnancy can predispose pregnant women, in particular, to GERD. Treatment for GERD-related esophagitis includes proton pump inhibitors (PPIs) and diet modification.

CRITICAL DECISION

How does esophageal anatomy affect the location of esophageal pathologies?

How foreign bodies become impacted in the esophagus is affected by esophageal anatomy. The esophagus is divided into three regions — cervical, thoracic, and abdominal — and three layers — inner mucosa, submucosa, and muscle. The muscle layers differ depending on the region of the esophagus. The upper third of the esophagus is made of striated muscle, the middle third is both smooth and striated muscle, and the distal third is GI smooth muscle. Innervation of the esophagus also varies by region: Spinal nerves innervate the cervical esophagus and provide sympathetic innervation, while the vagus nerve innervates the remainder of the esophagus and provides parasympathetic innervation.[10] The esophagus also receives its blood supply from three different arteries (from proximal to distal): the inferior thyroid artery, aorta, and left gastric artery.

The esophagus has three anatomic locations where impaction is likely. The cricopharyngeal muscle at vertebra C6 is the most common location in children younger than 4 years. Another common site is adjacent to the aortic arch, around vertebra T4. Rarely, a condition known as dysphagia lusoria can occur when a congenitally aberrant right subclavian artery (Bayford-Autenrieth syndrome) or a double aortic arch leads to impaction at T4.

The site of impaction can vary by age. The LES and diaphragmatic hiatus at vertebrae T10 and T11 are the most common impaction sites in adults. Patients younger than 16 years generally have impactions in the proximal esophagus that present with vomiting, gagging, choking, and neck or throat pain.[11] By contrast, patients older than 16 years tend to have impactions in the distal esophagus that present with anxiety, foreign body sensation, substernal chest pain, progressive dysphagia, and an inability to handle secretions.[12]

Other esophageal pathologies are also associated with certain anatomical sites of the esophagus. Diverticula are common near the esophageal sphincters due to uneven pressure on the esophageal wall. Zenker diverticula occur above the upper esophageal sphincter, Laimer diverticula occur in the upper esophagus just below the circular esophageal muscle, and epiphrenic diverticula occur just above the LES. Zenker, Laimer, and epiphrenic diverticula are caused by motor abnormalities, whereas midesophageal diverticula are usually caused by traction on the esophagus from an outside object.[13]

CRITICAL DECISION

What are common causes of esophageal perforation?

Esophageal perforations are generally caused by mechanical injury (eg, an ingested bone) or chemical corrosion (eg, an ingested button battery) (*Table 2*). Esophageal rupture, or Boerhaave syndrome, classically occurs in the left midthoracic esophagus. Although the textbook etiology for esophageal perforation or rupture is forceful vomiting, emergency physicians are more likely to encounter iatrogenic ruptures, most commonly from endoscopy for dilation or biopsy. Nasogastric (NG) tube placement and esophageal intubation are also common iatrogenic causes and are arguably more likely to occur in the emergency department given their frequent use. Transesophageal echocardiography and mediastinal surgery can also increase the risk of esophageal perforation. A high index of suspicion should be maintained for patients with recent lung, cervical and thoracic spinal, or cardiac surgeries. Thoracic or cervical spine trauma is another leading mechanical cause of esophageal perforation. Although this trauma is more commonly penetrating, it can cause significant blunt trauma injuries that rupture the esophagus. Unsurprisingly, performance-based occupations that include sword swallowing are also associated with esophageal rupture.

Foreign body impaction can lead to both mechanical and chemical perforations of the esophagus. In adults, hard objects or bones in food are commonly implicated. Dentures, retainers, and other dental protheses that contain wires or other sharp objects can also cause esophageal damage when accidentally swallowed.[14]

Caustic or chemical agents are another fairly common cause of esophageal perforation. In the United States, alkali materials are ingested more often, but in countries where hydrochloric and sulfuric acids are commonly available, acidotic esophagitis is slightly more common. Alkali, rather than acidic, agents are more damaging to the esophagus because they liquify its tissue.

Also included as a cause of chemical esophageal perforations is extremely severe reflux, although this is an uncommon occurrence. Perforations can also occur due to severe infections. In untreated

TABLE 1. Common infectious causes of esophagitis

immunocompromised patients, *Candida* and herpetic infections have reportedly caused esophageal perforations and subsequent mediastinitis.

Chest pain is the most common presenting symptom of esophageal perforation, and many patients are able to localize the site based on the pain. Other common symptoms include vomiting, hematemesis, dysphagia, tachypnea, cough, and if patients present late, fever. A history of esophageal instrumentation should raise suspicion for a rupture. If patients have a recent history of foreign body or caustic ingestion and symptoms of perforation, their condition should be treated as an emergency until proven otherwise. On physical examination, subcutaneous emphysema can sometimes be felt but requires at least 1 hour to develop. Spontaneous esophageal perforation presents with the classic Mackler triad that includes vomiting, chest pain, and subcutaneous emphysema in around 50% of cases. A delayed presentation of an esophageal perforation often presents as florid sepsis.[14]

CRITICAL DECISION

How should esophageal food impactions be managed?

When assessing for esophageal food impactions and determining the need for intervention, the airway should be assessed and the type of object or food ingested should be identified, if possible. The length of time since ingestion and any previously attempted treatments should also be determined. Indications for emergent endoscopy include airway compromise; complete esophageal obstruction (pooling of secretions that leads to aspiration); ingestion of sharp, long, or large objects (eg, bones or toothpicks); evidence of perforation; or an object that has been impacted for more than 24 hours.[15,16]

✔ Pearls

- Patients with suspected esophageal impaction should have their airways assessed first. If drooling is present, an urgent endoscopy is indicated. If esophageal disimpaction is not urgent, other treatment modalities like effervescents and medications can be considered.

- Consider the age and anatomy of patients when determining where a foreign body may be lodged in the esophagus. More proximal foreign bodies are more imminent airway threats.

- Esophagitis is a common cause of dysphagia and chest pain and can be infectious or noninfectious. HIV, steroid use, and antibiotic use are common culprits of infectious esophagitis. Common causes of noninfectious esophagitis include pills that get lodged in the esophagus, chemical ingestions, eosinophilic esophagitis, and GERD-related esophagitis.

Attempting to dislodge small food boluses is reasonable if patients are able to jump and firmly land on their heels. Effervescent or carbonated beverages are also a reasonable treatment for esophageal food impactions in stable patients because the gas from the drinks will dilate the distal esophagus. Up to 79% of patients have had their impactions dislodged by gas-forming agents alone. Interestingly, some food boluses have reportedly been treated with barium during imaging.

Current data do not show that medications are a clearly superior treatment for food impactions. In fact, a review of treatment methods for esophageal impaction found watchful waiting to be most effective for avoiding procedural disimpaction. However, treating impactions with medications is preferred over endoscopic or surgical removal because medications carry fewer risks.

The anticholinergic hyoscine butylbromide has been widely used to manage esophageal soft food impactions. However, despite its widespread use, multiple studies have concluded that there is no significant difference in disimpaction rates between hyoscine butylbromide treatment and watchful waiting. Additionally, the medication is not widely available in the United States for human use, so the alternative methscopolamine bromide would need to be used instead. For these reasons, hyoscine butylbromide is not an ideal esophageal smooth muscle relaxer for US-based physicians. Because it is on the WHO's list of essential medicines, hyoscine butylbromide is better suited to be used in low-resource settings, where other options are not readily available.[15]

More commonly used in the United States, glucagon can relax the LES in a dose-dependent fashion. Like hyoscine butylbromide, glucagon has not been found to have a significant advantage over placebo in noninterventional food disimpaction.[17] Despite the lack of evidence, many sources continue to recommend 1 to 2 mg of intravenous or intramuscular glucagon to attempt to avoid procedural disimpaction. Glucagon's major side effect is severe vomiting, so a prophylactic antiemetic should also be administered in these patients.[18] Benzodiazepines, opioids, calcium channel blockers, nitrates, and proteolytic enzymes (such as papain) are not recommended in food disimpaction due to their lack of efficacy in trials and their significant side effects.[15]

A small percentage of patients have a persistent globus sensation and are diagnosed with functional globus. These patients must have a nonpainful sensation of throat fullness with any of the following symptoms for diagnosis: dysphagia, odynophagia, sore throat, unexplained iron deficiency anemia, unintentional weight loss, palpable cervical lymphadenopathy on examination, or persistent vomiting. Functional globus can be diagnosed by using the Rome IV diagnostic criteria for globus.[6]

CRITICAL DECISION

What are the common complications of NG tube placement?

NG and orogastric tubes are commonly used in the emergency department to decompress the stomach and gain gastric access to deliver medications and nutrients. The only absolute contraindication to NG tube placement is severe facial trauma, which can be worsened by the procedure and can increase the risk of the tube being misplaced intracranially through the cribriform plate. Relative contraindications include severe coagulopathy (due to the risk of bleeding), gastric bypass or lap band procedures, known varices or structures without active bleeding, and a history of alkali or other caustic ingestion.

Common complications of NG tube placement include pulmonary placement, which can be avoided by taking a chest x-ray. This is especially necessary if activated charcoal will be administered via the tube because charcoal is extremely caustic to pulmonary tissue. Listening to the stomach while insufflating it with air is a common

Etiologies of Esophageal Perforation
Iatrogenic

- Endoscopic
  - Diagnostic endoscopy
    - Biopsy
    - Direct visualization
    - Transesophageal echocardiogram
  - Therapeutic endoscopy
    - Dilations
    - Variceal banding
    - Sclerotherapy
    - Laser therapy
    - Stent placement
- NG tube placement
- Endotracheal intubation
- Cervical and thoracic surgeries

Mechanical

- Traumatic
  - Penetrating
  - Blunt
  - Sword swallowing
- Spontaneous/Boerhaave syndrome
- Foreign bodies
  - Dentures
  - Button batteries
  - Food impaction

Caustic

- Alkali
- Acids

Infectious

- Fungal
- Viral

Malignancy

- Esophageal
- Lung
- Squamous cell carcinoma of the head and neck

TABLE 2. Common causes of esophageal perforation

technique to confirm correct placement; however, one study has shown that this technique catches only 6% of tube misplacements. Another confirmation technique that is fairly accurate is checking the pH of the gastric tube aspirate and confirming that it is less than 5.5. Epistaxis or variceal bleeding should be considered as possible complications when placing NG tubes in patients who are coagulopathic or anticoagulated. NG tubes can also induce gagging or vomiting that can increase intracranial pressures in patients who are not appropriately sedated and anesthetized. Be wary of this complication in patients with intracranial lesions or elevated intracranial pressure.[19]

Summary

Dysphagia can be a difficult and atypical symptom to address in the emergency department. Recognizing the emergent diagnoses that present with this chief complaint is a requirement of all emergency physicians. A detailed history that includes risk factors for malignancy and recent procedures can help differentiate emergent esophageal pathologies from those that are less serious. In cases of ingested foreign bodies, emergency physicians must know the indications for emergent endoscopy. Esophagitis, perforation, spasms, achalasia, and esophageal webs are other esophageal pathologies emergency physicians are likely to encounter. Finally, although a common procedure, NG tube placement is not without risks; therefore, emergency physicians must consider the indications and contraindications each time they order it.

REFERENCES

1. Jung H-K, Hong SJ, Lee OY, et al. 2019 Seoul consensus on esophageal achalasia guidelines. *J Neurogastroenterol Motil.* 2020 Apr 30;26(2):180-203.
2. Vaezi MF, Pandolfino JE, Vela MF. ACG clinical guidelines: diagnosis and management of achalasia. *Am J Gastroenterol.* 2013 Aug;108(8):1238-1249.

CASE RESOLUTIONS

CASE ONE

Given the patient's complex history and the physician's concern for a recurrent esophageal fistula at the site of the prior repair, an esophagram was ordered. While the patient was at radiology, the imaging technician called to say that the scout image had concerning findings. After reviewing the image, the physician canceled the esophagram (*Figure 2*).

The physician determined that the swallowed foreign body was likely a US penny due to its size. Based on its orientation, the penny was thought to be an esophageal foreign body; if it had been in the trachea, it would likely have presented as round on lateral view because this orientation helps it pass through the vocal cords. The patient's mother did not witness any foreign body ingestions but stated that the patient places small objects in his mouth from time to time.

Pediatric gastroenterology performed an upper endoscopy to retrieve the coin and found small superficial esophageal erosions after retrieval. The patient's previous surgical site appeared intact without signs of strictures or webbing. The patient tolerated the procedure well and was discharged the following day after tolerating full feeds by mouth.

CASE TWO

This patient's presentation was concerning for a complete obstruction of the esophagus from a food impaction, and he was diagnosed

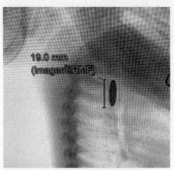

FIGURE 2. Esophagram scout image showing a US penny swallowed by a toddler with a history of esophageal atresia and associated tracheoesophageal fistula repair. *Credit:* Zachary Hagen, MD; and Jerrah Pickle, MD.

clinically based on his constant pooling of saliva. Although the patient was alert and speaking normally, he was at high risk of aspiration without urgent treatment of the obstruction. The time frame for disimpaction of uncomplicated obstructions is approximately 12 to 24 hours, but because this patient was at risk of aspiration, an urgent gastroenterology consultation and preprocedural laboratory tests were ordered. Gastroenterology successfully removed a large piece of meat lodged in the mid esophagus. The patient was discharged the next morning after an uncomplicated observation.

CASE THREE

This patient presented with symptoms consistent with infectious esophagitis. Her history of HIV put her at risk for the condition, especially in light of the questionable compliance with antiretroviral therapy. The most likely culprit for her infectious esophagitis was *Candida albicans*. Esophageal candidiasis is most common in HIV patients with a CD4 count less than 100 and is considered an AIDS-defining illness. It is also seen, albeit rarely, in immunocompetent patients who take steroids. Because the patient was stable, she was treated with a loading dose of oral fluconazole 400 mg followed by 200 mg daily for 2 weeks. Recommendations were to follow up with infectious disease and gastroenterology for reevaluation if her symptoms did not improve.[20] Treatment failure in this patient would warrant further workup for less common viral causes of esophagitis.

3. Coss-Adame E, Rao SSC. A review of esophageal chest pain. *Gastroenterol Hepatol (N Y).* 2015 Nov;11(11):759-766.
4. Novacek G. Plummer-Vinson syndrome. *Orphanet J Rare Dis.* 2006 Sep 15;1:36.
5. Hossain SMN, de Caestecker J. Acute oesophageal symptoms. *Clin Med (Lond).* 2015 Oct;15(5):477-481.
6. Rome IV diagnostic criteria for FGIDs. The Rome Foundation. https://theromefoundation.org/rome-iv/rome-iv-criteria/
7. O'Rourke A, Tansel A. Esophageal disorders: evaluation and management. In: Rosen CA, Gray S, Ha P, Limb C, Park S, Richter G, eds. *Bailey's Head and Neck Surgery: Otolaryngology.* Vol. 1. 6th ed. Wolters Kluwer; 2022:846-871.
8. Ahmad M, Soetikno RM, Ahmed A. The differential diagnosis of eosinophilic esophagitis. *J Clin Gastroenterol.* 2000 Apr;30(3):242-244.
9. Dellon ES, Rusin S, Gebhart JH, et al. A clinical prediction tool identifies cases of eosinophilic esophagitis without endoscopic biopsy: a prospective study. *Am J Gastroenterol.* 2015 Sep;110(9):1347-1354.
10. Patti MG, Gantert W, Way LW. Surgery of the esophagus: anatomy and physiology. *Surg Clin North Am.* 1997 Oct;77(5):959-970.
11. Kay M, Wyllie R. Pediatric foreign bodies and their management. *Curr Gastroenterol Rep.* 2005 Jun;7(3):212-218.
12. Ikenberry SO, Jue TL, Anderson MA, et al; ASGE Standards of Practice Committee. Management of ingested foreign bodies and food impactions. *Gastrointest Endosc.* 2011 Jun;73(6):1085-1091.
13. Schofer JM, Mattu A, Kessler C, et al, eds. *Emergency Medicine: A Focused Review of the Core Curriculum.* 2nd ed. AAEM Resident and Student Association, Inc; 2015.
14. Kaman L, Iqbal J, Kundil B, Kochhar R. Management of esophageal perforation in adults. *Gastroenterology Res.* 2010 Dec;3(6):235-244.
15. Leopard D, Fishpool S, Winter S. The management of oesophageal soft food bolus obstruction: a systematic review. *Ann R Coll Surg Engl.* 2011 Sep;93(6):441-444.
16. Chirica M, Kelly MD, Siboni S, et al. Esophageal emergencies: WSES guidelines. *World J Emerg Surg.* 2019 May 31;14(1):26.
17. Khayyat YM. Pharmacological management of esophageal food bolus impaction. *Emerg Med Int.* 2013;2013:924015.
18. Hardman J, Sharma N, Smith J, Nankivell P. Conservative management of oesophageal soft food bolus impaction. *Cochrane Database Syst Rev.* 2020 May 11;5(5):CD007352.
19. Sigmon DF, An J. Nasogastric tube. *StatPearls [Internet].* StatPearls Publishing; 2022. https://www.ncbi.nlm.nih.gov/books/NBK556063/
20. Pappas PG, Kauffman CA, Andes DR, et al. Clinical practice guideline for the management of candidiasis: 2016 update by the Infectious Diseases Society of America. *Clin Infect Dis.* 2016 Feb 15;62(4):e1-50.

MDCALC REFERENCES

Shah S. Diagnosis and management of achalasia. MDCalc. https://www.mdcalc.com/guidelines/505/acg/diagnosis-management-achalasia

Drossman D, Chang L; the Rome Foundation. Rome IV diagnostic criteria for functional dysphagia. MDCalc. https://www.mdcalc.com/calc/10283/rome-iv-diagnostic-criteria-functional-dysphagia

Drossman D, Chang L; the Rome Foundation. Rome IV diagnostic criteria for globus. MDCalc. https://www.mdcalc.com/calc/10284/rome-iv-diagnostic-criteria-globus

✖ Pitfalls

- Ruling out *Candida* esophagitis based on the absence of thrush. Patients with no oropharyngeal signs of candidiasis can still have *Candida* esophagitis.
- Placing an NG tube on a trauma patient without first carefully assessing for maxillofacial trauma. Severe maxillofacial trauma is the only absolute contraindication to placing an NG tube.
- Failing to consider esophageal perforation as a cause of acute chest pain. The differential diagnosis for chest pain focuses on cardiopulmonary origins, but the esophagus can also be a source of thoracic pathology.

CME Questions

Reviewed by **Amal Mattu, MD, FACEP**

Qualified, paid subscribers to *Critical Decisions in Emergency Medicine* may receive CME certificates for up to 5 ACEP Category I credits, 5 *AMA PRA Category 1 Credits*™, and 5 AOA Category 2-B credits for completing this activity in its entirety. Submit your answers online at acep.org/cdem; a score of 75% or better is required. You may receive credit for completing the CME activity any time within 3 years of its publication date. Answers to this month's questions will be published in next month's issue.

1 A patient presents with chest pain. What is most suggestive of pericarditis?

- A. Elevated troponin levels
- B. Fever
- C. Preceding urinary tract infection
- D. Triphasic friction rub

2 Which ECG findings suggest pericarditis rather than STEMI?

- A. Diffuse ST elevations and PR depressions without any ST depressions
- B. PR depressions with ST elevation in lead III that is greater than in lead II
- C. PR depressions with widespread ST elevations and ST depression in the lateral leads
- D. ST elevations only in the anterior leads

3 Which imaging modality should be used to evaluate for cardiac tamponade?

- A. Chest x-ray
- B. CT
- C. Echocardiography
- D. MRI

4 A 70-year-old woman presents with chest pain and is diagnosed with an acute myocardial infarction. She undergoes percutaneous intervention for placement of two stents. She then develops new chest pain and a friction rub, which lead to the diagnosis of post–myocardial infarction pericarditis. Which medication is considered first line for this condition?

- A. Aspirin
- B. Colchicine
- C. Ibuprofen
- D. Prednisone

5 According to the 2015 European Society of Cardiology guidelines, what can be used to diagnose pericarditis?

- A. Cough and elevated erythrocyte sedimentation rate and C-reactive protein values
- B. Pleuritic chest pain and leukocytosis
- C. Pleuritic chest pain and pericardial friction rub
- D. Widespread ST elevation and an enlarged heart on chest x-ray

6 A 65-year-old man presents with altered mental status and chest pain. Laboratory studies find severe uremia, and his chest x-ray shows an enlarged heart. A bedside echocardiogram is obtained and shows mild pericardial effusion. Which treatment would be contraindicated for treating his pericarditis?

- A. Aspirin
- B. Colchicine
- C. Dialysis
- D. Indomethacin

7 Tuberculous pericarditis should be suspected in which of these patients?

- A. 22-year-old male college student from Norway who had a recent GI infection
- B. 22-year-old man who recently immigrated from India and reports 3 months of cough, fatigue, and night sweats
- C. 63-year-old woman from the United Kingdom who is on immunosuppression medications for rheumatoid arthritis and reports chest pain and shortness of breath
- D. 63-year-old man with a recent myocardial infarction who has new chest pain

8 In which patient would cardiac MRI be most effective?

- A. 19-year-old man who presents with pleuritic chest pain, stable vital signs, and appears well overall
- B. 54-year-old man with muffled heart sounds, elevated jugular venous pressure, and low blood pressure
- C. 72-year-old woman with multiple episodes of recurrent pericarditis who now presents with dyspnea on exertion and peripheral edema
- D. 82-year-old woman with altered mental status and ECG findings that are consistent with pericarditis

9 What cardiac MRI findings are expected in patients with constrictive pericarditis?

- A. Delayed early filling and enhanced late filling
- B. Pericardial thickening and ventricular chamber flattening with septal flattening
- C. Right atrial collapse during diastole
- D. Water bottle–shaped heart

10 In which patient population should fungal pericarditis be suspected?

- A. Patients with a recent myocardial infarction
- B. Patients who are dependent on total parenteral nutrition
- C. Patients who are immunocompetent
- D. Patients who have an overall benign presentation

11 A 68-year-old woman presents with chest pain and a foreign body sensation in her chest after taking a large bite of chicken. Since symptoms started, she immediately vomits any food or liquids that she consumes. Her vital signs are stable. What is the most appropriate first-line treatment for this condition in the emergency department?

- A. Fluconazole
- B. Glucagon
- C. Hydromorphone
- D. Papain

12 What is an absolute contraindication to nasogastric tube placement?

    A.   Esophageal varices or strictures
    B.   History of an alkali ingestion
    C.   History of gastric bypass or lap band procedure
    D.   Severe facial trauma

13 What is the most common level for esophageal impaction of a foreign body in young children?

    A.   C4
    B.   C6
    C.   C8
    D.   T4

14 Which duo correctly pairs the diverticulum with its location?

    A.   Epiphrenic diverticulum: lower esophageal sphincter
    B.   Laimer diverticulum: middle third of the esophagus
    C.   Traction diverticulum: upper esophageal sphincter
    D.   Zenker diverticulum: cricopharyngeus

15 A 58-year-old woman with a medical history of hypertension and gastroesophageal reflux disease presents with dysphagia to solids that seems to have worsened over the past year. Her medical records state that she has lost 17 lb over that time. She initially had no symptoms with liquids but now notices worsening symptoms with colloids like yogurt. She has been a heavy smoker for 32 years. Her physical examination shows no abnormalities in the mouth or posterior oropharynx. What is the most likely diagnosis?

    A.   Achalasia
    B.   Esophageal carcinoma
    C.   Eosinophilic esophagitis
    D.   Esophageal food impaction

16 A toddler ingests an unknown solution from under his parents' kitchen sink. Which pH would cause the greatest esophageal injury?

    A.   5.0
    B.   7.0
    C.   9.0
    D.   12.0

17 A 32-year-old woman with a past medical history of menorrhagia and anemia presents for difficulty swallowing. She has presented many times in the past with similar complaints. Her symptoms are worse with solids than with liquids and have slowly worsened over the course of months. She admits to noncompliance with her iron supplementation. What is her likely diagnosis?

    A.   Achalasia
    B.   *Candida* esophagitis
    C.   Esophageal web
    D.   Pill esophagitis

18 What is the most common cause of esophageal perforation?

    A.   Caustic ingestion
    B.   Iatrogenic source
    C.   Nausea and vomiting
    D.   Trauma

19 What would be a normal change during pregnancy?

    A.   Decreased esophageal peristalsis
    B.   Decreased lower esophageal tone
    C.   Increased risk of esophageal food impaction
    D.   Increased risk of esophageal perforation due to nausea and vomiting

20 Which disease process is associated with esophageal dysfunction, acute kidney injury, and elevated liver enzymes?

    A.   Eosinophilic esophagitis
    B.   HIV
    C.   Plummer-Vinson syndrome
    D.   Scleroderma

ANSWER KEY FOR MAY 2023, VOLUME 37, NUMBER 5

1	2	3	4	5	6	7	8	9	10	11	12	13	14	15	16	17	18	19	20
A	A	B	A	A	A	C	B	D	B	D	C	D	A	B	C	A	B	C	B

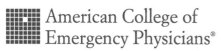

American College of
Emergency Physicians®

ADVANCING EMERGENCY CARE

Post Office Box 619911
Dallas, Texas 75261-9911

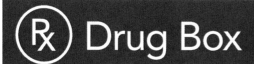

Off-Label Tizanidine

Frank LoVecchio, DO, MPH, FACEP
Valleywise Health Medical Center and ASU, Phoenix, Arizona

Objective
On completion of this column, you should be able to:
- Explain the indications for off-label utilization of tizanidine and its associated side effects.

Tizanidine is an FDA-approved drug for managing spasticity. It has been utilized off-label for acute skeletal pain with muscle spasms, usually combined with NSAIDs or acetaminophen. In general, tizanidine and other muscle relaxants should be used temporarily (eg, for a few days or intermittently when needed). Although studies are not robust, they show tizanidine to be clinically effective for patients with chronic neck and lumbosacral pain with a myofascial component. Patients should be warned of the possible side effects of sedation and orthostatic hypotension.

Kinetics
Metabolism: extensively hepatic via the CYP1A2 enzyme to inactive metabolites
Half-life elimination: ~2.5 hr
Time to peak, serum:
- *Fasting state:* capsule or tablet — 1 hr
- *Fed state:* capsule — 3 to 4 hr; tablet — 1.5 hr

Side Effects
- Asymptomatic, reversible increased liver enzymes and severe hepatotoxicity have been reported.
- Reversible hypotension has been demonstrated in 7% to 12% of patients who receive tizanidine.[1] Orthostatic hypotension has also been reported.
- A non–life-threatening, reversible sedated state occurs in 24% to 50% of patients who receive ≤36 mg/day of tizanidine.

Dosing
Oral: initial dose of 2 to 4 mg every 8 to 12 hr as needed or at bedtime; some patients may benefit from scheduling doses initially. Doses may increase based on response and tolerability up to a maximum dose of 24 mg/day (eg, 4-8 mg every 8 hr as needed).

Pediatric and Pregnancy Categories
Tizanidine has been used in case reports but not studied in these populations.

REFERENCE
Wallace JD. Summary of combined clinical analysis of controlled clinical trials with tizanidine. *Neurology.* 1994 Nov;44(11) (suppl 9):S60-S68.

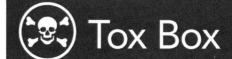

Pyrethroid Toxicity

By Christian A. Tomaszewski, MD, MS, MBA, FACEP
University of California San Diego Health

Objective
On completion of this column, you should be able to:
- State the presentation and treatment of pyrethroid toxicity.

Introduction
Pyrethroid insecticides are widely used for home pest control. Modern synthetic pyrethroids, such as permethrin for head lice, are similar to the natural pyrethrum that comes from chrysanthemums. Human toxicity is rare except in cases of massive ingestions or potential allergic symptoms if inhaled.

Mechanism of Action
- Strong lipophilicity allows for penetration and paralysis of insects' nervous systems.
- Delayed closure of voltage-sensitive sodium channels leads to hyperexcitation.

Kinetics
- *Absorption:* inhalation, ingestion, and dermal contact (less common)
- *Metabolism:* short plasma half-life (<8 hr); but when combined with piperonyl butoxide, metabolism is decreased

Clinical Manifestations (usually in massive ingestions)
- *Mucous membranes:* allergic symptoms with irritation
- *Dermal:* irritation, urticaria
- *GI:* vomiting, cramps, diarrhea post ingestion
- *Cardiac:* tachydysrhythmias, hypotension
- *Pulmonary:* cough, bronchospasm, pulmonary edema (especially with Type II pyrethroids)
- *Neuro:* headache, dizziness
  - Type I (eg, permethrin) — tremor, hyperreflexia, paresthesia
  - Type II (eg, deltamethrin) — coarse tremor, hyperreflexia, choreoathetosis, seizures

Diagnostics
- Routine screening of glucose and acetaminophen levels for intentional overdoses
- Chest x-ray if patient exhibits respiratory issues

Treatment
- Wash skin
- Activated charcoal usually not indicated due to mild symptoms and potential for seizures with massive ingestions
- Hypotension
  - IV fluid bolus for hypotension
  - Norepinephrine for fluid-unresponsive hypotension
- Benzodiazepines or barbiturates for seizures

Disposition
- Can medically clear if no respiratory issues and no neurologic symptoms 4 to 6 hr post exposure or ingestion

Critical decisions
in emergency medicine

Volume 37 Number 7: **July 2023**

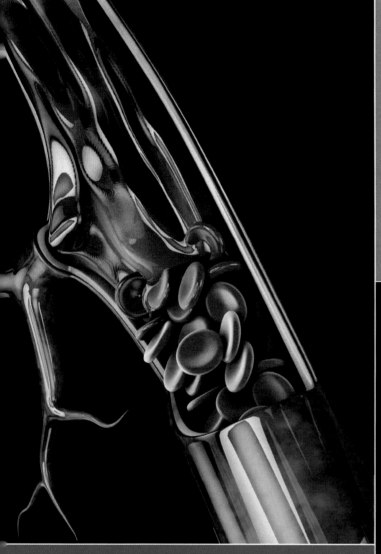

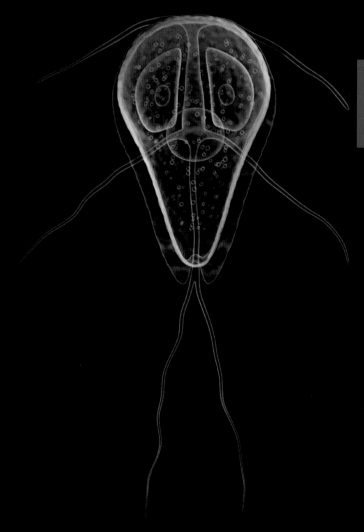

Leg Work

Deep vein thrombosis and pulmonary embolism, together known as venous thromboembolism, are responsible for up to 100,000 deaths per year. They can restrict blood flow, damage tissues, and lead to organ dysfunction. Emergency physicians, however, can provide prompt diagnosis and treatment of deep vein thombosis to avoid the sequelae-associated morbidity and mortality of this relatively common malady.

Gut Wrenching

Giardiasis is the most common intestinal protozoal infection worldwide, visits for Crohn disease have increased by more than 50% in recent years, and Meckel diverticulum is the most common cause of pediatric lower GI tract bleeding. To provide appropriate care, emergency physicians must be versed in the presentation, diagnosis, and treatment of these small bowel diseases.

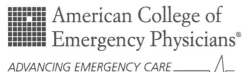

American College of Emergency Physicians®

ADVANCING EMERGENCY CARE

Critical decisions
in emergency medicine

Critical Decisions in Emergency Medicine is the official CME publication of the American College of Emergency Physicians. Additional volumes are available.

EDITOR-IN-CHIEF

Michael S. Beeson, MD, MBA, FACEP
Northeastern Ohio Universities,
Rootstown, OH

SECTION EDITORS

Joshua S. Broder, MD, FACEP
Duke University, Durham, NC

Andrew J. Eyre, MD, MS-HPEd
Brigham and Women's Hospital/
Harvard Medical School, Boston, MA

John Kiel, DO, MPH, FACEP, CAQSM
University of Florida College of Medicine,
Jacksonville, FL

Frank LoVecchio, DO, MPH, FACEP
Valleywise, Arizona State University, University of Arizona,
and Creighton Colleges of Medicine, Phoenix, AZ

Sharon E. Mace, MD, FACEP
Cleveland Clinic Lerner College of Medicine/
Case Western Reserve University, Cleveland, OH

Amal Mattu, MD, FACEP
University of Maryland, Baltimore, MD

Christian A. Tomaszewski, MD, MS, MBA, FACEP
University of California Health Sciences,
San Diego, CA

Steven J. Warrington, MD, MEd, MS
MercyOne Siouxland, Sioux City, IA

ASSOCIATE EDITORS

Tareq Al-Salamah, MBBS, MPH, FACEP
King Saud University, Riyadh, Saudi Arabia/
University of Maryland, Baltimore, MD

Wan-Tsu Chang, MD
University of Maryland, Baltimore, MD

Ann M. Dietrich, MD, FAAP, FACEP
University of South Carolina College of Medicine,
Greenville, SC

Kelsey Drake, MD, MPH, FACEP
St. Anthony Hospital, Lakewood, CO

Walter L. Green, MD, FACEP
UT Southwestern Medical Center, Dallas, TX

John C. Greenwood, MD
University of Pennsylvania, Philadelphia, PA

Danya Khoujah, MBBS, MEHP, FACEP
University of Maryland, Baltimore, MD

Nathaniel Mann, MD
Greenville Health System, Greenville, SC

George Sternbach, MD, FACEP
Stanford University Medical Center, Stanford, CA

EDITORIAL STAFF

Suzannah Alexander, Editorial Director
salexander@acep.org

Joy Carrico, JD
Managing Editor

Alex Bass
Assistant Editor

Kyle Powell
Graphic Artist

ISSN2325-0186 (Print)   ISSN2325-8365 (Online)

Contents

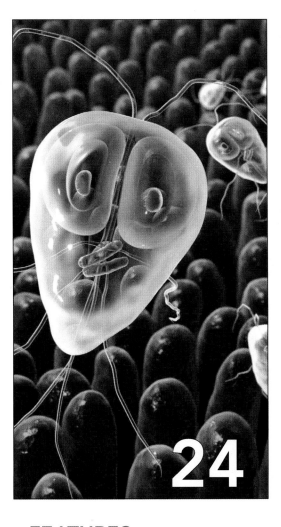

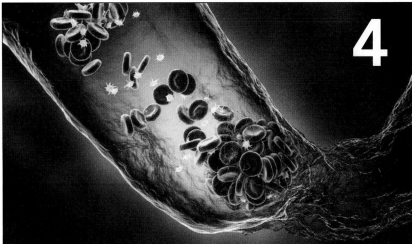

FEATURES

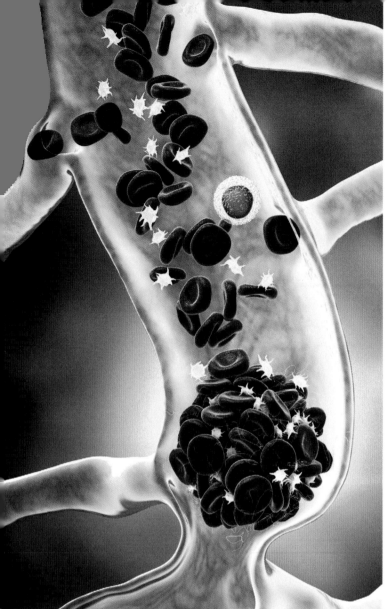

Leg Work

Emergency Diagnosis and Treatment of Deep Vein Thrombosis

LESSON **13**

By Richard Jean-Louis, MD, MA; and
Kinjal N. Sethuraman, MD, MPH
Dr. Jean-Louis is a resident at the University of Maryland Medical
Center, and Dr. Sethuraman is an associate professor in the
Department of Emergency Medicine and medical director of the
Center for Hyperbaric and Dive Medicine at the University of
Maryland School of Medicine in Baltimore.

Reviewed by Tareq Al-Salamah, MBBS, MPH, FACEP

Objectives

On completion of this lesson, you should be able to:

1. Describe the etiology of DVT.
2. List the risk factors associated with DVT.
3. Discuss the complications associated with DVT.
4. Name the tests and scoring tools used to diagnose DVT.
5. Explain the treatment of DVT.

From the EM Model

3.0 Cardiovascular Disorders
    3.3   Disorders of Circulation
        3.3.2 Venous
            3.3.2.1 Thromboembolism

CRITICAL DECISIONS

■ When should a diagnosis of DVT be considered?

■ What are the associated complications and sequelae of DVT?

■ What is the emergency department workup for DVT?

■ When should treatment for DVT be started in the emergency department?

■ What are the treatments for DVT?

Deep vein thrombosis (DVT) and pulmonary embolism (PE), together known as venous thromboembolism (VTE), affect up to 900,000 Americans annually and are responsible for up to 100,000 deaths per year. They can restrict blood flow, damage tissues, and lead to organ dysfunction. Emergency physicians, however, can provide prompt diagnosis and treatment of deep vein thrombosis to avoid the sequelae-associated morbidity and mortality of this relatively common malady.

■ CASE ONE

A 42-year-old woman presents with complaints of left leg pain. She reports that today she noticed a significant amount of pain in her left calf after driving several hours to visit a family member. Initially, she thought it was a muscle cramp, but over the past several hours, she has noticed swelling from her left ankle to the middle of her thigh. During the assessment, the patient denies fever, chills, itchiness, known bug bites, leg trauma, discharge, and open wounds. Her medical history includes acute myeloid leukemia, which was treated with chemotherapy several years ago. Aside from hormonal contraceptives, she takes no other medications. She denies drug and alcohol use but states that she smokes one to two cigarettes weekly.

On examination, the patient is well appearing and has a warm, tender, and erythematous left leg. She has 1+ nonpitting edema and erythema that spans from her Achilles area to the posterior and anterior portions of her mid thigh. No fluctuation, crepitus, hyperesthesia, swelling at the joints, or overlying bullae are found. Other findings include 2+ dorsalis pedis and posterior tibial pulses in the left lower extremity and full hip, knee, and ankle range of motion without any signs of bony tenderness. Sensation is intact throughout, and her right lower extremity is unremarkable.

■ CASE TWO

A 25-year-old man presents with unilateral upper extremity discomfort. Over the past 2 months, he has visited the emergency department for complaints ranging from dizziness to chest pain, but all workups were unremarkable. Intravenous access in this patient has been primarily ultrasound guided due to severe skin scars and sclerotic veins. Today, he reports that over the past 4 days, he has had gradually worsening pain, swelling, and redness of his left upper arm near the area where he typically injects heroin. His medical history also includes alcohol and fentanyl use. He denies any recent blunt trauma to the area, denies taking prescribed medications, and has no other findings on review of systems. His vital signs are within normal limits. Examination reveals a swollen left upper extremity from the antecubital fossa to the proximal humerus, predominantly in the medial portions; neurovascular examination is normal both proximally and distally.

■ CASE THREE

A 37-year-old woman presents with left inner thigh discomfort and an associated painful bulge. The pain and redness developed over several days before the mass on her inner thigh appeared. She denies vaginal pain and discharge and has not noticed any abnormal skin changes in her genital area. Her medical history includes HIV, for which she is compliant with emtricitabine and tenofovir. She also takes the oral contraceptive ethinyl estradiol. Her vital signs are normal. Her physical examination reveals a left medial thigh erythema, warmth, and tenderness with a palpable snake-like firmness that elicits discomfort. No induration, fluctuation, pulsatile mass, or crepitus is found.

Introduction

DVT has affected humans for at least 9 centuries. The first documented case comes from the late 1200s, when medieval documents report that the Norman cobbler Raoul sustained unilateral swelling of the leg with distal to proximal extension. Ever since, documentation of similar presentations has increased, namely in peripartum and postpartum women.[1]

The CDC reports that an estimated 900,000 US adults are affected by VTE each year, for an annual incidence of approximately 200/100,000 people, or 0.2% of the population. DVT and PE combined cause death in approximately 100,000 Americans annually.[2] Furthermore, both conditions cost the United States almost $10 billion in annual health care expenditures.[3] Although the incidence of VTE varies by country, VTE is estimated to affect nearly 10 million people worldwide every year.[4]

DVT is well characterized in the scientific literature, but research continues into diagnostic and therapeutic approaches. The simultaneous evolution of medicine and technology has significantly improved DVT management. When appropriately suspected, emergency physicians can accurately identify and treat DVTs, thereby reducing morbidity and mortality.

CRITICAL DECISION

When should a diagnosis of DVT be considered?

DVT should be considered in patients who complain of limb swelling, pain, erythema, and warmth.[5] The presence of these signs and symptoms are best assessed by comparing the affected extremity with the unaffected one (*Figure 1*). Findings of DVT are nonspecific and typically unilateral; however, bilateral DVTs are possible — they are estimated

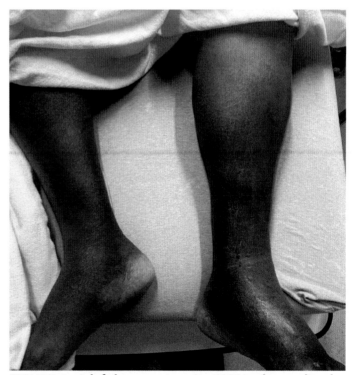

FIGURE 1. A left lower-extremity DVT in the popliteal vein of a patient with HIV. *Credit:* Richard Jean-Louis, MD.

to occur in around 7% of all DVT cases.[6] When possible, the history of the presenting illness should be obtained in the emergency department, including the onset, duration, and aggravating and alleviating factors. The context of the complaints should also be gathered, including a history of trauma, recent wounds, bug bites, systemic symptoms, the degree of pain, and the speed of spread for any redness of the skin. Importantly, risk factors for DVTs can be determined by asking questions that target the Virchow triad: the presence of stasis, hypercoagulable disease, and endothelial damage. Originally described in 1856, these three entities continue to be pathophysiologic themes to explore when obtaining a medical history for cases of suspected DVT.[5]

When assessing for stasis, emergency physicians should ask about any surgeries in the last 3 months. Some procedures, particularly orthopedic surgeries, can carry up to a 20-fold increased risk of DVT.[7] Similarly, general immobility, congestive heart failure, and recent long travel also contribute to venous stasis. In the literature, long travel is considered any distance greater than 10,000 km (≈6,200 miles). An Australian study reported that the incidence of VTE is highest during the first 2 weeks of long travel, termed the "hazard period." On average, people who travel long distances have an estimated 12% annual increased risk of DVT.[8]

Next, emergency physicians should inquire about hypercoagulable states. Common causes of hypercoagulability include iatrogenic modalities (ie, exogenous hormones, aprotinin, aminocaproic acid, chemotherapy), malignancy, a personal or family history of coagulopathy, pregnancy status, and smoking.

The relationship between cigarette smoking and DVT development has been well described for over 2 decades.[9] Toxins from cigarette smoke encourage endothelial damage by proinflammatory cytokines and reactive oxygen species, which negatively affects both arterial and venous systems throughout the body. One study found the overall hazard ratio of VTE in current smokers to be 1.19.[9]

Oral contraceptives and hormone replacement therapy are also two major independent risk factors for VTE. Combination estrogen-progesterone medications alter the coagulation cascade by increasing plasma fibrinogen and the activity of multiple coagulation factors. They may also reduce production of anticoagulation factors while upregulating platelet aggregation.[10]

Several diseases have also been linked to an increased occurrence of DVT. These include, but are not limited to, factor V Leiden thrombophilia, congenital and acquired antithrombin III deficiency (AT III), protein C or protein S deficiency, May-Thurner syndrome (MTS), HIV, and systemic lupus erythematosus (SLE).[11-15]

Factor V Leiden thrombophilia is one of the most common inherited thrombophilias in the United States — heterozygous prevalence is estimated to be between 3% and 7%. It is primarily found in White populations and affects less than 1% of African Americans. The pathophysiology is caused by a nucleotide mutation that renders factors V and Va resistant to inactivation by protein C, enhancing the procoagulant effects of factor Va and reducing the anticoagulant effects of factor V. This manifests as venous thrombosis, which carries high rates of mortality when undiagnosed. A retrospective cohort study found that the prevalence of the factor V Leiden mutation among patients with DVT was 21% compared to 5% of healthy subjects. Furthermore, patients with factor V Leiden were more likely to develop large DVTs.[15] A large population-based study examined the joint effects of (1) factor V Leiden and smoking and (2) oral contraceptive use and smoking on the risk of VTE. The researchers reported that the two factors of smoking and oral contraceptive use had the greatest synergistic effect, putting women who smoked and used oral contraceptives at an eight-fold increased risk of VTE compared to women who did neither. The joint effect of smoking and factor V Leiden led to a five-fold increased risk of VTE compared to women who were nonsmokers and did not carry the mutation.[16]

Congenital AT III is an autosomal dominant hereditary condition caused by a genetic mutation that alters the function and production of antithrombin, a glycoprotein produced by the liver. Defective antithrombin is unable to prevent clot formation and leads to thrombotic disease like DVT, PE, and ischemic cerebrovascular accidents. Up to 50% of affected individuals are estimated to experience thrombosis in their lifetime, usually during adolescence when hormones increase.[17,18] This condition should be suspected in patients who have had unexplained spontaneous abortions and thrombotic events.[19] Acquired AT III can occur from liver failure, malnutrition, or nephrotic syndrome.[20] Nephrotic syndrome most likely causes DVTs through proteinuria and loss of anticoagulating proteins.

Protein C and protein S are glycoproteins that function as natural anticoagulants. They are produced by the liver and maintain physiologic homeostasis by preventing thrombin production. When a mutation occurs in these proteins or hepatic production becomes impaired, the clot cascade can go unchecked and lead to thrombosis. Clinically significant venous thrombosis occurs in an estimated 1/20,000 individuals with protein C deficiency.[21]

MTS is a condition in which iliofemoral DVTs occur from a compressed right iliac common artery (RICA). Anatomic variants of the RICA predispose certain individuals to MTS.

✔ Pearls

- DVT risk factors include stasis, hypercoagulable states, and endothelial damage. These factors can be brought on by recent surgeries, immobility, recent long travel, pregnancy, smoking, exogenous hormones, coagulopathic medications, chemotherapy, malignancy, congestive heart failure, SLE, and congenital disorders that affect clotting abilities.

- Duplex ultrasonography is a safe and effective imaging modality with a high sensitivity for diagnosing DVT.

- The location and size of a DVT are important in dictating management and treatment.

- Large DVTs can lead to venous ischemia and gangrenous infection, which are associated with high mortality and morbidity.

The persistent pressure of the RICA on the iliofemoral veins as it branches off the abdominal aorta pushes the RICA against bony vertebrae, which prompts venous spur formation. The spurs formed under mechanical compression gradually develop into venous vascular obstructions that lead to DVTs. MTS is estimated to be present in 2% to 5% of all DVT cases, with autopsy studies predicting an even higher prevalence. Women, typically during their second and third decades of life, have a two-fold increase in MTS compared to men.[14]

HIV is also linked to increased rates of thrombosis. Studies have suggested a 7% annual incidence of DVT in patients with HIV. HIV is thought to impair thrombin regulation by directly affecting protein C and protein S function. Additionally, HIV leads to opportunistic infections that can cause endothelial damage and generate antibodies toward endogenous anticoagulants.[22]

SLE is an autoimmune condition that occurs nine times more often in women than in men.[23] It can cause a myriad of complications due to its multiorgan involvement. A cohort study found that thrombosis in patients with SLE was one of the main causes of death at the end of a 10-year period.[24] The production of antiphospholipid antibodies (APLAs) in SLE is one of the key factors that predisposes these patients to thrombosis. Two of the most common APLAs associated with DVTs in patients with SLE are anticardiolipin and lupus anticoagulant antibodies. These antibodies target plasma proteins and bind to their phospholipid surface to alter the coagulation cascade and cause disequilibrium in procoagulation and anticoagulation signaling mechanisms.[25] More recently, SARS-CoV-2 has been suggested to be a potential risk factor for VTE, but a clear relationship has yet to be established.[26]

A fat embolism should also be considered on the differential for VTE. This disease process typically has distinct risk factors, presents differently, and is treated differently. An uncommon disease, it occurs in approximately 0.5% to 2% of long-bone fractures. The classic triad associated with a fat embolism, usually from orthopedic trauma, is petechiae, dyspnea, and altered mental status.[27] Its diagnosis is clinical, but because of the difficulty in diagnosing it, physicians often follow the typical diagnostic pathway for VTE in patients with this condition. Treatment for a fat embolism is primarily supportive as opposed to the medications and surgical management characteristic of VTE treatment.

A focused, comprehensive physical examination of the extremity should be performed when assessing for DVT. After comparing the affected limb to the contralateral unaffected one, the affected limb's neurovascular status should be assessed, and the limb should be palpated to assess for warmth, fluctuation, and crepitus. The degree of discomfort can be gauged during the examination to determine if the patient experiences tenderness and out-of-proportion pain. Findings can help differentiate between DVT, various soft tissue infections, and septic arthritis. DVT can occur alongside cellulitis, venous stasis ulcers, and necrotizing fasciitis, albeit rarely.[28]

An examination maneuver known as Homans sign can be performed when suspecting DVT as a cause of lower-extremity pain. First described in a 1930s paper by Dr. John Homans, a positive Homans sign is calf pain caused by dorsiflexion of the foot.[29,30] Calf pain in a leg with DVT after this maneuver

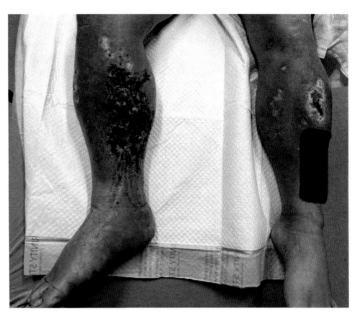

FIGURE 2. **Phlegmasia cerulea dolens in the right lower extremity of a patient with a history of multiple PEs.** *Credit:* Richard Jean-Louis, MD.

is purported to be caused by mechanical traction of the posterior tibial vein. Although easy to perform, the sensitivity of a positive Homans signs is estimated to be 10% to 50% and the specificity 30% to 90%.[31] Less common findings in cases of DVT of the lower leg are phlegmasia alba dolens and phlegmasia cerulea dolens. Phlegmasia alba dolens translates to "milk leg syndrome" because the complication causes the leg to be pale in addition to painful and edematous; it indicates that a large DVT has occurred in a large vein while sparing the collateral vessels. Phlegmasia cerulea dolens, or "copper leg," presents as limb cyanosis with pain and swelling and occurs when a large DVT affects both a large vein and its associated collateral vessels (*Figure 2*).[32]

CRITICAL DECISION

What are the associated complications and sequelae of DVT?

DVTs are associated with complications that increase morbidity and mortality.[1] In a Danish retrospective cohort analysis of nearly 130,000 patients published in 2014, the cohort's mortality risk from DVT within 30 days, 1 year, 10 years, and 30 years was found to be 3%, 13%, 42%, and 68%, respectively.[33,34] In isolation, DVTs can cause post-thrombotic syndrome (formerly known as post-phlebetic syndrome) that leads to vascular damage and venous insufficiency. Post-thrombotic syndrome develops in up to 50% of patients with DVT, irrespective of appropriate anticoagulation treatment.[35] The postulated pathophysiology of this condition is that venous hypertension causes limb muscle hypoperfusion, which reduces tissue integrity, increases tissue permeability, and ultimately leads to inflammation-mediated edema.[36] Symptom severity ranges from mild, chronic pain to enfeebling limb swelling and persistent venous ulcers.

The DVT complications of phlegmasia alba dolens and phlegmasia cerulea dolens both have mortality rates of around 20% to 50%. Although rare, these conditions are incredibly fatal:

They cause tissue ischemia, which when severe can progress to venous gangrene and septic shock that necessitate amputation to prevent death.[37] DVTs are especially lethal when they dislodge and navigate from the periphery into the central vasculature.

From the venous system, a DVT can access the right side of the heart and travel into the pulmonary arteries. The severity of a PE varies depending on the degree and location of the pulmonary artery occlusion. Segmental and subsegmental PEs are unlikely to induce cardiovascular collapse, whereas saddle emboli are more likely to cause sudden death at the estimated rates of 2.6% to 5.4%. The terms segmental and subsegmental PEs describe PEs that occur in the arterial branches that descend from the respective main pulmonary artery, interlobar artery, and lobar artery. A saddle PE, by contrast, is a thrombus that occurs at the main pulmonary artery bifurcation point.[38] The clot burden of a saddle PE can cause retrograde blood flow into the right heart. The relatively lower pressures of the right atrium and ventricle make them more susceptible to harmful increased filling pressures, contractile weakening, and myocardial stress. Continued regurgitation can lead to right ventricular (RV) failure, which impairs systolic function and can ultimately lead to cardiac arrest.[39] Point-of-care ultrasound (POCUS) allows the degree of cardiac dysfunction to be assessed with a tricuspid annular plane systolic excursion less than 17 mm, 60/60 echo sign (pulmonary acceleration time <60 ms, tricuspid regurgitation jet <60 mm Hg), D sign (straightening of the interventricular septum), or McConnell sign (RV wall motion abnormality with apical sparing).[39,40]

Furthermore, when a complete blockage of blood occurs in a pulmonary artery, the lungs are deprived of oxygen because of impaired gas exchange. This cascade causes a ventilation-perfusion (V/Q ratio) mismatch that can perpetuate hypoxemia, cardiac dysfunction, and tissue hypoperfusion. The long-term sequelae after PE survival include cardiac dysfunction and pulmonary hypertension, which can detrimentally affect physical activity and the overall quality of life.

CRITICAL DECISION

What is the emergency department workup for DVT?

Multiple pathways have been proposed for guiding the diagnosis of DVTs. Some of the most common pathways include a combination of D-dimer laboratory testing and the clinical assessment of pretest probability. Several pretest probability scoring tools exist including the Padua score for DVT risk, the Caprini score for predicting DVT in surgical patients, and both the original and modified Wells criteria for DVT.[41-43]

The original Wells DVT score had nine parameters, excluding the parameter for "previously diagnosed DVT." The modified Wells score employs 10 different parameters ranging from points −2 to +1 (*Table 1*). A score of −2 to 0 corresponds with "low risk/unlikely" and indicates a DVT prevalence of up to 5%; a score of 1 to 2 corresponds with "moderate risk" and indicates a DVT prevalence of up to 17%; and a score of 3 or more corresponds with "high risk/likely" and indicates a prevalence of up to 53%. The Wells criteria recommends obtaining a D-dimer test for patients in the moderate risk category as part of the DVT workup: Data have shown that a negative D-dimer test is sufficient to rule out DVT in over 99% of moderate-risk patients. Furthermore, the Wells criteria also

Wells Score for DVT Criteria Description	Points
Active malignancy (treatment within the last 6 months or palliative)	+1
Bedridden 3+ days or major surgery within 12 weeks	+1
Calf swelling 3+ cm compared to the other leg (measured below tibial tuberosity)	+1
Collateral (nonvaricose) superficial veins present	+1
Entire leg swollen	+1
Localized tenderness along the deep venous system	+1
Pitting edema, confined to the symptomatic leg	+1
Paralysis, paresis, or recent plaster immobilization of the lower extremity	+1
Previously documented DVT	+1
Alternative diagnosis more likely	−2

−2-0 = low risk/unlikely
1-2 = moderate risk
3+ = high risk/likely

TABLE 1. **Modified Wells score for DVT**

recommends obtaining an ultrasound in all patients in the high-risk category to properly rule out DVT.[44]

In patients 50 years or younger who are in the moderate-risk category, a high-sensitivity D-dimer assay level less than 500 ng/mL is sufficient to rule out DVT, whereas a level greater than 500 ng/mL requires ultrasonography to rule out a DVT.[44] D-dimer assays vary in their specificity and predictive values, so physicians must know which one is used at their institution. The three tiers of D-dimer sensitivity assays are moderate, high, and highest. Moderate-sensitivity D-dimer assays are measured by whole blood D-dimer (83% sensitivity) and latex semiquantitative assays (85% sensitivity). High-sensitivity assays include immunoturbidimetric assays (93% sensitivity); D-dimer assays with the highest sensitivity are enzyme-linked immunosorbent assays (96% sensitivity). Modern, high-sensitivity assays have high enough negative predictive values for D-dimer levels to effectively rule out DVT in moderate-risk populations.[45] In patients older than 50 years, an age-adjusted D-dimer level can be calculated (age × 10) to determine the normal upper limit (eg, a D-dimer level in an 89 year old can be considered normal up to 890 ng/mL).[46]

The type of ultrasonography used to rule out lower-extremity DVT varies by institution. The two major ultrasound modality types used in most developed countries are compression and duplex ultrasound. Compression ultrasonography classically uses a 5 to 10 MHz linear array transducer to scan proximal deep veins, including the common femoral, femoral, and popliteal veins. Duplex whole-leg ultrasonography also uses a 5 to 10 MHz linear array probe but relies on a Doppler mode and a B-mode to obtain defined images of the vessel being analyzed.[28] Compression ultrasonography is quicker than duplex because it visualizes only proximal veins, but its accuracy can be limited by habitus and vascular variance. Although duplex ultrasound is relatively more time-consuming, it is more accurate and successful at ruling out DVTs and, therefore, is the preferred method for evaluating for DVTs. If compression ultrasonography does not reveal a DVT but clinical suspicion remains high, patients should have a requisite follow-up ultrasound in 1 week.[47]

When should treatment for DVT be started in the emergency department?

Once a DVT is confirmed on ultrasonography, its location and severity are considered. Most cases of DVT can be managed with anticoagulation, but some may require surgical or thrombolytic intervention. In 2021, the American College of Chest Physicians (CHEST) released updated guidelines and recommendations on the treatment of venous thromboembolism. One of their strong recommendations is that distal lower-extremity DVTs (distal to the popliteal vein) be managed by serial imaging without anticoagulation unless follow-up imaging shows extension in proximal veins or distal progression.[48] They also strongly recommend that a patient with an acute DVT who has a history of antiphospholipid syndrome be treated with adjusted-dose vitamin K antagonists, like warfarin, instead of direct factor Xa inhibitors.

Initiation of anticoagulation depends on the VTE size, location, and accompanying symptoms. In some patients, laboratory workup such as hemoglobin and hematocrit levels, platelet function, a coagulation profile, and both liver and renal function tests may be necessary. These results can aid in risk stratification for bleeding when anticoagulation is deemed necessary. If patients are at a high risk of bleeding (ie, a 1+ on the HAS-BLED score for major bleeding risk) or have severe pain, poor follow-up ability, anemia, thrombocytopenia, or liver or kidney disease, they should be admitted for further workup and be started on anticoagulation during observation (*Table 2*). A study demonstrated that the HAS-BLED score adapted for patients with acute DVT can predict the risk of bleeding when starting anticoagulation.[49]

Several studies have also examined the feasibility of safely discharging patients with acute VTE from the emergency department, when appropriate.[50,51] Physicians should have a low threshold for admitting patients with VTE, especially those with a PE, because of the potential for worsening disease and an increased risk of bleeding. However, low-risk PE patients, as defined by Hestia and pulmonary embolism severity index scores, can safely be discharged. Low-risk patients are otherwise healthy individuals who are younger than 65 years, are not pregnant, are clinically stable, and have a low bleeding risk, normal vital signs, reliable follow-up, no comorbidities, and no active cancer.[51,52]

When anticoagulation is unfeasible, inferior vena cava (IVC) filter placement can be a viable option. In cases of iliac DVTs, approaches such as interventional radiology–guided aspiration or mechanical thrombectomy and catheter-guided thrombolysis have been shown to be safe and effective management methods.[53]

What are the treatments for DVT?

When possible, anticoagulation should be used to manage DVTs and prevent associated sequelae. Anticoagulation is not intended to lyse the thrombus but rather to prevent extension and embolization to the pulmonary arteries. Traditionally, the standard therapy was heparin with a bridge to vitamin K antagonists. However, with the advent of direct oral

HAS-BLED Criteria	Points
Hypertension	+1
Abnormal liver or renal function	+1 or +2
History of stroke	+1
History of GI bleed	+1
Labile INR	+1
Elderly (>65 years old)	+1
Drugs and alcohol	+1 or +2

TABLE 2. HAS-BLED criteria for 1-year bleeding risk stratification for anticoagulation

anticoagulants (DOACs), outpatient treatment regimens have become more varied. DOACs do not require frequent, routine laboratory testing — their effects on commonly used coagulation laboratory tests are negligible compared to medications like warfarin. Furthermore, studies have demonstrated that DOACs, including rivaroxaban and apixaban, are noninferior to the combination of low-molecular-weight heparin (LMWH) and vitamin K antagonists.[54,55] Additionally, DOACs are associated with less recurrence of thromboembolism and major bleeding events. Because the safety of DOACs in pregnant patients has not been reliably investigated thus far, the American College of Obstetricians and Gynecologists recommends treating pregnant patients with heparin when anticoagulation is indicated.[55] CHEST recommends that cancer patients with DVT be managed with LMWH.[48] The American Society of Hematology's 2021 guidelines for VTE treatment in patients with cancer include strong recommendations for LMWH as the initial VTE treatment and conditional recommendations for LMWH or DOACs for initial VTE treatment, DOACs for short-term treatment, and LMWH or DOACs for long-term treatment.[56]

The recommended dosing for initiating DOACs and LMWH in DVT patients in the emergency department is:
- Rivaroxaban: 15 mg PO twice a day for 21 days, followed by 20 mg daily for a minimum of 90 days[43];
- Apixaban: 10 mg PO twice a day for 7 days, followed by 5 mg twice a day for a minimum of 90 days[43]; and
- Enoxaparin: 1 mg/kg SC twice a day or 1.5 mg/kg SC daily while tracking anti-Xa levels. Activated partial thromboplastin time can be used when anti-Xa is unavailable.[37]

Summary

DVT affects over 300,000 Americans annually. As described by the Virchow triad, certain precipitants and risk factors can increase the likelihood of developing DVTs. Prompt diagnosis and management are integral to preventing extension and associated complications that can lead to high mortality and morbidity. Several scoring tools have been developed to augment clinical gestalt and medical decision-making and assist in appropriately risk stratifying patients. With the advancement in duplex ultrasonography, diagnosis has become more accurate. Additionally, multiple treatment options exist for managing patients with DVT. Physicians should consider each clinical scenario and let factors specific to each patient guide their diagnostic and treatment approach.

REFERENCES

1. Galanaud J-P, Laroche J-P, Righini M. The history and historical treatments of deep vein thrombosis. *J Thromb Haemost.* 2013 Mar;11(3):402-411.

2. Data and statistics on venous thromboembolism. CDC. Last reviewed June 28, 2023. https://www.cdc.gov/ncbddd/dvt/data.html

3. Raskob GE, Silverstein R, Bratzler DW, Heit JA, White RH. Surveillance for deep vein thrombosis and pulmonary embolism: recommendations from a national workshop. *Am J Prev Med.* 2010 Apr;38(suppl 4):S502-S509.

4. Khan F, Tritschler T, Kahn SR, Rodger MA. Venous Thromboembolism. *Seminar.* 2021 Jul 3;398(10294):64-77.

5. Kumar DR, Hanlin E, Glurich I, Mazza JJ, Yale SH. Virchow's contribution to the understanding of thrombosis and cellular biology. *Clin Med Res.* 2010 Dec;8(3-4):168-172.

6. Casella IB, Bosch MA, Sabbag CRD. Incidence and risk factors for bilateral deep venous thrombosis of the lower limbs. *Angiology.* 2009 Feb-Mar;60(1):99-103.

7. Kaboli P, Henderson MC, White RH. DVT prophylaxis and anticoagulation in the surgical patient. *Med Clin North Am.* 2003 Jan;87(1):77-110, viii.

8. Kelman CW, Kortt MA, Becker NG, et al. Deep vein thrombosis and air travel: record linkage study. *BMJ.* 2003 Nov 8;327(7423):1072.

9. Anand SS. Smoking: a dual pathogen for arterial and venous thrombosis. *Circulation.* 2017 Jan 3;135(1):17-20.

10. Bonnar J. Coagulation effects of oral contraception. *Am J Obstet Gynecol.* 1987 Oct;157(4 pt 2):1042-1048.

11. Chung, WS. Systemic lupus erythematosus increases the risks of deep vein thrombosis and pulmonary embolism: a nationwide cohort study. *J of Thromb and Haemost.* 2014 Apr;12(4):452-458.

12. Saber AA, Aboolian A, LaRaja RD, Baron H, Hanna K. HIV/AIDS and the risk of deep vein thrombosis: a study of 45 patients with lower extremity involvement. *Am Surg.* 2001 Jul;67(7):645-647.

13. May R, Thurner J. The cause of the predominantly sinistral occurrence of thrombosis of the pelvic veins. *Angiology.* 1957 Oct;8(5):419-427.

14. Harbin MM, Lutsey PL. May-Thurner syndrome: history of understanding and need for defining population prevalence. *J Thromb Haemost.* 2020 Mar;18(3):534-542.

15. Arsov T, Miladinova D, Spiroski M. Factor V Leiden is associated with higher risk of deep venous thrombosis of large blood vessels. *Croat Med J.* 2006 Jun;47(3):433-439.

16. Pomp ER, Rosendaal FR, Doggen CJ. Smoking increases the risk of venous thrombosis and acts synergistically with oral contraceptive use. *Am J Hematol.* 2008 Feb;83(2):97-102.

17. Pabinger I, Schneider B. Thrombotic risk in hereditary antithrombin III, protein C, or protein S deficiency. *Atherosclerosis, Thrombosis, and Vascular Biology.* 1996;16(6):742-748.

18. Morena-Barrio B, Orlando C, Morena-Barrio M, Vicente V, Jochmans K, Corral J. Incidence and features of thrombosis in children with inherited antithrombin deficiency. *Hematologica.* 2019 Dec;104(12):2512-2518.

19. White K, Hunt B. Inherited antithrombin deficiency in pregnancy. *Thrombosis Update.* 2022 Mar;6(100094).

20. Găman AM, Găman GD. Deficiency of antithrombin III (AT III) - case report and review of the literature. *Curr Health Sci J.* 2014 Apr-Jun;40(2):141-143.

21. Padda IS, Patel P, Sridhar DC. Protein C and S. *StatPearls [Internet].* StatPearls Publishing. Updated April 23, 2023. https://www.ncbi.nlm.nih.gov/books/NBK557814/

22. Bibas M, Biava G, Antinori A. HIV-associated venous thromboembolism. *Mediterr J Hematol Infect Dis.* 2011;3(1):e2011030.

23. Dall'Era M, Wofsy D. Clinical features and treatment of systemic lupus erythematosus. In: Firestein GS, Kelley WN, eds. *Textbook of Rheumatology.* 11th ed. Elsevier; 2009:1413-1437.

24. Cervera R, Khamashta MA, Font J, et al; European Working Party on Systemic Lupus Erythematosus. Morbidity and mortality in systemic lupus erythematosus during a 10-year period: a comparison of early and late manifestations in a cohort of 1,000 patients. *Medicine (Baltimore).* 2003 Sep;82(5):299-308.

25. Love PE, Santoro SA. Antiphospholipid antibodies: anticardiolipin and the lupus anticoagulant in systemic lupus erythematosus (SLE) and in non-SLE disorders. Prevalence and clinical significance. *Ann Intern Med.* 1990 May 1;112(9):682-698.

26. Ahuja NA, Bhinder J, Nguyen J, et al. Venous thromboembolism in patients with COVID-19 infection: risk factors, prevention, and management. *Semin Vasc Surg.* 2021 Sep;34(3):101-116.

27. Fat embolism syndrome. Cleveland Clinic. Reviewed July 31, 2022. https://my.clevelandclinic.org/health/diseases/23995-fat-embolism-syndrome

28. Lensing AW, Doris CI, McGrath FP, et al. A comparison of compression ultrasound with color Doppler ultrasound for the diagnosis of symptomless postoperative deep vein thrombosis. *Arch Intern Med.* 1997 Apr 14;157(7):765-768.

29. Levi M, Hart W, Büller HR. Physical examination — the significance of Homan's sign. *Ned Tijdschr Geneeskd.* 1999 Sep 11;143(37):1861-1863.

30. Homans J. Thrombophlebitis of the lower extremities. *Ann Surgery.* 1928 May;87(5):641-651.

31. Baker, WF Jr. Diagnosis of deep venous thrombosis and pulmonary embolism. *Med Clin North Am.* 1998 May 1;82(3):459-476.

32. Kou CJ, Batzlaff C, Bezzant ML, Sjulin T. Phlegmasia cerulea dolens: a life-threatening manifestation of deep vein thrombosis. *Cureus.* 2020 Jun 12;12(6):e8587.

33. Søgaard KK, Schmidt M, Pedersen L, Horváth-Puhó E, Sørensen HT. 30-year mortality after venous thromboembolism: a population-based cohort study. *Circulation.* 2014 Sep 2;130(10):829-836.

34. Naess IA, Christiansen SC, Romundstad P, Cannegieter SC, Rosendaal FR, Hammerstrøm J. Incidence and mortality of venous thrombosis: a population-based study. *J Thromb Haemost.* 2007 Apr;5(4):692-699.

35. Kahn SR. The post-thrombotic syndrome. *Hematology Am Soc Hematol Educ Program.* 2016 Dec 2;2016(1):413-418.

36. Visonà A, Quere I, Mazzolai L, et al; European Society of Vascular Medicine. Post-thrombotic syndrome. *Vasa.* 2021 Sep;50(5):331-340.

37. Chinsakchai K, Ten Duis K, Moll FL, de Borst GJ. Trends in management of phlegmasia cerulea dolens. *Vasc Endovascular Surg.* 2011 Jan;45(1):5-14.

38. Alkinj B, Pannu BS, Apala DR, Kotecha A, Kashyap R, Iyer VN. Saddle vs nonsaddle pulmonary embolism: clinical presentation, hemodynamics, management, and outcomes. *Mayo Clin Proc.* 2017 Oct; 92(10):1511-1518.

39. Shah BR, Velamakanni SM, Patel A, Khadkikar G, Patel TM, Shah SC. Analysis of the 60/60 sign and other right ventricular parameters by 2D transthoracic echocardiography as adjuncts to diagnosis of acute pulmonary embolism. *Cureus.* 2021 Mar 10;13(3):e13800.

40. Cativo Calderon EH, Mene-Afejuku TO, Valvani R, et al. D-shaped left ventricle, anatomic, and physiologic implications. *Case Rep Cardiol.* 2017;2017:4309165.

41. Barbar S, Noventa F, Rossetto V, et al. A risk assessment model for the identification of hospitalized medical patients at risk for venous thromboembolism: the Padua Prediction Score. *J Thromb Haemost.* 2010 Nov;8(11):2450-2457.

✖ Pitfalls

- Overlooking the fact that DVTs can coexist with other pathologies, including cellulitis, venous stasis ulcers, and necrotizing fasciitis. A delayed DVT diagnosis can cause PE to occur.

- Failing to recognize phlegmasia cerulea dolens and phlegmasia alba dolens. These conditions can be catastrophic — they have high mortality rates and may require immediate catheter-based thrombolysis or surgical decompression.

- Forgetting that post-thrombotic syndrome can cause significant morbidity in patients by impairing function and leading to chronic illness.

CASE ONE

The emergency physician suspected this patient had a DVT based on her lower-extremity pain and swelling and multiple risk factors. The physical examination revealed a tender left calf with erythema that encompassed the posterior popliteal fossa down to the Achilles tendon. No crepitus, fluctuation, or induration were noted. The patient did not exhibit hyperesthesia and had intact proximal and distal pulses throughout the extremity. No signs of bony deformities, trauma, or joint swelling were present. Range of motion throughout the lower extremities and capillary refill were normal. A duplex ultrasound was ordered and confirmed the diagnosis of a DVT in the popliteal vein. The patient had no other complaints outside of extremity pain and swelling, was hemodynamically stable, and had no comorbidities. Her laboratory results returned normal. After shared decision-making and appropriate bleeding risk stratification, she was started on apixaban and was discharged with outpatient follow-up at a hematology clinic for medication management and a hypercoagulable workup.

CASE TWO

The patient's complaint of severe pain near the site where he injects drugs was concerning for infection, inflammatory reaction to a foreign body, and a DVT. Given this differential, the emergency physician obtained x-rays of the upper humerus and forearm, which were negative for bone and joint abnormalities and radiopaque foreign bodies. A duplex ultrasound revealed a nonocclusive superficial venous thrombosis in the medial cubital vein and an occlusive DVT in the brachial vein. Laboratory tests did not show any abnormalities in his CBC, liver and renal function, or coagulation profile. Given the patient's severe pain and likelihood for poor follow-up, he was admitted to the hospital and started on anticoagulation. After pain control and initiation of anticoagulation, his symptoms improved, and he was discharged to a rehabilitation facility with a 3-month course of rivaroxaban and an outpatient follow-up appointment.

CASE THREE

The patient's physical examination revealed ipsilateral erythema from the proximal thigh to the mid calf. A palpable 4-inch cord-like structure without fluctuation or erythema was present in the groin. POCUS was performed and revealed cobblestoning without a fluid collection. An official duplex ultrasound demonstrated superficial phlebitis with extension into the iliofemoral deep venous system. Given the extent of the venous thrombus, a CT angiography of the chest and a CT of the abdomen and pelvis with intravenous contrast were performed; they revealed no evidence of a PE, but a nonocclusive thrombus was visualized in the IVC. The patient was started on a heparin drip and eventually underwent an interventional radiology–guided thrombectomy with successful debulking. Her hormonal contraceptives were stopped, and her gynecologist switched her to a copper intrauterine device. She refused an IVC filter, was discharged on enoxaparin, and was scheduled for follow-up.

42. Caprini JA, Arcelus JI, Hasty JH, Tamhane AC, Fabrega F. Clinical assessment of venous thromboembolic risk in surgical patients. *Semin Thromb Hemost.* 1991;17(suppl 3):304-312.

43. Engelberger RP, Aujesky D, Calanca L, Staeger P, Hugli O, Mazzolai L. Comparison of the diagnostic performance of the original and modified Wells score in inpatients and outpatients with suspected deep vein thrombosis. *Thromb Res.* 2011 Jun;127(6):535-539.

44. Wells PS, Owen C, Doucette S, Fergusson D, Tran H. Does this patient have deep vein thrombosis? *JAMA.* 2006;295(2):199-207.

45. Bates SM, Jaeschke R, Stevens S, et al. Diagnosis of DVT: antithrombotic therapy and prevention of thrombosis, 9th ed: American College of Chest Physicians Evidence-Based Clinical Practice Guidelines. *Chest.* 2012 Feb;141(suppl 2):e351S-e418S.

46. Righini M, Van Es J, Den Exter PL, et al. Age-adjusted D-dimer cutoff levels to rule out pulmonary embolism: the ADJUST-PE study. *JAMA.* 2014 Mar 19;311(11):1117-1124.

47. Cogo A, Lensing AW, Koopman MM, et al. Compression ultrasonography for diagnostic management of patients with clinically suspected deep vein thrombosis: prospective cohort study. *BMJ.* 1998 Jan 3;316(7124):17-20.

48. Stevens SM, Woller SC, Kreuziger LB, et al. Antithrombotic therapy for VTE disease: second update of the CHEST guideline and expert panel report. *Chest.* 2021 Dec;160(6):e545-e608.

49. Brown JD, Goodin AJ, Lip GYH, Adams VR. Risk stratification for bleeding complications in patients with venous thromboembolism: application of the HAS-BLED bleeding score during the first 6 months of anticoagulant treatment. *J Am Heart Assoc.* 2018 Mar 7;7(6):e007901.

50. Frank Peacock W, Coleman CI, Diercks DB, et al. Emergency department discharge of pulmonary embolus patients. *Acad Emerg Med.* 2018 Sep;25(9):995-1003.

51. Kabrhel C, Vinson DR, Mitchell AM, et al. A clinical decision framework to guide the outpatient treatment of emergency department patients diagnosed with acute pulmonary embolism or deep vein thrombosis: results from a multidisciplinary consensus panel. *J Am Coll Emerg Physicians Open.* 2021 Dec 15;2(6):e12588.

52. Elias A, Mallett S, Daoud-Elias M, Poggi JN, Clarke M. Prognostic models in acute pulmonary embolism: a systematic review and meta-analysis. *BMJ Open.* 2016 Apr 29;6(4):e010324.

53. Mühlberger D, Wenkel M, Papapostolou G, et al. Surgical thrombectomy for iliofemoral deep vein thrombosis: patient outcomes at 8.5 years. *PLoS One.* 2020 Jun 18;15(6):e0235003.

54. Cohen AT, Bauersachs R. Rivaroxaban and the EINSTEIN clinical trial programme. *Blood Coagul Fibrinolysis.* 2019 Apr;30(3):85-95.

55. American College of Obstetricians and Gynecologists' Committee on Practice Bulletins — Obstetrics. ACOG practice bulletin no. 196: thromboembolism in pregnancy. *Obstet Gynecol.* 2018 Jul;132(1):e1-e17.

56. Lyman GH, Carrier M, Ay C, et al. American Society of Hematology 2021 guidelines for management of venous thromboembolism: prevention and treatment in patients with cancer. *Blood Adv.* 2021 Feb 23;5(4):927-974.

57. Enoxaparin: US Food and Drug Administration — approved indications, dosages, and treatment durations. Centers for Medicare and Medicaid Services. https://www.cms.gov/Medicare-Medicaid-Coordination/Fraud-Prevention/Medicaid-Integrity-Education/Pharmacy-Education-Materials/Downloads/enox-dosingchart11-14.pdf

MD CALC

https://www.mdcalc.com/calc/362/wells-criteria-dvt
https://www.mdcalc.com/calc/807/has-bled-score-major-bleeding-risk

An Adolescent With New-Onset Seizure

By Abigail Marcom, MD; and
Zachary Burroughs, MD
Prisma Health-Upstate Children's Emergency
Center, Greenville, South Carolina

Reviewed by Sharon E. Mace, MD, FACEP

Objective

On completion of this article, you should be able to:
- Discuss the diagnosis and treatment of subdural empyema.

CASE PRESENTATION

A 14-year-old boy with autism spectrum disorder and selective mutism presents with altered mental status and a first-time seizure. The patient has a recent history of an uncomplicated COVID-19 infection. Four days ago, he developed redness in his right eye that worsened over the next 24 hours; however, no pain with extraocular movements or vision changes occurred. Two days ago, a persistent fever also developed. The only other associated symptom was a decreased appetite. His parents contacted EMS on day 4 of his symptoms after they found him lethargic and minimally responsive — EMS rated him a score of 5 on the Glasgow Coma Scale (GCS). EMS gave the patient supplemental oxygen via a nonrebreather mask and 5 mg of IV midazolam for an en-route seizure event with eye rolling and limb jerking.

On arrival, the patient's vital signs include P 146, R 34, and T 38.8°C (101.9°F); SpO_2 is 99% on 6 L nasal cannula. His neurologic examination reveals a GCS score of 10 (ie, eyes open to verbal commands and localized pain) and 2-mm pupils bilaterally that are round and reactive. Examination of his face shows mild swelling and redness to the right upper and lower eyelids, without proptosis or purulence; he has no gaze deviation. He has clear and equal breath sounds bilaterally; tachycardia without any murmurs, rubs, or gallops; and warm and well-perfused extremities with a capillary refill time of 2 to 3 seconds.

Discussion

Seizures and other serious complications can occur after the rather common condition of sinusitis. The 2013 American Academy of Pediatrics (AAP) guidelines recommend this diagnosis in children with an acute upper respiratory tract infection who present with persistent illness (ie, nasal discharge of any quality, daytime cough, or both, lasting >10 days without improvement), a worsening course (ie, worsening or new onset of nasal discharge, daytime cough, or fever after initial improvement), or severe onset (ie, concurrent fever [temperature ≥39°C (102.2°F)] and purulent nasal discharge for at least 3 consecutive days).[1]

Sinusitis symptoms are often similar to those of other common illnesses such as allergic rhinitis or a viral upper respiratory infection.[2] Physical examination findings are unhelpful in distinguishing between sinusitis and uncomplicated upper respiratory infections because they are nonspecific: erythema and swelling of the nasal turbinates and pain with percussion of the sinuses.[3] The presentation of symptoms often varies between patients of different ages. Younger children typically present with a cough and mucopurulent nasal secretions, while older children present with nasal congestion, facial pressure, and headaches.[2] Antibiotic treatment is the mainstay of therapy and is often initiated after 10 or more days of unimproved illness or worsening illness after an initial improvement (ie, second sickening).

In neurodivergent patients who have difficulty describing their symptoms, diagnosing sinusitis becomes more challenging. Complications of sinusitis are divided into three categories — orbital, osseous, and intracranial — and can be serious. Orbital complications are the most common

(60%-75% of patients) and range from preseptal cellulitis to cavernous sinus thrombosis.[2] Osseous complications include conditions such as osteomyelitis of the frontal or maxillary bones (ie, Pott puffy tumor).[2,4] Intracranial complications include meningitis, intracranial abscess, subdural empyema, and epidural abscess. Subdural empyema is the most common intracranial complication of sinusitis.[4,5] Patients who develop intracranial complications from sinusitis have a high incidence of morbidity and mortality — from 3.7% to 11% in general and 25% to 35% from subdural empyema when considered alone. Although antibiotics have reduced the incidence of subdural empyema, they do not absolutely prevent it from developing.[6]

Patients with subdural empyema classically present with frontal sinusitis, a rapidly progressive headache, and persistent fevers. The 2013 AAP guidelines list the following as indications for CT in patients with suspected complications from sinusitis: suspicion of orbital complications (eg, a swollen eye, especially when accompanied by proptosis or impaired extraocular muscles) or intracranial complications (eg, a very severe headache, photophobia, seizures, or other focal neurologic findings).[3,7] The condition of the patient in the case presentation warranted immediate stabilization and CT imaging because of his recent upper respiratory infection and current signs of orbital cellulitis, a persistent fever, an altered mental status, and seizure activity. Before neurologic symptoms arise, the presentation of subdural empyema is a constellation of subtle symptoms; however, physicians should keep this diagnosis on the differential when evaluating any child with suspected sinusitis.

Subdural empyema is a collection of purulence in the potential space between the dura mater and the arachnoid

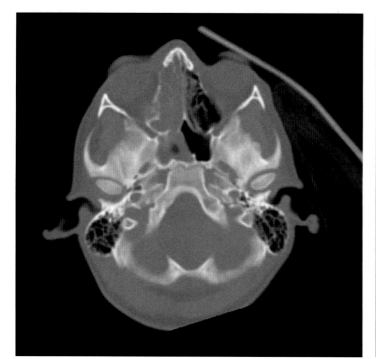

FIGURE 1. CT showing a right-sided paranasal sinus opacification. *Credit:* Abigail Marcom, MD; and Zachary Burroughs, MD.

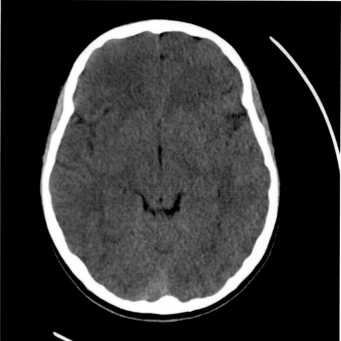

FIGURE 2. CT brain showing edema with loss of gray-white differentiation in the right frontal lobe. *Credit:* Abigail Marcom, MD; and Zachary Burroughs, MD.

membrane.[6] The most common antecedent of this condition is bacterial sinusitis. The pediatric population is at greater risk of developing complications from bacterial sinusitis because of the increased vascularity in their sinuses. Subdural empyema most often develops in teenage boys and young men.[4] Although the reason remains unclear, boys are thought to be more likely to develop subdural empyema because of an anatomical predisposition.[6] Sinusitis in the frontal sinus is most likely to cause intracranial complications, followed by sinusitis in the ethmoid, sphenoid, and maxillary sinuses.[7] Organisms spread into the subdural space through direct extension due to the close proximity of these sinuses to the potential space. Specific mechanisms of spread include hematogenous spread and direct inward spread through haversian canals in bone. Bacteria can more easily migrate if patients had a previous head trauma or previous neurosurgery.[4] The most common organisms isolated in subdural empyema are polymicrobial: anaerobes, aerobic streptococci, staphylococci, *Haemophilus influenzae*, *Streptococcus pneumoniae*, and other gram-negative bacteria. Although *Staphylococcus epidermidis* is considered normal skin flora, it has been implicated in some cases of subdural empyema.

Of all intracranial complications of sinusitis, subdural empyema is associated with more neurologic sequelae. Patients with subdural empyema are more likely to present with neurologic deficits and an altered mental status. In a study of children with this condition, Patel et al found that they have longer hospital stays and multiple neurosurgical procedures. These children are also more likely to have long-term morbidity such as cognitive problems, hemiparesis, and expressive dysphasia more than 6 months after initial illness. A worse outcome is associated with subdural empyema because infections spread more rapidly within the subdural space compared to the epidural and intracranial spaces.[7] Sing et al reported a 37% incidence of extracranial complications such as preseptal and orbital cellulitis in patients who had a subdural empyema.[4] Prompt recognition of symptoms, rapid imaging, and prompt treatment are essential to preventing long-term, devastating consequences and to improving clinical outcomes in these patients.

As an early screening tool, laboratory studies should be obtained, including a WBC count, erythrocyte sedimentation rate, and C-reactive protein levels.[4] Signs and symptoms of subdural empyema share characteristics with several other diagnoses like bacterial meningitis, brain abscesses, epidural abscesses, and cerebral thrombophlebitis; they are differentiated from one another by laboratory studies *and* imaging. Imaging should precede a lumbar puncture if there are focal neurologic deficits or suspected increased intracranial pressure. Lumbar puncture is not indicated for subdural empyema but can be useful if meningitis is also suspected. The CSF in patients with subdural empyema may indicate a bacterial infection through an elevated WBC count, increased protein level, and decreased glucose level. Sometimes, however, their CSF is normal, without any signs of bacterial growth.[4]

Imaging is recommended in every patient with a suspected subdural empyema. MRI with contrast is the gold standard and is more sensitive than CT for identifying subdural collections of purulence.[4,5] If MRI is unavailable, CT is the next choice. An identified subdural empyema is considered a neurosurgical emergency and warrants immediate intravenous antibiotics and a multiteam approach of urgent consultations with pediatric neurosurgery, infectious disease, and otolaryngology.[4] No specific antibiotic guidelines exist, but most studies suggest starting empiric therapy with a third-generation cephalosporin, metronidazole, and vancomycin. Corticosteroids are often added to the regimen to decrease intracranial swelling, but their addition is controversial because they could dampen the host's immune response and affect antibiotic penetration; improved outcomes through the use of steroids have yet to be shown.[7]

Despite adequate intravenous antibiotics, some infections still require surgical intervention. Surgical drainage is thought to be the most important factor for improving outcomes.[6] The most common surgical interventions for subdural empyema are craniectomy and burr hole surgery. Some studies indicate that surgical intervention within the first 72 hours is of the utmost importance to decrease the rate of any associated disabilities. A nonsurgical approach with intravenous antibiotics is appropriate only in patients who do not have a significant midline shift on imaging, who have a subdural abscess less than 1 cm, or who are clinically stable.[5] Endoscopic sinus surgery is typically indicated in cases of direct extension through a bony defect located near the abscess. Some reports indicate that the sinus infection can be cleared adequately with intravenous antibiotics alone and that neurosurgical intervention is necessary only to drain the subdural empyema. Other studies refute this idea and state that skipping early sinus drainage is associated with repeat craniectomies. Ideally, otolaryngology management with simultaneous neurosurgical invention leads to the best outcomes, but this specialty combination is not always possible and should not delay neurosurgical intervention.[7]

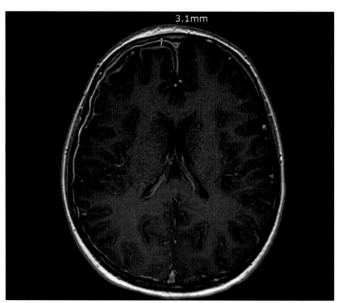

FIGURE 3. MRI of the brain with contrast showing a 3-mm fluid collection in the subdural space, consistent with a subdural empyema. *Credit:* Abigail Marcom, MD; and Zachary Burroughs, MD.

CASE RESOLUTION

A head CT without contrast was completed after the patient's seizure activity subsided; it revealed edema with loss of gray-white differentiation in the right frontal lobe and a right paranasal sinus opacification (*Figures 1* and *2*). A subsequent MRI with contrast showed leptomeningeal enhancement over the right cerebral hemisphere and right-sided pansinusitis with complete opacification. A 3-mm fluid collection was seen in the subdural space, consistent with a subdural empyema, but no midline shift was visualized (*Figure 3*). A lumbar puncture was performed because of the evidence of meningitis on imaging. The patient's CSF revealed leukocytosis (131 cells/μL or 0.131 x 10^9/L) but normal protein and glucose levels; a culture of the fluid was negative.

The patient's case was discussed with a pediatric neurosurgical team; the team did not pursue initial intracranial intervention because there was no midline shift and only a small subdural empyema collection (<3 mm) on MRI. The patient was started on intravenous ceftriaxone, metronidazole, and vancomycin. He was urgently seen by otolaryngology and taken to the operating room for a sinus endoscopy with an ethmoidectomy and maxillary antrostomy. The culture obtained from the sinus washout grew microaerophilic *Streptococcus* and methicillin-sensitive *Staphylococcus aureus*.

The patient remained hospitalized for 6 days on intravenous antibiotics, dexamethasone, and levetiracetam. He was then discharged home with a peripherally inserted central catheter line to complete a course of intravenous ceftriaxone and metronidazole. He was also discharged on oral levetiracetam and sinus nasal rinses, with close follow-up with all involved subspecialties (ie, neurosurgery, otolaryngology, neurology, and infectious disease).

The patient presented again 4 days later for breakthrough seizures and a return of fever. A repeat MRI showed a larger right subdural empyema of up to 13 mm with a leftward midline shift of 2 mm. Pediatric neurosurgery performed a burr hole surgery for evacuation of the empyema, and otolaryngology performed an additional sinus washout. Repeat cultures obtained at that time were sterile.

The patient was then discharged 4 days post operation with intravenous antibiotics (ceftriaxone) and seizure prophylaxis (levetiracetam). Four months after the subdural empyema evacuation, the patient was reported to be doing well and at his neurologic baseline. He continued on seizure prophylaxis. Repeat imaging from neurosurgery suggested typical postoperative changes without residual or recurrent subdural fluid collection.

REFERENCES

1. Wald ER, Applegate KE, Bordley C, et al; American Academy of Pediatrics. Clinical practice guideline for the diagnosis and management of acute bacterial sinusitis in children aged 1 to 18 years. *Pediatrics*. 2013 Jul;132(1):e262-e280.
2. Ramadan HH. Chronic rhinosinusitis in children. *Int J Pediatr*. 2012;2012:573942.
3. Chow AW, Benninger MS, Brook I, et al; Infectious Diseases Society of America. IDSA clinical practice guideline for acute bacterial rhinosinusitis in children and adults. *Clin Infect Dis*. 2012 Apr;54(8):e72-e112.
4. Arifianto MR, Ma'ruf AZ, Ibrahim A, Bajamal AH. Interhemispheric and infratentorial subdural empyema with preseptal cellulitis as complications of sinusitis: a case report. *Pediatr Neurosurg*. 2018;53(2):128-133.
5. Ziegler A, Patadia M, Stankiewicz J. Neurological complications of acute and chronic sinusitis. *Curr Neurol Neurosci Rep*. 2018 Feb 5;18(2):5.
6. Calik M, Iscan A, Abuhandan M, Yetkin I, Bozkuş F, Torun MF. Masked subdural empyema secondary to frontal sinusitis. *Am J Emerg Med*. 2012 Oct;30(8):1657.e1-1657.e4.
7. Meshref M, Nourelden AZ, Elshanbary AA, et al. Subdural empyema due to mixed infections successfully treated medically: a case report with review literature. *Clin Case Rep*. 2022 Jul 14;10(7):e6049.

The Critical Procedure
Emergency Needle Decompression

By Steven J. Warrington, MD, MEd, MS; and
Courtney Johnson

MercyOne Siouxland in Sioux City and Buena
Vista University in Storm Lake, Iowa

Objective

On completion of this article, you should be able to:

- Explain the process of performing a needle decompression on patients with a suspected tension pneumothorax.

Introduction

Patients with blunt or penetrating trauma can develop a tension pneumothorax that causes them to become unstable. A needle decompression may be necessary in these situations, especially if no other procedure can be immediately performed, and patients will usually need further definitive care following the needle decompression.

Contraindications

- No complete contraindications

Benefits and Risks

An emergency needle decompression is a rapid method of evacuating a tension pneumothorax. Additionally, it provides a technique to stabilize a patient when the physician regards an emergent tube thoracostomy as inappropriate.

Failure is possible when performing a needle decompression, most commonly due to chest wall thickness. Risks include bleeding, infection, injury to the lung or nearby structures (eg, neurovascular bundle), and compromise to other structures (eg, spleen, liver, and diaphragm) due to incorrect needle placement. Additionally, if the patient who undergoes needle decompression does not actually have a pneumothorax, there is a risk of causing a pneumothorax or hemothorax.

Alternatives

The primary alternative procedure is a tube thoracostomy. If the patient will need an emergent thoracotomy, it may make sense to skip the needle decompression and go straight to the thoracostomy, depending on equipment availability, the patient's clinical status, and the staff's skill level.

Alternative locations for where to perform the needle decompression also exist. The technique presented suggests placing the needle at the ipsilateral midclavicular line of the second intercostal space (ie, above the third rib). An alternative approach is to use the ipsilateral anterior axillary line at the fourth or fifth intercostal space.

Reducing Side Effects and Risk

Choosing the second intercostal space as the point of injection increases the success rate because the chest wall is less thick and the diaphragm and other organs are less likely to be damaged. Keeping the needle at the midclavicular line reduces the risk of injuring the internal mammary artery, which runs parallel and close to the sternum.

A needle or angiocath longer than 5 cm is recommended because that length exceeds the average chest wall thickness at the second intercostal space. It is possible to attach a syringe to the needle and aspirate during advancement to be certain when the space is reached, thus reducing the risk of not advancing the needle far enough, which would ruin the procedure. Advancing the angiocath and removing the needle after entering the space reduces the risk of pleural injury. Advancing the needle over the superior aspect of the rib avoids injuring neurovascular structures.

Special Considerations

The patient's size is the biggest consideration in a needle decompression. In small children, the literature recommends using the fourth intercostal space anterior axillary line as the primary injection site due to chest wall thickness and the location of the heart and thymus. An adult patient's size will also determine whether a longer or shorter needle should be used. Chest wall thickness varies more in women and overweight individuals. Although the most common location to perform needle decompression is in the second intercostal space midclavicular line, when that fails, the literature suggests that a needle decompression at the fifth intercostal space anterior axillary line may render effective results.

— TECHNIQUE (SECOND INTERCOSTAL APPROACH) —

1. **Obtain** consent from the patient as situationally appropriate. Verbal consent is suitable when the patient is unstable or there is no time for a traditional signed consent.
2. **Assemble** the necessary equipment of needle, syringe, and cleanser. An 8-cm 14- or 16-gauge needle is commonly used.
3. **Identify** the site by palpating the sternomanubrial joint, which represents the second rib, and go to the midclavicular line. The site of needle introduction is the space under the second rib and above the third rib (ie, the second intercostal space).
4. **Prepare** the site for a sterile procedure.
5. **Insert** the needle at a 90° angle with the syringe attached.
6. **Advance** the needle until air is aspirated.
7. **Detach** the syringe and advance the angiocath; then remove the needle. Attach a three-way stopcock, if available, with suction or a syringe to allow for aspiration of the pleural space and airflow stoppage.
8. **Provide,** or arrange for, definitive care.

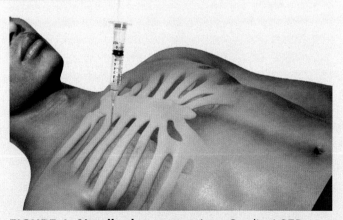

FIGURE 1. Needle decompression. *Credit:* ACEP.

Sinus Rhythm With PVCs, a Run of NSVT, and LA-LL Lead Reversal

By Jeremy Berberian, MD; William J. Brady, MD, FACEP; and Amal Mattu, MD, FACEP

Dr. Berberian is the associate director of emergency medicine residency education at ChristianaCare and assistant professor of emergency medicine at Sidney Kimmel Medical College, Thomas Jefferson University in Philadelphia, Pennsylvania. Dr. Brady is a professor of emergency medicine, medicine, and nursing, and vice chair for faculty affairs in the Department of Emergency Medicine at the University of Virginia School of Medicine in Charlottesville. Dr. Mattu is a professor, vice chair, and codirector of the Emergency Cardiology Fellowship in the Department of Emergency Medicine at the University of Maryland School of Medicine in Baltimore.

Objectives

On completion of this article, you should be able to:

■ Describe the ECG findings seen with VT.

■ Define the ECG criteria for premature ventricular contractions.

■ Describe the ECG findings seen with LA-LL lead reversal.

CASE PRESENTATION

A 76-year-old man presents with intermittent palpitations (*Figure 1*).

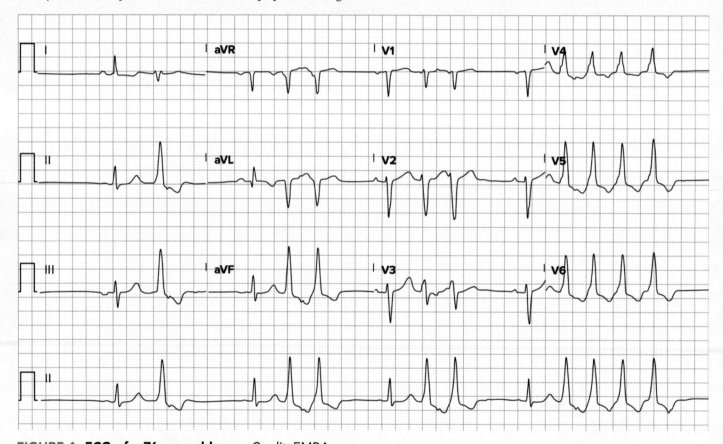

FIGURE 1. ECG of a 76-year-old man. *Credit:* EMRA.

ECG Findings

His ECG shows a sinus bradycardia with an irregular pattern of premature ventricular contractions (PVCs) followed by a run of ventricular tachycardia (VT), normal axis, and left arm-left leg (LA-LL) lead reversal.

Using the lead II rhythm strip, the rhythm in this ECG is as follows (*Figure 2*):

- Sinus beat
- PVC with retrograde P wave
- Sinus beat

- Unifocal PVC couplet (ie, two PVCs in a row with the same morphology)
- Sinus beat
- Unifocal PVC couplet (ie, two PVCs in a row with the same morphology)
- Sinus beat
- Four-beat run of VT

The retrograde P waves are best visualized in leads V_1 through V_3, where they clearly point in the opposite direction of the sinus P waves, which is expected with retrograde P waves.

This patient had an unremarkable workup and was admitted to the cardiology service for telemetry and evaluation for automatic implantable cardioverter defibrillator (AICD) placement.

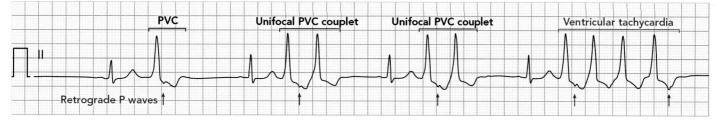

FIGURE 2. The lead II rhythm strip shows frequent PVCs, a run of VT, and retrograde P waves. *Credit:* EMRA.

Notably, the four-beat run of VT at the end of the ECG cannot be further differentiated into sustained or nonsustained without knowing whether there was any hemodynamic instability at that time (this patient remained hemodynamically stable, so this was nonsustained VT [NSVT]). Short runs of VT (ie, three to five PVCs) are often referred to as "bursts" or "salvos" of VT.

His ECG also shows LA-LL lead reversal. A notable finding in this ECG that should prompt concern for LA-LL lead reversal is the prominent P wave in lead I compared to lead II (*Figure 3*). In general, the P wave should be more prominent in lead II than in lead I in normal sinus rhythm with correct lead placement.

ECG findings seen with LA-LL lead reversal include (*Table 1*):
- In comparison to normal P-QRS-T complexes (ie, normal sinus rhythm with normal lead placement), leads I and II "switch places," meaning that the normal findings in lead I are noted in lead II and vice versa.
- In comparison to normal P-QRS-T complexes (ie, normal sinus rhythm with normal lead placement), leads aVL and aVF switch places, so the normal findings in lead aVL are noted in lead aVF and vice versa.
- Lead III is inverted, meaning that the P-QRS-T complexes are all oriented in the opposite direction from the normal P-QRS-T complexes (ie, normal sinus rhythm with normal lead placement).
- Lead aVR is unchanged.

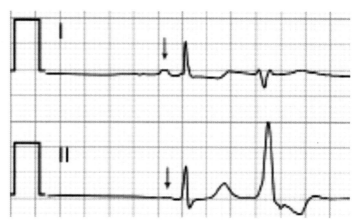

FIGURE 3. A more prominent P wave in lead I than in lead II in the setting of a normal sinus rhythm suggests LA-LL lead reversal. *Credit:* EMRA.

ACKNOWLEDGMENT

This case is reprinted from *Emergency ECGs: Case-Based Review and Interpretations,* available at www.emra.org/amazon or by scanning the QR code.

	I	II	III	aVR	aVL	aVF	V₁-V₆
LA-RA	Inverted	Switches with III	Switches with II	Switches with aVL	Switches with aVR	No change	No change
LA-LL	Switches with II	Switches with I	Inverted	No change	Switches with aVF	Switches with aVL	No change
LA-RL	Looks like II	Unchanged	Flatline	Looks like inverted II	Looks identical to aVF	Looks identical to aVL	No change
RA-LL	Switches with inverted III	Inverted	Switches with inverted I	Switches with aVF	No change	Switches with aVR	No change
RA-RL	Looks like inverted III	Flatline	Unchanged	Looks identical to aVF	Looks like inverted III	Looks identical to aVR	No change
LA-LL + RA-RL	Flatline	Looks like inverted III	Inverted	Looks identical to aVL	Looks identical to aVR	Looks like inverted III	No change
Dextrocardia	Inverted	Switches with III	Switches with II	Switches with aVL	Switches with aVR	No change	Dominant S-wave and poor R-wave progression

Note: RL is a ground lead, so RL-LL reversal does not result in any significant changes.

TABLE 1. Characteristics of lead reversal. *Credit:* EMRA.

Outpatient Treatment for Low-Risk Pulmonary Embolism

By Nikita R. Paripati, MD; and Michael E. Abboud, MD, MSEd
University of Pennsylvania in Philadelphia

Reviewed by Andrew J. Eyre, MD, MS-HPEd

Objective

On completion of this article, you should be able to:

■ Explain when outpatient treatment for pulmonary embolism is appropriate.

Maughan BC, Frueh L, McDonagh MS, Casciere B, Kline JA. Outpatient treatment of low-risk pulmonary embolism in the era of direct oral anticoagulants: a systematic review. *Acad Emerg Med.* 2021 Feb;28(2):226-239.

KEY POINTS

■ Risk assessment models, including the PESI, sPESI, and Hestia criteria, can be beneficial for identifying low-risk patients with newly diagnosed PE.

■ Outpatient treatment for low-risk PE patients is associated with a low risk of mortality and adverse outcomes.

■ Published data on the use of DOACs to treat acute PE is limited; however, the few controlled studies that exist show a very low rate of major adverse outcomes with this treatment.

■ No statistically significant association exists between anticoagulant treatment class (DOAC, LMWH, vitamin K antagonists) and the rate of major adverse events.

The presentation of pulmonary embolism (PE) varies considerably, ranging from an asymptomatic, incidental finding to a massive clot that causes hemodynamic instability or immediate death. As such, the mortality associated with PE is highly variable and the data unclear. Historically, patients with a new PE diagnosis were admitted to the inpatient setting, mostly because treatment required intravenous or injectable anticoagulant medications (ie, heparin or low-molecular-weight heparin [LMWH]) and titration of vitamin K antagonists (ie, warfarin) to therapeutic levels. However, this treatment practice has changed since direct oral anticoagulants (DOACs) were introduced. Additionally, data suggest that most patients who present with an acute PE are hemodynamically stable and may meet the criteria for outpatient management. The mortality in this subgroup of patients is low, ranging from 0.5% to 2.5%. Several risk assessment models — the pulmonary embolism severity index (PESI), the simplified PESI (sPESI), and the Hestia criteria — are used to help identify short-term mortality in hemodynamically stable patients with acute PE.

Treatment for an acute PE includes anticoagulants such as LMWH, warfarin, and DOACs. In recent years, DOACs have surpassed vitamin K antagonists such as warfarin in effectiveness and are now the leading outpatient therapy for venous thromboembolism (VTE). Robust data do not exist for the outpatient management of PE, so the researchers in the discussed LLSA article sought to systematically analyze the existing studies. The studies analyzed included randomized controlled trials and prospective nonrandomized controlled trials of adults with acute, symptomatic PE who were discharged directly from the emergency department or within 48 hours of hospital admission. These studies were found by searching several databases that contained studies published between 1980 and 2019. Four major adverse outcomes — all-cause mortality, PE-related mortality, recurrent VTE, and major bleeding — and

three minor adverse outcomes — clinically relevant nonmajor bleeding (CRNMB), return visit to the emergency department, and hospital readmission — were identified. A subgroup analysis was used to determine the association between anticoagulant class and the rate of the four major adverse events. Twelve studies that were determined to have low to moderate bias were included as high-quality studies in the analysis. Overall, 1,814 patients who were treated in the outpatient setting had less than a 1% risk of the four major adverse outcomes. The rate of CRNMB was 0.2% to 5.1%. The rate of return visits ranged from 14.9% to 16%; the rate of hospital readmissions at 30 days ranged from 1.5% to 3%.

The selection process of PE patients for outpatient management varies. Using an approach that integrates a risk stratification model (eg, PESI, sPESI, or Hestia criteria) can help identify PE patients at a lower mortality risk. Notably, however, these criteria alone are not definitive; the physician's clinical judgment and the patient's presentation should take priority.

Generally, patients with PE are at a lower risk of mortality if they have normal vital signs and no respiratory distress; oxygen requirement; or comorbidities, including malignancy, thrombocytopenia, heart disease, chronic lung disease, and kidney or liver failure. Once patients are identified as low risk, they can be evaluated for high-risk features by undergoing an echocardiogram and laboratory tests for troponin and BNP levels. If right ventricular dilation or hypokinesis or bowing of the interventricular septum is identified, hospital discharge should be promptly reconsidered. Physicians should also evaluate for concomitant lower-extremity deep vein thrombosis because a higher clot burden can cause clinical worsening and increase the risk of recurrence.

Patients should also be educated on their PE diagnosis and the risks and benefits of anticoagulation therapy. Stable patients with dementia, altered mental status, medical illiteracy or poor medical literacy, poor social support, or a history of medication nonadherence should be more readily admitted. Physicians should also consider admitting patients who will have difficulty with follow-up, like those with no fixed residence or limited access to transportation.

Before an anticoagulant is selected for treatment, patients should be confirmed to have no contraindications to treatment. Contraindications include conditions that increase the risk of bleeding, like thrombocytopenia, active bleeding, recent major surgery, trauma, stroke, and malignancy (especially intracranial, spinal, or oropharyngeal). A patient's fall risk, especially for older adults, should be considered as well in determining bleeding risk. There is no definitive consensus on selecting an anticoagulant for outpatient therapy. The researchers who published this study found no statistically significant association between anticoagulant class and the rate of adverse events. Overall, outpatient management of PE has a low risk of major adverse events at 90 days post discharge and has many advantages when patients are appropriately selected, including an improved quality of life and reduced hospital costs.

Critical Decisions in Emergency Medicine's LLSA literature reviews feature articles from ABEM's 2023 Lifelong Learning and Self-Assessment Reading List. Available online at acep.org/moc/llsa and on the ABEM website.

Critical Cases in Orthopedics and Trauma

Bilateral Patellar Tendon Rupture

By Ian Benjamin, MD, MS
University of Washington in Seattle

Reviewed by John Kiel, DO, MPH, FACEP, CAQSM

Objective

On completion of this article, you should be able to:

■ Describe how to manage bilateral patellar tendon ruptures in the emergency department.

CASE PRESENTATION

A 42-year-old woman with a medical history of bilateral patellar tendon injuries presents with increased knee pain, swelling, and an inability to ambulate since yesterday. After she is evaluated for other injuries, the physician notes swollen knees without clear evidence of infection or trauma. Her sensorimotor examination is notable for an inability to extend her right knee against gravity and limited active range of motion of her left knee. X-rays identify high-riding patellas (ie, patella alta) bilaterally. An MRI is ordered.

Discussion

Bilateral patellar tendon tears are rare, debilitating injuries characterized by the complete rupture of the patellar tendons and loss of knee extension bilaterally. These injuries most often occur from high-energy trauma, such as falls from height, sports-related accidents, or motor vehicle collisions. However, nontraumatic or spontaneous patellar tendon tears can occur.[1]

An accurate history and thorough physical examination are typically sufficient to diagnose bilateral patellar tendon ruptures. The clinical presentation often includes swelling; sudden, severe knee pain; and an inability to extend the knee. Patients may have experienced a popping or tearing sensation at the time of injury. Emergency physicians should palpate for the tendon at the inferior pole of the patella and ensure that the patient can independently perform a straight leg raise test while lying horizontally. Cases of tendon rupture may have a palpable or visible defect where the tendon normally lies (*Figure 1*). Bilateral involvement should raise suspicion for a systemic disorder, such as systemic lupus erythematosus (SLE) or chronic renal failure.[1] After the physical examination, the next step in diagnosis is lateral knee x-rays; they can detect patella alta, which is associated with complete tendon rupture (*Figure 2*).

The pathophysiology that predisposes patients to patellar tendon tears is generally multifactorial. Aging, fluoroquinolone use, corticosteroid injections, or prolonged systemic steroids change tendon composition and morphology. Changes observed in old age include the hardening of tendon fibers (ie, tendinosclerosis), fatty degeneration of fibers, a decrease in collagen and proteoglycan coupled with an increase in elastin, and replacement of the wavy collagen fibers bound in fascicles by linear hyalinized fibrils.[2] Testosterone administration can reduce tendon elasticity and can increase fibrosis over time. Fluoroquinolones are theorized to be directly toxic to tendons — they affect the vascular supply and lead to collagenous degenerative changes.

Reduced blood to the patellar tendon is a major contributor to tears and is most often associated with chronic microtrauma. Vascular abnormalities are also seen in disease states, such as obesity, SLE, and renal disease, in which abnormal neovascularization forms immature and fragile blood vessels that are more susceptible to bleeding. Reduced blood flow and chronic inflammation impede the tendon's ability to heal, predisposing it to injury.[3]

Knee x-rays should be supplemented by either ultrasound or MRI because abnormalities associated with incomplete patellar tendon tears may not be visualized on x-rays. Ultrasound is a safe, timely, and low-cost point-of-care imaging modality with a high sensitivity and specificity for assessing patellar tendon injuries in the emergency department.[4] It is typically performed using a linear array transducer that is arranged sagittally to the tendon at center

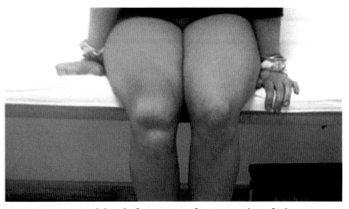

FIGURE 1. Visible defect on inferior pole of the patella. *Credit:* De Giorgi S, Notanicola A, Vicenti G, Moretti B. Patellar tendon rupture after lateral release without predisposing systemic disease or steroid use. *Case Rep Orthop.* 2015;2015:215796. (CC BY [https://www.ncbi.nlm.nih.gov/pmc/articles/PMC4413034/]; https://openi.nlm.nih.gov/detailedresult?img=PMC4413034_CRIOR2015-215796.002).

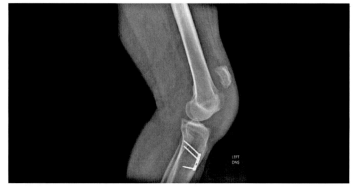

FIGURE 2. Lateral knee x-ray showing the patella alta associated with a patellar tendon rupture. Note the bone anchors from previous petalla tendon repair. *Credit:* Ian Benjamin, MD, MS.

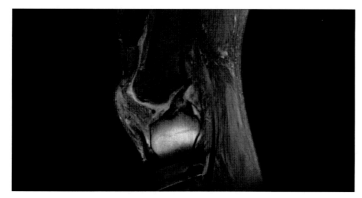

FIGURE 3. MRI showing full-thickness tendon rupture.
Credit: Ian Benjamin, MD, MS.

frequencies of 7 to 10 mHz.[5] The patient in the case presentation underwent an MRI in addition to an ultrasound because of the extent of the occult knee injury; however, MRI is more costly and not always available in the emergency department (*Figure 3*).

A complete tendon rupture is characterized by a gap or interruption in the continuity of the tendon fibers and appears as a hypoechoic (dark) region within the tendon substance on ultrasound (*Figure 4*). Ruptured tendons often exhibit altered morphology compared to intact tendons. The normal smooth, parallel fibrillar pattern can be disrupted, and the torn edges can appear frayed or irregular, particularly at the rupture site.[5] In some cases, tendon rupture is accompanied by surrounding tissue edema or inflammation that leads to tendon thickening or swelling, which can be visualized as an increased tendon diameter or hyperechoic (light) halo around the tendon.

Real-time ultrasound also allows for dynamic assessment of tendon movement during joint motion. In tendon rupture, abnormal movement or a lack of tendon excursion compared to the contralateral side during active or passive joint motion may be noted.[4] Doppler ultrasound can assess the vascularity of the tendon and surrounding tissues. Immediately after tendon rupture, increased vascularity at the site of injury can occur due to the inflammatory response and neovascularization. As healing progresses, the vascularity seen on ultrasound typically decreases.

Importantly, ultrasound findings can vary depending on the rupture's chronicity, any associated injuries, and individual patient factors. Additionally, the skill and experience of the ultrasound operator play a crucial role in accurately identifying and interpreting findings. In cases of a unilateral patellar tendon

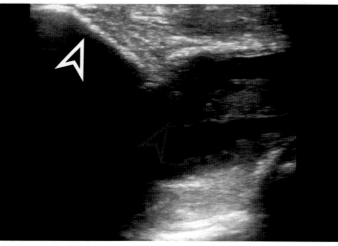

FIGURE 4. Ultrasound (*long-axis view*) of the patella (*white arrow*) with a complete patellar tendon rupture (*red arrow*) and an associated hypoechogenicity indicating a tear. *Credit:* Ian Benjamin, MD, MS.

tear, the injured leg should always be compared to the unaffected leg for reference.

Treatment options for bilateral patellar tendon tears include surgical repair or conservative management. Surgical repair is recommended for most patellar tendon tears to restore the extensor mechanism, improve knee function, and minimize poor outcomes. The surgical technique involves primary tendon repair with or without augmentation using autograft or allograft materials. The choice of technique depends on various factors, including the degree of tendon retraction, the quality of the remaining tendon tissue, and the surgeon's preference and experience.[6] Conservative management, by contrast, is typically reserved for partial tears or for patients with significant comorbidities. It involves immobilization of the knees in a fully extended position, crutches for support, and aggressive rehabilitation. The conservative approach is associated with prolonged immobilization and functional limitations that often lead to poorer outcomes and delayed return to activities.[5,6]

Complications associated with patellar tendon repair include postoperative infection, knee stiffness, patella baja (low-riding patella), and persistent quadricep weakness. Despite appropriate management, some patients can experience persistent functional limitations and difficulty with activities that require significant knee extension strength.[5]

CASE RESOLUTION

The patient's MRI showed a full-thickness tendon rupture. She was discharged in bilateral knee immobilizers and was scheduled for outpatient follow-up in the sports medicine clinic. A subsequent MRI of the left knee showed a complete patellar tendon tear, partial medial joint capsule rupture, grade 2 medial collateral ligament sprain, tears of the lateral meniscus anterior horn and medial meniscus posterior horn, and a partially ruptured Baker cyst. Unfortunately, after obtaining these images, the patient was lost to follow-up.

REFERENCES

1. Saragaglia D, Pison A, Rubens-Duval B. Acute and old ruptures of the extensor apparatus of the knee in adults (excluding knee replacement). *Orthop Traumatol Surg Res.* 2013 Feb;99(suppl 1):S67-S76.
2. Kannus P, Józsa L. Histopathological changes preceding spontaneous rupture of a tendon. A controlled study of 891 patients. *J Bone Joint Surg Am.* 1991 Dec;73(10):1507-1525.
3. Loehr J, Welsh RP. Spontaneous rupture of the quadriceps tendon and patellar ligament during treatment for chronic renal failure. *Can Med Assoc J.* 1983 Aug 1;129(3):254-256.
4. Lee D, Stinner D, Mir H. Quadriceps and patellar tendon ruptures. *J Knee Surg.* 2013 Oct;26(5):301-308.
5. Matava MJ. Patellar tendon ruptures. *J Am Acad Orthop Surg.* 1996 Nov;4(6):287-296.
6. Greis PE, Holmstrom MC, Lahav A. Surgical treatment options for patella tendon rupture, part I: acute. *Orthopedics.* 2005 Jul;28(7):672-679.

The Critical Image

Urinary Retention in a Child

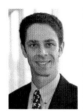

By Joshua S. Broder, MD, FACEP

Dr. Broder is a professor and the residency program director in the Department of Emergency Medicine at Duke University Medical Center in Durham, North Carolina.

Objectives

On completion of this article, you should be able to:

- State the diverse differential diagnosis of urinary retention in children.
- Describe the limits of plain x-rays in the diagnosis of constipation.
- Recognize ultrasound findings of uterine and vaginal fluid.

CASE PRESENTATION

A 12-year-old girl without a previous medical or surgical history presents with urinary retention for the past 12 hours. Two weeks ago, she developed dysuria and urinary frequency accompanied by lower abdominal cramping and pain. One week ago, she developed constipation, with no large bowel movements since that time. She denies fever, back pain, nausea, and vomiting. She is premenarchal and is not sexually active. Her vital signs are BP 129/80, P 83, R 15, and T 36.5°C (97.7°F); SpO$_2$ is 100% on room air. She weighs 47.8 kg (105.4 lbs), and her body mass index is 18.19 kg/m^2.

The patient appears uncomfortable. Her pupils are round and reactive. She has normal cardiovascular and pulmonary examinations. Her lower abdomen is distended with a palpable suprapubic mass. Her neurologic examination shows normal strength, sensation, and lower-extremity reflexes. She denies perineal numbness.

Her urinalysis is normal except for 2+ ketones, and her creatinine level is 0.6 mg/dL. X-rays are obtained (*Figure 1*). At shift change, a repeat physical examination is performed, and ultrasound images are obtained (*Figure 2*).

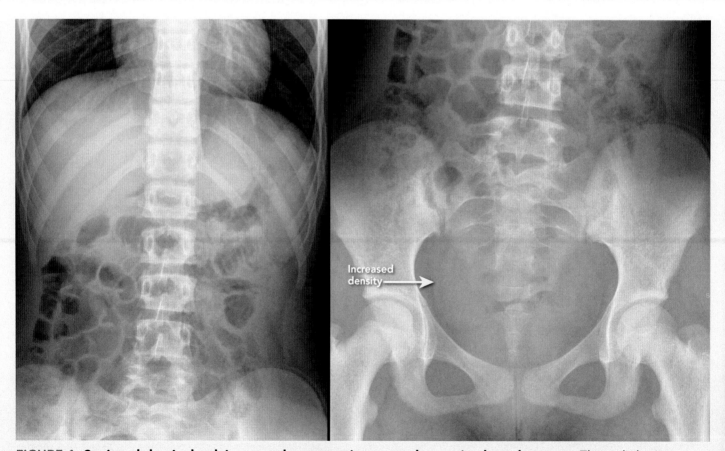

Increased density

FIGURE 1. Supine abdominal-pelvic x-rays demonstrating a nonobstructive bowel pattern. The radiologist remarked on a "modest stool burden." Not noted by the radiologist but visible in retrospect is a pelvic soft tissue or fluid density mass, better seen on ultrasound images (see *Figure 2*).

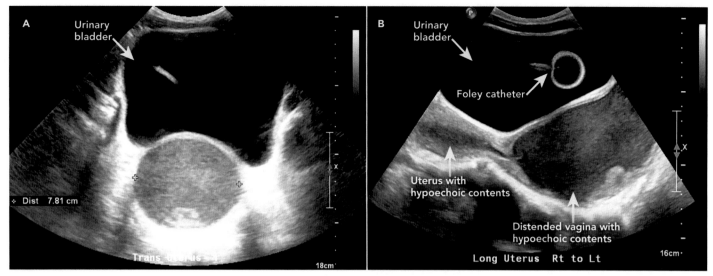

FIGURE 2. Transabdominal ultrasound demonstrating a distended bladder and an enlarged lower uterine segment and vagina filled with hypoechoic fluid. A Foley catheter was placed before the examination but clamped to provide an acoustic window through the bladder. **A.** Transverse view. **B.** Sagittal view.

Discussion

Acute urinary retention, defined as an inability to void lasting longer than 12 hours, is rare in children. Causes of urinary retention in children include neurologic, infectious, structurally obstructive, and medication-induced (eg, anticholinergic) etiologies. A retrospective review found that 17% of pediatric urinary obstruction cases were related to neurologic conditions, 13% to urinary tract infections, 13% to drug use, 7% to local inflammatory processes, 6% to locally invasive neoplasms, 6% to benign obstructive causes, and 2% to incarcerated hernias. Constipation was associated with obstruction in 13% of cases.[1]

Emergency physicians should consider a wide differential diagnosis and include a thorough history (including medication use and red flags for neoplasm) and examination (including a careful neurologic assessment) to evaluate for the myriad causes. Imaging may play a role — potentially ultrasound, CT, or MRI — depending on the suspected etiology.

Although abdominal x-rays are commonly used to evaluate children, their diagnostic accuracy for constipation is poor. A retrospective study of 1,116 pediatric patients undergoing abdominal x-rays found that the sensitivity of x-ray for constipation was 73.8%, specificity was 26.8%, positive predictive value was only 46.4%, and negative predictive value was 54.3%.[2] A 2014 practice guideline of the North American Society for Pediatric Gastroenterology, Hepatology and Nutrition and the European Society for Pediatric Gastroenterology, Hepatology and Nutrition concluded that "evidence supports not using abdominal radiography to diagnose functional constipation."[3] Emergency physicians should avoid attributing urinary retention to constipation without considering other causes and should be particularly guarded in using x-rays to substantiate a diagnosis of constipation.

CASE RESOLUTION

The repeat examination of the patient revealed Tanner stage 3 external genitalia with pubic hair. Based on these findings, the physician suspected that the patient should have begun menstruation, so the ultrasound was ordered. A gynecologist performed an examination under anesthesia and discovered an imperforate hymen, which was excised. Retained uterine and vaginal blood was released, and the urinary obstruction was relieved.

REFERENCES

1. Gatti JM, Perez-Brayfield M, Kirsch AJ, Smith EA, Massad HC, Broecker BH. Acute urinary retention in children. *J Urol.* 2001 Mar;165(3):918-921.
2. Anwar Ul Haq MM, Lyons H, Halim M. Pediatric abdominal x-rays in the acute care setting — are we overdiagnosing constipation? *Cureus.* 2020 Mar 15;12(3):e7283.
3. Tabbers MM, DiLorenzo C, Berger MY, et al; European Society for Pediatric Gastroenterology, Hepatology, and Nutrition; North American Society for Pediatric Gastroenterology. Evaluation and treatment of functional constipation in infants and children: evidence-based recommendations from ESPGHAN and NASPGHAN. *J Pediatr Gastroenterol Nutr.* 2014 Feb;58(2):258-274.

Feature Editor: Joshua S. Broder, MD, FACEP. See also *Diagnostic Imaging for the Emergency Physician* (Winner of the 2011 Prose Award in Clinical Medicine, the American Publishers Award for Professional and Scholarly Excellence) and *Critical Images in Emergency Medicine* by Dr. Broder.

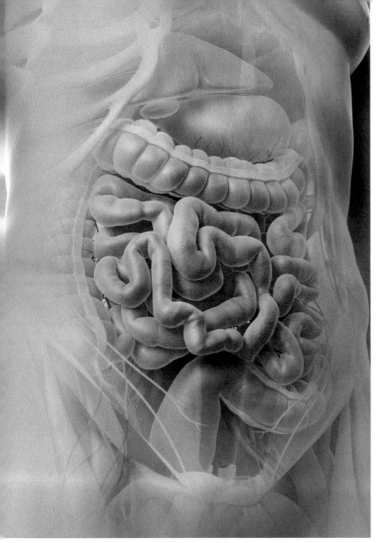

Gut Wrenching

Small Bowel, Big Problems

LESSON 14

 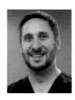

By Tyler Stannard, MD, FAWM; Stephen Rogers, MD; and Rebecca Kernen, MD

Dr. Stannard is an assistant professor, Dr. Rogers is a medical education fellow, and Dr. Kernen is a resident at the University of Texas Southwestern Medical Center in Dallas.

Reviewed by Walter L. Green, MD, FACEP

Objectives

On completion of this lesson, you should be able to:

1. Describe the history and presenting symptoms of giardiasis.
2. Compare the diagnostic modalities for *Giardia*.
3. Identify the most appropriate treatment for giardiasis.
4. Recognize complications and adverse events associated with Crohn disease.
5. Explain treatment options for Crohn disease flares.
6. Discuss when to consider a diagnosis of Meckel diverticulum.
7. Compare imaging approaches and treatment options for Meckel diverticulum.

From the EM Model

2.0 Abdominal and Gastrointestinal Disorders
    2.8   Small Bowel
        2.8.1   Infectious Disorders
        2.8.2   Inflammatory Sisorders
            2.8.2.1   Regional Enteritis/Crohn Disease
        2.8.4   Structural Disorders
            2.8.4.4   Meckel Diverticulum

▬ CRITICAL DECISIONS ▬

- What are the most common risk factors and presenting symptoms of giardiasis, and how is the disease diagnosed?

- How should giardiasis be treated?

- How should emergency physicians approach Crohn disease flares?

- How is Crohn disease treated in the emergency department?

- What are the most common presentations of symptomatic Meckel diverticulum?

- What are the best imaging options for Meckel diverticulum?

- What are the treatment options for Meckel diverticulum?

Familiar emergency department presentations such as abdominal pain, diarrhea, and rectal bleeding are often caused by diseases of the small bowel. Giardiasis is the most common intestinal protozoal infection worldwide, visits for Crohn disease have increased by more than 50% in recent years, and Meckel diverticulum is the most common cause of pediatric lower GI tract bleeding. To provide appropriate care, emergency physicians must be versed in the presentation, diagnosis, and treatment of these small bowel diseases.

■ CASE ONE

A 6-year-old girl presents with a 3-day history of worsening, colicky right lower quadrant pain. She has also had two episodes of nonbilious vomiting. Her parents are concerned because she has a prior history of intussusception, which was successfully treated with an air-contrast enema. On examination, the patient's vital signs are notable for tachycardia and low-grade fever. A mass is palpable in the right lower quadrant.

■ CASE TWO

A 30-year-old man with a history of Crohn disease presents with 3 days of crampy abdominal pain that became sharp this morning. He reports some bright red blood from his rectum as well as diarrhea, which is common for him. He denies any nausea or vomiting but does disclose 2 days of subjective fever.

■ CASE THREE

An otherwise healthy 50-year-old man presents with abdominal cramping and diarrhea of 12 days' duration. He went on a week-long camping trip in the western United States 4 weeks ago and filtered his water for most of the trip. He was seen in an emergency department 6 days ago and was diagnosed with a viral gastroenteritis. He continues to have abdominal cramping and foul-smelling stools.

Introduction

Emergency physicians must be able to recognize, understand, and treat parasitic infections. With increasing travel and immigration across the globe and ongoing parasitic endemics in the rural United States, the number of patients who present to emergency departments with parasitic diseases continues to grow.[1] Parasitic infections encompass a broad range of eukaryotic organisms, which can be divided into unicellular protozoa and multicellular helminths. *Giardia duodenalis* (also known as *G. intestinalis* and *G. lamblia*), which causes the disease giardiasis, is the world's most common intestinal protozoal parasite.[2]

There are roughly 1.2 million annual cases of giardiasis in the United States, with an estimated annual hospitalization cost of $34 million.[3,4] Its most common presenting symptom is diarrhea. Given that there are an estimated 179 million annual cases of all-cause diarrhea in the United States, it is prudent to keep parasitic disease on the differential diagnosis.[5] As such, emergency physicians should be apprised of the various diagnostic modalities and the appropriate treatment for giardiasis.`

Every year, emergency physicians encounter more cases of inflammatory bowel disease (IBD), including Crohn disease. From 2006 to 2014, the number of emergency department visits for patients suffering from IBD increased by more than 50%.[6] Therefore, it is imperative that emergency physicians be able to recognize and manage the most common complications of Crohn disease.

Unlike ulcerative colitis, Crohn disease can occur at any point along the GI tract; lesions (often described as "skip lesions") can be found at any point from the mouth to the anus, including the small bowel. Because it is a transmural disease, Crohn disease can lead to many complications that are seen less often with other IBDs. Crohn disease is also frequently accompanied by extraintestinal manifestations and symptoms, which can include arthritis, uveitis, erythema nodosum, renal stones, and venous thromboembolism.[7]

Pediatric rectal bleeding is a concerning presentation for parents and physicians, especially when it is accompanied by unstable vital signs. When patients present with hematochezia, physicians should consider the most common causes of pediatric lower GI tract bleeding, including Meckel diverticulum. Knowing the common presentations, imaging modalities, and treatment options facilitates appropriate investigation and management of lower GI tract bleeding.

Meckel diverticulum is an outpouching of the small bowel (*Figure 1*). It is a true diverticulum, consisting of all three layers of the intestinal wall and a persistent remnant of the embryologic omphalomesenteric or vitelline duct (the connection between the yolk sac and midgut normally obliterates during the 5th and 6th weeks of development).[8] Meckel diverticulum is the most common congenital malformation of the GI tract. The "rule of twos" is used to describe Meckel diverticulum: It occurs in about 2% of infants, usually measures 2 inches long, is located in the ileum approximately 2 feet from the ileocecal valve, is twice as common in boys and men, and often contains two types of tissue (ie, native intestinal tissue and ectopic tissue). Additionally, Meckel diverticulum accounts for approximately 50% of all cases of lower GI tract bleeding in children younger than 2 years.[9]

CRITICAL DECISION

What are the most common risk factors and presenting symptoms of giardiasis, and how is the disease diagnosed?

Risk Factors

To determine which patients are at risk of a *Giardia* infection, physicians must understand the parasite's life cycle and pathophysiology. *Giardia* exists in two forms: trophozoite and cyst. The cyst is the infectious form; it is passed through feces by its typical reservoirs of humans, beavers, cats, dogs, and cattle. It can be transmitted through waterborne (most common), foodborne, and other fecal-oral routes. Thus, the most significant risk factors include drinking from unfiltered water sources (eg, while hiking), traveling internationally to endemic areas, ingesting raw or

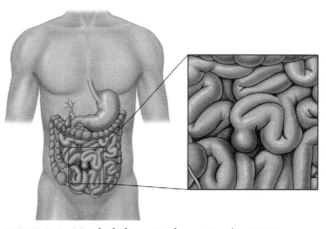

FIGURE 1. Meckel diverticulum. *Credit:* ACEP.

uncooked food, immunosuppression, and being in environments with fecal incontinence or poor hand hygiene (eg, at a day care). After the cyst is ingested, excystation occurs in the duodenum. Motile trophozoites are released, and subsequent symptoms occur from functional and structural damage of the small intestine and from host immune responses. After the trophozoites travel to the colon, encystation occurs; cysts are then excreted into the environment, and the cycle repeats.[10]

Symptoms

Symptoms occur after an incubation period of 1 to 3 weeks. Although 50% of cases are asymptomatic, symptomatic patients who present to the emergency department most commonly have diarrhea, abdominal cramps, greasy stools, flatulence, nausea, vomiting, weight loss, and dehydration. Giardiasis typically does not cause fever, hematochezia, or mucus-tinged stools. However, it may lead to chronic illness, resulting in malabsorption, chronic diarrhea, and failure to thrive in children.[10,11]

Giardia is a common pathogen found in patients who present with persistent or chronic diarrhea. The WHO defines diarrhea as the passage of three or more loose or liquid stools in a 24-hour period, or more frequently than normal for an individual. The American College of Gastroenterology (ACG) classifies diarrhea as acute (lasting <14 days), persistent (lasting 14-30 days), and chronic (lasting >30 days). Because of the incubation period, symptoms that present less than 1 week after exposure should not be attributed to *Giardia*. Rather, parasitic infections should be considered after 7 to 10 days of ongoing diarrhea along with the relevant risk factors.[12,13]

Diagnosis

It may be appropriate for emergency physicians to diagnose giardiasis based on history and symptom presentation. However, stool microscopy with ova and parasite examination is the traditional method of detecting *Giardia* and remains the gold standard for evaluating cysts and trophozoites. The advantages of the ova and parasite examination are its ease and low cost. However, it has poor sensitivity because shedding is intermittent. When the examination is limited to one stool sample, only 60% to 80% of infections are diagnosed. Examining two samples increases detection to 80% to 90%; if three samples are examined, detection exceeds 90%.[14] These stool samples are typically collected on consecutive days, which is impractical from an emergency medicine standpoint.

Other methods of detecting *Giardia* include enzyme immunoassay techniques and rapid antigen detection tests. These tests are 95% to 100% sensitive and 100% specific. Some commonly available kits include direct immunofluorescent assays, immunochromatographic assays, and enzyme-linked immunosorbent assays. These studies tend to be expensive and are not readily available in all clinical settings.[15] Fecal leukocytes and peripheral eosinophilia are typically absent and do not add diagnostic value. Although the decision to treat is not always based on definitive test results, physicians must know the diagnostic modalities available and understand their associated benefits and limitations.

CRITICAL DECISION

How should giardiasis be treated?

The mainstays of treatment for giardiasis are supportive care and antimicrobials. Patients must be rehydrated, and any electrolyte abnormalities from diarrhea must be corrected. The

	Age <1 year	Age 1-3 years	Age ≥3 years
Treatment	Metronidazole	Nitazoxanide	Tinidazole or nitazoxanide
Alternative agent		Metronidazole	Metronidazole
Coinfection suspected	Anthelmintic (eg, albendazole or mebendazole)		

TABLE 1. Recommended treatments for giardiasis

choice of antimicrobial is based on age (*Table 1*). For patients at least 3 years old, a single dose of tinidazole or a 3-day course of nitazoxanide is the recommended first-line agent; alternatively, metronidazole can be used.[15,16] In a meta-analysis of 60 randomized controlled trials, tinidazole was more effective than albendazole or metronidazole.[17] However, because the safety of tinidazole in patients younger than 3 years is unstudied, nitazoxanide is the preferred agent for patients aged 1 to 3 years. The alternative agent in this age group is metronidazole. For infants, metronidazole is the preferred agent. Anthelmintics such as albendazole or mebendazole are reasonable alternatives if coinfection with another parasite is suspected.

CRITICAL DECISION

How should emergency physicians approach Crohn disease flares?

The initial assessment of a patient who presents with a Crohn disease flare must be guided by the clinical presentation. Most patients who present with a Crohn disease flare complain of increased diarrhea, abnormal pain, or systemic symptoms that are atypical for them. Physicians must also consider specific patients' previous presentations and history of complications.[18] For example, the physician must be aware if a patient with Crohn disease has a history of small bowel obstruction or fistula.

Because patients who present with Crohn disease flares often know how their flares typically feel, they can also describe whether the present flare feels different. Physicians

— ✔ Pearls

- When a patient presents with abdominal pain and diarrhea that last longer than 7 days, expand the differential diagnosis to include parasitic infections.

- The best antimicrobial for giardiasis depends on the patient's age; a one-time dose of tinidazole is the best agent for patients who are at least 3 years old.

- Consider all possible complications of Crohn disease and use physical examination findings and patient history to guide imaging and treatment.

- Young children with Meckel diverticulum most commonly present with GI tract bleeding, and older children and adults more often present with symptoms of small bowel obstruction or Meckel diverticulitis.

must note any abnormal vital signs, including fever, and be confident in their physical examination skills when examining for peritonitis. A common workup would include a CBC, comprehensive metabolic panel, lipase test, type and screen for significant bleeding, and possibly an erythrocyte sedimentation rate or C-reactive protein test for monitoring. Anemia and an elevated platelet count are common findings.[19] If there is a secondary concern for infectious diarrhea, stool cultures may also be sent, including a *Clostridioides difficile* (formerly *Clostridium difficile*) test. Finally, a CT scan of the abdomen must be ordered if there is concern for small bowel obstruction, infection, or peritonitis.[7]

CRITICAL DECISION

How is Crohn disease treated in the emergency department?

Much of the outpatient management of Crohn disease consists of glucocorticoids and immunomodulators, and much of the symptomatic control is achieved through oral 5-aminosalicylates.[20] Primary emergency department treatment options for patients with Crohn disease emphasize symptom control and stabilization. Fluids with electrolyte repletion must be initiated, and all patients need adequate analgesia. Current ACG guidelines discourage the use of antidiarrheal medications for acute treatment of Crohn disease.[7,19]

Emergency physicians frequently encounter complications of Crohn disease, which are also outlined in the ACG guidelines. For patients who present with constipation and abdominal distension concerning for small bowel obstruction, a nasogastric tube should be placed while adequate analgesia and bowel rest are provided. Patients with symptoms of an infection, such as abdominal tenderness and fever, should be started on antibiotics, either broad-spectrum or ciprofloxacin and metronidazole. Finally, because of the increased risk of venous thromboembolism, any hospitalized patient with Crohn disease must be started on enoxaparin sodium.[7,18] Finally, during a mild Crohn flare that does not require admission, starting a steroid burst of methylprednisolone or prednisone and possibly budesonide may be beneficial. However, the dose or type of immunomodulator must not be adjusted without the input of the gastroenterology team.[7,19]

✖ Pitfalls

- Relying on negative results of an ova and parasite examination of a single stool sample for diagnosing giardiasis.
- Failing to order CT imaging in patients with Crohn disease flares when concerned for small bowel obstruction, infection, or peritonitis.
- Discounting the possibility of Meckel diverticulum when CT imaging is nondiagnostic.
- Trusting negative Meckel scan results when rectal bleeding is absent and clinical suspicion of Meckel diverticulum is high.

CRITICAL DECISION

What are the most common presentations of symptomatic Meckel diverticulum?

Lower GI Bleeding

Meckel diverticulum accounts for approximately 50% of all lower GI tract bleeding in children younger than 2 years. The outpouching can contain several types of ectopic tissue. The most common of these is gastric tissue, followed by pancreatic tissue. When there is ectopic gastric mucosa in the diverticulum, gastrin cells secrete acidic enzymes, resulting in ulceration and lower GI tract bleeding. Typically, the pancreatic bicarbonate in the duodenum neutralizes the acid secreted by the normal gastric mucosa. However, in a Meckel diverticulum, the ectopic gastric mucosa secretes acid that is not neutralized, resulting in ulceration of the adjacent mucosa and painless rectal bleeding. The ulcerations are generally more prominent downstream of the diverticulum where the enzymes are secreted.[10] Notably, the blood supply to the diverticulum is provided by a branch from the superior mesenteric artery, known as the vitelline artery.[9,21] Ulceration into branches of this vessel causes the painless rectal bleeding and anemia seen in pediatric patients.

Bowel Obstruction

Small bowel obstruction from internal volvulus or intussusception can also be a presenting symptom of Meckel diverticulum. Fibrous bands connecting the diverticulum to the umbilicus (or to the base of the mesentery because of incomplete involution of embryologic structures) can predispose to twisting around the focal point. This twisting causes a secondary volvulus. Additionally, the outpouching can act as a lead point for an enteroenteric or enterocolic intussusception, which often cannot be reduced hydrostatically.[9,22] In children, recurrent or atypical intussusception should raise clinical suspicion for Meckel diverticulum. Additionally, volvulus or intussusception may lead to incarceration and symptoms of small bowel obstruction, including abdominal pain and progressive nonbilious to bilious vomiting.

Meckel Diverticulitis

Inflammation in the diverticulum, known as Meckel diverticulitis, can cause acute abdominal pain as well. Enteroliths or foreign bodies (or rarely, parasites) can obstruct the pouch and cause local inflammation, progressing to perforation and peritonitis. Importantly, Meckel diverticulitis may resemble acute appendicitis and is often misdiagnosed preoperatively. Right lower quadrant pain in patients with a history of appendectomy can be a symptom of Meckel diverticulitis.[9] Fever, vomiting, abdominal pain, and bloody stools can represent many different pathologies; Meckel diverticulum is often a diagnostic challenge that is discovered incidentally during workup for other potential etiologies.

CRITICAL DECISION

What are the best imaging options for Meckel diverticulum?

Depending on the clinical presentation, a definitive diagnosis of Meckel diverticulum is generally made one of three ways:

with a Meckel scan, mesenteric angiography, or abdominal exploration. In the case of abdominal exploration, a Meckel diverticulum is often found incidentally during an exploratory laparotomy for alternative diagnoses. A Meckel diverticulum can also be identified by CT in the presence of acute inflammation or obstruction at the diverticulum. However, CT can have unreliable results in the absence of acute inflammation, an ultrasound, or an upper GI series, and the diverticulum can be easily confused with other abdominal structures.

Meckel Scan

A Meckel scan, often called a ^{99m}Tc sodium pertechnetate scan, is the most sensitive diagnostic test for Meckel diverticulum. It has a sensitivity of 85% in children but only 60% in adults. It has a specificity of 95% and accuracy of 90%.[22] Radionuclide ^{99m}Tc pertechnetate is taken up by the stomach and the mucin-producing cells of the gastric mucosa in the diverticula and is secreted into the lumen of the gut (*Figure 2*). This study captures multiple images over time and may be enhanced using pentagastrin, which stimulates uptake of pertechnetate by the gastric cells.[23] Histamine blockers can also be administered to inhibit pertechnetate secretion by the gastric cells. The disadvantage of using a Meckel scan is that diverticula with pancreatic or duodenal tissue rather than gastric mucosa are not visualized. Therefore, because of the ulceration associated with the gastric mucosa, patients who present with rectal bleeding are more likely to have positive test results.

Mesenteric Angiography

In cases of active and ongoing bleeding, contrast extravasation is evident using a ^{99m}Tc-RBC scan or a superior mesenteric angiogram. Conventional contrast mesenteric arteriography may be appropriate if the source of GI tract bleeding is brisk enough (generally >0.5 mL/min) to require transfusion and the source has not been identified using another imaging modality.[10] When used correctly in the setting of brisk GI tract bleeding, mesenteric angiography is an effective method of detecting Meckel diverticulum with a sensitivity and specificity of approximately 100%.

What are the treatment options for Meckel diverticulum?

Treatment options depend on whether patients are symptomatic. In patients who are hypotensive from bleeding, resuscitation with blood transfusion takes priority over diagnostic imaging and definitive management. In asymptomatic cases, if the outpouching is found incidentally on imaging, observation is generally preferred. Although these patients should be referred to outpatient surgery, resection is not typically recommended. If the diverticulum is found incidentally during surgery, the surgeon may or may not resect it. In many cases, surgeons opt for resection in otherwise healthy patients who are younger than 50 years and have anatomic risk factors (ie, length >2 cm, palpable abnormality, or fibrous bands).[9,22] In asymptomatic cases, surgeons typically leave the diverticulum and follow the patient with close observation.

In symptomatic patients, the treatment of choice is usually surgery by simple diverticulectomy or segmental small bowel resection and primary anastomosis. Most symptomatic patients are found to have ectopic mucosa within the diverticulum. Therefore, the diverticulum is resected carefully to ensure complete removal of all ectopic tissue, which can be confirmed with histologic examination of frozen tissue.

Summary

Abdominal pain with diarrhea is a common presenting complaint in the emergency department. If diarrhea has lasted longer than 7 days and the patient history includes associated risk factors, parasitic infection should be considered on the differential diagnosis. Patients with giardiasis typically present with nonspecific GI complaints, diarrhea being the predominant symptom. Diagnosis can be made using an ova and parasite examination or a *Giardia*-specific test, but it may also be appropriate to diagnose the condition based on history and presenting symptoms. Treatment includes supportive care and age-appropriate antimicrobials.

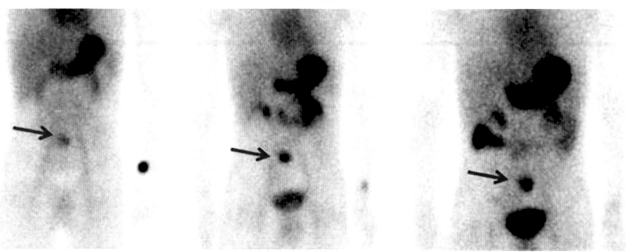

FIGURE 2. Meckel scan. Radionuclide ^{99m}Tc-pertechnetate is taken up by the mucin-producing cells of the gastric mucosa in the diverticulum and is secreted into the lumen of the gut (*red arrow*). *Credit:* Xie Q, Ma Q, Ji B, Gao S, Wen Q. Incremental value of SPECT/CT in detection of Meckel's diverticulum in a 10-year-old child. *SpringerPlus.* 2016 Aug 5;5:1270 (license info [https://www.springernature.com/gp/open-research/about/the-fundamentals-of-open-access-and-open-research]; https://springerplus.springeropen.com/articles/10.1186/s40064-016-2928-4/figures/1).

CASE RESOLUTIONS

CASE ONE

An ultrasound was obtained; it demonstrated an intussusception. An air-contrast enema was performed and was able to reduce the intussusception. However, because this visit was the patient's second presentation with similar symptoms, a Meckel scan was obtained. Her scan showed enhanced uptake in the ileum, confirming Meckel diverticulum. The patient underwent a diverticulectomy and recovered fully.

CASE TWO

Laboratory findings were remarkable for slight leukocytosis and elevated inflammatory markers. A CT scan showed an abscess that required broad-spectrum antibiotics and drainage using interventional radiology, but no further surgical intervention was needed. Following drainage, the patient continued on oral antibiotics as an outpatient and made a full recovery. He followed up with his gastroenterologist, and his immunomodulators were adjusted.

CASE THREE

An ova and parasite examination was ordered; laboratory results were nondiagnostic. Based on history and presenting symptoms, the patient was treated with a one-time dose of tinidazole for presumed giardiasis. By the time of his follow-up appointment 2 weeks later, his diarrhea and abdominal cramping had resolved.

Crohn disease is responsible for a large percentage of abdominal pain complaints in the emergency department. When patients with known Crohn disease present with abdominal pain, both the current clinical picture and the prior history of complications must be considered. Physicians must also remember to treat infections, control pain, and provide adequate fluid hydration and electrolyte repletion. Mild, uncomplicated exacerbations can be treated on an outpatient basis, but serious complications must be ruled out first.

Although most patients with Meckel diverticulum are asymptomatic, 2% of patients have symptoms. Symptomatic cases usually present with one of three scenarios: lower GI tract bleeding, intestinal obstruction, or Meckel diverticulitis. Pediatric patients most often present with painless rectal bleeding and anemia in the first 10 years of life, with an average age of 2.5 years. In adults, the most common complication is small bowel obstruction; however, Meckel diverticulum is also considered in adults with GI tract bleeding from an unclear source. When clinical suspicion is high, obtaining a Meckel scan is generally preferred. In many cases, management of Meckel diverticulum consists of symptom observation.

REFERENCES

1. Cahill JD, Becker BM. Parasites. In: Walls RM, Hockberger RS, Gausche-Hill M, et al, eds. *Rosen's Emergency Medicine: Concepts and Clinical Practice*. Vol 2. 10th ed. Elsevier; 2023:1654-1673.
2. Leung AKC, Leung AAM, Wong AHC, Sergi CM, Kam JKM. Giardiasis: an overview. *Recent Pat Inflamm Allergy Drug Discov*. 2019;13(2):134-143.
3. Collier SA, Stockman LJ, Hicks LA, Garrison LE, Zhou FJ, Beach MJ. Direct healthcare costs of selected diseases primarily or partially transmitted by water. *Epidemiol Infect*. 2012;140(11):2003-2013.
4. Zylberberg HM, Green PH, Turner KO, Genta RM, Lebwohl B. Prevalence and predictors of Giardia in the United States. *Dig Dis Sci*. 2017;62(2):432-440.
5. DuPont HL. Acute infectious diarrhea in immunocompetent adults. *N Engl J Med*. 2014;370(16):1532-1540.
6. Ballou S, Hirsch W, Singh P, et al. Emergency department utilisation for inflammatory bowel disease in the United States from 2006 to 2014. *Aliment Pharmacol Ther*. 2018;47(7):913-921.
7. Swartz J, Singh M, Donaldson R, et al. Crohn's disease. WikiEM. Updated September 7, 2022. https://wikem.org/wiki/Crohn%27s_disease
8. Stallion A, Shuck JM. Meckel's diverticulum. In: Holzheimer RG, Mannick JA, eds. *Surgical Treatment: Evidence-Based and Problem-Oriented*. Munich: Zuckschwerdt; 2001. https://www.ncbi.nlm.nih.gov/books/NBK6918/
9. An J, Zabbo CP. Meckel diverticulum. *StatPearls [Internet]*. StatPearls Publishing. Updated January 30, 2023. https://www.ncbi.nlm.nih.gov/books/NBK499960/
10. Leder K, Weller PF. Giardiasis: epidemiology, clinical manifestations, and diagnosis. UpToDate. Updated May 26, 2021. https://www.uptodate.com/contents/giardiasis-epidemiology-clinical-manifestations-and-diagnosis
11. Conners EE, Miller AD, Balachandran N, Robinson BM, Benedict KM. Giardiasis outbreaks - United States, 2012-2017. *MMWR Morb Mortal Wkly Rep*. 2021 Mar 5;70(9):304-307.
12. Riddle MS, DuPont HL, Connor BA. ACG clinical guideline: diagnosis, treatment, and prevention of acute diarrheal infections in adults. *Am J Gastroenterol*. 2016;111(5):602-622.
13. Thielman NM, Guerrant RL. Acute infectious diarrhea. *N Engl J Med*. 2004;350(1):38-47.
14. Hooshyar H, Rostamkhani P, Arbabi M, Delavari M. Giardia lamblia infection: review of current diagnostic strategies. *Gastroenterol Hepatol Bed Bench*. 2019;12(1):3-12.
15. Bartelt LA. Giardiasis: treatment and prevention. UpToDate. Updated September 6, 2022. https://www.uptodate.com/contents/giardiasis-treatment-and-prevention
16. Shane AL, Mody RK, Crump JA, et al. 2017 Infectious Diseases Society of America clinical practice guidelines for the diagnosis and management of infectious diarrhea. *Clin Infect Dis*. 2017;65(12):e45-e80.
17. Ordóñez-Mena JM, McCarthy ND, Fanshawe TR. Comparative efficacy of drugs for treating giardiasis: a systematic update of the literature and network meta-analysis of randomized clinical trials. *J Antimicrob Chemother*. 2018;73(3):596-606.
18. Al Hashash J, Regueiro M. Overview of medical management of high-risk, adult patients with moderate to severe Crohn disease. UpToDate. Updated October 17, 2022. https//www.uptodate.com/contents/medical-management-of-moderate-to-severe-crohn-disease-in-adults
19. Lichtenstein GR, Loftus EV, Isaacs KL, Regueiro MD, Gerson LB, Sands BE. ACG clinical guideline: management of Crohn's disease in adults. *Am J Gastroenterol*. 2018;113(4):481-517.
20. Regueiro M, Al Hashash J. Overview of the medical management of mild (low risk) Crohn disease in adults. UpToDate. Updated August 8, 2022. https://www.uptodate.com/contents/overview-of-the-medical-management-of-mild-low-risk-crohn-disease-in-adults
21. Kovacs M, Botstein J, Braverman S. Angiographic diagnosis of Meckel's diverticulum in an adult patient with negative scintigraphy. *J Radiol Case Rep*. 2017 Mar 31;11(3):22-29.
22. Javid PJ, Pauli EM. Meckel's Diverticulum. UpToDate. Updated February 1, 2022. https://www.uptodate.com/contents/meckels-diverticulum
23. Titley-Diaz WH, Aziz M. Meckel scan. In: *StatPearls [Internet]*. StatPearls Publishing. Updated July 25, 2022. https://www.ncbi.nlm.nih.gov/books/NBK560500/

CME Questions

Reviewed by **Tareq Al-Salamah, MBBS, MPH, FACEP**; and **Walter L. Green, MD, FACEP**

Qualified, paid subscribers to *Critical Decisions in Emergency Medicine* may receive CME certificates for up to 5 ACEP Category I credits, 5 *AMA PRA Category 1 Credits*™, and 5 AOA Category 2-B credits for completing this activity in its entirety. Submit your answers online at acep.org/cdem; a score of 75% or better is required. You may receive credit for completing the CME activity any time within 3 years of its publication date. Answers to this month's questions will be published in next month's issue.

1 **Which component is not part of the Virchow triad for assessing deep vein thrombosis risk?**
  A. Endothelial damage
  B. Hypercoagulable state
  C. Inflammation
  D. Stasis

2 **Which organ produces antithrombin?**
  A. Kidneys
  B. Liver
  C. Lungs
  D. Spleen

3 **Nephrotic syndrome most likely causes deep vein thrombosis by which mechanism?**
  A. Hydrostatic and oncotic pressure gradient change that causes venous swelling
  B. Hyperlipidemia that causes atherosclerosis
  C. Hypertension that causes turbulent venous flow
  D. Proteinuria that leads to a loss of anticoagulating proteins

4 **A 52-year-old obese woman presents with left leg swelling. Her medical history includes hypertension, hyperlipidemia, coronary artery disease with drug-eluting stents, and opioid use disorder. She reports that she smokes 30 packs of cigarettes a year. Her D-dimer level is 990 ng/mL, and ultrasonography reveals a noncompressible proximal femoral vein. What is her greatest risk factor for deep vein thrombosis?**
  A. Cigarette smoking
  B. Coronary artery disease
  C. Hyperlipidemia
  D. Opioid use

5 **Which test is most sensitive in diagnosing lower-extremity deep vein thrombosis?**
  A. Compression ultrasonography
  B. D-dimer
  C. Duplex ultrasonography
  D. Homans sign test

6 **Which combination of conditions poses the highest risk of venous thromboembolism?**
  A. Cigarette smoking and oral contraceptive use
  B. HIV and factor V Leiden
  C. Oral contraceptive use and factor V Leiden
  D. Oral contraceptive use and HIV

7 **A 31-year-old man presents with right calf pain. He returned to California from China 2 days ago. His D-dimer level is 632 ng/mL, and his ultrasound reveals an occlusive popliteal deep vein thrombosis. What is the goal of initiating anticoagulation in this patient?**
  A. Control pain
  B. Lyse the thrombus
  C. Prevent extension of the thrombus
  D. Prevent platelet aggregation

8 **A patient with systemic lupus erythematosus is diagnosed with acute right popliteal deep vein thrombosis. During workup, they are found to have high-risk antiphospholipid syndrome. Based on the American College of Chest Physicians' recommendations, what anticoagulant should this patient be started on?**
  A. Apixaban
  B. Aspirin
  C. Rivaroxaban
  D. Warfarin

9 **Which scoring tool can be used to risk stratify low pretest probability patients for deep vein thrombosis?**
  A. Emergency department assessment of chest pain score
  B. Geneva score
  C. HAS-BLED score for deep vein thrombosis
  D. Wells score for deep vein thrombosis

10 **A previously healthy 34-year-old man presents with left arm pain. He has been donating plasma every month for the past year as an extra source of income. On examination, his vital signs are within normal limits; his left upper extremity is erythematous, tender, swollen, and warm in the skin area from the antecubital fossa to the medial portion of his upper arm. His history and physical examination do not suggest anemia, a bleeding disorder, or liver or renal disease. A duplex ultrasound reveals superficial vein thrombosis of the medial cubital vein and brachial deep vein thrombosis. What is the best next step?**
  A. Discharge and repeat ultrasound in a week for surveillance
  B. Order a CT angiography of the left upper extremity
  C. Order laboratory tests
  D. Start the patient on a direct oral anticoagulant and discharge him

11 **A 2-year-old boy presents with 10 days of abdominal cramping and diarrhea. His mother was recently informed of a *Giardia* outbreak at the day care he attends. What is the best choice of antimicrobial?**
  A. Albendazole
  B. Metronidazole
  C. Nitazoxanide
  D. Tinidazole

12 **What is the most common initial symptom of giardiasis?**
  A. Diarrhea
  B. Fever
  C. Hematochezia
  D. Malabsorption

13 **What is the most sensitive test for *Giardia*?**
  A. Eosinophilia
  B. Fecal leukocyte
  C. Microscopy with direct fluorescence antibody
  D. One-time ova and parasite examination

14 An 8-year-old boy presents with chronic diarrhea, anal fissures, and oral ulcers. His parents deny any recent travel or antibiotic use. What is the most likely diagnosis?

- A. Cholera
- B. *Clostridioides difficile* infection
- C. Crohn disease
- D. Ulcerative colitis

15 A well-appearing patient presents with a Crohn disease flare. There is mild leukocytosis and fever but no evidence of abscess or perforation on CT. What is the most appropriate antibiotic choice?

- A. Amoxicillin
- B. Ceftriaxone
- C. Ciprofloxacin and metronidazole
- D. Oral vancomycin

16 What is a common extraintestinal manifestation of Crohn disease?

- A. Encephalitis
- B. Erythema marginatum
- C. Erythema nodosum
- D. Vitreous hemorrhage

17 What is the best diagnostic modality when there is concern for Meckel diverticulum in a stable pediatric GI tract bleed?

- A. ^{99m}Tc sodium pertechnetate scan
- B. Abdominal x-ray
- C. Stool culture
- D. Ultrasound

18 Meckel diverticulitis often mimics which common pathology?

- A. Appendicitis
- B. Colitis
- C. Gastritis
- D. Pyelonephritis

19 What is the next step after incidental diagnosis of asymptomatic Meckel diverticulum in a child?

- A. Admission for consideration of abdominal exploration
- B. Emergent exploratory laparotomy
- C. Placement of a nasogastric tube
- D. Referral to outpatient pediatric surgery

20 A 2-year-old boy presents with brisk, painless lower GI tract bleeding. His vital signs are BP 70/40, P 150, R 24, and T 37°C (98.6°F); SpO$_2$ is 98% on room air. What is the best first step in treatment?

- A. Abdominal ultrasound
- B. Blood transfusion
- C. Meckel scan
- D. Surgical exploration

ANSWER KEY FOR JUNE 2023, VOLUME 37, NUMBER 6

1	2	3	4	5	6	7	8	9	10	11	12	13	14	15	16	17	18	19	20
D	A	C	A	C	B	B	C	B	B	B	D	B	A	B	D	C	B	B	D

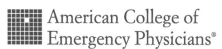
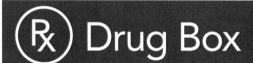
Drug Box

Contrast Allergy and Pretreatment

Frank LoVecchio, DO, MPH, FACEP
Valleywise Health Medical Center and ASU, Phoenix, Arizona

Objective

On completion of this column, you should be able to:
- Explain how to manage contrast allergies in the emergency department.

Rates of contrast allergy have varied dynamically. The early hyperosmolar agents were associated with rates of allergic and physiologic reactions as high as 15%. These agents are no longer in use, and current low-osmolality agents have a much lower likelihood of adverse reactions (0.2%-0.7%).[1]

The two basic types of contrast allergies are physiologic and allergic-like reactions. Physiologic reactions often occur secondary to pain or the infusion sensation and can be vasovagal, inotropic, or neurologic. Although often benign and dose dependent, physiologic reactions can be deadly if seizures or life-threatening hypotension and arrhythmia occur. Other symptoms include nausea, vomiting, flushing, chills, warmth, headaches, dizziness, anxiety, a metallic taste, and hypertension.

Allergic-like reactions are not thought to be from the typical IgE-mediated response of most allergies because of a low rate of positive skin tests in these patients. A histamine-dependent response is thought to be more likely. Severe reactions include diffuse edema, facial edema with dyspnea, erythema with hypotension, laryngeal edema with stridor, wheezing, or bronchospasm with significant hypoxia or anaphylactic shock.[2]

Differentiating the two types of contrast allergies guides pretreatment and treatment regimens. Presenting symptoms determine the type of treatment, and treatment paradigms are in the American College of Radiology (ACR) Manual on Contrast Media.[3]

A prior allergic-like reaction is the single greatest risk factor for a reaction. Pretreatment should be considered in patients with a prior mild to moderate reaction (pretreatment has limited data to show efficacy in patients with prior severe reactions). Pretreatment algorithms from the ACR guidelines recommend a combination of antihistamines and corticosteroids. Although most pretreatment protocols require a time delay between pretreatment administration and contrast administration, this time delay is not practical in the emergency department. Emergency physicians, instead, avoid the time delay between the two and follow patients closely after imaging. Examples of pretreatment include:
- Prednisone 50 mg PO 13, 7, and 1 hour before the scan. Diphenhydramine 50 mg PO/IV/IM 1 hour before the scan.
- Methylprednisolone 40 mg IV or hydrocortisone 200 mg IV every 4 hours or at least two doses of diphenhydramine 50 mg IV 1 hour before the scan.
Even with pretreatment, 12% of patients with prior reactions have breakthrough reactions, but the severity is typically similar to or less than prior responses.[4]

REFERENCES
1. Beckett KR, Moriarity AK, Langer JM. Safe use of contrast media: what the radiologist needs to know. *Radiographics.* 2015 Oct;35(6):1738-1750.
2. Wang CL, Cohan RH, Ellis JH, Caoili EM, Wang G, Francis IR. Frequency, outcome, and appropriateness of treatment of nonionic iodinated contrast media reactions. *AJR Am J Roentgenol.* 2008 Aug;191(2):409-415.
3. Kodzwa R. ACR Manual on Contrast Media: 2018 updates. *Radiol Technol.* 2019 Sep;91(1):97-100.
4. Davenport MS, Mervak BM, Ellis JH, Dillman JR, Dunnick NR, Cohan RH. Indirect cost and harm attributable to oral 13-hour inpatient corticosteroid prophylaxis before contrast-enhanced CT. *Radiology.* 2016 May;279(2):492-501.

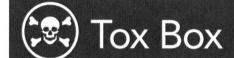
Tox Box

Selenious Acid Toxicity

By Christian A. Tomaszewski, MD, MS, MBA, FACEP
University of California San Diego Health

Objective

On completion of this column, you should be able to:
- State the symptoms and treatment of selenious acid toxicity.

Introduction

Selenious acid is found in gun-bluing agents that are used to enhance the color of steel. It also has industrial uses (eg, metallurgy, glass, and pigments). Although ingestions are rare, the extreme amount of selenium, normally an essential trace element, can cause severe, rapid toxicity with small ingestions (<1 mg/kg). For instance, a toddler died in under 4 hours after ingesting 15 mL of 9% selenious acid.

Mechanism of Action
- Inhibits sulfhydryl-containing enzymes
- Is a corrosive acid

Kinetics
- Rapidly absorbed after oral ingestion or dermal exposure
- Half-life is days

Clinical Manifestations (usually in massive ingestions)
- **Triphasic pattern:** (1) GI, (2) muscle weakness, and (3) cardiovascular
- **GI:** nausea, vomiting (foul garlic smell), diarrhea, burns, and hemorrhagic gastritis
- **Muscle:** weakness and respiratory failure
- **Cardiac:** chest pain, hypotension, prolonged QT interval, and ventricular dysrhythmias
- **Pulmonary:** dyspnea, hypoxia, edema, and pneumonitis (if inhaled)

Diagnostics
- Routine screening of glucose and acetaminophen levels if intentional overdose
- Chest x-ray if respiratory issues
- Selenium serum concentration for confirmation
- Electrolytes to check for hyperkalemia or metabolic acidosis

Treatment
- IV fluid bolus and norepinephrine for hypotension
- Endoscopy to evaluate for symptomatic burns post stabilization
- Hypothetical treatments (limited success and questionable efficacy)
  - Chelation (dimercaprol or calcium disodium EDTA)
  - Dialysis

Disposition
- Can medically clear if no GI or other symptoms at 6 hr post ingestion

Critical decisions
in emergency medicine

Volume 37 Number 8: **August 2023**

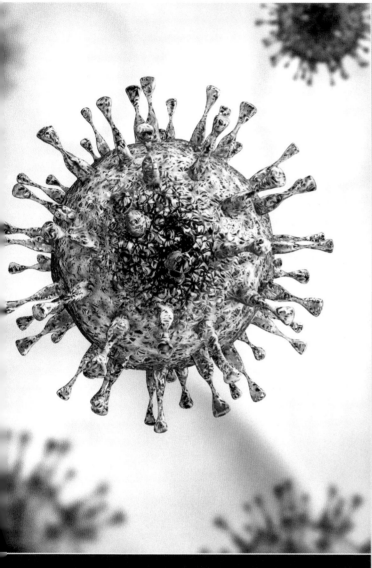

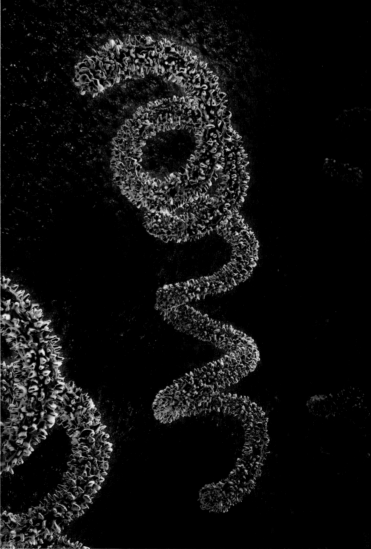

Yellow-Bellied

Liver disease is seen daily in the emergency department — roughly 25% of people in the United States have some form of it. Diagnosing liver conditions can be challenging because symptoms vary widely in type and severity. Emergency physicians must understand the pathophysiology and etiology of the different types of liver disease to manage both acute and chronic cases.

Striking Back

Historically called the *great imitator*, syphilis is a complex and dynamic disease with diverse presentations and a serious risk of long-term sequelae. Improved testing and treatment in the 20th century reduced the incidence of syphilis and decreased exposure to its varied clinical presentations. Unfortunately, recent years have seen a dramatic increase in its incidence.

THE OFFICIAL CME PUBLICATION OF THE AMERICAN COLLEGE OF EMERGENCY PHYSICIANS

Individuals in Control of Content

1. Jeremy Berberian, MD – Faculty
2. William J. Brady, MD, FACEP – Faculty
3. Bryanna Carpenter, MD, MPH – Faculty
4. Geoffrey Froehlich, MD – Faculty
5. Matthew Johnson, MD – Faculty
6. AJ Kirk, MD – Faculty
7. Mary McHugh, MD – Faculty
8. Samuel Parnell, MD – Faculty
9. Brittney Rooney, MD – Faculty
10. Ariana Shaari, BA – Faculty
11. Sharon A. Swencki, MD, FACEP – Faculty
12. Laura Welsh, MD – Faculty
13. Michael S. Beeson, MD, MBA, FACEP – Faculty/Planner
14. Joshua S. Broder, MD, FACEP – Faculty/Planner
15. Andrew J. Eyre, MD, MS-HPEd – Faculty/Planner
16. Walter L. Green, MD, FACEP – Faculty/Planner
17. John Kiel, DO, MPH, FACEP, CAQSM – Faculty/Planner
18. Frank LoVecchio, DO, MPH, FACEP – Faculty/Planner
19. Sharon E. Mace, MD, FACEP – Faculty/Planner
20. Amal Mattu, MD, FACEP – Faculty/Planner
21. Christian A. Tomaszewski, MD, MS, MBA, FACEP – Faculty/Planner
22. Steven J. Warrington, MD, MEd, MS – Faculty/Planner
23. Tareq Al-Salamah, MBBS, MPH, FACEP – Planner
24. Wan-Tsu Chang, MD – Planner
25. Ann M. Dietrich, MD, FAAP, FACEP – Planner
26. Kelsey Drake, MD, MPH, FACEP – Planner
27. John C. Greenwood – Planner
28. Danya Khoujah, MBBS, MEHP, FACEP – Planner
29. Nathaniel Mann, MD – Planner
30. George Sternbach, MD, FACEP – Planner
31. Joy Carrico, JD – Planner/Reviewer

Contributor Disclosures. In accordance with the ACCME Standards for Integrity and Independence in Accredited Continuing Education, all relevant financial relationships, and the absence of relevant financial relationships, must be disclosed to learners for all individuals in control of content 1) before learners engage with the accredited education, and 2) in a format that can be verified at the time of accreditation. The following individuals have reported relationships with ineligible companies, as defined by the ACCME. These relationships, in the context of their involvement in the CME activity, could be perceived by some as a real or apparent conflict of interest. All relevant financial relationships have been mitigated to ensure that no commercial bias has been inserted into the educational content. Joshua S. Broder, MD, FACEP, is a founder and president of OmniSono Inc, an ultrasound technology company, and a consultant on the Bayer USA Cardiac Imaging Advisory Board. Sharon E. Mace, MD, FACEP, performs contracted research funded by Biofire Corporation, Genetesis, Quidel, and IBSA Pharma. Frank LoVecchio, DO, MPH, FACEP, receives speaking fees from ABBVIE for antibiotics. Christian A. Tomaszewski, MD, MS, MBA, FACEP, performs contracted research for Roche, Pfizer, and AstraZeneca (site PI with financial support provided to institution). William J. Brady, MD, FACEP, holds an ownership interest in Medical Decisions. All remaining individuals with control over content have no relevant financial relationships to disclose.

This educational activity consists of two lessons, eight feature articles, a post-test, and evaluation questions; as designed, the activity should take approximately 5 hours to complete. The participant should, in order, review the learning objectives for the lesson or article, read the lesson or article as published in the print or online version until all have been reviewed, and then complete the online post-test (a minimum score of 75% is required) and evaluation questions. Release date: August 1, 2023. Expiration date: July 31, 2026.

Accreditation Statement. The American College of Emergency Physicians is accredited by the Accreditation Council for Continuing Medical Education to provide continuing medical education for physicians.

The American College of Emergency Physicians designates this enduring material for a maximum of 5 *AMA PRA Category 1 Credits™*. Physicians should claim only the credit commensurate with the extent of their participation in the activity.

Each issue of *Critical Decisions in Emergency Medicine* is approved by ACEP for 5 ACEP Category I credits. Approved by the AOA for 5 Category 2-B credits.

Commercial Support. There was no commercial support for this CME activity.

Target Audience. This educational activity has been developed for emergency physicians.

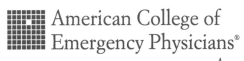
American College of Emergency Physicians®

ADVANCING EMERGENCY CARE

Critical decisions
in emergency medicine

Critical Decisions in Emergency Medicine is the official CME publication of the American College of Emergency Physicians. Additional volumes are available.

EDITOR-IN-CHIEF
Michael S. Beeson, MD, MBA, FACEP
Northeastern Ohio Universities,
Rootstown, OH

SECTION EDITORS
Joshua S. Broder, MD, FACEP
Duke University, Durham, NC

Andrew J. Eyre, MD, MS-HPEd
Brigham and Women's Hospital/
Harvard Medical School, Boston, MA

John Kiel, DO, MPH, FACEP, CAQSM
University of Florida College of Medicine,
Jacksonville, FL

Frank LoVecchio, DO, MPH, FACEP
Valleywise, Arizona State University, University of Arizona,
and Creighton Colleges of Medicine, Phoenix, AZ

Sharon E. Mace, MD, FACEP
Cleveland Clinic Lerner College of Medicine/
Case Western Reserve University, Cleveland, OH

Amal Mattu, MD, FACEP
University of Maryland, Baltimore, MD

Christian A. Tomaszewski, MD, MS, MBA, FACEP
University of California Health Sciences,
San Diego, CA

Steven J. Warrington, MD, MEd, MS
MercyOne Siouxland, Sioux City, IA

ASSOCIATE EDITORS
Tareq Al-Salamah, MBBS, MPH, FACEP
King Saud University, Riyadh, Saudi Arabia/
University of Maryland, Baltimore, MD

Wan-Tsu Chang, MD
University of Maryland, Baltimore, MD

Ann M. Dietrich, MD, FAAP, FACEP
University of South Carolina College of Medicine,
Greenville, SC

Kelsey Drake, MD, MPH, FACEP
St. Anthony Hospital, Lakewood, CO

Walter L. Green, MD, FACEP
UT Southwestern Medical Center, Dallas, TX

John C. Greenwood, MD
University of Pennsylvania, Philadelphia, PA

Danya Khoujah, MBBS, MEHP, FACEP
University of Maryland, Baltimore, MD

Nathaniel Mann, MD
Greenville Health System, Greenville, SC

George Sternbach, MD, FACEP
Stanford University Medical Center, Stanford, CA

EDITORIAL STAFF
Suzannah Alexander, Editorial Director
salexander@acep.org

Joy Carrico, JD
Managing Editor

Alex Bass
Assistant Editor

Kyle Powell
Graphic Artist

ISSN2325-0186 (Print)   ISSN2325-8365 (Online)

Contents

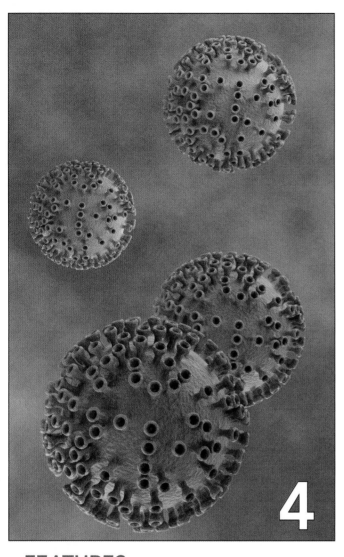

4

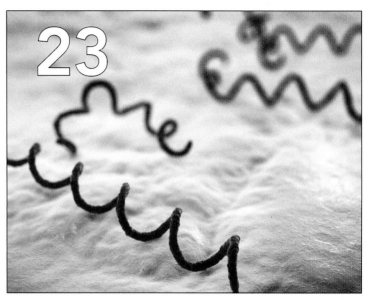

23

FEATURES

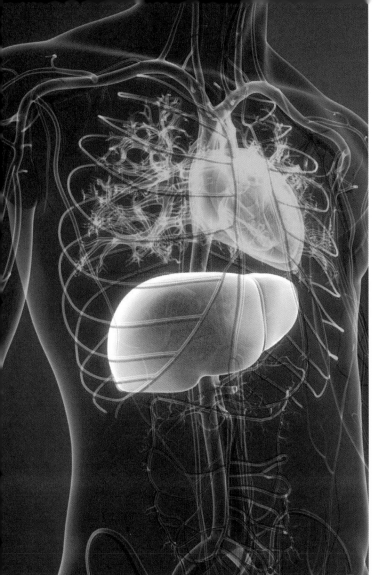

Yellow-Bellied

Liver Disease in the Emergency Department

LESSON 15

By Sharon A. Swencki, MD, FACEP; Geoffrey Froehlich, MD; and Matthew Johnson, MD

Dr. Swencki is an attending physician with MedStar Emergency Physicians at Medstar Harbor Hospital and Medstar Union Memorial Hospital in Baltimore, Maryland. Dr. Froehlich is an attending physician with Medstar Emergency Physicians at Medstar Union Memorial Hospital and Medstar Franklin Square Medical Center in Rossville, Maryland. Dr. Johnson is an emergency medicine resident at Medstar Georgetown University Hospital and Medstar Washington Hospital Center in Washington, DC.

Reviewed by Michael S. Beeson, MD, MBA, FACEP

Objectives

On completion of this lesson, you should be able to:

1. Identify infectious causes of ALD and CLD.
2. Describe the management of acetaminophen overdose.
3. Name the liver diseases that are associated with pregnancy.
4. Recall the management of acute hepatic failure.
5. Explain the management strategies for common complications of cirrhosis.
6. Discuss the management of liver transplant patients in the emergency department.

From the EM Model

2.0   Abdominal and Gastrointestinal Disorders
    2.3   Liver
          2.3.1   Noninfectious Hepatitis/Cirrhosis
          2.3.3   Infectious Disorders
          2.3.5   Hepatic Encephalopathy
13.0   Obstetrics and Gynecology
    13.3   Complications of Pregnancy

■ CRITICAL DECISIONS ■

- What clinical findings should raise suspicion for acute viral hepatitis, and how is the condition managed?
- What therapies are available for infectious causes of liver disease?
- What medications are usually involved in drug-induced liver failure, and what antidotes should be given?
- What are the unique causes of liver disease in pregnancy, and how are they diagnosed?
- What treatments are indicated for patients with acute liver failure?
- What are the most common complications of CLD, and how are they managed?
- How should coagulopathy be approached in patients with CLD?
- How should post–liver transplant patients be managed in the emergency department?

Liver disease is seen daily in the emergency department — roughly 25% of people in the United States have some form of it. Diagnosing liver conditions can be challenging: Symptoms vary widely in type and severity. Emergency physicians must understand the pathophysiology and etiology of the different types of liver disease to manage both acute and chronic cases.

CASE PRESENTATIONS

■ CASE ONE

A 28-year-old man presents with nausea, vomiting, mild abdominal pain, and jaundice. He states that he has been using intravenous drugs for the past 6 months but denies a history of hepatitis. His vital signs include BP 110/72, P 115, R 22, and T 38.4°C (101.1°F). His scleras are icteric, and his mucous membranes are dry. The patient's lungs are clear, and his heart sounds are tachycardic but regular. The abdomen is soft, with mild right upper quadrant tenderness. Hepatomegaly is present, with palpable, firm liver edges. Laboratory tests reveal mild dehydration. ALT and AST levels are more than 1,000 units/L; the serum total bilirubin concentration is elevated at 6.4 mg/dL.

■ CASE TWO

A 35-year-old pregnant woman at 33 weeks' twin gestation presents with dizziness and abdominal pain. She reports acute epigastric pain, nausea, and vomiting that started about 2 hours ago. The patient's pregnancy had been going well until recently, when she began experiencing headaches and swelling in her hands and face.

A physical examination reveals a gravid patient who is pale and diaphoretic; she is in obvious pain. Her vital signs include BP 75/46, P 136, R 28, and T 37.2°C (98.9°F). Her head and neck examination is unremarkable. The woman's lungs are clear; her heart is tachycardic; and her abdomen is gravid, with a palpable fundus well above the umbilicus. The abdomen is somewhat rigid and extremely tender. Laboratory abnormalities include a platelet count of 68,000/μL, an AST concentration of 870 units/L, an ALT concentration of 300 units/L, a bilirubin level of 18 mg/dL, and an INR of 2.6; her urinalysis shows proteinuria. A bedside sonogram reveals free fluid in the abdomen and two fetuses with heart rates of 113 and 105 bpm.

■ CASE THREE

A 51-year-old man presents with a 24-hour history of an acute mental status change. The patient is accompanied by his daughter, who states that her father began vomiting yesterday and then became disoriented. Over the next 24 hours, he became more agitated, confused, and aggressive. The patient has a history of a hepatitis C infection and sometimes takes lactulose for inattention, trouble sleeping, and disorientation.

In the emergency department, he is diaphoretic, yelling, and grabbing at the air. His vital signs include BP 147/99, P 109, R 20, and T 36.4°C (97.5°F). His scleras are icteric, and his mucous membranes are moist. The neck is supple, lungs are clear, and heart sounds are tachycardic. The abdomen is soft but distended, with a positive fluid wave. Engorged superficial vessels are noted on the abdomen. A rectal examination shows heme-negative brown stool. The patient is alert but does not follow commands. He is moving all four extremities, and asterixis is present. A CBC reveals a hematocrit measurement of 38.8% and a platelet count of 90,000/μL. Electrolyte studies are notable for the following concentrations: sodium 135 mEq/L, potassium 5.2 mEq/L, chloride 109 mEq/L, CO_2 16 mEq/L, BUN 42 mg/dL, and creatinine 2.2 mg/dL. Liver function tests show only minor abnormalities. The blood ammonia level is 162 μg/dL.

Introduction

Liver disease can be acute or chronic. Acute liver disease (ALD) can result from infection, metabolic disturbances, toxic injury, or hepatic perfusion abnormalities, all of which lead to hepatic inflammation or injury with hepatocyte necrosis and potential scarring in the liver. The clinical spectrum of disease ranges from asymptomatic infections to acute liver failure.

Chronic liver disease (CLD) is the 12th leading cause of death in the United States — the American Liver Foundation estimates that roughly 25% of people in the United States live with some form of liver disease. CLD leads to cirrhosis. The most common causes of cirrhosis are viral hepatitis, alcoholic liver disease, and nonalcoholic fatty liver disease.[1] Many patients are asymptomatic during the period of compensated cirrhosis and may be diagnosed only because of their history and abnormal laboratory findings (eg, increased bilirubin levels, elevated PTT and INR, decreased albumin levels, and decreased platelet counts). These patients should be referred for further workup if the condition is discovered in the emergency department.[2]

CRITICAL DECISION

What clinical findings should raise suspicion for acute viral hepatitis, and how is the condition managed?

Most patients with viral hepatitis present during the symptomatic phase of the illness. Common initial complaints that should raise suspicion for ALD include right upper quadrant pain, fatigue, anorexia, aversion to strong odors, and dark urine or pale stools. A history of travel, consumption of undercooked foods, intravenous drug use, sexual contacts, and exposure to another person with viral hepatitis are important risk factors to assess. The physical examination may reveal jaundice or a firm, enlarged liver with palpable margins. Dehydration can also be present secondary to nausea and vomiting.[3]

When viral hepatitis is suspected, laboratory studies to order include a full set of liver function tests; a coagulation profile; and alkaline phosphatase, creatinine, electrolyte, and fractionated serum bilirubin levels. Elevated conjugated or direct bilirubin concentrations are predominant in acute viral hepatitis; markedly elevated aminotransferases to the hundreds to thousands and an AST:ALT ratio of less than 1 are to be expected.[4]

The mainstay of emergency department management of acute viral hepatitis is supportive care, including intravenous rehydration and treatment of nausea and pain. Signs and symptoms that should raise concern for more severe disease include an altered mental status, hypoglycemia, severe hyperbilirubinemia, renal insufficiency, and prolonged coagulation tests. Hospital admission should be considered in patients with any of these ominous indicators of acute liver failure.[3]

Serologic tests for viral antibodies should be requested if acute viral hepatitis is suspected based on clinical findings. Although the results usually do not affect how acute hepatitis is managed in the emergency department, they will aid in the patient's inpatient or follow-up care. Ammonia levels can also be elevated and should be assessed in any patient with an altered mental status from presumed acute hepatitis.[3]

Admission Guidelines

Most patients with viral hepatitis do not require hospital admission (*Table 1*). Patients with clinical and laboratory indicators of acute liver failure should be admitted to the ICU.[4] For those discharged home, a primary care physician should be enlisted to provide additional monitoring, education, follow-up for hepatitis serologic tests, and any necessary treatment.

CRITICAL DECISION

What therapies are available for infectious causes of liver disease?

Infectious hepatitis is a significant burden worldwide and a frequent cause of both ALD and CLD. Numerous viruses are known to cause liver inflammation. However, the hepatotropic viruses, termed A to E, are the most common culprits.[5] Less common infectious causes of liver disease include liver abscesses and sexually transmitted infections. Various therapies are available for both prevention and treatment of these infections.

Hepatitis A, B, and D are vaccine-preventable diseases. The hepatitis A vaccine should be administered to any patient diagnosed with the hepatitis A virus (HAV) who has not already been immunized, preferably within 14 days of exposure. Along with the first dose of the hepatitis A vaccine, a single intramuscular injection of hepatitis A immune globulin is preferred in children older than 1 year, adults older than 40 years, and immunocompromised patients.[6] The hepatitis B vaccine is protective against both the hepatitis B virus (HBV) and hepatitis D virus (HDV). In patients with known exposure to HBV and no history of vaccination, both hepatitis B immune globulin and the first dose of the hepatitis B vaccine should be given within 2 weeks of exposure, preferably within the first 24 to 48 hours.[7] Generally, the therapy for infection with HBV is supportive, although symptomatic patients and those who develop complications (bilirubin level >3 mg/dL, coagulopathy, and acute liver failure) may benefit from antiretroviral therapy.[8]

No vaccine exists for the hepatitis C virus (HCV); however, direct-acting antivirals are the treatment of choice for HCV infections. The major liver societies agree in recommending that all treatment-naïve and treatment-experienced individuals who are infected with HCV should be started on targeted antiviral therapy with a goal of achieving an undetectable viral load at 12 or 24 weeks. Although various antiviral cocktails exist, ultimately all require genotype testing prior to initiating therapy; these antiviral treatments are beyond the scope of this lesson.[9]

Various other viruses can cause liver inflammation. The most common are cytomegalovirus (CMV), Epstein-Barr virus (EBV), and herpes simplex virus (HSV). However, varicella-zoster virus, adenovirus, influenza, human herpesvirus 6, chikungunya, dengue, and even Ebola have been implicated in viral liver disease. These infections have a wide range of presentations. They typically cause a relatively mild primary infection but can cause acute and, possibly, severe liver disease in immunocompromised hosts. Targeted therapy is often available, including ganciclovir for CMV and acyclovir for HSV and EBV.

Bacteria, fungi, and pathogenic amoebas can also cause a variety of hepatic infections. These infections typically cause liver abscesses and mostly occur in immunocompromised patients and patients with underlying malignancies. The prototypic examples include pyogenic abscesses caused by *Escherichia coli*

Acute Viral Hepatitis Admission Criteria
• Severe dehydration
• Significant electrolyte abnormalities
• Intractable vomiting
• Significant comorbid disease
• Immunocompromise
• Age >50 years
• Acute liver failure (altered mental status, hypoglycemia, elevated INR, severe bilirubinemia, renal insufficiency)

TABLE 1. Admission criteria for acute viral hepatitis

and *Klebsiella pneumoniae*. *Entamoeba histolytica* causes amebic liver abscesses. Fungal abscesses, primarily due to *Candida albicans*, often occur in patients with prolonged antibiotic exposure, hematologic malignancies, solid organ transplants, or other immunodeficiencies.[10] Fitz-Hugh–Curtis syndrome is an uncommon perihepatic complication of pelvic inflammatory disease and is caused by *Neisseria gonorrhoeae* or *Chlamydia trachomatis*.[11] Therapies for each of these conditions target the underlying infectious agent.

CRITICAL DECISION

What medications are usually involved in drug-induced liver failure, and what antidotes should be given?

Drug-induced liver injury (DILI) can range from mild elevations in liver enzymes to fulminant liver failure. DILI is the most common cause of acute liver failure in the United States and many other western countries.[12] Acetaminophen is the most common offending agent, accounting for up to 42% of cases.[13,14] Antimicrobial drugs (eg, amoxicillin-clavulanate, trimethoprim-sulfamethoxazole, isoniazid, and nitrofurantoin) remain the most common cause of nonacetaminophen DILI. Antiepileptics, antiarrhythmics (amiodarone), chemotherapeutic drugs (methotrexate), and, increasingly, herbal and dietary supplements are other causes.[15-17]

Acetaminophen is a dose-dependent toxin.[14] Therapeutic doses are defined as less than 4 g/day for adults and less than 75 mg/kg/day for children. For single-dose ingestions, drug levels are measured relative to the time of ingestion, and the concentrations are applied to the Rumack-Matthews nomogram to assess for toxicity. Levels should be measured at least 4 hours after acute ingestion. Serial measurements up to 12 hours after ingestion may be needed to fully exclude significant overdose with extended-release preparations. Serum acetaminophen levels above 150 mg/L at 4 hours are considered toxic. However, the United Kingdom decreased its treatment threshold to 100 mg/L at the 4-hour mark in 2012.[13] Chronic or staggered acetaminophen ingestions cannot be applied to this nomogram and should be considered for treatment regardless of the initial drug levels.[13]

Acetylcysteine therapy is the antidote for acetaminophen overdose. It targets the hepatotoxic metabolite of acetaminophen, N-acetyl-p-benzoquinone imine. Acetylcysteine is most effective when administered within 8 to 10 hours after ingestion, but its beneficial effects can be extended.[14] If there is any possibility a patient was exposed to a toxic level of acetaminophen, the emergency physician should initiate treatment, either orally (with a loading dose of 140 mg/kg; then 70 mg/kg every 4 hours for a total of 17 doses over 3 days) or intravenously (with a loading dose of 150 mg/kg; then 50 mg/kg for 4 hours; then 100 mg/kg over

	Hyperemesis Gravidarum[18]	HELLP Syndrome[19]	AFLP[20]	ICP[21]
Frequency	0.3%-3.0%	0.05%-0.7%	<0.1%	0.3%-0.5%
Etiology	Unknown, likely multifactorial	Continuum with eclamptic diseases	Possibly related to deficiencies in fatty acid metabolism	Unknown
Risk factors	Increased placental mass, motion sickness, migraines, family or personal history	Nulliparity, multigestation, hypertension, diabetes mellitus, preeclampsia, chronic kidney disease, autoimmune disease, etc.	Multigestation, obesity, diabetes mellitus, hepatic disorders, nulliparity, a male fetus, fetal fatty acid oxidation disorders	Hepatitis, nonalcoholic liver disease, gallstones, cholecystitis, pancreatitis
Timing	1st trimester	3rd trimester, rarely 2nd	3rd trimester	2nd and 3rd trimesters
Symptoms	Persistent vomiting, weight loss	Right upper quadrant pain, malaise, nausea and vomiting	Nausea and vomiting, jaundice, hypoglycemia, abdominal pain, encephalopathy, polyuria/polydipsia	Pruritus
Diagnostics	Weight loss >5% pre-pregnancy weight	Elevated LDH 2/2 hemolysis, low platelet count, hypertension, proteinuria	Swansea criteria can help stratify; liver biopsy is diagnostic	Elevated bile acid levels (>10 mmol/L)
AST/ALT	<300 units/L	<500 units/L	<500 units/L	Minimal increase
Bilirubin	<4 mg/dL	Typically normal	Elevated	<6 mg/dL
Treatment	1st trimester: doxylamine and vitamin B$_6$ 2nd trimester: serotonin antagonists and phenothiazine products IV hydration +/– dextrose	Airway, breathing, and circulation; blood pressure control; obstetrics consult for delivery	Airway, breathing, and circulation; coagulopathy correction; obstetrics consult for delivery	1st trimester: ursodeoxycholic acid
Disposition	Admission if unable to tolerate oral intake	Best managed at a referral center	Best managed at a referral center	No maternal risks but need close outpatient follow-up due to fetal risks

TABLE 2. Comparison of various pregnancy-related liver disorders

the next 16 hours).[14] Treatment can be stopped if further evaluation reveals the patient was not exposed to a toxic amount of the drug.

Treatment for hepatotoxicity secondary to nonacetaminophen drug use requires cessation of the offending agent and supportive care; no targeted treatments have yet been found.[15,17] Using acetylcysteine in nonacetaminophen acute liver failure has shown some benefit in early stages of the disease in adult patients but, unfortunately, has not shown benefit in pediatric patients.[17]

CRITICAL DECISION

What are the unique causes of liver disease in pregnancy, and how are they diagnosed?

Pregnancy-related liver disorders are uncommon. They can lead to death but can be prevented with timely recognition and management. Although the previously discussed liver disorders can occur in pregnancy, there are several that specifically affect pregnant women. These include hyperemesis gravidarum; hemolysis, elevated liver enzymes, and low platelets (HELLP) syndrome; acute fatty liver disease of pregnancy (AFLP); and intrahepatic cholestasis of pregnancy (ICP) (*Table 2*). Given their significant clinical and laboratory overlap, these diseases often present a diagnostic dilemma.

CRITICAL DECISION

What treatments are indicated for patients with acute liver failure?

The current, most widely accepted definition of acute liver failure comes from the American Association for the Study of Liver Diseases (AASLD): an INR ≥1.5, neurologic dysfunction with any degree of hepatic encephalopathy, no prior evidence of

liver disease, and a course of disease ≤26 weeks.[22,23] This relatively rare but serious disease process is diagnosed in an estimated 2,000 US patients each year and leads to multiorgan dysfunction with neurologic, renal, pulmonary, and hemodynamic sequelae.[23]

Specific targeted therapy exists for only a handful of conditions that cause acute liver failure (*Table 3*). For the remainder, supportive care is the mainstay of treatment. This includes providing volume expansion, correcting acid or base status and electrolyte levels, maintaining normothermia and normoglycemia, avoiding fluid overload, correcting hypoxia and protecting the airway, controlling fever, avoiding nephrotoxic medications, and closely monitoring the patient for infections to ensure rapid diagnosis and treatment.[24,25] Although it is one of the diagnostic criteria for acute liver failure, coagulopathy is generally not corrected unless patients are actively bleeding or undergoing invasive procedures.[24]

Patients with acute liver failure are at a high risk of fungal and bacterial infections (up to 80%).[26] Worsening of hepatic

Cause	Therapy
Infectious causes	Antibiotics, antivirals, antifungals
Acetaminophen overdose Nonacetaminophen drug ingestion	Acetylcysteine may be considered
Amanita muscaria mushroom	Penicillin or silibinin
Pregnancy-related liver disorders	Delivery of fetus
Autoimmune hepatitis	Corticosteroids
Acute ischemic liver injury ("shock liver")	Cardiovascular support

TABLE 3. Specific therapies for acute liver failure

Grade	Signs
I	Changes in behavior with minimal change in level of consciousness
II	Gross disorientation, drowsiness, possibly asterixis, inappropriate behavior
III	Marked confusion, incoherent speech, sleeping most of the time but arousable to vocal stimuli
IV	Comatose, unresponsive to pain, decorticate or decerebrate posturing

TABLE 4. Grades of encephalopathy

Acetaminophen-Induced Acute Liver Failure
Arterial pH <7.3 after resuscitation Lactate >3.0 mmol/L after adequate fluid resuscitation Or all three within a 24-hr period: • Hepatic encephalopathy (grade III or IV) • INR >6.5 • Creatinine level >3.4 mg/dL

Nonacetaminophen Acute Liver Failure

INR >6.5 and any grade of encephalopathy
Or any grade of encephalopathy plus three of the following:
• Age <10 or >40 years
• Jaundice for >7 days before onset of encephalopathy
• INR ≥3.5
• Serum bilirubin ≥17 mg/dL
• Unfavorable etiology, such as:
  • Wilson disease
  • Idiosyncratic drug reaction
  • Seronegative hepatitis

TABLE 5. King's College criteria (AASLD guidelines – acute liver failure)

encephalopathy or renal function may be the only sign of infection. Surveillance for infectious complications with chest x-rays and periodic cultures of urine, sputum, and blood are warranted, and prophylactic antibiotics are often administered.[23,26] A low threshold should be maintained to start antibiotics and antifungals in these patients, especially if they are encephalopathic or have evidence of acute organ failure.[24]

Cerebral edema and intracranial hypertension (ICH) are the most severe complications of acute liver failure and can lead to uncal herniation.[25] An altered mental status warrants ICU admission because altered patients can rapidly deteriorate, and the change in mental status indicates a poor prognosis.[23,25] Hepatic encephalopathy is graded from I to IV (*Table 4*). The risk of cerebral edema and ICH increases with an increasing grade of encephalopathy.[26] Exposure to sustained elevation of circulating plasma ammonia is felt to play a role in the pathophysiology of cerebral edema and ICH; treatment is aimed at lowering cerebral ammonia uptake.[23] Oral or rectal lactulose therapy holds a role in the treatment of hepatic encephalopathy in acute liver failure.[22] Other supportive therapies (which are similar to those used to treat traumatic brain injury) can be utilized (eg, head of bed elevation, maintenance of blood pressure and normoglycemia, and the use of hypertonic saline).[24]

Early referral of patients with acute liver failure to specialty centers that perform transplantation can aid in preventing and limiting the progression of acute liver failure and in increasing the chance of survival.[24] The King's College criteria can help guide referral for a liver transplant in both acetaminophen and nonacetaminophen cases of acute liver failure (*Table 5*).

CRITICAL DECISION

What are the most common complications of CLD, and how are they managed?

In chronic viral hepatitis, caused primarily by HBV and HCV, liver damage is mostly from immunologically driven hepatocellular necrosis. An estimated 2.4 million Americans are thought to be infected with HCV and another 850,000 with HBV. Most of these patients are unaware of their infections; both viruses typically cause indolent infections, with minimal symptoms, if any, although some patients with HBV have more acute disease with more rapid progression.[27,28] Currently, potential treatments for HBV include a number of medications that slow progression of the disease; curative treatment does not yet exist. For HCV, recently developed medications have shown a high degree of success in clearing infections, although access to these medications can be challenging.

In both alcoholic and nonalcoholic fatty liver disease, fatty infiltration of hepatocytes, called steatosis, is associated with hepatocellular injury and inflammation (although mechanisms differ between the two). The final common pathway in cirrhosis is persistent inflammation that leads to fibrosis and distorted liver architecture, with development of impaired organ function and sequelae such as portal hypertension. Treatment of alcoholic liver disease focuses on abstinence from alcohol intake, while treatment of nonalcoholic fatty liver disease focuses on the metabolic processes that lead to steatosis. Although some fibrosis is potentially reversible, treatment of the offending processes early in their course before the development of cirrhosis and its associated complications is a key individual and public health goal.

Ascites

Ascites is the most frequent complication of cirrhosis — it is experienced by roughly 60% of patients within 10 years of a cirrhosis diagnosis. However, ascites can occur in other disease processes as well. If patients without cirrhosis present with ascites, evaluation for alternative causes such as right heart failure, malignancy, pancreatic disease, tuberculosis, and renal pathology should be considered. Diagnostic paracentesis should be performed in patients with ascites.

The pathophysiology of ascites in patients with cirrhosis is complex but is related to portal hypertension and increased retention of sodium and water. Portal hypertension leads to a higher splanchnic blood volume and increased production of nitric oxide, which causes splanchnic vasodilation and further increases portal hypertension. Collateral circulation allows vasodilatory molecules to enter the systemic circulation and causes arterial vasodilation. These changes lead to effective hypovolemia that prompts the kidneys, sensing a relative malperfusion, to activate the renin-angiotensin-aldosterone system (RAAS), which increases sodium and water retention. Increased splanchnic hydrostatic pressure subsequently overwhelms the oncotic pressure, allowing transudative fluid to leak into the peritoneum.[29] Bacterial translocation and systemic inflammation are theorized to play a role as well.[30]

Medical therapy for ascites should be guided by moderate salt restriction and a sequential addition of aldosterone antagonists such as spironolactone, followed by loop diuretics. Adverse effects of loop diuretics are common, and doses must frequently be adjusted. Fluid restriction is reserved only for patients with substantial hyponatremia. NSAID use should be avoided to evade acute kidney injury (AKI), as should angiotensin-converting enzyme (ACE) inhibitors or angiotensin receptor blockers (ARB) to prevent relative hypovolemia from worsening. The addition of midodrine has been suggested to improve refractory ascites, but data quality is weak.[30]

A significant number of patients can become refractory to diuretic treatment, or adverse effects may limit its use, leaving large-volume paracentesis as the treatment of choice. In patients who undergo large-volume paracentesis (>5 L), administration of albumin at 6 to 8 g/L of ascites removed is recommended to prevent postparacentesis circulatory dysfunction (PPCD), worsened renal function, and rapid reaccumulation of ascites. Despite comorbid coagulopathy and thrombocytopenia frequently occurring in patients with ascites, these comorbidities are not a contraindication to paracentesis. Routine laboratory measurements and the prophylactic transfusion of blood products for reversal are discouraged.[30]

Patients who become refractory to medical therapy should be referred for procedures such as transjugular intrahepatic portosystemic shunt (TIPS), peritoneovenous shunt, or liver transplantation because these patients have a 6-month mortality rate as high as 20%. Patients with refractory ascites who are not being considered for a liver transplant should be offered a palliative care referral.[31]

Spontaneous Bacterial Peritonitis

Spontaneous bacterial peritonitis (SBP) is a feared complication of ascites because it carries a mortality rate of 20% per episode. Patients often present with localizing abdominal symptoms (eg, pain, tenderness, nausea, and vomiting), signs of systemic inflammation (eg, fever, leukocytosis, tachycardia, tachypnea, and shock), or other symptoms such as worsening encephalopathy, renal failure, or acute liver decompensation. A significant percentage of patients (10%-40%) are asymptomatic, so fluid removed by paracentesis should be analyzed. The incidence of SBP in hospitalized patients with ascites approaches 30%; thus, diagnostic paracentesis should be performed on all such patients, regardless of the admitting diagnosis.[30]

If SBP is suspected, a cell count and culture of the peritoneal fluid should be obtained. Patients with a peritoneal fluid polymorphonuclear leukocyte (PMN) count greater than 250/mm³ are at risk of SBP and should receive antibiotic treatment. Antibiotics should also be initiated for any patient who has signs or symptoms of SBP, regardless of the peritoneal fluid PMN count. Infections are typically monobacterial, mostly with enteric organisms and more than half the time with gram-negative bacteria. When cultures are positive, they can help confirm the diagnosis, but importantly, they may be negative in as many as 60% of patients. Typically, third-generation cephalosporins such as ceftriaxone and cefotaxime have been first-line treatments, but real consideration should be given to the risk of multidrug-resistant organisms. Carbapenems should be used in patients at risk of a nosocomial infection.[31]

In patients with a suspected secondary source of peritonitis, CT along with peritoneal cell counts should be obtained. Other testing of the peritoneal fluid for protein, glucose, lactate dehydrogenase (LDH), carcinoembryonic antigen (CEA), and alkaline phosphatase levels has been suggested to distinguish primary from secondary peritonitis, but no clear consensus exists.[30]

Albumin infusion should also be added to the treatment regimen at 1.5 g/kg in patients with SBP and a creatinine level greater than 1 mg/dL, BUN level greater than 30 mg/dL, or total bilirubin level greater than 5 mg/dL. Treatment with albumin infusion in patients with cirrhosis and non-SBP infections is not recommended.[31]

Hepatic Hydrothorax

Portal hypertension can also cause pleural effusions. These pleural effusions most commonly occur on the right side. Left-sided effusions or effusions in the absence of ascites should trigger a search for alternative causes. Treatment is like that of ascites, with sodium restriction, diuresis, and thoracentesis with albumin infusion as necessary. Reaccumulation is frequent, and referral for evaluation for TIPS or a liver transplant should be made for these patients.[31]

Hepatorenal Syndrome With AKI

Hepatorenal syndrome is a type of AKI that is specific to patients with cirrhosis, after exclusion of hypovolemia, other shock states, nephrotoxins, and anatomic factors. A rise in the serum creatinine level greater than 0.3 mg/dL or 50% from baseline in 48 hours is seen. This rise is thought to be caused by impaired renal perfusion via renal artery vasoconstriction that occurs after activation of the RAAS from decompensated splanchnic vasodilation. Hepatorenal syndrome can be associated with SBP or can occur spontaneously. These patients are best managed in the ICU, where hemodynamic parameters and fluid balance can be closely monitored. Patients should be treated with a combination of albumin and vasoconstrictors like terlipressin, an FDA-approved medication for this syndrome.[32] Available outside of the emergency department for some time, terlipressin is now the drug of choice for hepatorenal syndrome with AKI; norepinephrine is an alternative. These patients should also be considered for transfer to a transplant-capable center given the condition's high short-term mortality.[30]

✔ Pearls

- The mainstay of treatment for both ALD and CLD is general supportive care.

- Unstable gravid women with pregnancy-related liver diseases require delivery of the fetus as soon as possible.

- Acetylcysteine is the therapy of choice for ALD that is caused by acetaminophen toxicity but should be considered for all cases of ALD.

- Consult liver transplant centers early for patients with acute liver failure.

- All patients with variceal bleeding should be given antibiotics, which reduce mortality.

Hyponatremia

Hyponatremia is a frequent complication of cirrhosis. Hyponatremia (sodium level <130 mEq/L) is seen in almost a quarter of patients with cirrhosis. Patients are frequently asymptomatic, and treatment of chronic hyponatremia is often unnecessary.[31]

Hyponatremia can be either hypovolemic or hypervolemic. Hypovolemic hyponatremia tends to be more acute and is often due to aggressive diuresis. Treatment involves discontinuing diuretics and gently replacing intravascular volume with intravenous fluids.

Hypervolemic hyponatremia shares a pathogenesis with cirrhosis complications: activation of the RAAS axis and an increase in antidiuretic hormone secretion. Hypervolemic hyponatremia is almost always a chronic process, and overzealous correction runs the risk of precipitating osmotic demyelination syndrome. Fluid restriction of 1 to 1.5 L/day is the first-line treatment for severe hyponatremia (<125 mEq/L). Active treatment with hypertonic saline should be reserved for patients who have acute hyponatremia and severe symptoms such as encephalopathy or seizures. The goal rate for repletion is 4 to 6 mEq/L/24-hour period. Albumin infusion and ICU admission should be considered for these patients.[30]

Hepatic Encephalopathy

Hepatic encephalopathy is defined by the AASLD and the European Association for the Study of the Liver (EASL) as "brain dysfunction caused by liver insufficiency and/or portosystemic shunting; it manifests as a wide spectrum of neurological or psychiatric abnormalities ranging from subclinical alterations to coma." Like with acute liver failure, hepatic encephalopathy is staged from minimal impairment (recognized only with psychometric or neuropsychological testing) to stage IV (defined as comatose). Grades II through IV, referred to as overt hepatic encephalopathy, represent decompensated cirrhosis. An estimated 30% to 40% of patients with cirrhosis experience hepatic encephalopathy, with 20% to 80% experiencing minimal impairment and 5% to 25% experiencing overt hepatic encephalopathy within 5 years of diagnosis.[33]

The pathogenesis of hepatic encephalopathy is complex and not well understood. Increased portosystemic shunting is frequently associated, and patients with TIPS have a higher risk of hepatic encephalopathy. Ammonia is one of the chief substances implicated in this process, but blood ammonia levels are neither diagnostic nor prognostic. A normal ammonia level, however, should prompt a search for alternative causes of an altered mental status.

Acute decompensations can be triggered by a number of processes, including (but not limited to) GI bleeding (especially variceal bleeding), infection, medication effects, constipation, dietary changes, or worsening of hepatic or renal function. Because there is no definitive test for hepatic encephalopathy in the emergency department, a broad differential must be maintained, with particular attention paid to electrolyte abnormalities such as hyponatremia, hypoglycemia, ketoacidosis, infection, medication or intoxicant effects, or intracranial events such as stroke or hemorrhage.[33]

Treatment should be initiated for any patient with hepatic encephalopathy. In patients with grade III or IV encephalopathy, management of the airway and ICU admission should be strongly considered. Identification and control of the precipitating factor should be the primary focus; these strategies may be effective in up to 90% of patients. First-line therapy for hepatic encephalopathy is nonabsorbable disaccharides, including lactulose. Antibiotics such as rifaximin can also be added. These treatments can be given via a nasogastric tube in patients who are at risk for aspiration.[33]

Variceal Bleeding

Variceal bleeding is one of the most feared emergent complications of cirrhosis, and unfortunately, the development of upper GI tract varices is quite common in patients with liver disease. The prevalence of esophageal varices in patients with cirrhosis is 30% to 70% and is generally correlated with the severity of liver disease. Thirty percent of patients with esophageal varices have bleeding within the first year of this diagnosis.[34]

The treatment of acute bleeding from varices should start with resuscitation with blood products. Intubation should be considered to decrease the risk of blood aspiration. A restrictive transfusion strategy that targets a hemoglobin concentration of 7 g/dL versus 9 g/dL has been shown to decrease rebleeding in patients with variceal bleeding and reduce mortality in patients with milder cirrhosis. Higher transfusion thresholds should be considered in patients with other comorbidities or ongoing bleeding. Transfusion of platelets should be performed if the platelet count is below 50,000/μL or multiple units of blood products are being transfused. Fresh frozen plasma (FFP), plasma products such as cryoprecipitate and prothrombin complex concentrate (PCC), and recombinant factor VIIa should be used on a case-by-case basis and may be best employed with goal-directed strategies such as thromboelastography. Use of tranexamic acid is specifically discouraged in the 2022 EASL guidelines.[35]

Octreotide is the first-line treatment for variceal bleeds in the United States, but terlipressin has been the drug of choice in other countries, and recent FDA approval may increase its availability. Patients should be treated endoscopically with banding or sclerotherapy as soon as possible and should be considered for TIPS if banding or sclerotherapy is unsuccessful. In patients with severe bleeding, balloon tamponade with a Sengstaken-Blakemore, Minnesota, or similar tube should be attempted only when endoscopy or TIPS is unavailable.[35]

All patients with variceal bleeding should be treated with antibiotics; ceftriaxone is the typical drug of choice, although the possibility of multidrug-resistant organisms should be considered as well. Early treatment with antibiotics is shown to decrease rebleeding, reduce bacterial translocation and SBP, and improve survival.[35]

CRITICAL DECISION

How should coagulopathy be approached in patients with CLD?

Synthetic function of the hepatocytes is impaired in CLD. The liver produces proteins that possess both procoagulant and anticoagulant factors, potentially altering clotting hemostasis. It was long assumed that the increased INR seen in CLD shifted this balance in favor of coagulopathy. However, growing evidence suggests that this assumption may not always be true. This balance is extremely brittle, however, and subtle upsets of the tenuous equilibrium can push patients toward coagulopathy or hypercoagulability. Additionally, the frequent comorbidity of decreased platelet counts can make the assessment of bleeding risk in cirrhotic patients exceedingly difficult.[35]

The EASL's 2022 guidelines recommend against the use of traditional hemostatic and viscoelastic tests to gauge the risk of bleeding in patients with cirrhosis, although they can be used for benchmarking. In patients with cirrhosis, correction of INR with FFP before invasive procedures is strongly discouraged because it exposes patients to transfusion risks and the possibility of increased portal hypertension without a demonstrated effect on bleeding risk. Routine use of PCCs is also discouraged. Platelet transfusion is not recommended with counts above 50,000/μL. Consideration of platelet transfusion at lower counts should be done on a case-by-case basis.[35]

There is growing evidence that an increased INR does not preclude the development of venous thromboembolism (VTE) in patients with cirrhosis and that patients with CLD may be at a higher risk of VTE. Clinical prediction scores such as the Padua prediction score and the IMPROVE risk score were developed to determine which patients with cirrhosis are at a high risk of thromboembolic disease. Thromboprophylaxis with low-molecular-weight heparin (LMWH) is currently the first-line treatment, and treatment of VTE should be done with heparins rather than vitamin K antagonists. Current data on the use of direct oral anticoagulants (DOACs) is reassuring for patients with mild liver disease. Safety data on DOACs for patients with more severe cirrhosis is incomplete; DOACs should be used cautiously or avoided in these patients.[35]

CRITICAL DECISION

How should post–liver transplant patients be managed in the emergency department?

Because CLD is progressive, a number of patients ultimately undergo liver transplantation. Although transplantation may reduce some of the complications, a host of other aspects must be considered in the post-transplant patient. Coordination with their transplant team is important, and contact should be initiated early.

At one large US transplant center, despite aggressive follow-up interventions, roughly 45% of liver transplant patients sought care in the emergency department within the first postoperative year; 80% of them required hospital admission.[36] Another center in Korea reported a similar frequency of admission, with liver function test abnormalities and a fever as the most frequent specific causes for readmission.[37]

Investigation of abnormal liver function tests should include evaluation for ischemia, biliary obstruction, drug toxicity, and

hypersensitivity. Ultrasound and CT should be used liberally to identify structural abnormalities. Concern for transplant rejection may require biopsy.

Infectious complications in transplant patients are frequent — immunosuppression is most intense in the first year after transplantation. Culturing broadly in patients with a suspected infection is prudent; fungal and protozoal infections like *Pneumocystis jiroveci* pneumonia (PJP) may not typically be a concern in immunocompetent patients but should be considered in patients with liver transplants.

Summary

ALD arises from hepatic injury caused by infections, toxins, and other metabolic or perfusion abnormalities. Infectious hepatitis viruses — specifically HAV, HBV, and HCV — are the most common infectious causes of liver disease. Toxin-induced acute liver injury can result from many different medications; however, acetaminophen toxicity is one of the most common causes of ALD worldwide. Overdose with acetaminophen is treated with acetylcysteine therapy, both orally and intravenously. Several pregnancy-specific liver diseases exist and must be quickly recognized to ensure positive outcomes for both the mother and fetus. In cases of acute liver failure, care is mostly supportive and often requires ICU-level monitoring.

Cirrhosis of the liver is most often caused by chronic alcohol use or viral hepatitis (specifically HBV and HCV). Emergency physicians often manage the complications of CLD, including ascites, SBP, variceal bleeds, hepatorenal syndrome, hyponatremia, coagulopathy, and encephalopathy. Although general supportive care is the main management strategy for these patients, a thorough understanding of related complications and their causes can help guide specific targeted therapies.

Liver transplant patients are being seen more often in the emergency department. Their care should be coordinated with their transplant center. Liberal laboratory and imaging studies should be obtained in these patients.

REFERENCES

1. Younossi ZM, Koenig AB, Abdelatif D, Fazel Y, Henry L, Wymer M. Global epidemiology of nonalcoholic fatty liver disease — meta-analytic assessment of prevalence, incidence, and outcomes. *Hepatology.* 2016 Jul;64(1):73-84.

2. Marsano LS, Mendez C, Hill D, Barve S, McClain CJ. Diagnosis and treatment of alcoholic liver disease and its complications. *Alcohol Res Health.* 2003;27(3):247-256.

3. Samji NS. Viral hepatitis treatment and management. Medscape Drugs and Diseases. Updated July 7, 2023. https://emedicine.medscape.com/article/775507-treatment

4. O'Mara SR, Wiesner L. Hepatic disorders. In: Tintinalli JE, Ma O, Yealy DM, et al, eds. *Tintinalli's Emergency Medicine: A Comprehensive Study Guide.* 9th ed. McGraw-Hill Education; 2020:516-523.

5. Zarrin A, Akhondi H. Viral hepatitis. *StatPearls [Internet].* StatPearls Publishing; 2022. Last updated August 8, 2022. https://www.ncbi.nlm.nih.gov/books/NBK556029/

6. Foster MA, Haber P, Nelson NP. Hepatitis A. *Epidemiology and Prevention of Vaccine-Preventable Diseases.* 14th ed. CDC; 2021. Last updated August 18, 2021. https://www.cdc.gov/vaccines/pubs/pinkbook/hepa.html

7. Haber P, Schilie S. Hepatitis B. *Epidemiology and Prevention of Vaccine-Preventable Diseases.* 14th ed. CDC; 2021. Last updated August 18, 2021. https://www.cdc.gov/vaccines/pubs/pinkbook/hepb.html

─────── ✖ **Pitfalls** ───────

- Diagnosing hepatic encephalopathy based on abnormal ammonia levels.

- Using FFP to normalize INR as a bleeding prophylaxis.

- Failing to consider the various causes of decompensation in post-transplant patients and failing to involve their transplant specialists.

- Overlooking an altered mental status in patients with acute liver failure as a harbinger of higher morbidity and the need for a higher level of care.

■ CASE ONE

The young man who used intravenous drugs was given antiemetic agents and intravenous fluids in the emergency department. He was able to tolerate oral hydration and was discharged home. Serology test results indicated that the patient had an acute HBV infection.

■ CASE TWO

A diagnosis of hepatic rupture was considered in the pregnant woman with HELLP syndrome because of her severe abdominal pain, acute abdominal examination findings, hypotension, and free fluid on abdominal ultrasonography. The patient underwent an immediate emergency cesarean delivery and packing of the liver. Her postoperative course was complicated by disseminated intravascular coagulation and renal failure; however, after a long hospitalization, she was discharged home. After an uneventful course in the neonatal ICU, both babies were discharged in good condition.

■ CASE THREE

The disoriented middle-aged man was admitted to the hospital. Lactulose was given via a nasogastric tube, and the patient was hydrated with intravenous fluids and treated prophylactically with antibiotics. Diagnostic paracentesis showed no evidence of SBP. The patient's mental status improved, and he signed out against medical advice. He is currently awaiting a liver transplant.

8. Wu YL, Shen CL, Chen XY. Antiviral treatment for chronic hepatitis B: safety, effectiveness, and prognosis. *World J Clin Cases.* 2019 Jul 26;7(14):1784-1794.

9. Spearman CW, Dusheiko GM, Hellard M, Sonderup M. Hepatitis C. *Lancet.* 2019 Oct 19;394(10207):1451-1466.

10. Czerwonko ME, Huespe P, Bertone S, et al. Pyogenic liver abscess: current status and predictive factors for recurrence and mortality of first episodes. *HPB (Oxford).* 2016 Dec;18(12):1023-1030.

11. Theofanakis CP, Kyriakidis AV. Fitz-Hugh–Curtis syndrome. *Gynecol Surg.* 2011;8:129-134.

12. Ye H, Nelson LJ, Gómez Del Moral M, Martínez-Naves E, Cubero FJ. Dissecting the molecular pathophysiology of drug-induced liver injury. *World J Gastroenterol.* 2018 Apr 7;24(13):1373-1385.

13. Lancaster EM, Hiatt JR, Zarrinpar A. Acetaminophen hepatotoxicity: an updated review. *Arch Toxicol.* 2015 Feb;89(2):193-199.

14. Bunchorntavakul C, Reddy KR. Acetaminophen-related hepatotoxicity. *Clin Liver Dis.* 2013 Nov;17(4):587-607.

15. Reuben A, Koch DG, Lee WM; Acute Liver Failure Study Group. Drug-induced acute liver failure: results of a U.S. multicenter, prospective study. *Hepatology.* 2010 Dec;52(6):2065-2076.

16. Björnsson HK, Björnsson ES. Drug-induced liver injury: pathogenesis, epidemiology, clinical features, and practical management. *Eur J Intern Med.* 2022 Mar;97:26-31.

17. Alempijevic T, Zec S, Milosavljevic T. Drug-induced liver injury: do we know everything? *World J Hepatol.* 2017 Apr 8;9(10):491-502.

18. Committee on Practice Bulletins-Obstetrics. ACOG practice bulletin no. 189: nausea and vomiting of pregnancy. *Obstet Gynecol.* 2018 Jan;131(1):e15-e30.

19. Gestational hypertension and preeclampsia: ACOG practice bulletin, number 222. *Obstet Gynecol.* 2020 Jun;135(6):e237-e260.

20. Nelson DB, Byrne JJ, Cunningham FG. Acute fatty liver of pregnancy. *Obstet Gynecol.* 2021 Mar 1;137(3):535-546.

21. Lee RH, Greenberg M, Metz TD, Pettker CM; Society for Maternal-Fetal Medicine. Society for Maternal-Fetal Medicine Consult Series #53: intrahepatic cholestasis of pregnancy: replaces consult #13, April 2011. *Am J Obstet Gynecol.* 2021 Feb;224(2):B2-B9.

22. Montrief T, Koyfman A, Long B. Acute liver failure: a review for emergency physicians. *Am J Emerg Med.* 2019 Feb;37(2):329-337.

23. Polson J, Lee WM; American Association for the Study of Liver Disease. AASLD position paper: the management of acute liver failure. *Hepatology.* 2005 May;41(5):1179-1197.

24. Jayalakshmi VT, Bernal W. Update on the management of acute liver failure. *Curr Opin Crit Care.* 2020 Apr;26(2):163-170.

25. Bernal W, Wendon J. Acute liver failure. *N Engl J Med.* 2013 Dec 26;369(26):2525-2534.

26. Singanayagam A, Bernal W. Update on acute liver failure. *Curr Opin Crit Care.* 2015 Apr;21(2):134-141.

27. Edlin BR, Eckhardt BJ, Shu MA, Holmberg SD, Swan T. Toward a more accurate estimate of the prevalence of hepatitis C in the United States. *Hepatology.* 2015 Nov;62(5):1353-1363.

28. Roberts H, Kruszon-Moran D, Ly KN, et al. Prevalence of chronic hepatitis B virus (HBV) infection in U.S. households: National Health and Nutrition Examination Survey (NHANES), 1988-2012. *Hepatology.* 2016;63(2):388-397.

29. Moore KP, Wong F, Gines P, et al. The management of ascites in cirrhosis: report on the consensus conference of the International Ascites Club. *Hepatology.* 2003 Jul;38(1):258-266.

30. Biggins SW, Angeli P, Garcia-Tsao G, et al. Diagnosis, evaluation, and management of ascites, spontaneous bacterial peritonitis and hepatorenal syndrome: 2021 practice guidance by the American Association for the Study of Liver Diseases. *Hepatology.* 2021 Aug;74(2):1014-1048.

31. Aithal GP, Palaniyappan N, China L, et al. Guidelines on the management of ascites in cirrhosis. *Gut.* 2021 Jan;70(1):9-29.

32. FDA approves treatment to improve kidney function in adults with hepatorenal syndrome. U.S. Food & Drug Administration. Updated September 14, 2022. https://www.fda.gov/drugs/news-events-human-drugs/fda-approves-treatment-improve-kidney-function-adults-hepatorenal-syndrome

33. Vilstrup H, Amodio P, Bajaj J, et al. Hepatic encephalopathy in chronic liver disease: 2014 Practice Guideline by the American Association for the Study of Liver Diseases and the European Association for the Study of the Liver. *Hepatology.* 2014 Aug;60(2):715-735.

34. LaBrecque D, Khan AG, Sarin SK, et al. World Gastroenterology Organisation global guidelines esophageal varices. World Gastroenterology Organisation. Published January 2014. https://www.worldgastroenterology.org/guidelines/esophageal-varices/esophageal-varices-english

35. European Association for the Study of the Liver. EASL Clinical Practice Guidelines on prevention and management of bleeding and thrombosis in patients with cirrhosis. *J Hepatol.* 2022 May;76(5):1151-1184.

36. McElroy LM, Schmidt KA, Richards CT, et al. Early postoperative emergency department care of abdominal transplant recipients. *Transplantation.* 2015 Aug;99(8):1652-1657.

37. Oh SY, Lee JM, Lee H, et al. Emergency department visits and unanticipated readmissions after liver transplantation: a retrospective observational study. *Sci Rep.* 2018 Mar 6;8(1):4084.

MDCALC

https://www.mdcalc.com/calc/568/acetaminophen-overdose-nac-dosing

https://www.mdcalc.com/guidelines/507/acg/liver-disease-pregnancy

https://www.mdcalc.com/calc/674/hepatic-encephalopathy-grades-stages

https://www.mdcalc.com/calc/532/kings-college-criteria-acetaminophen-toxicity

https://www.mdcalc.com/guidelines/10365/acg/evaluation-abnormal-liver-chemistries

https://www.mdcalc.com/calc/2023/padua-prediction-score-risk-vte

https://www.mdcalc.com/calc/10349/improve-risk-score-venous-thromboembolism-vte

Intrauterine Device Removal

By Steven J. Warrington, MD, MEd, MS
MercyOne Siouxland in Sioux City, Iowa

Objective

On completion of this article, you should be able to:
- Discuss the steps to remove an IUD.

Introduction

Although uncommon, patients sometimes present to emergency departments for removal of intrauterine devices (IUDs). The procedure for removal is generally quick and simple, without the need for additional equipment. For a patient who is unable to tolerate an IUD, removal can significantly improve and resolve symptoms.

Contraindications
- Concern for extrauterine location
- Pregnancy

Benefits and Risks

The primary benefit of IUD removal is usually symptomatic relief. However, some patients request removal at the emergency department to end contraception.

Patients with intact and well-positioned devices and who are not yet pregnant have minimal risks with the procedure. Some patients, however, may feel discomfort, have a vasovagal reaction, or experience symptoms of pain, nausea, dizziness, cramping, and spotting that can last for a few days. If the device's strings are lost, more invasive instrumentation is needed for removal; rare complications such as bleeding, infection, or perforation can occur in these situations. If a patient is pregnant with the IUD in place, there is a risk of abortion; a specialist generally manages this type of situation.

Alternatives

The primary alternative to IUD removal in the emergency department is referral for removal by a specialist, which is generally done in the outpatient or operative setting. Sometimes, however, these specialists remove IUDs in the emergency department, depending on the patient's situation.

Reducing Side Effects

There are minimal side effects to IUD removal, although pretreatment can reduce patient discomfort. Pretreatment may include NSAIDs or local or regional anesthetics such as a paracervical block.

Special Considerations

Although IUD removal is generally a mild procedure, some patients experience significant discomfort or have a vasovagal reaction. Individuals at a higher likelihood of these reactions are those who have had prior reactions during IUD placement or cervical procedures and those who are nulliparous or require cervical dilation.

If the patient believes the IUD is in place but no strings are visible, the device may have migrated. A single plain x-ray of the pelvis should be able to demonstrate if there is an IUD present and can be quicker than other diagnostic routes. Alternatively, an ultrasound can help identify an IUD's presence and location (in the case of extrauterine IUDs). If the device is extrauterine, surgical removal is necessary. After removing an IUD, patients should receive education on alternative contraceptive therapy.

TECHNIQUE

1. **Consider** if the IUD may be extrauterine and decide if investigation of its location is needed prior to the device's removal.

2. **Obtain** the patient's consent and discuss the procedure.

3. **Set up** the speculum and ring forceps or other instrument to grasp the IUD strings and place the patient in the lithotomy position.

4. **Insert** the speculum and visualize the cervix; strings should be exiting from it.

5. **Grasp** the strings using the instrument of choice (eg, ringed forceps) and pull firmly toward the vaginal opening until the device is delivered.

6. **Discuss** potential symptoms and alternative methods of contraception with the patient. If there is concern for infection, consider culturing the IUD.

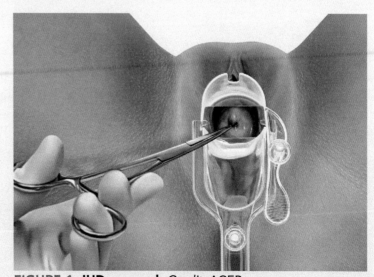

FIGURE 1. IUD removal. *Credit: ACEP.*

Flutter With Variable Block and Left Anterior Fascicular Block

By Jeremy Berberian, MD; William J. Brady, MD, FACEP; and Amal Mattu, MD, FACEP

Dr. Berberian is the associate director of emergency medicine residency education at ChristianaCare and assistant professor of emergency medicine at Sidney Kimmel Medical College, Thomas Jefferson University in Philadelphia, Pennsylvania. Dr. Brady is a professor of emergency medicine, medicine, and nursing, and vice chair for faculty affairs in the Department of Emergency Medicine at the University of Virginia School of Medicine in Charlottesville. Dr. Mattu is a professor, vice chair, and codirector of the Emergency Cardiology Fellowship in the Department of Emergency Medicine at the University of Maryland School of Medicine in Baltimore.

Objectives

On completion of this article, you should be able to:

- Describe the ECG findings seen with atrial flutter.
- Identify the ratio of flutter waves to QRS complexes in an ECG with atrial flutter.
- Define the ECG characteristics of an LAFB.

CASE PRESENTATION

A 70-year-old woman presents with exertional dyspnea (*Figure 1*).

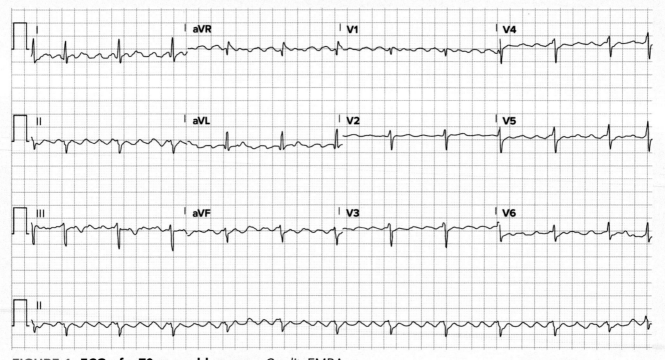

FIGURE 1. ECG of a 70-year-old woman. *Credit:* EMRA.

ECG Findings

The patient's ECG shows atrial flutter with variable block and an average ventricular rate of 68 bpm, left axis deviation, and a left anterior fascicular block (LAFB). Flutter waves, also called F waves, are best seen in the inferior leads and are diagnostic of atrial flutter. Atrial flutter is typically due to a right atrial reentry circuit around the tricuspid ring. It is classified as a macro-reentry tachycardia because it revolves around a large obstacle, the right atrium, as opposed to a small obstacle like the atrioventricular (AV) node. This patient's ECG shows atrial flutter with both 4:1 and 3:1 conduction (*Figures 2 and 3*). The flutter waves have a consistent FF interval of 220 ms, which equates to approximately 272 bpm. Most of the ECG

shows 4:1 conduction, with an RR interval of 880 ms, which is exactly four times the FF interval of 220 ms (*Figure 4*).

The presence of an LAFB in this patient's ECG is not clinically important but is worth reviewing for the times when it can be. Any time there is a right bundle branch block (RBBB) with an axis deviation, there may be a concurrent fascicular block. A new RBBB + fascicular block + first or second AV block is concerning for an incomplete trifascicular block and, when seen in the setting of syncope, can warrant admission for cardiac monitoring. Patients with trifascicular blocks can have transient episodes of third-degree AV block and may require pacemaker placement.

The characteristic findings in an LAFB include (*Figure 5*):
- Left axis deviation between −45° and −90°

CASE RESOLUTION

The patient had a history of atrial flutter and was on chronic oral anticoagulation medication. She was admitted to the internal medicine service for pneumonia and a new oxygen requirement.

- qR complex in lead aVL +/– lead I
- rS complex in leads II, III, and aVF
- Prolonged R-wave peak time greater than or equal to 45 ms in lead aVL
- QRS complex duration less than 120 ms in the absence of a concurrent conduction delay

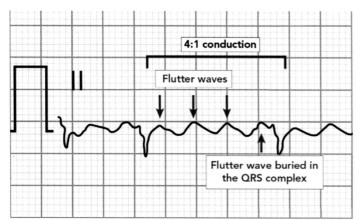

FIGURE 2. Atrial flutter with 4:1 conduction seen in the initial portion of the lead II rhythm strip. *Credit:* EMRA.

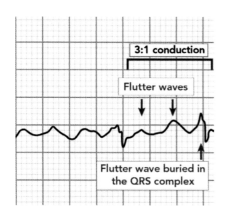

FIGURE 3. Atrial flutter with 3:1 conduction seen at the end of the lead II rhythm strip (the last and second-to-last QRS complexes are shown here). *Credit:* EMRA.

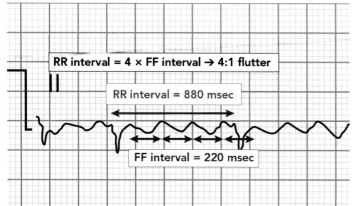

FIGURE 4. The initial portion of the lead II rhythm strip shows an atrial rate exactly four times the ventricular rate, consistent with atrial flutter with 4:1 conduction. *Credit:* EMRA.

ATRIAL FLUTTER LEARNING POINTS

- It occurs from a reentrant circuit in the right atrium.

- The stereotypical sawtooth pattern of P waves is seen best in the inferior leads.

- There is an absence of isoelectric baseline (eg, TP segment) in lead II.

- The atrial rate is 250 to 350 bpm and is typically fixed over time.

- The ventricular rate is a fraction of the atrial rate (ie, for an atrial rate of 300 bpm, 2:1 conduction produces a ventricular rate of 150 bpm, 3:1 conduction produces a ventricular rate of 100 bmp, 4:1 conduction produces a ventricular rate of 75 bpm, etc).

- When the ventricular rate is consistently around 150 bpm, atrial flutter should be considered.

- Vagal maneuvers or adenosine slow the ventricular rate but have no effect on flutter waves.

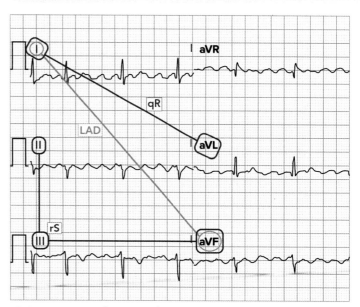

FIGURE 5. Findings in this ECG are consistent with an LAFB, including qR complexes in leads I and aVL (*red box*); rS complexes in leads II, III, and aVF (*purple box*); and left axis deviation (*green line*). *Credit:* EMRA.

ACKNOWLEDGMENT

This case is reprinted from *Emergency ECGs: Case-Based Review and Interpretations*, available at www.emra.org/amazon or by scanning the QR code.

Clinical Pediatrics

Ultrasound of a Pediatric Skin Abscess

By Brittney Rooney, MD; and
Sharon E. Mace, MD, FACEP
Cleveland Clinic; and Cleveland Clinic Lerner
College of Medicine at Case Western Reserve
University, Cleveland, Ohio

Objective

On completion of this article, you should be able to:

■ Explain the significance of ultrasound in evaluating SSTIs in the pediatric population.

CASE PRESENTATION

A 4-year-old girl with a medical history of Crohn disease presents with worsened skin cellulitis on her right lower leg. Her Crohn disease is treated with adalimumab and methotrexate. Her pediatrician started her on trimethoprim-sulfamethoxazole 7 days ago for the skin cellulitis; however, she was switched to clindamycin yesterday after the lesion increased in size. Her pediatrician sent her to the emergency department after purulent drainage was noted from the lesion.

On arrival, her vital signs include P 95, R 18, and T 37.1°C (98.7°F); SpO_2 is 100% on room air. The patient is awake, alert, and appears in no acute distress. Her eyes are nonicteric. She has no mouth or throat lesions and no exudate. Her lungs are clear, and she has a regular heart rhythm without murmurs. Her abdomen is soft, nontender, and nondistended. The area of erythema and induration in the right lower leg has two areas of fluctuance. Laboratory studies, including a CBC, basic metabolic panel, and C-reactive protein test, are all within normal limits. Bedside ultrasound using a linear probe to examine the skin of the right lower extremity shows cellulitis with a small focal fluid collection, which is consistent with an abscess (*Figure 1*).

Discussion

Skin and soft tissue infections (SSTIs) are a frequent complaint of pediatric patients in the emergency department and have increased in incidence in recent years.[1-3] The pathogens most frequently responsible for cellulitis are *Staphylococcus aureus* and group A streptococci. Other pathogens, like *Pseudomonas aeruginosa*, are also implicated in patients who are immunocompromised or have diabetes mellitus.[4-6] Cellulitis and abscesses must be differentiated from other skin infections such as necrotizing fasciitis for appropriate treatment.

Studies have found that ultrasound is better than physical examination at diagnosing abscesses in both adults and children.[1,7,8] In adults, ultrasound detects abscesses with a sensitivity of 98% and specificity of 88% compared to a sensitivity of 86% and specificity of 70% for physical examination.[7] In children with abscesses, ultrasound has a sensitivity between 96% and 97.5% and a specificity between 69.2% and 87% compared to the physical examination's sensitivity of 78.7% to 84% and specificity of 60% to 66.7%.[1,8]

In studies of adults, ultrasound changed how cellulitis was managed in the emergency department for approximately one-half of patients with the condition.[9] In pediatric studies, ultrasound was discordant with the clinical examination and changed management for 13.8% to 25% of patients.[1,8,10]

Overall, ultrasound can help detect subclinical abscesses, avoid more invasive procedures, and increase the success rate of abscess incisions.[10] A multicenter study of emergency department pediatric patients with suspected soft tissue abscesses reported decreased clinical failure rates for patients who underwent drainage with ultrasound (4.4%) compared to patients who underwent drainage without ultrasound (15.6%).[2]

Point-of-care ultrasound (POCUS) has an advantage over radiology-performed ultrasound — it is faster, resulting in a significantly shorter length of stay. POCUS is associated with

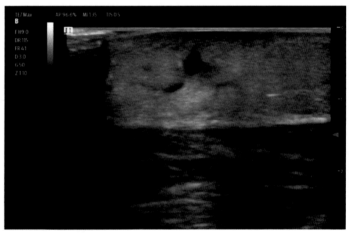

FIGURE 1. Ultrasound of skin on lower leg demonstrating a hypoechoic circular structure consistent with an abscess. *Credit: Brittney Rooney, MD.*

a –73-minute adjusted median difference in length of stay compared to the radiology-performed ultrasound group.[11]

Transducer Selection

Because abscesses are usually superficial, a linear array, high-frequency (7-12 MHz) transducer should be used. In the uncommon situation of a deep abscess, a low-frequency linear array transducer or a curvilinear transducer should be used.

Differential Diagnosis of Skin Infections by Ultrasound Appearance

SSTIs vary in appearance on ultrasound, which aids in proper diagnosis. An abscess appears as a mainly anechoic (black without internal echoes) or hypoechoic (darker than surrounding structures) spherical or oblong structure because it does not reflect or bounce back ultrasound waves as well as the other structures around it (see *Figure 1*). Color Doppler can be used when evaluating an abscess and is especially helpful for ascertaining blood vessels in the vicinity of the abscess (*Figure 2*).

A cyst on ultrasound is also a spherical or oblong structure but is uniformly anechoic throughout. Early cellulitis on ultrasound is characterized by generalized swelling and increased echogenicity of the skin and subcutaneous tissues. Late cellulitis can have a characteristic cobblestone appearance that occurs from an increased amount of fluid in subcutaneous tissues.[3] Ultrasound can also be used to diagnose necrotizing fasciitis; its findings include subcutaneous thickening, air, and fascial fluid (STAFF).[12]

Summary

Bedside ultrasound can be used to distinguish an abscess from cysts, cellulitis, and other SSTIs and increases diagnostic accuracy compared to a physical examination alone. Ultrasound can be especially useful for determining whether an abscess needs to be drained and for monitoring treatment. POCUS is readily available in emergency departments, easy to use, noninvasive, painless, rapid, and efficient. For the pediatric

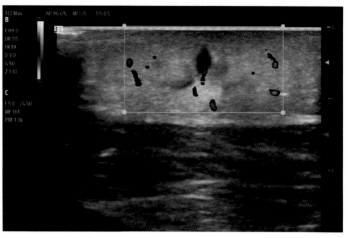

FIGURE 2. Color Doppler ultrasound demonstrating a hypoechoic oval structure consistent with an abscess with hyperemia. The presence of a color Doppler signal indicates hyperperfusion of the area surrounding the abscess. *Credit:* Brittney Rooney, MD.

population in particular, ultrasound has the added benefit of avoiding radiation exposure.

CASE RESOLUTION

Because the patient was immunocompromised and did not respond to outpatient therapy, she was admitted to the pediatrics service for intravenous antibiotics. She received intravenous clindamycin for 24 hours before being switched to oral clindamycin. Pediatric surgery was consulted and recommended a repeat ultrasound to evaluate the results of antibiotic therapy and the need for incision and drainage.

Ultrasound performed by radiology revealed diffuse soft tissue thickening of the skin and subcutaneous tissues over the right calf muscles, which corresponded to the area of abnormality. An irregular hypoechoic small fluid collection in the subcutaneous tissue measured 0.8 × 0.9 × 0.6 cm and appeared to communicate with the skin. An additional tiny fluid collection was also noted in the skin and measured 3 × 1 × 3 mm. The surrounding subcutaneous fat appeared echogenic and edematous, the underlying fascia was intact, and there was moderate regional hyperemia. The findings were consistent with cellulitis and two areas of fluid collection that were likely abscesses.

Surgical drainage was not recommended for the abscesses because of their small size and the patient's marked clinical improvement after spontaneous drainage. A wound culture was obtained from the drainage, but no growth occurred (the patient had been on antibiotics for about a week prior to obtaining the culture). The patient was discharged home with a full 10-day course of clindamycin. At her 1-month follow-up appointment, the examination of her lower extremity was normal, without any signs of infection.

REFERENCES

1. Adams CM, Neuman MI, Levy JA. Point-of-care ultrasonography for the diagnosis of pediatric soft tissue infection. *J Pediatr.* 2016 Feb;169:122-127.
2. Gaspari RJ, Sanseverino A. Ultrasound-guided drainage for pediatric soft tissue abscesses decreases clinical failure rates compared to drainage without ultrasound: a retrospective study. *J Ultrasound Med.* 2018 Jan;37(1):131-136.
3. Ramirez-Schrempp D, Dorfman DH, Baker WE, Liteplo AS. Ultrasound soft-tissue applications in the pediatric emergency department: to drain or not to drain? *Pediatr Emerg Care.* 2009 Jan;25(1):44-48
4. Yuoh CM, Chi H, Chiu NC, et al. Etiology, clinical features, management and outcomes of skin and soft tissue infections in hospitalized children: a 10-year review. *J Microbiol Immunol Infect.* 2022 Aug;55(4):728-739.
5. Mistry RD, Scott HF, Zaoutis TE, Alpern ER. Emergency department treatment failures for skin infections in the era of community-acquired methicillin-resistant *Staphylococcus aureus*. *Pediatr Emerg Care.* 2011 Jan;27(1):21-26.
6. Kim, WE. Diseases of subcutaneous tissue. In: Kliegman RM, ed. *Nelson Textbook of Pediatrics.* 21st ed. Elsevier; 2020:3531-3535.
7. Squire BT, Fox JC, Anderson C. ABSCESS: applied bedside sonography for convenient evaluation of superficial soft tissue infections. *Acad Emerg Med.* 2005 Jul;12(7):601-606.
8. Iverson K, Haritos D, Thomas R, Kannikeswaran N. The effect of bedside ultrasound on diagnosis and management of soft tissue infections in a pediatric ED. *Am J Emerg Med.* 2012 Oct;30(8):1347-1351.
9. Tayal VS, Hasan N, Norton HJ, Tomaszewski CA. The effect of soft-tissue ultrasound on the management of cellulitis in the emergency department. *Acad Emerg Med.* 2006 Apr;13(4):384-388.
10. Sivitz AB, Lam SH, Ramirez-Schrempp D, Valente JH, Nagdev AD. Effect of bedside ultrasound on management of pediatric soft-tissue infection. *J Emerg Med.* 2010 Nov;39(5):637-643.
11. Lin MJ, Neuman M, Rempell R, Monuteaux M, Levy J. Point-of-care ultrasound is associated with decreased length of stay in children presenting to the emergency department with soft tissue infection. *J Emerg Med.* 2018 Jan;54(1):96-101.
12. Castleberg E, Jenson N, Dinh VA. Diagnosis of necrotizing fasciitis with bedside ultrasound: the STAFF exam. *West J Emerg Med.* 2014 Feb;15(1):111-113.

Triplane Fracture in a 14-Year-Old Athlete

By Ariana Shaari, BA; and John Kiel, DO, MPH, FACEP, CAQSM
New Jersey Medical School in Newark; and University of Florida
College of Medicine, Jacksonville

Objective

On completion of this lesson, you should be able to:

■ Describe how to identify and manage a triplane fracture in the emergency department.

CASE PRESENTATION

A 14-year-old boy with no medical history presents with left ankle pain after being kicked during a soccer match. He reports that although he did not initially notice any pain, his ankle eventually gave out and prevented him from continuing to play. He reports that he now has pain that is progressive, dull, and radiates to the left leg. He denies any prior injury to the area. Physical examination reveals swelling of the medial and lateral aspects of his left ankle. No abrasions, lacerations, or ecchymosis are noted. A dorsalis pedis pulse is present. The left lower-extremity compartments are soft and compressible. No pain is present on passive stretching of the big toe. Sensation to light touch is present in the superficial fibular, deep fibular, and tibial nerve distributions of the left lower extremity. Ankle and great toe plantar- and dorsiflexion are intact. The remaining physical examination is reassuring. Imaging of the left ankle reveals a Salter-Harris type IV fracture of the tibial plafond with intra-articular swelling (*Figure 1*).

Definition of Triplane Fractures

Triplane fractures are rare, clinically significant pediatric orthopedic injuries. They account for 5% to 15% of ankle fractures in the pediatric population and are often associated with fibular fractures.[1-3] Triplane fractures are most common in adolescents — usually between the ages of 12 and 15 years — due to the vulnerability of the physis and incomplete physeal closure. They are also slightly more prevalent in boys.[2,4] Management depends on the level of displacement. Without proper treatment, patients are at risk of disturbed physeal growth and joint incongruity.

Triplane ankle fractures are distal tibial physeal Salter-Harris IV fractures and make up 25% of distal tibial fractures.[4-7] These fractures can be either entirely extra-articular or intra-articular.[3] More specifically, they occur in the sagittal, transverse, and frontal planes.[2] The Salter-Harris classification system is often used to guide appropriate management and to evaluate

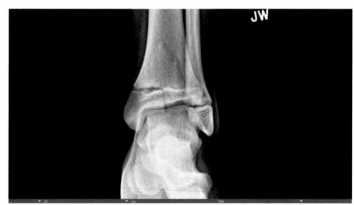

FIGURE 1. Posterior-anterior ankle x-ray demonstrating a Salter-Harris type IV fracture of the tibial plafond with intra-articular extension.

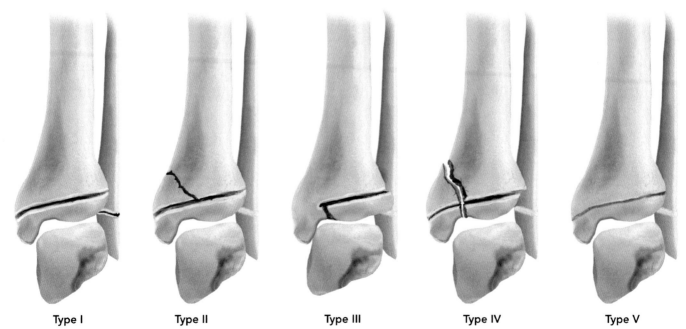

| Type I | Type II | Type III | Type IV | Type V |

FIGURE 2. Salter-Harris classification system. *Credit:* ACEP.

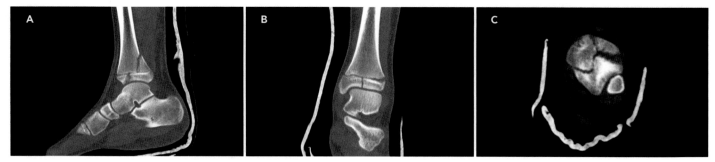

FIGURE 3. Ankle CT (**A.** *sagittal view*, **B.** *coronal view*, **C.** *axial view*) showing the fracture extending from the distal tibial metaphysis through the physis and epiphysis.

prognosis (*Figure 2*). Type I Salter-Harris fractures extend through the growth plate; type II involve the physis and metaphysis; type III involve the physis and epiphysis; type IV involve the epiphysis, physis, and metaphysis; and type V are physis crush injuries.[5]

Presentation and Imaging

The typical etiology of a triplane fracture includes a twisting force to the lower extremity, especially during sports or when an external rotation force is applied to a supinated foot.[5,8] The clinical presentation typically includes tenderness to palpation over the physis, ecchymosis, edema, and deformity.[5]

Regarding imaging, x-rays do not reliably display the number of fracture fragments, so CT is needed to further investigate fracture lines and for operative planning.[9] Previous literature reports that this particular fracture resembles a three-pointed star on CT.[10] Performing CTs rather than relying solely on x-rays before management has also been shown to improve accuracy with the point of insertion and direction of the screw during an open reduction and internal fixation (ORIF).[11]

Management

The management of a triplane fracture depends on the level of fracture displacement. Triplane fractures that are displaced more than 2 mm on CT are managed with ORIF, which reduces the chance of articular incongruity.[5] For fixation, one or two screws are generally placed parallel to the physis in the metaphysis, epiphysis, or both.[4]

Nondisplaced or minimally displaced fractures with a less than 2-mm displacement can be managed with cast immobilization in a long leg cast.[5] During closed reduction, the foot is moved into internal rotation for lateral fractures and into external rotation for medial fractures. After closed reduction, CT and serial x-rays are used to evaluate the positioning of the reduction.[2]

When identified and managed promptly, triplane fractures have a good prognosis.[4] Without proper management, however, patients are at risk of disrupted physeal growth.[12] Patients should be monitored for ankle deformity for 2 years following the injury.[5]

CASE RESOLUTION

The patient was placed in a short leg splint. CT without intravenous contrast further characterized the triplane Salter-Harris type IV fracture of the tibial plafond with associated ankle joint effusion and soft tissue swelling (*Figure 3*). The patient was directed to maintain the splint on the left lower extremity.

Because of the fracture's nature, the patient underwent ORIF. At 1-, 2-, and 3-month follow-up appointments, x-rays demonstrated an intact internal fixation of the screw in the distal tibial epiphysis. Alignment at the Salter-Harris IV fracture of the distal tibia remained unchanged and near-anatomic. Early healing at the fracture site was noted; no dislocations were seen. Disuse osteopenia and mild ankle soft tissue swelling were reported. The patent was subsequently lost to follow-up.

REFERENCES

1. Spiegel PG, Cooperman DR, Laros GS. Epiphyseal fractures of the distal ends of the tibia and fibula. A retrospective study of two hundred and thirty-seven cases in children. *J Bone Joint Surg Am.* 1978 Dec;60(8):1046-1050.
2. Schnetzler KA, Hoernschemeyer D. The pediatric triplane ankle fracture. *J Am Acad Orthop Surg.* 2007 Dec;15(12):738-747.
3. Venkatadass K, Sangeet G, Prasad VD, Rajasekaran S. Paediatric ankle fractures: guidelines to management. *Indian J Orthop.* 2020 Oct 6;55(1):35-46.
4. Shamrock AG, Varacallo M. Triplane ankle fracture. *StatPearls [Internet].* StatPearls Publishing; 2023. Updated March 6, 2023. https://www.ncbi.nlm.nih.gov/books/NBK547737/
5. Wuerz TH, Gurd DP. Pediatric physeal ankle fracture. *J Am Acad Orthop Surg.* 2013 Apr;21(4):234-244.
6. Caterini R, Farsetti P, Ippolito E. Long-term followup of physeal injury to the ankle. *Foot Ankle.* 1991 Jun;11(6):372-383.
7. Barmada A, Gaynor T, Mubarak SJ. Premature physeal closure following distal tibia physeal fractures: a new radiographic predictor. *J Pediatr Orthop.* 2003 Nov-Dec;23(6):733-739.
8. Feldman DS, Otsuka NY, Hedden DM. Extra-articular triplane fracture of the distal tibial epiphysis. *J Pediatr Orthop.* 1995 Jul-Aug;15(4):479-481.
9. Jones S, Phillips N, Ali F, Fernandes JA, Flowers MJ, Smith TWD. Triplane fractures of the distal tibia requiring open reduction and internal fixation. Pre-operative planning using computed tomography. *Injury.* 2003 May;34(4):293-298.
10. Rapariz JM, Ocete G, González-Herranz P, et al. Distal tibial triplane fractures: long-term follow-up. *J Pediatr Orthop.* 1996 Jan-Feb;16(1):113-118.
11. Cutler L, Molloy A, Dhukuram V, Bass A. Do CT scans aid assessment of distal tibial physeal fractures? *J Bone Joint Surg Br.* 2004 Mar;86(2):239-243.
12. Cooperman DR, Spiegel PG, Laros GS. Tibial fractures involving the ankle in children. The so-called triplane epiphyseal fracture. *J Bone Joint Surg Am.* 1978 Dec;60(8):1040-1046.

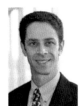

The Critical Image
Thumb Pain After a Scuffle

By Joshua S. Broder, MD, FACEP
Dr. Broder is a professor and the residency program director in the Department of Emergency Medicine at Duke University Medical Center in Durham, North Carolina.

Objectives

On completion of this article, you should be able to:

- Recognize an important x-ray finding of a thumb injury.
- Discuss the key associated soft tissue injury that is not visible on x-ray.
- Describe the emergency department management and follow-up of patients with thumb injuries.

CASE PRESENTATION

A 14-year-old boy presents with pain in his right thumb after an altercation earlier that day. He reports that his hand may have been stepped on. He denies numbness or weakness but has avoided moving his thumb because of pain. His vital signs are BP 111/71, P 73, R 15, and T 37.3°C (99.1°F); SpO$_2$ is 99% on room air. On examination, the patient has swelling and tenderness at the right thumb metacarpophalangeal (MCP) joint, with limited range of motion due to pain. Distal sensation and capillary refill time are normal. X-rays are obtained; the radiologist notes a Salter-Harris type IV fracture of the medial aspect of the right proximal phalanx of the thumb (*Figures 1, 2,* and *3*).

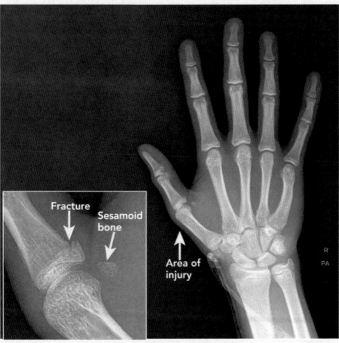

FIGURE 1. Posterior-anterior x-ray. On this view, the bony injury is subtle — a cortical defect of the proximal metaphysis that intersects the growth plate. From this image alone, the injury would be classified as a Salter-Harris type II injury.

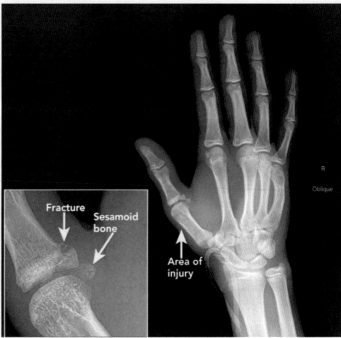

FIGURE 2. An oblique x-ray demonstrating a more apparent fracture line that passes through a small portion of the metaphysis, growth plate, and epiphysis. This classifies the injury as a Salter-Harris type IV fracture. The joint space is also involved, making this an intra-articular fracture.

Discussion

Hyperextension or hyperabduction of the thumb's MCP joint can result in a radiographically apparent injury: an avulsion fracture of the proximal medial aspect of the proximal phalanx. However, the accompanying radiographically occult soft tissue injury — rupture of the ulnar collateral ligament (UCL) of the thumb — can create greater long-term morbidity. UCL injuries can occur with or without an avulsion fracture. Therefore, fractures should raise suspicion for a ligamentous injury, but the injury should still be suspected in the absence of fractures. Complete UCL tears require surgical repair to avoid laxity of the thumb's grip and chronic pain.[1]

Thumb MCP joint injuries carry monikers that are associated with historical injury mechanisms. *Gamekeeper's thumb* refers to a rupture of the UCL that happened when gamekeepers intentionally broke the necks of small game animals. Skiers can experience this same hyperextension injury when they pass a

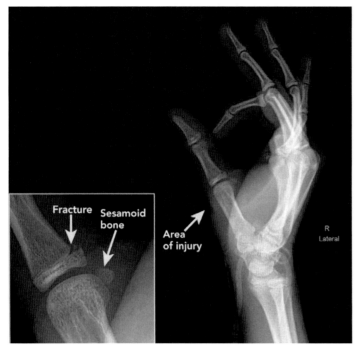

FIGURE 3. **On this lateral view, the injury again appears to pass only through a tiny portion of the distal metaphysis and into the growth plate (physis).** The articular involvement is not evident.

firmly planted ski pole, earning the injury the name *skier's thumb* in these situations. However, the injury should be suspected after other activities that lead to hyperextension. In one series of 127 patients who underwent surgical repair of acute thumb UCL rupture, falls were the most common cause (49%), while skiing represented only 2.4% of the injuries.[2] In acute injuries, assessment of the UCL may be intolerable to patients because of associated pain. Local anesthesia can be administered, or a digital block can be performed, to improve patient tolerance and allow for detection of ligamentous injury. Comparing the degree of joint laxity between the injured and the uninjured side can be helpful; 35° to 40° of joint opening or an opening of the joint without a clear endpoint suggests significant ligamentous disruption. If examination results are uncertain, ultrasound of the ligament can be performed and has a reported sensitivity of 92% for UCL rupture.[2]

For the patient in the case presentation, several factors could lead to a missed injury:
- He does not report a classic injury mechanism for UCL injury.
- A normal finding (sesamoid bone) is present in the region and could distract from the injury.

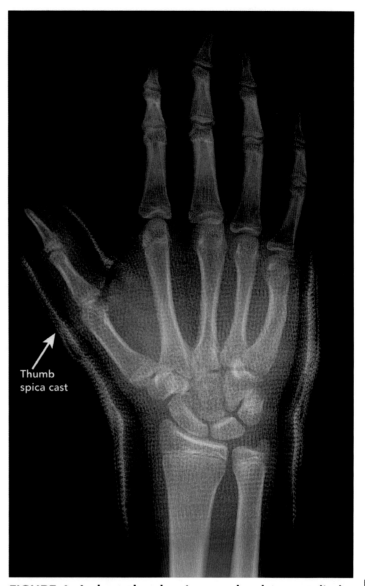

FIGURE 4. **A short thumb spica cast has been applied.**

- The radiographically visible injury itself is subtle and could be overlooked. It is more visible on some image views than on others, emphasizing the importance of obtaining and reviewing multiple views.
- The radiology report notes another potentially important element of the injury — a growth plate injury — but does not note the common anatomic location of gamekeeper's or skier's thumb. Focusing on the growth plate injury could cause the soft tissue injury to be overlooked.

CASE RESOLUTION

The patient was treated with thumb spica casting (*Figure 4*). He was referred for rapid surgical evaluation.

REFERENCES
1. Agout C, Bacle G, Brunet J, Marteau E, Charruau B, Laulan J; Orthopedics and Traumatology Society of Western France. Chronic instability of the thumb metacarpo-phalangeal joint: seven-year outcomes of three surgical techniques. *Orthop Traumatol Surg Res.* 2017 Oct;103(6):923-926.
2. Chuter GS, Muwanga CL, Irwin LR. Ulnar collateral ligament injuries of the thumb: 10 years of surgical experience. *Injury.* 2009 Jun;40(6):652-656.

Feature Editor: Joshua S. Broder, MD, FACEP. See also *Diagnostic Imaging for the Emergency Physician* (Winner of the 2011 Prose Award in Clinical Medicine, the American Publishers Award for Professional and Scholarly Excellence) and *Critical Images in Emergency Medicine* by Dr. Broder.

The LLSA Literature Review

Emerging and Re-emerging STIs

By Bryanna Carpenter, MD, MPH; and Laura Welsh, MD
Boston University in Massachusetts

Reviewed by Andrew J. Eyre, MD, MS-HPEd

Objective

On completion of this article, you should be able to:

■ List prevalent STIs and their recommended treatments.

Williamson DA, Chen MY. Emerging and reemerging sexually transmitted infections. *N Engl J Med.* 2020 May 21;382(21):2023-2032.

KEY POINTS

■ Rates are rising for the STIs *N. meningitidis* and *M. genitalium*.

■ A different strain of *C. trachomatis* has given rise to LGV and proctitis, which can be severe.

■ Syphilis rates have significantly increased in MSM in the last decade, especially among those who receive pre-exposure prophylaxis against HIV. Infection rates have also increased generally, leading to an increase in congenital syphilis infections.

■ Rising rates of drug-resistant *N. gonorrhoeae* infections are of increasing concern.

Since the 1990s when sexually transmitted infections (STIs) reached their lowest levels, STI rates have been increasing, especially in men who have sex with men (MSM). This increase has been especially prevalent in high-income countries. Outbreaks of nonclassic STIs have also become more common, including infections with *Shigella*, hepatitis A virus (HAV), and *Neisseria meningitidis*. Antibiotic resistance accompanies these increased outbreaks.

Sexually transmitted *Shigella* infections can range from self-limiting gastroenteritis to severe bloody dysentery. They are associated with HIV, are most prevalent in MSM, and are often seen in populations that engage in direct oral-anal contact, have condomless sex, attend sex parties, use dating apps, and use drugs to enhance sex (also known as *chemsex*). *Shigella* is often resistant to multiple antibiotics, with some areas reporting up to 93% resistance to azithromycin. Susceptibility testing is needed to determine the best course of treatment.

HAV is known to be transmitted by contaminated water. High-income countries have fewer incidents of HAV via contaminated water, which has led to large populations of nonimmune adults and, in turn, several outbreaks, particularly in MSM. Phenotyping these outbreaks confirmed that most outbreaks worldwide are tied to one of three strains of HAV, demonstrating the role international travel has had in its spread. Recent efforts to control these outbreaks have focused on education and vaccination, especially in those coinfected with HIV.

Sexually transmitted *N. meningitidis*, typically thought to colonize the nasopharynx, has been identified more recently in mucosal sites such as the cervix, urethra, and rectum. It has recently been linked to two conditions: urethritis in men who have sex with women and invasive meningococcal disease in MSM. These outbreaks have so far been seen in small clusters and have been successfully treated by a one-time dose of intramuscular ceftriaxone and a one-time oral dose of azithromycin.

Rising rates of *N. gonorrhoeae* infections are also accompanied by a rise in antibiotic resistance. In the United States alone, 550,000 drug-resistant infections are estimated to occur annually. Resistance to ceftriaxone and azithromycin is of increasing concern. Recent clinical trials have examined the efficacy of newer antibiotics such as solithromycin, zoliflodacin, and gepotidacin.

Recently, a different strain of the *Chlamydia trachomatis* infection has given rise to a less common infection that spreads through the lymphatics: lymphogranuloma venereum (LGV). LGV often causes inguinal lymphadenopathy. Rectal LGV infections can cause a painful proctitis that is associated with rectal discharge or, in severe cases, proctocolitis. In MSM, the infection has been linked to high-risk sexual practices. The recommended treatment length for LGV is 21 days with doxycycline (the usual course for the more common *C. trachomatis* infection is 7 days).

STIs with *Mycoplasma genitalium* have also increased recently. Screening is recommended only in symptomatic individuals and should include susceptibility testing. Resistance to azithromycin and moxifloxacin, both standard treatments, has increased in recent years.

Zika virus has been recognized as an STI since its emergence in 2008. Infections with Zika have shown maternal-fetal transmission; the fetal infection causes microcephaly and other brain anomalies. The WHO recommends that people infected with Zika use condoms or refrain from sex for at least 3 months for men and 2 months for women and that women of reproductive age avoid pregnancy for 2 months after a suspected or confirmed infection. Similarly, the Ebola virus can be sexually transmitted through the semen of male survivors. The WHO recommends that male survivors of Ebola be offered monthly semen testing and that those with positive tests abstain from sex or use condoms until testing is negative on two separate occasions.

Syphilis remains a global problem. Rates have significantly increased in MSM in the last decade, especially among those receiving pre-exposure prophylaxis against HIV. Syphilis rates have also increased generally, increasing the rate of congenital infections. Because of the potentially similar appearance of the anogenital ulcerations in primary syphilis to other infections, cotesting should be performed. To avoid congenital infections, testing should be completed during the first trimester of pregnancy.

New or re-emerging STIs represent an ongoing health problem. With increases in travel, online connections, and technology, controlling the spread of STIs will continue to be a challenge. Access to health care and testing is a priority for controlling these infections. A multi-pronged approach is also needed to control emerging STIs and should include testing, education, and the development of new vaccines and treatments, with cooperation between governments, the private sector, and health care communities.

Critical Decisions in Emergency Medicine's LLSA literature reviews feature articles from ABEM's 2023 Lifelong Learning and Self-Assessment Reading List. Available online at acep.org/moc/llsa and on the ABEM website.

22 *Critical Decisions in Emergency Medicine*

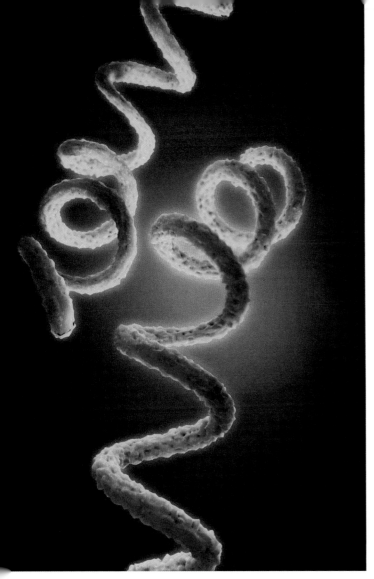

Striking Back
Diagnosing and Managing Syphilis

LESSON 16

By AJ Kirk, MD; Mary McHugh, MD; and Samuel Parnell, MD
Dr. Kirk is an associate professor of emergency medicine at UT Southwestern and the chief and medical/surgical director of the Parkland emergency department in Dallas, Texas. Dr. McHugh is an assistant professor of emergency medicine and the clerkship director for the emergency medicine clerkship at UT Southwestern. Dr. Parnell is an assistant professor of emergency medicine and assistant program director of the emergency medicine resident program at UT Southwestern.

Reviewed by Walter L. Green, MD, FACEP

Objectives

On completion of this lesson, you should be able to:

1. Recognize the presenting features of the diverse stages of syphilis.
2. Explain syphilis transmission and how to protect staff from exposure.
3. Describe the most appropriate approach for evaluating and diagnosing syphilis in the emergency department.
4. Define the recommended treatment regimens for syphilis and list the indications for each.
5. Identify the nuances of clinical presentations that warrant admission.

From the EM Model

10.0 Systemic Infectious Disorders
    10.1   Bacterial
        10.1.8 Spirochetes
            10.1.8.1 Syphilis

▬ CRITICAL DECISIONS ▬

- What clinical signs and symptoms should raise suspicion for a syphilitic infection?

- How should health care workers protect against syphilis?

- How is syphilis diagnosed in the emergency department?

- How should syphilis be managed, and what are potential treatment complications?

- What are the special considerations for diagnosing pediatric patients with syphilis?

- What follow-up care is appropriate, and when is admission warranted?

Historically called the *great imitator*, syphilis is an ancient, complex, and dynamic disease with diverse presentations and a serious risk of long-term sequelae. Improved testing and treatment in the 20th century reduced the incidence of syphilis and decreased exposure to its varied clinical presentations. Unfortunately, recent years have seen a dramatic increase in its incidence. Once again, physicians must prepare themselves to face off against this ancient disease.

CASE ONE

A 21-year-old man without a significant medical history presents with a sore on his genitals. The patient says he had unprotected sexual intercourse with a woman 4 weeks earlier and now has a painless ulcer on his penis; the ulcer erupted about 1 week ago.

The physical examination reveals a solitary, indurated, nontender ulcer without drainage. Inguinal lymphadenopathy and penile discharge are absent, and vital signs are normal. The physician diagnoses the wound as a chancre, treats the patient for primary syphilis, and counsels the patient to encourage his recent sexual partners to seek medical care.

The patient is discharged home but returns within hours with complaints of fever, headache, and muscle aches. His vital signs now include BP 95/60, P 115, R 14, and T 38.5°C (101.3°F).

CASE TWO

A 32-year-old man presents with flu-like symptoms, including 3 days of subjective fever, body aches, and intermittent headaches. He has no associated chest pain, shortness of breath, cough, or nasal congestion. The patient has a history of hypertension, which is well controlled with a single medication. The patient also mentions a rash that started on his chest 1 week ago and has now spread to his arms, legs, hands, and feet.

He says he is sexually active with multiple partners and inconsistently uses condoms. His vital signs include BP 130/85, P 89, R 14, and T 37.8°C (100°F). A head, eyes, ears, nose, and throat examination is normal, as are cardiac, respiratory, and abdominal evaluations.

A diffuse, erythematous, maculopapular rash covers the palms of the hands and soles of the feet. Cervical and inguinal lymphadenopathy, both of which are nontender, are also noted. The patient casually mentions the presence of a penile ulcer that developed 3 months ago but resolved without treatment.

CASE THREE

A 48-year-old woman with a medical history of hypertension, diabetes mellitus, and rheumatoid arthritis presents with 4 months of progressively worsening sharp, shooting pains in different areas of her body. Acetaminophen and ibuprofen have had no effect, nor has hydrocodone. The patient states that her level of discomfort exceeds the arthritis-related joint pains she normally experiences and has been accompanied by a slow decrease in sensation, especially in the fingers. She also reports feeling wobbly when she walks, especially at night. This unsteadiness has resulted in two falls. She reports no fever, chest pain, shortness of breath, nausea, or vomiting. The patient denies ever being diagnosed with an STI but reports that she "got around" in her early years. The cardiac, respiratory, and abdominal examinations are normal, as are the patient's vital signs.

A full neurologic examination shows intact extraocular movements. Her ocular examination, however, is significant for small bilateral pupils that constrict to accommodation but not to light. The patient also has a reduced sensitivity to light touch and decreased proprioception of the great toes bilaterally. She has decreased patellar reflexes bilaterally, a positive Romberg test, and an ataxic and jerky gait. Given the woman's extensive neurologic symptoms and examination findings, the physician initiates a head CT, lumbar puncture, and broad laboratory analysis.

Introduction

Although the prevalence and incidence of syphilis has undulated over the course of US history, the rate of the most infectious forms of syphilis (primary and secondary) has increased almost every year in both male and female patients since a recorded historic low in 2001. According to the CDC, syphilis cases have increased by 68% since 2017, and these primary and secondary syphilis cases have affected a wide swath of the population.[1] Although syphilis rates in men who have sex with men (MSM) have slowed in recent years, this patient population is still disproportionately affected, accounting for the majority of all male primary and secondary syphilis cases.[1]

These troubling statistics elucidate the importance of physician awareness, recognition, and appropriate treatment of this serious disease, particularly where its incidence is on the rise. Even more pressing, the national congenital syphilis rate continues to rise; the latest data from 2020 reveals a 15% increase relative to 2019 and a 254% increase relative to 2016, both of which mirror increases in the syphilis diagnosis rates among women of reproductive age.[2,3] Mortality rates for congenital syphilis are estimated to be as high as 16.3/100,000 live births, with concerns for massive underreporting.

Past penicillin treatment and testing advances decreased the prevalence of syphilis while also lowering physician clinical exposure and, at times, expertise. Limited health care resources for vulnerable populations, the stigma of sexually transmitted infections (STIs), and the natural disease course (which often includes a period of regression) have all complicated the battle against the disease's propagation. As a result, the incidence of syphilis has dramatically risen over the past few years. Understanding the diverse manifestations of syphilis in adult and pediatric patients, using appropriate pathways for diagnosis, following published guidelines for treatment, and encouraging patients to refer at-risk contacts for treatment are all necessary to help curb this ongoing public health threat. By gaining clinical knowledge and adopting appropriate diagnostic and management strategies, emergency physicians can effectively treat, and hopefully reduce, the spread of syphilis.

CRITICAL DECISION

What clinical signs and symptoms should raise suspicion for a syphilitic infection?

Treponema pallidum, an exclusively human pathogen, is the causative infectious organism of the diseases syphilis, yaws, and pinta.[4] There are four well-defined stages of syphilis: primary, secondary, latent, and tertiary. However, the natural course and clinical presentation of syphilis are complex. Syphilis is dynamic; regression and latency are common. Additionally, patients can present with neurologic and CNS manifestations at any time during their infection.[4]

Physicians also frequently divide syphilis into early and late stages of disease. The early stages occur in the days to months after initial infection and include primary, secondary, and early latent syphilis. Patients who do not receive appropriate treatment can then develop late syphilis. Late syphilis frequently occurs at least 1 year after initial exposure and includes late latent and tertiary syphilis.

Primary Syphilis

Primary syphilis, which represents the initial infection, is characterized by a solitary painless ulcer with indurated borders (ie, chancre), typically on the genitals. Approximately 5% of syphilis chancres are extragenital, erupting on the oral mucosa after unprotected orogenital contact.[5] The ulcer appears after an average incubation period of 21 days and generally regresses spontaneously in approximately 3 to 6 weeks. Nonsuppurative regional lymphadenopathy generally develops within 30 days of the lesion's appearance. Unlike a chancre, this symptom can persist for months.[2,6]

Secondary Syphilis

A clinically asymptomatic period (typically 3 to 6 weeks) follows resolution of the primary chancre. Development of a generalized rash and lymphadenopathy define secondary syphilis. The classic rash is dull red-pink and variable with papular lesions, although macules and papulosquamous eruptions may also be present (*Figure 1*).[7]

The rash commonly starts on the trunk and flexor surfaces of the extremities with generalized progression to the palms and soles (*Figures 2* and *3*). However, papulosquamous reactions can be limited to the palms of the hands and soles of the feet.[6,7] These symptoms are often accompanied by systemic, infection-induced symptoms such as fever, malaise, headache, and sore throat.

Condylomata lata (painless, wart-like mucosal lesions) may erupt in moist areas such as the mouth, perineum, axilla, and between the toes (*Figure 4*).[4] Like the chancre of primary syphilis, all lesions at this stage are highly infectious and saturated with spirochetes. Alopecia may be found on examination, and hepatitis may be noted on laboratory tests.[8] As in primary syphilis, this stage of the disease spontaneously regresses.[4]

Emergency physicians should do a thorough review of systems in patients who present with other risk factors for STIs to ascertain if these patients are within the period of regression after a primary or secondary infection. Emergency physicians should also consider including syphilis screenings or, if this is not possible, should encourage the patient to follow up with a primary care physician or the local health authority.

Latent Syphilis

Latent syphilis is diagnosed when patients have serologic evidence of infection but no signs or symptoms of disease. A clinical latency period that ranges from months to years can occur following resolution of the primary or secondary stage of syphilis.[6] Milder relapses of secondary syphilis can occur during this latent period. Latent syphilis is further divided into early and late periods. Early latent syphilis is defined as an infection acquired within 12 months of serologic testing and late latent syphilis as an infection acquired more than 12 months before serologic testing. If the infection duration is unknown, patients are usually presumed to have late latent syphilis. After a symptomatic hiatus,

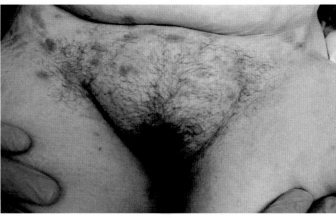

FIGURE 1. Secondary syphilis rash with faint erythematous macules on the abdomen and prominent, raised papules near the perineum and inguinal folds. *Credit:* Walter L. Green, MD, FACEP.

approximately one-third of cases progress to tertiary syphilis; cases that do not progress are halted by host immunologic disease clearance.[4]

Tertiary Syphilis

Tertiary syphilis is characterized by widespread gummata (ie, granulomatous lesions), which can affect any organ system. Rectal gummata can resemble fungating masses that are similar to neoplasms and may require surgical intervention.[9] More often, however, tertiary syphilis is discovered secondary to neurologic and cardiovascular involvement.

Clinical manifestations of tertiary syphilis can include meningitis, dementia, neuropathy, and thoracic aneurysm. An intracranial gumma can imitate a neoplastic cerebral mass such as a glioma or glioblastoma. Historically, intracranial gummata were thought to require years to develop, but formation in only a few months has been described.[10] During the tertiary stage, patients are not considered infectious with *T. pallidum*.[4]

Neurosyphilis

Neurosyphilis is characterized by meningovasculitis and degenerative parenchymal changes in any part of the CNS. Findings include mental status and personality changes, progressive dementia,

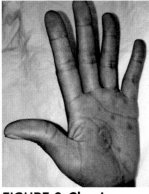

FIGURE 2. Classic erythematous papules on the palm with one central area of desquamation. *Credit:* Walter L. Green, MD, FACEP.

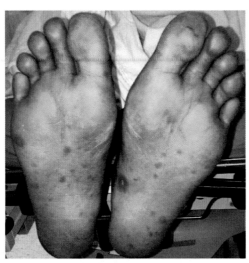

FIGURE 3. Erythematous papules on the feet. *Credit:* Walter L. Green, MD, FACEP.

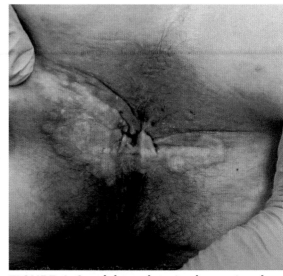

FIGURE 4. Condyloma lata in the perianal region. *Credit:* Walter L. Green, MD, FACEP.

demyelination of the posterior column's dorsal roots and dorsal root ganglia (ie, tabes dorsalis), and syphilitic paresis (eg, personality, affect, reflexes, eyes, sensorium, intellect, and speech changes).[11]

Neurosyphilis usually begins as meningitis. Although patients often present with no physical symptoms, diagnostic findings will be present on CSF analysis.[11] Patients frequently present with CNS manifestations of syphilis late in the disease course. However, neurosyphilis can occur at any time. Distinct clinical variants of neurologic involvement include the following:

- **Asymptomatic neurosyphilis:** An Argyll Robertson pupil is occasionally found on examination, even in otherwise asymptomatic patients. In such cases, the pupil will be dilated and possibly irregular; it will not react to light but will constrict with accommodation.[11,12]
- **Meningeal neurosyphilis:** Irritation of the meninges and increased intracranial pressure result in clinical symptoms.[11]
- **Ocular syphilis:** Signs and symptoms include iritis, uveitis, chorioretinitis, and painless vision loss.[13,14]
- **Otosyphilis:** Sensorineural hearing loss, tinnitus, and vertigo can occur. Hearing loss can be unilateral or bilateral, have a sudden onset, and progress rapidly.[14]
- **Meningovascular neurosyphilis:** Multiple, generally small cerebrovascular infarctions can occur; the presentation can imitate ischemic cerebral infarction.[15]
- **Paretic neurosyphilis:** Signs and symptoms include progressive dementia, dysarthria, myoclonic jerks, action tremors, seizures, hyperreflexia, positive Babinski sign, Argyll Robertson pupils, and progressive physical dissolution.[11]
- **Tabetic neurosyphilis:** Signs and symptoms include lancinating (lightning) pains, paresthesia, ataxia (secondary to sensory loss), urinary overflow incontinence, constipation or megacolon, absent knee and ankle deep tendon reflexes, impaired vibration and proprioception, positive Romberg sign, Argyll Robertson pupils, optic atrophy, and Charcot joints.[11]

Cardiovascular Syphilis

Classically, and of most concern, cardiac syphilis involves the aorta and causes arteritis of the vasa vasorum. However, the disease can involve any part of the cardiovascular system. This pathology results in medial necrosis and loss of elastic fibers, a process that manifests as an ascending thoracic aortic aneurysm, root dilation, and aortic valve regurgitation. The onset is usually gradual, and patients present with an asymptomatic murmur or heart failure. The disease can ultimately lead to subsequent aortic valve incompetence and aortic rupture.[4]

CRITICAL DECISION

How should health care workers protect against syphilis?

The COVID-19 pandemic and the subsequent mpox (formerly called monkeypox) outbreak have certainly underscored the importance of staff safety in the emergency department. *T. pallidum* enters the host through mucous membranes, nonintact skin, or transplacental and hematologic routes.[4] The chancre of primary syphilis and the condyloma of secondary syphilis are known for their infectious capability. Contact precautions must be maintained to protect health care staff, and universal protocols for preventing disease transmission through bodily fluids should be included in routine care.

CRITICAL DECISION

How is syphilis diagnosed in the emergency department?

The key components of syphilis testing in the emergency department include knowing the testing protocols of a particular facility and knowing the department's process for notifying the public health department.

As the incidence of syphilis has continued to rise, the approach to testing has become more nuanced. An institution's protocols may vary depending on local disease incidence. Testing for syphilis is challenging because *T. pallidum* does not grow on laboratory media. Direct spirochete visualization using dark-field microscopy can detect syphilis at all stages of the disease, but a negative test does not rule out syphilis.[4,16]

Because identifying *T. pallidum* is challenging, the diagnosis is commonly made by identifying antibodies that form when *T. pallidum* reacts with cardiolipin.[17] Nonspecific cardiolipin antibodies, which flocculate in the presence of the *T. pallidum* antibody, can be detected by venereal disease research laboratory (VDRL) and rapid plasma reagin (RPR) blood tests.[4] Syphilis screening in the United States has traditionally involved this labor-intensive nontreponemal test (RPR or VDRL) with subsequent confirmation of positive results by a specific treponemal test (eg, *T. pallidum* particle agglutination [TP-PA] or the fluorescent treponemal antibody absorption test [FTA-ABS]). In both North America and Europe, the testing paradigm is shifting toward reverse algorithm testing that uses treponemal-specific enzyme immunoassays (EIA) and chemiluminescence immunoassays for initial syphilis screening and a nontreponemal test (RPR or VDRL) on specimens with a positive result (*Figure 5*).[18]

The traditional process of nontreponemal testing followed by specific treponemal testing leads to less false-positive testing. However, because the initial nontreponemal tests can take up to 6 weeks to be positive, this increases the risk of false-negative testing. The nontraditional process of treponemal testing followed by nontreponemal testing identifies more patients earlier in the disease process, but patients with a positive EIA test and negative nontreponemal test will need to be counseled to best understand their next steps. The complexity of syphilis testing worsens when considering that more and more patients have access to results on their patient portals that do not include their physician's interpretation. When ordering syphilis testing, physicians should explain to patients that interpreting the results can be complex and that they should seek follow-up care with a primary care physician, an infectious disease specialist, or the public health department.

In suspected neurosyphilis cases, a CSF analysis and serologic syphilis testing are indicated.[19] Because HIV and other STIs are associated with an increased risk of syphilis, patients with a positive syphilis screen should have additional STI testing.[8]

✔ Pearls

- Optimal management of syphilis requires confirmatory testing; treatment with penicillin or, rarely, alternative antibiotics according to CDC guidelines; treating sexual partners; and testing for concomitant STIs.
- Recommending follow-up care to monitor treatment response is imperative for patients with syphilis. Admission is warranted for patients with neurosyphilis, pregnant patients, or patients with other severe complications.
- Patients should be warned to expect the Jarisch-Herxheimer reaction after treatment starts and should be educated on the difference between this reaction and a penicillin allergy.

How should syphilis be managed, and what are potential treatment complications?

How syphilis is treated depends on the clinical stage in which the patient presents (*Table 1*). In general, treatment regimens can be divided into three groups: early syphilis; late syphilis; and neurologic, otologic, and ocular syphilis.[20]

Primary syphilis, secondary syphilis, and early latent syphilis should be treated with benzathine penicillin G (2.4 million units IM).[20] Data to support the use of penicillin alternatives for primary and secondary syphilis are limited. In nonpregnant patients, doxycycline (100 mg PO 2 times/day for 14 days) or tetracycline (500 mg PO 4 times/day for 14 days) can be used to treat penicillin-allergic patients with early disease. Patients with early syphilis require close outpatient monitoring and repeat serologic testing at 6 and 12 months post treatment.

Given benzathine penicillin G's proven effectiveness and the high prevalence of mistaken penicillin allergy reporting, physicians should try to establish the validity of the allergic reaction.[8] Any pregnant woman with a penicillin allergy must be desensitized and treated with the agent.[6] Because of increasing resistance in certain regions, azithromycin is no longer recommended.[17] The patient's sexual partners within the past 90 days should also be tested and treated with penicillin or doxycycline.[14]

Tertiary syphilis and late latent syphilis should be treated with three doses of benzathine penicillin G (ie, 2.4 million units IM weekly for 3 weeks). These patients should be followed closely by a primary care physician or the local department of public health to ensure compliance, and disease regression should be monitored through repeat serologic testing at 6 and 12 months.[6]

Neurologic, otologic, and ocular syphilis require admission and management with aqueous crystalline penicillin G (3-4 million units IV every 4 hours or 18-24 million units continuously by IV infusion for 10-14 days).[11,21] Ceftriaxone (2 g IV daily for 10-14 days) can be used as a second-line treatment in patients with a true penicillin allergy.[19] These patients can have significant morbidity and mortality and require follow-up with neurologic examination, serologic testing, and lumbar puncture at 3 and 6 months after treatment.

The CDC recommends managing infants and children with benzathine penicillin G (50,000 units/kg IM) up to the suggested adult dose (2.4 million units IM).[22]

Syphilis treatment is not without complications. Anywhere from 55% to 95% of patients with primary or secondary syphilis can experience an acute, febrile inflammatory response, known as the Jarisch-Herxheimer reaction, after appropriate treatment due to the lysis of spirochetes.[20] Symptoms include fever, headache, exacerbation of skin lesions, and myalgia. This reaction typically occurs within hours of treatment.[20] Patients should be told to expect this apparent worsening of symptoms and should be specifically counseled on how this is different from an allergic response to penicillin. Care is supportive with the coadministration of antipyretics and fluids, which may diminish symptoms but will not prevent this systemic response. Symptoms usually resolve within 12 to 24 hours.[20]

Unfortunately, a syphilis infection only leads to partial immunity. Subsequent syphilis infections after a previous infection and treatment are not only possible, they are common. Furthermore, because of the immune response attenuation, reinfection can present with the same or different symptoms than the initial infection.[20] This underscores the importance of repeat serologic testing after treatment and continued monitoring of high-risk individuals.

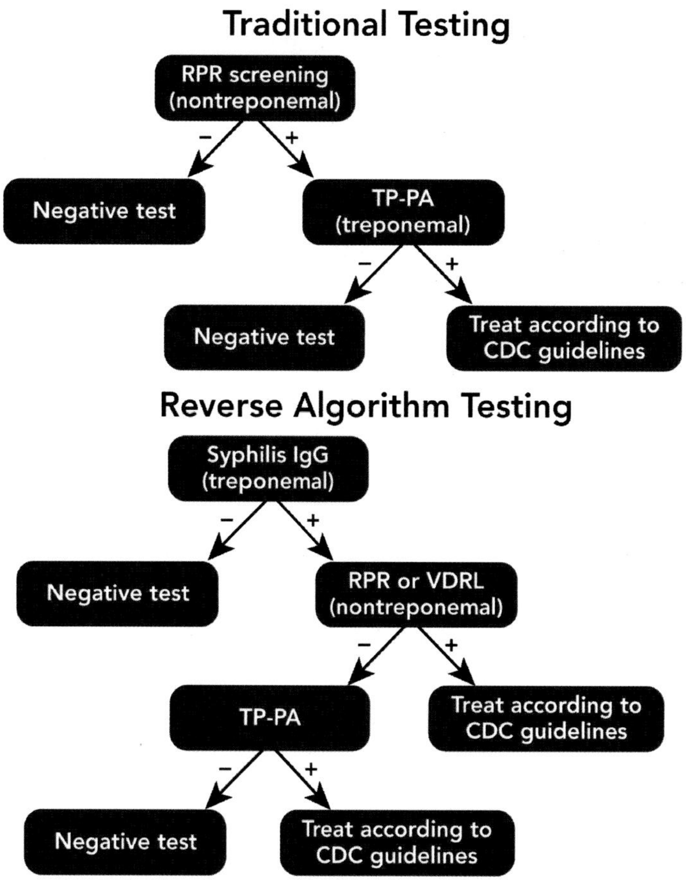

FIGURE 5. Traditional testing versus reverse algorithm testing for syphilis. *Credit:* ACEP.

What are the special considerations for diagnosing pediatric patients with syphilis?

Children can acquire syphilis through sexual contact or transplacental infection. Congenital syphilis is defined as disease transmission from a pregnant woman to a fetus. A fetus is susceptible to transplacental infection only after the fourth month of pregnancy, underscoring the importance of early pregnancy testing, treatment, and repeat evaluations in high-risk patients.[4]

Manifestations of congenital syphilis vary depending on the age of the patient. Signs and symptoms are unpredictable and can occur immediately or years later. Most babies born with syphilis are asymptomatic at birth but can develop complications later in life. Some common clinical manifestations are:

- **Newborn:** often asymptomatic; can include jaundice, anemia, thrombocytopenia, reticulocytosis, hepatosplenomegaly, edema, subclinical CNS infection, and overt meningitis[21]
- **Young infants (3-12 weeks):** moist mucocutaneous lesions, pseudoparalysis of the arms or legs, shotty lymphadenopathy, hepatomegaly, splenomegaly (50%), anemia, "snuffles" (syphilitic rhinitis characterized by profuse mucopurulent discharge), and a syphilitic rash (raised, bright red maculopapular lesions commonly on the palms and soles)[21]
- **Older children (6-12 years):** bilateral interstitial keratitis (photophobia, lacrimation, corneal vascularization), chorioretinitis, optic atrophy, meningovascular syphilis, deafness, saber shins (thickening of the periosteum of the anterior tibias), knee joint effusions, and disseminated gummata[21]

Syphilis Stage	Treatment	Follow-Up and Monitoring
Early syphilis Primary syphilis Secondary syphilis Early latent syphilis	**First-line treatment** • Benzathine penicillin G 2.4 million units IM once **Alternative treatment** • Doxycycline 100 mg PO twice daily for 14 days • Ceftriaxone 1 g daily IM or IV for 10-14 days	Follow-up appointment and serologic testing with a nontreponemal test (ie, RPR or VDRL) at 6 and 12 months
Late syphilis Late latent syphilis Tertiary syphilis	**First-line treatment** • Benzathine penicillin G 2.4 million units IM once weekly for 3 weeks **Alternative treatment** • Doxycycline 100 mg PO twice daily for 4 weeks • Ceftriaxone 2 g daily IM or IV for 10-14 days	Follow-up appointment and serologic testing with a nontreponemal test (eg, RPR or VDRL) at 6, 12, and 24 months
Neurologic/ otologic/ocular syphilis	**First-line treatment** • Aqueous penicillin G 3-4 million units IV every 4 hours (or 18-24 million units continuously by IV infusion) for 10-14 days • Patients with a reported mild to moderate penicillin allergy should be desensitized and treated with IV penicillin. **Alternative treatment** • Procaine penicillin G 2.4 million units IM daily plus probenecid 500 mg PO 4 times daily, both for 10-14 days • Ceftriaxone 2 g IV daily for 10-14 days **Special considerations** • Adjunctive oral or topical glucocorticoids are often used with antibiotics for otologic and ocular syphilis.	Follow-up appointment with neurologic examination, serologic testing, and lumbar puncture at 3 and 6 months after treatment and every 6 months after until the CSF WBC count is normal and the CSF VDRL is nonreactive; normalization of the RPR test can also help predict successful treatment.

TABLE 1. Treatment and monitoring of patients with syphilis based on disease stage

Sequelae of pediatric syphilis, especially from congenital or infantile infection, include rhagades (scarring of the mouth or nose), saddle nose deformity (depressed nasal bridge), a high forehead (secondary to CNS infection), Hutchinson teeth (peg-shaped upper central incisors with a central notch), and mulberry molars (lobulated mulberry appearance of the 6th-year molars). The Wimberger sign, which is nearly pathognomonic, is defined by bilateral, symmetric osteomyelitis with pathologic fractures of the medial tibial metaphyses.[21]

Any child who is diagnosed with a syphilis infection should be evaluated for sexual abuse, neglect, and nonaccidental trauma. Children with syphilis should also be screened for other STIs. If there is any concern for abuse, child protective services should be contacted.

CRITICAL DECISIONS

What follow-up care is appropriate, and when is admission warranted?

Given the complexity of testing for syphilis and the potential sequelae of untreated disease, follow-up for patients with suspected syphilis is imperative. Because syphilis must be reported to the local public health department, protocols should be in place to help treat any sexual partners within the last 90 days and to arrange for repeat serology.[8] Patients with treated syphilis should follow up and obtain repeat serologic testing at 6 and 12 months after treatment because an appropriate serologic response can take up to that length of time to appear. A fourfold or greater decline in the nontreponemal titer indicates an adequate response to syphilis treatment.[20] Patients without an adequate response should be evaluated for reinfection, which is common, or treatment failure, which is uncommon and likely related to poor treatment adherence, treatment with an alternative agent, an immunocompromised status, or an undiagnosed CNS disease.

Admission should be considered for pregnant women because the Jarisch-Herxheimer reaction can potentially increase the risk of preterm labor. Additionally, pregnant patients who are allergic to penicillin may require admission for penicillin desensitization therapy.

Patients being treated for otologic, ocular, or neurologic syphilis also require admission, as do those with suspected cardiovascular involvement, who may require monitoring for emergent complications.[23]

Summary

The incidence of syphilis has significantly increased over the past decade, and unfortunately, the rise of the great imitator shows no signs of slowing. Untreated syphilis is associated with significant morbidity. Congenital syphilis can be especially catastrophic for the developing fetus. Patients can present with a wide variety of signs and symptoms depending on the clinical stage of the disease. Most cases are associated with sexual activity; in patients at a high risk of STIs, physicians should highly suspect syphilis and have a low threshold for testing. MSM and people living with HIV infection are at an especially high risk of a syphilis infection and reinfection and should have regular syphilis screenings.[20]

Transmission can occur through direct contact with infectious lesions. Health care workers should protect themselves and prevent disease transmission when caring for patients with suspected syphilis. Prevention is especially important for workers who are pregnant or may become pregnant; congenital syphilis is associated with significant morbidity and mortality.

Although penicillin is the mainstay of treatment, there are subtleties to managing different stages of the disease, and patients who require additional penicillin dosing should be identified. It is also important to remember that true penicillin allergy, although frequently reported, is present in less than 1% of patients. In rare circumstances, physicians will need to employ alternative therapies for penicillin-allergic patients.

Patients and physicians should be aware of the potential for the self-limited Jarisch-Herxheimer reaction that occurs in response to appropriate treatment of a syphilis infection. Patients with this reaction frequently have fever, myalgia, headache, and rash. Severe complications have been reported but are rare. The Jarisch-Herxheimer reaction can occur in 55% to 95% of cases, and patients with early syphilis are at an increased risk. Unfortunately, the reaction cannot be prevented.[20]

CASE RESOLUTIONS

■ CASE ONE

When the 21-year-old man with a painless penile ulcer returned with fever, tachycardia, and mild hypotension, the physician suspected an acute reaction to spirochete lysis (ie, Jarisch-Herxheimer reaction), which can occur within hours after receiving syphilis treatment. The patient was managed supportively with antipyretics and fluids and began to feel better almost immediately. He was observed and then discharged home with instructions to continue antipyretic medications for the next 24 hours.

■ CASE TWO

The 32-year-old man's flu-like symptoms raised red flags. Secondary syphilis jumped to the top of the differential diagnosis due to several clinical clues, including normal vital signs, body aches, a headache, and a progressive rash that involved the palms and soles.

Based on a positive RPR test, the patient was treated with benzathine penicillin G (2.4 million units IM) and was warned about the contagiousness of his lesions. He was also advised to follow up with his primary care physician for repeat serologic testing.

■ CASE THREE

The middle-aged woman with myalgia, decreased sensation, and ataxia underwent a head CT and basic laboratory tests, all of which were within normal limits. Despite the reassuring workup, the emergency physician still highly suspected neurosyphilis given the patient's Argyll Robertson pupils, ataxic gait, decreased lower-extremity reflexes, positive Romberg test, and loss of proprioception. Aware that nontreponemal measurements can be falsely negative in cases of neurosyphilis, the physician ordered an FTA-ABS test, which was positive. The diagnosis was confirmed with a lumbar puncture, which showed CSF pleocytosis, an elevated protein level, and a positive CSF VDRL test. The patient was admitted to the hospital and treated for 14 days with intravenous penicillin G. She improved clinically and was discharged after 14 days of treatment.

At discharge, she was instructed to undergo repeat CSF studies within 3 to 6 months and then every 6 months afterward for 2 years to ensure complete resolution of all abnormalities.

Most patients with syphilis can be treated in the emergency department and then discharged home. However, certain factors mandate admission including pregnancy and ocular, otologic, or neurosyphilitic infections. All confirmed cases of syphilis should be reported to the local health department, and all patients with syphilis need follow-up care for monitoring and serologic testing to ensure they respond appropriately to therapy.

REFERENCES

1. Sexually transmitted disease surveillance 2021. CDC. Last reviewed April 11, 2023. https://www.cdc.gov/std/statistics/2021
2. Su JR, Brooks LC, Davis DW, Torrone EA, Weinstock HS, Kamb ML. Congenital syphilis: trends in mortality and morbidity in the United States, 1999 through 2013. *Am J Obstet Gynecol.* 2016 Mar;214(3):381.e1-e9.
3. Newman L, Kamb M, Hawkes S, et al. Global estimates of syphilis in pregnancy and associated adverse outcomes: analysis of multinational antenatal surveillance data. *PLoS Med.* 2013;10(2):e1001396.
4. Pottinger P, Reller B, Ryan KJ, Vedantam G, Weissman S. Spirochetes. In: Ryan KJ, ed. *Sherris & Ryan's Medical Microbiology.* 8th ed. McGraw Hill; 2022:657-677.
5. Fueyo-Casado A, Pedraz-Muñoz J, Campos Muñoz L, López-Bran E. Photo quiz. Genital ulcers and rash in a male patient. *Am Fam Physician.* 2012 Oct 15;86(8):763-764.
6. Serrano KD. Sexually transmitted infections. In: Tintinalli JE, Ma OJ, Yealy DM, et al, eds. *Tintinalli's Emergency Medicine: A Comprehensive Study Guide.* 9th ed. McGraw-Hill Education; 2020:1013-1024.
7. Badri T, Jennet SB. Images in clinical medicine. Rash associated with secondary syphilis. *N Engl J Med.* 2011 Jan 6;364(1):71.
8. Belcher C, Dawson M. Infectious disease emergencies. In: Stone CK, Humphries RL, eds. *CURRENT Diagnosis & Treatment Emergency Medicine.* 8th ed. McGraw-Hill Education; 2017:771-809.
9. Bender Ignacio RA, Koch LL, Dhanireddy S, Charmie Godornes B, Lukehart SA, Marrazzo JM. Syphilis? An unusual case of surgical emergency in a human immunodeficiency virus–infected man. *Open Forum Infect Dis.* 2015 Jun 20;2(3):ofv094.
10. Sprenger K, Furrer H. Chameleons everywhere. *BMJ Case Rep.* 2014 Nov 24;2014:bcr2014205608.
11. Bacterial, fungal, spirochetal, and parasitic infections of the nervous system. In: Ropper AH, Samuels MA, Klein JP, Prasad S, eds. *Adams and Victor's Principles of Neurology.* 12th ed. McGraw Hill; 2023:696-738.
12. Aziz TA, Holman RP. The Argyll Robertson pupil. *Am J Med.* 2010 Feb;123(2):120-121.
13. Lee MI, Lee AWC, Sumsion SM, Gorchynski JA. Don't forget what you can't see: a case of ocular syphilis. *West J Emerg Med.* 2016 Jul;17(4):473-476.
14. Marra, CM. Neurosyphilis. UpToDate. Reviewed June 2023. https://www.uptodate.com/contents/neurosyphilis
15. Liu L-L, Zheng W-H, Tong M-L, et al. Ischemic stroke as a primary symptom of neurosyphilis among HIV-negative emergency patients. *J Neurol Sci.* 2012 Jun 15;317(1-2):35-39.
16. Levinson W, Chin-Hong P, Joyce EA, Nussbaum J, Schwartz B. Laboratory diagnosis. In: *Review of Medical Microbiology and Immunology: A Guide to Clinical Infectious Diseases.* 17th ed. McGraw Hill; 2022.
17. Chen JC. Update on emerging infections: news from the Centers for Disease Control and Prevention. Brief report: azithromycin treatment failures in syphilis infections — San Francisco, California, 2002-2003. *Ann Emerg Med.* 2004 Sep;44(3):232-234.
18. Yax JA, Niforatos JD, Summers DL, et al. A model for syphilis screening in the emergency department. *Public Health Rep.* 2021 Mar-Apr;136(2):136-142.
19. Disease management: syphilis. In: Esherick JS, Clark DS, Slater ED, eds. *CURRENT Practice Guidelines in Primary Care 2015.* McGraw-Hill Education; 2015:436-437.
20. Tiecco G, Antoni MD, Storti S, et al. A 2021 update on syphilis: taking stock from pathogenesis to vaccines. *Pathogens.* 2021 Oct 21;10(11):1364.
21. Gaensbauer J, Nomura Y. Infections: bacterial and spirochetal. In: Bunik M, Hay WW Jr, Levin MJ, Abzug MJ, eds. *Current Diagnosis & Treatment: Pediatrics.* 26th ed. McGraw Hill; 2022:1237-1300.
22. Workowski KA, Bachmann LH, Chan PA, et al. Sexually transmitted infections treatment guidelines, 2021. *MMWR.* 2021 Jul 23;70(4):1-184.
23. Phillip SS. Spirochetal infections. In: Papadakis MA, McPhee SJ, Rabow MW, McQuaid KR, eds. *Current Medical Diagnosis & Treatment 2023.* McGraw Hill; 2023:1480-1495.

✖ Pitfalls

- Treating tertiary syphilis with only a single dose of benzathine penicillin G 2.4 million units IM instead of the preferred regimen of 2.4 million units IM once weekly for 3 weeks.

- Assuming a secondary syphilitic rash is not contagious.

- Misinterpreting the serologic titer after syphilis treatment. A fourfold decline in the nontreponemal titer represents an appropriate treatment response.

CME Questions

Reviewed by **Michael S. Beeson, MD, MBA, FACEP**; and **Walter L. Green, MD, FACEP**

Qualified, paid subscribers to *Critical Decisions in Emergency Medicine* may receive CME certificates for up to 5 ACEP Category I credits, 5 *AMA PRA Category 1 Credits*™, and 5 AOA Category 2-B credits for completing this activity in its entirety. Submit your answers online at acep.org/cdem; a score of 75% or better is required. You may receive credit for completing the CME activity any time within 3 years of its publication date. Answers to this month's questions will be published in next month's issue.

1 A 41-year-old health care worker presents after accidentally sticking herself with a used needle. She has no history of a hepatitis vaccination. The source patient used intravenous drugs. What treatment should be given?

   A. Hepatitis B immune globulin and hepatitis B vaccine
   B. Hepatitis B immune globulin only
   C. Hepatitis C immune globulin and hepatitis C vaccine
   D. No treatment is necessary

2 A 17-year-old boy presents at 6 pm. He reports that he ingested a handful of over-the-counter pain relievers approximately 1 hour earlier. At what time should a blood sample be drawn to measure the acetaminophen level?

   A. 6 pm
   B. 8 pm
   C. 9 pm
   D. 10 pm

3 What is the treatment of choice for spontaneous bacterial peritonitis?

   A. Amoxicillin-clavulanic acid
   B. Cefotaxime
   C. Oral cephalexin
   D. Vancomycin

4 What percentage of patients with spontaneous bacterial peritonitis are asymptomatic?

   A. Less than 10%
   B. 10% to 40%
   C. 40% to 60%
   D. More than 60%

5 A 35-year-old pregnant woman presents with itching. She has elevated bile acids but no abdominal pain or jaundice. Which disease is likely the cause of her symptoms?

   A. Acute fatty liver of pregnancy
   B. HELLP syndrome
   C. Infectious hepatitis
   D. Intrahepatic cholestasis of pregnancy

6 Hepatic insufficiency with hypoglycemia, coagulopathy, jaundice, and encephalopathy is more common in which pregnancy-related disease?

   A. Acute fatty liver of pregnancy
   B. HELLP syndrome
   C. Hyperemesis gravidarum
   D. Intrahepatic cholestasis of pregnancy

7 A 72-year-old man presents with an acute variceal bleed. Which treatment is shown to decrease the rate of rebleeding and mortality?

   A. Proton pump inhibitors
   B. Transfusion of platelets and plasma
   C. Transfusion to a hemoglobin level of 10 g/dL
   D. Treatment with antibiotics such as ceftriaxone

8 In patients with a history suspicious for chronic liver disease, which laboratory abnormalities can indicate undiagnosed cirrhosis and the need for further workup?

   A. Decreased bilirubin level, decreased albumin level, decreased platelet count
   B. Elevated albumin level, elevated PTT and INR, elevated platelet count
   C. Elevated bilirubin level, decreased albumin level, decreased platelet count
   D. Elevated PTT and INR, elevated platelet count, elevated bilirubin level

9 What therapy is available for patients recently diagnosed with hepatitis C?

   A. Ceftriaxone
   B. Hepatitis C vaccine
   C. Rifaximin
   D. Targeted antiviral therapy

10 Compared to patients with chronic liver failure, patients with acute liver failure who present with hepatic encephalopathy are more likely to experience which complication?

   A. Cerebral edema
   B. GI hemorrhage
   C. Hemorrhagic stroke
   D. Spontaneous bacterial peritonitis

11 An otherwise healthy 23-year-old woman presents at 24 weeks' gestation with a confirmed case of syphilis. She is allergic to penicillin and reports hives and facial swelling after receiving amoxicillin in the past. What is the most appropriate disposition for this patient?

   A. Administer benzathine penicillin G and discharge home
   B. Admit for inpatient penicillin desensitization therapy
   C. Admit for inpatient treatment with doxycycline
   D. Discharge home with a prescription for doxycycline

12 **What medication is an appropriate alternative to penicillin therapy for managing primary and secondary syphilis?**

A. Azithromycin
B. Ciprofloxacin
C. Doxycycline
D. Vancomycin

13 **What should be considered when treating a Jarisch-Herxheimer reaction?**

A. It can be prevented by dividing the penicillin treatment into two doses
B. It can be prevented by pretreatment with diphenhydramine
C. It is an acute allergic response to penicillin
D. Treatment with antipyretics can diminish symptoms, but the reaction cannot be prevented

14 **A 14-year-old boy presents with classic symptoms of primary syphilis. Aside from the usual treatments, what additional intervention is warranted?**

A. Administer doxycycline instead of benzathine penicillin G
B. Admit for management of pediatric syphilis infection
C. Evaluate for sexual abuse and screen for other sexually transmitted infections
D. Screen urine for drugs of abuse

15 **A patient who was treated for primary syphilis with benzathine penicillin G returns 12 hours after discharge with fever, chills, and body aches. What is the most likely diagnosis?**

A. COVID-19
B. Influenza
C. Jarisch-Herxheimer reaction
D. Penicillin allergy

16 **A 58-year-old man with a history of hypertension, HIV, and an unknown sexually transmitted infection at an unspecified point in his past presents with a 2-cm ulcer with a necrotic center and surrounding erythema on his nose. The emergency physician is concerned for gummatous disease. What treatment should be prescribed?**

A. Benzathine penicillin G 2.4 million units IM once weekly for 3 weeks
B. Benzathine penicillin G IV for 14 days
C. Doxycycline 100 mg twice a day for 14 days
D. Single-dose benzathine penicillin G (2.4 million units IM)

17 **An 18-year-old man presents with concern for syphilis from a recent partner with known active, untreated disease. He was sexually active with this person for the first time 4 days ago and is currently asymptomatic. What is the best next management step?**

A. Order a rapid plasma reagin test and advise the patient to return in 1 to 2 weeks when the results will be more sensitive; administer treatment then if warranted
B. Order a rapid plasma reagin test; discharge home if negative
C. Order a treponemal test and admit while awaiting results; treat only if test results are positive
D. Treat the patient empirically, order a treponemal test, and discharge home

18 **A 71-year-old woman is diagnosed with neurosyphilis. She is allergic to penicillin. What treatment should be initiated in the emergency department prior to admission?**

A. Aqueous crystalline penicillin G (200,000-300,000 units/kg IV)
B. Ceftriaxone (2 g IV)
C. Doxycycline (100 mg PO)
D. Tetracycline (500 mg PO)

19 **What is an Argyll Robertson pupil?**

A. A normally reactive pupil that is unequal in size compared to the corresponding pupil
B. A pupil that reacts to accommodation but not to light
C. A pupil that reacts to light but not to accommodation
D. A pupil that reacts to neither light nor accommodation

20 **A 45-year-old woman was diagnosed with primary syphilis 6 months ago and was appropriately treated with intramuscular benzathine penicillin G. She presents today for repeat serologic testing. Her initial rapid plasma reagin level was 1:32. What rapid plasma reagin titer would indicate an appropriate treatment response?**

A. 1:8
B. 1:16
C. 1:32
D. 1:64

ANSWER KEY FOR JULY 2023, VOLUME 37, NUMBER 7

1	2	3	4	5	6	7	8	9	10	11	12	13	14	15	16	17	18	19	20
C	B	D	A	C	A	C	D	D	D	C	A	C	C	C	C	A	A	D	B

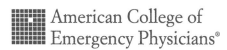
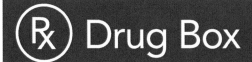

Drug Box

Fluid Management of Sepsis-Induced Hypotension

Frank LoVecchio, DO, MPH, FACEP
Valleywise Health Medical Center and ASU, Phoenix, Arizona

Objective
On completion of this column, you should be able to:
- State the results from a study comparing restrictive and liberal fluid resuscitation strategies for patients with sepsis-induced hypotension.

Intravenous fluids and vasopressor agents are often used in patients with sepsis. Vasopressors treat hypoperfusion by contracting blood vessels and increasing cardiac contractility; their risks include arrhythmia, increased myocardial demand, and vasoconstriction. As endorsed in the Society of Critical Care's 2021 guidelines, large volumes of fluid (30 mL/kg) are usually administered during the initial resuscitative stage of septic shock, but this strategy is based on poor evidence.[1]

The Crystalloid Liberal or Vasopressors Early Resuscitation in Sepsis (CLOVERS) trial was an NIH-sponsored unblinded superiority study that was undertaken to compare the effects of a restrictive fluid strategy (with early use of vasopressors) to those of a liberal fluid strategy. Ultimately, the researchers wanted to find out if restrictive fluid strategy during the first 24 hours of resuscitation for sepsis-induced hypotension would lessen mortality compared to a liberal fluid strategy.

Approximately 780 patients were randomly assigned to either a restrictive fluid group or a liberal fluid group. Randomization occurred within 4 hours of presentation if patients met the criteria for sepsis-induced hypotension that was refractory to initial treatment with 1 to 3 L of intravenous fluid. The primary outcome was all-cause mortality before a discharge home by day 90.

Compared to the liberal fluid group, the restrictive fluid group was administered less intravenous fluid (difference of medians of −2,134 mL; 95% confidence interval [CI], −2,318 to −1,949) and had an earlier, more prevalent, and longer duration of vasopressor use. Death from any cause before a discharge home by day 90 occurred in 109 patients (14%) in the restrictive fluid group and in 116 patients (14.9%) in the liberal fluid group (estimated difference of −0.9 percentage points; 95% CI, −4.4 to 2.6; $P = 0.61$). Five patients in the restrictive fluid group and four patients in the liberal fluid group had their data censored (lost to follow-up). The number of reported serious adverse events was similar in the two groups.[2] In summary, there was no difference in mortality before a discharge home by day 90 or in the number of serious adverse events between the restrictive fluid and liberal fluid strategies in patients with sepsis-induced hypotension.

REFERENCES
1. Oczkowski S, Alshamsi F, Belley-Cote E, et al. Surviving Sepsis Campaign Guidelines 2021: highlights for the practicing clinician. *Pol Arch Intern Med.* 2022 Aug 22;132(7-8):16290.
2. Shapiro NI, Douglas IS, Brower RG, et al; National Heart, Lung, and Blood Institute Prevention and Early Treatment of Acute Lung Injury Clinical Trials Network. Early restrictive or liberal fluid management for sepsis-induced hypotension. *N Engl J Med.* 2023 Feb 9;388(6):499-510.

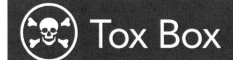

Tox Box

Acute DEET Poisoning

By Christian A. Tomaszewski, MD, MS, MBA, FACEP
University of California San Diego Health

Objective
On completion of this column, you should be able to:
- Describe the treatment for acute poisoning from DEET.

Introduction
Diethyltoluamide (DEET) is the most common and effective topical insect repellent; it is available in both creams and sprays, with concentrations of 5% to 100%. The repellent is usually considered safe but can, albeit rarely, cause toxicity after deliberately large ingestions (>1-2 mL/kg of ≥50% formulation) or excessive dermal applications (>10% formulation).

Mechanism of Action
- CNS toxicity
- Weak, reversible cholinesterase inhibition

Kinetics
- **Absorption:**
  - Dermal (50% is absorbed and levels peak at 1 hr)
  - Oral (levels peak at 30 min)
  - Inhalation (peak levels unknown)
- **Metabolism:** hepatic, with 70% renally excreted within 24 hr

Clinical Manifestations (usually in massive ingestions)
- **GI:** nausea and vomiting
- **Cardiac:** bradycardia and hypotension
- **Muscle:** weakness and respiratory failure
- **Neuro:** encephalopathy, myoclonus, and seizures
- **Dermal:** (rarely) erythema and urticaria

Diagnostics
- Routine screening of glucose and acetaminophen levels in intentional overdoses
- Comprehensive metabolic panel in symptomatic cases

Treatment
- **Decontamination:**
  - Wash skin
  - No activated charcoal due to rapid CNS symptoms in toxic ingestions
- **Hypotension:**
  - IV fluid bolus for hypotension
  - Norepinephrine for fluid-unresponsive hypotension
- **Seizures:** benzodiazepines or barbiturates

Critical decisions

in emergency medicine

Volume 37 Number 9: **September 2023**

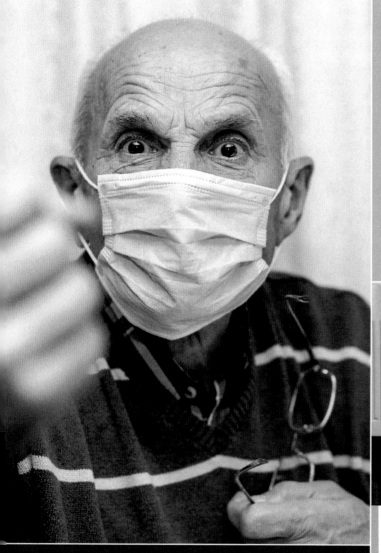

Worked Up

Acute agitation is a common presentation in the emergency department. Obtaining a history and physical examination in these circumstances is difficult, making the many possible etiologies of the agitation challenging to discern. Because agitated patients can endanger themselves and others, acute intervention is often required, and emergency physicians must be well versed in various techniques to protect all parties involved.

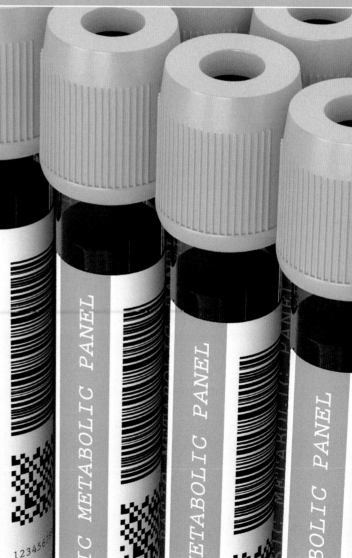

Balancing Act

Metabolic acidosis is common in acutely ill patients and has many potential causes. Treatment should be timely because the condition can lead to shock and respiratory failure. Further complicating matters, its potential presentations are numerous. Determining the cause of metabolic acidosis is the priority because treatment depends on the etiology and is integral to the successful management of these critically ill patients.

THE OFFICIAL CME PUBLICATION OF THE AMERICAN COLLEGE OF EMERGENCY PHYSICIANS

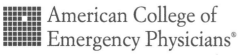

Critical decisions in emergency medicine

Critical Decisions in Emergency Medicine is the official CME publication of the American College of Emergency Physicians. Additional volumes are available.

EDITOR-IN-CHIEF
Michael S. Beeson, MD, MBA, FACEP
Northeastern Ohio Universities,
Rootstown, OH

SECTION EDITORS
Joshua S. Broder, MD, FACEP
Duke University, Durham, NC

Andrew J. Eyre, MD, MS-HPEd
Brigham and Women's Hospital/
Harvard Medical School, Boston, MA

John Kiel, DO, MPH, FACEP, CAQSM
University of Florida College of Medicine,
Jacksonville, FL

Frank LoVecchio, DO, MPH, FACEP
Valleywise, Arizona State University, University of Arizona,
and Creighton Colleges of Medicine, Phoenix, AZ

Sharon E. Mace, MD, FACEP
Cleveland Clinic Lerner College of Medicine/
Case Western Reserve University, Cleveland, OH

Amal Mattu, MD, FACEP
University of Maryland, Baltimore, MD

Christian A. Tomaszewski, MD, MS, MBA, FACEP
University of California Health Sciences,
San Diego, CA

Steven J. Warrington, MD, MEd, MS
MercyOne Siouxland, Sioux City, IA

ASSOCIATE EDITORS
Tareq Al-Salamah, MBBS, MPH, FACEP
King Saud University, Riyadh, Saudi Arabia/
University of Maryland, Baltimore, MD

Wan-Tsu Chang, MD
University of Maryland, Baltimore, MD

Ann M. Dietrich, MD, FAAP, FACEP
University of South Carolina College of Medicine,
Greenville, SC

Kelsey Drake, MD, MPH, FACEP
St. Anthony Hospital, Lakewood, CO

Walter L. Green, MD, FACEP
UT Southwestern Medical Center, Dallas, TX

John C. Greenwood, MD
University of Pennsylvania, Philadelphia, PA

Danya Khoujah, MBBS, MEHP, FACEP
University of Maryland, Baltimore, MD

Nathaniel Mann, MD
Greenville Health System, Greenville, SC

George Sternbach, MD, FACEP
Stanford University Medical Center, Stanford, CA

EDITORIAL STAFF
Suzannah Alexander, Editorial Director
salexander@acep.org

Joy Carrico, JD
Managing Editor

Alex Bass
Assistant Editor

Kyle Powell
Graphic Artist

ISSN2325-0186 (Print)   ISSN2325-8365 (Online)

Contents

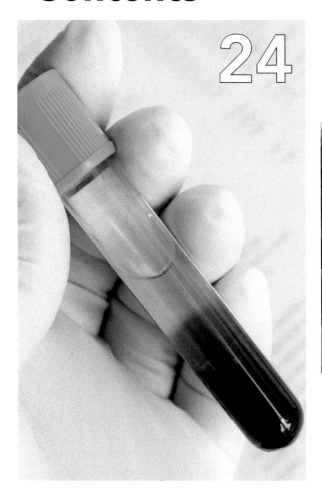

24

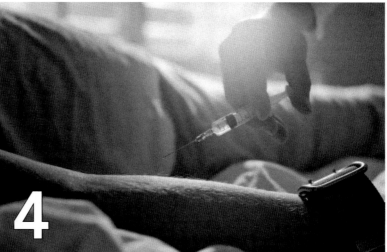

4

FEATURES

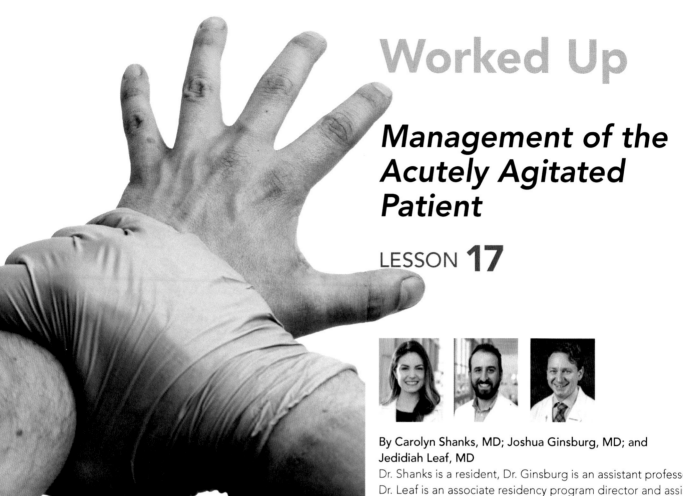

Worked Up

Management of the Acutely Agitated Patient

LESSON 17

By Carolyn Shanks, MD; Joshua Ginsburg, MD; and Jedidiah Leaf, MD

Dr. Shanks is a resident, Dr. Ginsburg is an assistant professor, and Dr. Leaf is an associate residency program director and assistant professor in the Department of Emergency Medicine at the University of Texas Southwestern Medical Center in Dallas.

Reviewed by Walter L. Green, MD, FACEP

Objectives

On completion of this lesson, you should be able to:

1. Recognize and quickly assess agitated patients.
2. Employ effective techniques to verbally de-escalate situations with agitated patients.
3. Compare the different medication options for treating agitated patients.
4. Describe the indications for and risks associated with physical restraint.
5. Determine which agitated patients should be admitted and which can be safely discharged.

From the EM Model

20.0 Other Core Competencies of the Practice of Emergency Medicine
   20.4 Systems-Based Practice
      20.4.3 Emergency Department Operations
         20.4.3.3 Safety, Security, and Violence in the Emergency Department

CRITICAL DECISIONS

■ What underlying etiologies can cause agitation?

■ How should physicians approach agitated patients and assess the severity of their agitation?

■ Which verbal de-escalation techniques are effective with agitated patients?

■ Which medications are most effective for managing agitation?

■ When and how can patients be safely restrained?

■ What is the appropriate disposition for agitated patients?

Acute agitation is a common presentation in the emergency department. Obtaining a history and physical examination in these circumstances is difficult, making the many possible etiologies of the agitation challenging to discern. Because agitated patients can endanger themselves and others, acute intervention — for which there are multiple techniques — is often required. The emergency physician should be well versed in these techniques to protect all parties involved in treating an agitated patient.

CASE ONE

A 22-year-old man is brought in by EMS after being found in the street behaving erratically. EMS responders report that the patient was seen smoking what was believed to be methamphetamine. His vital signs are BP 160/100, P 119, R 22, and T 37.6°C (99.7°F); SpO$_2$ is 100% on room air. The patient is yelling loudly and swinging his arms and legs violently. He does not answer questions appropriately or allow an examination. The emergency physician employs de-escalation techniques, but the patient remains agitated; therefore, pharmacologic intervention is deemed necessary.

CASE TWO

A 14-year-old girl is brought to the emergency department by her family after threatening to kill her mother with a kitchen knife. Her brother reports that she has been acting increasingly strange over the past 2 weeks. She is currently pacing around the room but has allowed the triage nurse to obtain vital signs, which are BP 135/95, P 105, R 18, and T 36.5°C (97.7°F); SpO$_2$ is 100% on room air. On the physician's arrival, the patient screams, "Get out!" She expresses concern that everyone is trying to hurt her.

CASE THREE

A 56-year-old man with a history of developmental delay presents from his group home after throwing items at his roommate. He is crying and combative, striking at any staff members who attempt to approach him. Vital signs are unobtainable, but the patient is noted to be moving all extremities spontaneously and has no clear external signs of trauma other than a bruise on his left arm. The nurse requests pharmacologic intervention.

Introduction

Agitation, defined as "an extreme form of arousal that is associated with increased verbal and motor activity," is often encountered in the emergency department.[1] It is estimated to constitute 2.6% of presentations. However, this is likely an underestimation because agitation can be a feature of many conditions.[2] Emergency departments encounter many agitated patients in part because they are accessible around the clock. The risk of agitation is compounded by patient stress regarding health concerns and frustration with respect to noise, overcrowding, and long wait times.[3-5]

Agitated patient presentations are likely to increase in the coming years. According to the Agency for Healthcare Research and Quality, emergency department visits for depression, anxiety, and stress reactions increased by 55.5% between 2006 and 2013. Visits for substance use disorders increased by 37%, and visits for psychoses and bipolar disorders increased by 52%. Although depression does not typically cause agitation on its own, depressed patients can have concomitant agitation. Overall, individuals suffering from psychiatric illness are more likely to present to the emergency department with agitation.[6]

Acute agitation is dangerous. A recent survey of 263 emergency physicians across 65 institutions found that 78% encountered violent patients in the prior year, with 21% reporting they were physically assaulted by a patient.[7] In some communities, this number is even higher — for example, residents surveyed from a single hospital system in New York City reported an assault rate of 66%.[8] Nurses have an even greater risk of assault than physicians because of their close contact with patients. One survey found that 70% of emergency department nurses had been hit or kicked by patients, as compared to 47% of emergency physicians.[9] Because acute agitation is highly prevalent and inherently dangerous to patients and staff, emergency physicians must be well versed in its management. This competency includes familiarity with verbal de-escalation techniques, understanding of pharmacologic treatment options, and knowledge of how and when to safely restrain patients.

CRITICAL DECISION

What underlying etiologies can cause agitation?

Various potentially life-threatening pathologies can cause agitation (*Table 1*). Although agitation may be secondary to an underlying psychiatric illness, a psychiatric disorder should be considered a diagnosis of exclusion. Red flags that can indicate a nonpsychiatric cause include extremes of age, lack of prior psychiatric history, vital sign abnormalities, immunosuppression, evidence or report of trauma, neurologic deficits, and abnormal examination findings. Agitation must be distinguished from delirium. Delirium presents as a waxing and waning of symptoms, often with confusion, impaired attention, and an altered level of consciousness.[10] Risk factors for delirium include older age, infection, critical illness, and certain medications.

Derangements in vital signs can aid in determining the cause of agitation. For example, hypoxia and hypercapnia can both lead to altered mentation. Mild hypoxia frequently presents as confusion and agitation. Hypercapnia traditionally leads to lethargy but can also cause confusion or agitation because of its cerebral vasodilatory effects. Hyperthermia can cause agitation (such as in the setting of heat stroke) or can be secondary to the effects of drugs or infection. Fever is also notable because infection is an important consideration in agitated patients. An infection of the CNS, such as encephalitis or meningitis, can cause agitation by directly affecting the brain or meninges. Moreover, even peripheral infections can lead to metabolic derangements that alter mentation.

Metabolic causes of agitation include hyperthyroidism, hyperglycemia or hypoglycemia, and electrolyte derangements. Specifically, rapid changes in sodium levels and hypercalcemia are

Mechanism	Conditions
Thermoregulatory	Hyperthermia and hypothermia
Respiratory	Hypercapnia and hypoxia
Infectious	Encephalitis, meningitis, and sepsis from other infections
Traumatic	Brain injury
Toxicologic	Adverse drug reaction, drug overdose or intoxication, and sedative-hypnotic agent withdrawal
Metabolic	Hyperglycemia, hypoglycemia, electrolyte abnormalities, and thyroid storm
Neurologic	Encephalitis, seizure (postictal), stroke, and subarachnoid hemorrhage

TABLE 1. **Life-threatening medical causes of acute agitation**

Score	Behavior
1	Difficult or unable to arouse
2	Asleep but responds normally to verbal or physical contact
3	Drowsy, appears sedated
4	Quiet and awake (normal level of activity)
5	Signs of overt (physical or verbal) activity, calms down with instructions
6	Extremely or continuously active, not requiring restraint
7	Violent, requiring restraint

TABLE 2. **Behavioral Activity Rating Scale**

associated with agitation. Hypercalcemia, which most often presents in the setting of malignancy or hyperparathyroidism, can lead to neuropsychiatric effects of possible dopaminergic and serotonergic dysfunction, including known cases of psychosis.[11] Hyponatremia and hypernatremia can both cause neuronal injury, which can lead to altered mentation. Hypokalemia, however, is less likely than other electrolyte derangements to cause agitation or altered mentation.

Trauma is another important cause of agitation to consider: One study found agitation in 10% of patients with severe traumatic brain injuries.[12] Drug use, medication side effects, polypharmacy, and drug withdrawal can also lead to neurologic changes, including agitation. For example, withdrawal from sedative-hypnotic agents or opioids can cause agitation, in contrast to the depressed mental status that these agents can cause in overdose.

CRITICAL DECISION

How should physicians approach agitated patients and assess the severity of their agitation?

To minimize the risk of injury and allow for safe management, an agitated patient should be placed in a room that limits additional stimulation and provides adequate space for clinical management. Unnecessary equipment should be removed from the room, along with any items that could be dangerous in the hands of an agitated patient. Continuous observation should be considered. There should be a low threshold to call law enforcement or security to keep the staff safe.

Once the scene is determined to be safe and adequate staffing is available, it is necessary to obtain vital signs and evaluate the patient's airway, breathing, and circulation. As with all critical patients, these initial steps are crucial. Physical examination can also offer valuable insight into possible medical, traumatic, or toxicologic etiologies. However, agitation can make it challenging to obtain a thorough history and examination. History-taking can be bolstered by chart review and discussions with family members or EMS. When possible, obtain a point-of-care glucose measurement in addition to the history and physical examination.

There are several validated scoring systems used to quantify the severity of agitation and guide the next steps. For example, the Behavioral Activity Rating Scale classifies agitation on a scale from 1 (difficult or unable to arouse) to 7 (a severely agitated state with violence that requires physical restraint); a score of 4 indicates a normal, calm state (*Table 2*).[13] Another scoring system is the Brøset Violence Checklist, which evaluates a patient's risk of violence over the next 24 hours based on the presence or absence of six behavioral variables (*Table 3*).[14] The risk of escalation to physical violence is greater in patients who verbally attack staff.[15] If verbal de-escalation fails, progression to pharmacotherapy or physical restraint may be necessary.

Behavior	Score
Confusion	Absent = 0 Present = 1
Irritability	Absent = 0 Present = 1
Boisterousness	Absent = 0 Present = 1
Physical threats	Absent = 0 Present = 1
Verbal threats	Absent = 0 Present = 1
Attacks on objects	Absent = 0 Present = 1

- 0 points = The risk of violence is low.
- 1-2 points = The risk of violence is moderate. Preventative measures should be taken.
- ≥3 points = The risk of violence is high. Preventative measures must be taken. Plans for handling an attack should be activated.

TABLE 3. **Brøset Violence Checklist**

CRITICAL DECISION

Which verbal de-escalation techniques are effective with agitated patients?

Verbal de-escalation is a powerful tool to employ when treating agitated patients. It consists of a three-step process: engaging the patient, establishing a collaborative relationship, and verbally defusing the situation. One primary physician should lead the de-escalation. Measures should be in place to ensure the safety of patients, physicians, and other team members. These measures include having security personnel available, maintaining a safe distance between the physician and patient, and positioning to allow for rapid egress.[16]

Physicians should act respectfully and empathetically when approaching agitated patients. They should address patients by name, ask affirmative and open-ended questions, and sincerely express that they are there to help. The conversation often takes the form of a loop in which the physician actively listens, responds in a way that validates any concerns, and states the next steps in terms of how they would like to help. This cycle must often be repeated as patients become calmer and more receptive. Simple gestures, such as providing a blanket or pillow or offering a snack or beverage, can also help build a therapeutic relationship.

Although de-escalation may take time and attention, it is a valuable investment that can ultimately prevent complications such

✔ Pearls

- Verbal de-escalation avoids the injuries and complications that can arise from pharmacologic intervention and physical restraint.

- There are many life-threatening causes of agitation, which must be identified and treated.

- Multiple pharmacologic agents are available to help calm agitated patients.

- Physicians should consider each patient individually and tailor medication choices based on age, medical history, and the suspected cause of agitation.

as oversedation and injury. However, physicians should also set clear boundaries to ensure patients understand that certain behaviors — such as assault — will not be tolerated. Physicians can help coach patients on how to stay in control, but there should be reasonable consequences if patients do not comply with the set limitations.[16] Unfortunately, some situations cannot be de-escalated. In these cases, additional interventions may be needed.

CRITICAL DECISION

Which medications are most effective for managing agitation?

Three classes of medication are commonly used to calm agitated patients: benzodiazepines, antipsychotics, and dissociative agents, such as ketamine. Each class has certain benefits and risks. Several populations — including pregnant, pediatric, and geriatric patients — require extra consideration with respect to pharmacologic intervention.

Benzodiazepines

Benzodiazepines work by binding to the γ-aminobutyric acid-A (ie, $GABA_A$) receptors that line the neuronal membranes, resulting in sedation and anxiolysis through CNS inhibition. Options for both intramuscular and intravenous administration are available, with variable time to onset and duration of action (*Table 4*). All benzodiazepines are metabolized by the liver. However, some benzodiazepines are safer than others for patients with liver disease. Compared to agents metabolized via hepatic CYP-mediated oxygenation, benzodiazepines metabolized through hepatic conjugation are less dependent on global liver function and maintain a stable half-life despite the presence of liver disease.[17] The benzodiazepines metabolized in this manner—lorazepam, oxazepam, and temazepam—can be remembered using the mnemonic *LOT*.

Benzodiazepines are the pharmacotherapy of choice for patients who are under the influence of any drug that causes a sympathomimetic response (eg, cocaine or methamphetamine) and for managing agitation secondary to withdrawal from alcohol and certain sedative-hypnotic drugs. They are also the treatment of choice for agitation of unknown etiology. The primary side effect of benzodiazepine use is respiratory depression, especially when combined with alcohol or other sedating drugs.[18]

Antipsychotics

First-generation antipsychotics (FGAs), also called typical antipsychotics, work by antagonizing dopamine receptors. Haloperidol and droperidol are commonly used FGAs because they act rapidly and are easily given intramuscularly (*Table 5*). The FDA issued a black box warning for droperidol in 2001, when it was thought to be associated with fatal arrhythmias. Since then, multiple studies have found that QTc-interval prolongation–related adverse events (eg, arrhythmias and death) following administration of droperidol are rare.[19-22] In a randomized double-blind trial that compared IM droperidol (5 mg), ziprasidone (10 mg and 20 mg), and lorazepam (2 mg), droperidol adequately sedated 64% of patients (compared to 25%, 35%, and 33%, respectively) and resulted in fewer episodes of respiratory depression.[23]

Second-generation antipsychotics (SGAs), or atypical antipsychotics, antagonize both dopamine and serotonin receptors.[19] SGAs are also more selective in the dopamine receptors they antagonize, which reduces the risk of side effects while maintaining

Drug	Dosage	Time to Onset	Duration	Metabolism
Lorazepam	2-4 mg IM / 2-4 mg IV	5-10 min	2-6 hr	Hepatic conjugation
Midazolam	5-10 mg IM / 2-5 mg IV	5-15 min	1-2 hr	Hepatic CYP-mediated oxygenation
Diazepam	5-10 mg IV	1 min	1-2 hr	Hepatic CYP-mediated oxygenation

TABLE 4. **Benzodiazepine dosages and characteristics**

similar efficacy to FGAs.[24] Because of their favorable side effect profile, SGAs are preferred over FGAs.[18] Olanzapine is FDA-approved for oral and intramuscular administration, but recent research has shown that intravenous administration is also safe and effective.[21,25,26] Recent expert consensus recommends risperidone (followed by olanzapine) as the agent of choice for agitated patients who are willing to take medication orally.[18]

Antipsychotics are preferred in agitated patients with suspected alcohol intoxication because benzodiazepines increase the risk of respiratory depression. In patients whose symptoms are thought to stem from underlying psychiatric illness, antipsychotics are also preferred because they can address the underlying psychosis.[18] However, antipsychotics carry a risk of QT-interval prolongation; the risk is greatest with ziprasidone (*Table 6*).[27] Cardiac monitoring should be considered with antipsychotics if large doses are given or intravenous administration is used.

Ketamine

The dissociative drug ketamine has recently gained traction for use in severe, uncontrolled agitation. It works by blocking N-methyl-D-aspartate (ie, NMDA) receptors, leading to pain control and dissociation. It can be given intravenously or intramuscularly and titrated from pain control doses to a dissociative dose that is effective for sedation. Recent studies have repeatedly demonstrated more rapid sedation from ketamine than other agents. In one blinded, randomized controlled trial of 80 patients, 5 mg/kg of IM ketamine was compared to a combination of 5 mg IM midazolam and 5 mg IM haloperidol. Ketamine led to adequate sedation more quickly by almost 10 minutes and with no statistically significant increase in adverse events.[28] Other research confirms that patients given ketamine are more likely to be sedated within 5 minutes (22% versus 0%) and within 15 minutes

Drug	Dosage	Time to Onset	Duration	Metabolization
Haloperidol	2-5 mg IM	5-20 min	4-6 hr	CYP2D6, CYP3A4, UGT-glucuronidation
	2-5 mg IV	1-5 min		
	2-10 mg PO	45-60 min		
Droperidol	2.5-5 mg IM	15-30 min	6-8 hr	Hepatic CYP-mediated oxygenation
	2.5-5 mg IV	3-10 min		
Olanzapine	5-10 mg IM	15-45 min	2-4 hr	CYP1A2, UGT-glucuronidation
	5-10 mg PO	15-45 min		
Risperidone	1-2 mg IM	15-30 min	2-3 hr	CYP2D6
	1-2 mg PO	30-60 min		
Ziprasidone	10-20 mg IM	15-20 min	2-4 hr	CYP1A2, CYP3A4

TABLE 5. **Antipsychotic dosages and characteristics**

	Anticholinergic Symptoms	Extrapyramidal Symptoms	Hyperglycemia	QT prolongation	Sedation
FGAs (typical)					
Haloperidol	Low incidence	High incidence	Moderate incidence	Low incidence	Low incidence
Droperidol	Low incidence	High incidence	Moderate incidence	Moderate incidence	Low incidence
SGAs (atypical)					
Olanzapine	High incidence	Low incidence	High incidence	Low incidence	High incidence
Quetiapine	Moderate incidence	Low incidence	High incidence	Low incidence	High incidence
Risperidone	Low incidence (rare)	Moderate incidence	Moderate incidence	Low incidence	Moderate incidence
Ziprasidone	Low incidence	Low incidence	Low incidence	Moderate incidence	Moderate incidence

TABLE 6. **Side effects of antipsychotics commonly used for agitation**[27]

(66% versus 7%) as compared to a combination of haloperidol and lorazepam.[29]

Side effects of ketamine include hypersalivation, emergence delirium, and laryngospasm. Laryngospasm is generally short-lived and can be managed by opening the airway with a jaw thrust and assisting oxygenation with bag-valve-mask ventilation. Other studies found high rates of subsequent intubation when ketamine is given by EMS, but ketamine use by physicians for agitation in the emergency department does not result in more intubations.[21,30,31]

Alternative Medications

Sublingual dexmedetomidine is a relatively recent formulation that has shown significant benefit over placebo in agitated patients with bipolar disorder, as reported in a 2022 randomized double-blind trial.[32] Research comparing the use of a single class of drugs to the use of multiple drug classes in agitated patients is limited. Some initial studies show that using multiple classes of medication can lead to more effective sedation but may be riskier, including increased risk of hypotension and respiratory depression.[18,33-35] Initial research also demonstrates an increased risk of hypotension and hypoxia when olanzapine IM and lorazepam IM are given within hours of each other, so this combination should be avoided until the interaction is investigated further.[36,37]

Pregnant Patients

Multiple studies have examined antipsychotic use during pregnancy. Results show a good overall safety profile and demonstrate that most typical and atypical antipsychotics are safe in pregnant people.[38-40] The exception is risperidone, which is associated with a slightly increased risk of birth malformations when given in the first and second trimesters.[40] Benzodiazepines are associated with a slightly increased risk of preterm birth and low birth weight when given in early pregnancy, but the teratogenic risk appears to be low.[41,42]

Children

According to a consensus statement from the American Association for Emergency Psychiatry, benzodiazepines, antipsychotics, and diphenhydramine are appropriate choices for treating agitation in the pediatric emergency department. However, benzodiazepines can paradoxically increase agitation in children with autism spectrum disorder or developmental delay and should be avoided in these patients. Experts also recommend against the use of ketamine, barbiturates, and opioids for agitation in children.[43]

Older Patients

In geriatric patients, all pharmacologic interventions have risks. With any medication, the best strategy is to "start low and go slow" with conservative initial dosing and small dose increases.

Antipsychotics are an appropriate first choice: FGAs and SGAs are both associated with improved symptom control. However, because older patients are particularly susceptible to the extrapyramidal and cardiovascular effects of antipsychotics, SGAs are recommended as the first-line therapy. Some initial studies show support for the use of olanzapine.[44-48] One double-blind randomized comparison of olanzapine IM (2.5 mg and 5 mg) to lorazepam IM (1 mg) found that olanzapine offered faster onset and longer duration of sedation without increased side effects.[46] Risperidone is also commonly used in older patients and has shown effectiveness with minimal side effects.[47,49] Daily use of antipsychotics for psychosis in patients with dementia is associated with increased mortality, but this trend is not seen with their emergent use in the emergency department.[24,48]

Benzodiazepines are as effective as antipsychotics in older patients, but they are associated with increased respiratory depression and falls, worsened and prolonged delirium, and paradoxical disinhibition with increased agitation.[44,47] For these reasons, benzodiazepines are not a first-line option for the geriatric population. Data are scant regarding ketamine in geriatric patients, but initial studies show its use is limited by adverse events.[44] Diphenhydramine should also be avoided because of side effects such as excessive sedation and the worsening of delirium.[44,50]

CRITICAL DECISION

When and how can patients be safely restrained?

Restraining patients is inherently risky. Restraints should be considered only after failure of less restrictive measures, such as verbal and pharmacologic interventions. Recent analysis has shown two groups of patients are more frequently restrained: (1) younger men and boys with histories of psychiatric illnesses and drug use and (2) older patients with medical complaints. A 2020 study found more use of restraints in Black patients than in White patients with similar presentations (with a risk ratio of 1.22), which suggests the decision to restrain is impacted by racial bias.[51]

Ideally, physical restraint should be implemented by a team of five people, including security officers trained to manage combative patients and the nurse responsible for administering medication. The physician in charge of the patient's care should be present but preferably not among the team of five physically restraining the patient. One person should be stationed at each limb, and a fifth should be available to hold the patient's head. If only two limbs can be tied down, the contralateral arms and legs should be secured, with the arm tied upward, which theoretically decreases the amount of force and momentum that struggling can generate. Meanwhile, the physician should continue to attempt verbal de-escalation while explaining what is happening. The correct position for restraint is supine. Prone positioning increases the risk of aspiration.[5] After restraints are placed, an intramuscular medication should be given promptly so that the restraints can be removed as soon as possible.

Restrained patients must be continuously monitored. The most common complication of physical restraint is skin breakdown at the site of the restraints. More severe outcomes can also occur, including rhabdomyolysis and acidosis in patients who continue to actively fight against the restraints. Patients should be restrained for only the minimum necessary duration, and the continued need for physical restraint should be re-evaluated every hour. In addition to continuous visual monitoring, restrained patients should have continuous cardiac monitoring, pulse oximetry, and end-tidal CO_2 monitoring.

CRITICAL DECISION

What is the appropriate disposition for agitated patients?

Patients who pose a threat to themselves or others or who cannot care for themselves because of mental illness are unsafe for discharge and should be admitted to inpatient psychiatry. If a patient's condition improves after correction or resolution of a medical cause, discharge can be considered. For example, if a patient is agitated secondary to intoxication and later clinically returns to baseline without other concerning medical findings, a safe discharge can be arranged. By contrast, most cases of delirium require medical management and admission.

Disposition becomes complicated when patients refuse admission or recommended treatments. In these cases, physicians must determine whether patients have decision-making capacity. Emergency physicians and psychiatrists are both qualified to make decisions regarding capacity. Capacity refers to the ability to make informed, logical choices based on the risks and benefits of certain interventions. There are four components of capacity: understanding the given information, appreciating how the information applies to oneself, reasoning through and reflecting on the information, and clearly expressing a choice.[52] Capacity is dynamic and can change as the clinical picture evolves. Although patients with capacity usually make decisions in their own best interest, they sometimes choose differently. Conversely, patients who lack decision-making capacity may require involuntary hospitalization.

Summary

Acutely agitated patients are at high risk because they can endanger themselves and others and because agitation can have life-threatening underlying causes. Emergency physicians must be able to identify potential causes of agitation and intervene on these causes while also providing symptom control. Possible interventions include verbal de-escalation, pharmacotherapy, and physical restraint.

✖ Pitfalls

- Failing to consider the risks or to monitor for side effects of medication used to calm an agitated patient.
- Attempting to restrain an agitated patient without a coordinated team approach.
- Failing to promptly administer an intramuscular medication after restraining a patient.
- Hindering the development of a therapeutic relationship through a lack of empathy and care for an agitated patient.

REFERENCES

1. Nordstrom K, Zun LS, Wilson MP, et al. Medical evaluation and triage of the agitated patient: consensus statement of the American Association for Emergency Psychiatry Project BETA Medical Evaluation Workgroup. West J Emerg Med. 2012 Feb;13(1):3-10.
2. Miner JR, Klein LR, Cole JB, Driver BE, Moore JC, Ho JD. The characteristics and prevalence of agitation in an urban county emergency department. Ann Emerg Med. 2018 Oct;72(4):361-370.
3. Kowalenko T, Walters BL, Khare RK, Compton S; Michigan College of Emergency Physicians Workplace Violence Task Force. Workplace violence: a survey of emergency physicians in the state of Michigan. Ann Emerg Med. 2005 Aug;46(2):142-147.
4. Gates DM, Ross CS, McQueen L. Violence against emergency department workers. J Emerg Med. 2006;31(3):331-337.
5. Rossi J, Swan MC, Isaacs ED. The violent or agitated patient. Emerg Med Clin North Am. 2010 Feb;28(1):235-256.
6. Weiss AJ, Barrett ML, Heslin KC, Stocks C. Trends in emergency department visits involving mental and substance use disorders, 2006-2013. Healthcare Cost and Utilization Project. Published December 1, 2016. https://www.hcup-us.ahrq.gov/reports/statbriefs/sb216-Mental-Substance-Use-Disorder-ED-Visit-Trends.jsp
7. Behnam M, Tillotson RD, Davis SM, Hobbs GR. Violence in the emergency department: a national survey of emergency medicine residents and attending physicians. J Emerg Med. 2011 May;40(5):565-579.
8. Schnapp BH, Slovis BH, Shah AD, et al. Workplace violence and harassment against emergency medicine residents. West J Emerg Med. 2016 Sep;17(5):567-573.
9. Omar H, Yue R, Amen AA, Kowalenko T, Walters BL. Reassessment of violence against emergency physicians. Ann Emerg Med. 2018 Oct;72(4)(supp):S144.
10. Mattison MLP. Delirium. Ann Intern Med. 2020 Oct 6;173(7):ITC49-ITC64.
11. Nagy L, Mangini P, Schroen C, Aziz R, Tobia A. Prolonged hypercalcemia-induced psychosis. Case Rep Psychiatry. 2020 Feb 1;2020:6954036.
12. Brooke MM, Questad KA, Patterson DR, Bashak KJ. Agitation and restlessness after closed head injury: a prospective study of 100 consecutive admissions. Arch Phys Med Rehabil. 1992 Apr;73(4):320-323.
13. Swift RH, Harrigan EP, Cappelleri JC, Kramer D, Chandler LP. Validation of the behavioural activity rating scale (BARS)™: a novel measure of activity in agitated patients. J Psychiatr Res. 2002 Mar-Apr;36(2):87-95.
14. Woods P, Almvik R. The Brøset violence checklist (BVC). Acta Psychiatr Scand Suppl. 2002;(412):103-105.
15. Lanza ML, Zeiss RA, Rierdan J. Non-physical violence: a risk factor for physical violence in health care settings. AAOHN J. 2006 Sep;54(9):397-402.
16. Richmond JS, Berlin JS, Fishkind AB, et al. Verbal de-escalation of the agitated patient: consensus statement of the American Association for Emergency Psychiatry Project BETA De-Escalation Workgroup. West J Emerg Med. 2012 Feb;13(1):17-25.
17. Mihic SJ, Mayfield J. Hypnotics and sedatives. In: Brunton LL, Knollmann BC, eds. Goodman & Gilman's The Pharmacological Basis of Therapeutics. 14th ed. McGraw-Hill; 2022:427-441.
18. Wilson MP, Pepper D, Currier GW, Holloman GH Jr, Feifel D. The psychopharmacology of agitation: consensus statement of the American Association for Emergency Psychiatry Project BETA Psychopharmacology Workgroup. West J Emerg Med. 2012 Feb;13(1):26-34.
19. Chokhawala K, Stevens L. Antipsychotic medications. StatPearls [Internet]. StatPearls Publishing; 2023. Last updated February 26, 2023. https://www.ncbi.nlm.nih.gov/books/NBK519503
20. Gaw CM, Cabrera D, Bellolio F, Mattson AE, Lohse CM, Jeffery MM. Effectiveness and safety of droperidol in a United States emergency department. Am J Emerg Med. 2020 Jul;38(7):1310-1314.
21. Cole JB, Lee SC, Martel ML, Smith SW, Biros MH, Miner JR. The incidence of QT prolongation and torsades des pointes in patients receiving droperidol in an urban emergency department. West J Emerg Med. 2020 Jul 2;21(4):728-736.
22. Calver L, Page CB, Downes MA, et al. The safety and effectiveness of droperidol for sedation of acute behavioral disturbance in the emergency department. Ann Emerg Med. 2015 Sep;66(3):230-238.e1.
23. Martel ML, Driver BE, Miner JR, Biros MH, Cole JB. Randomized double-blind trial of intramuscular droperidol, ziprasidone, and lorazepam for acute undifferentiated agitation in the emergency department. Acad Emerg Med. 2021 Apr;28(4):421-434.

CASE ONE

Two doses of intramuscular midazolam were given, but the patient remained aggressive, punching at nurses and pulling at equipment. He was placed in physical restraints and given intramuscular ketamine, after which his agitation resolved. His restraints were then removed. After several hours of monitoring, his vital signs normalized, and he became calm and cooperative. The patient was evaluated by the psychiatry team, who knew him from previous visits. He was ultimately cleared for discharge with outpatient resources.

CASE TWO

Verbal de-escalation was attempted, but the patient continued pacing and yelled, "I will do what must be done to protect myself from you!" Oral medication was offered to help calm her, and she begrudgingly agreed to take 5 mg of sublingual olanzapine. She later became calm enough to allow collection of the necessary laboratory studies and talk with the psychiatry team, who arranged for inpatient admission.

CASE THREE

Instead of pharmacologic intervention, the physician used verbal de-escalation. While making eye contact and addressing the patient by name, the physician explained that they were there to help and requested to know what had happened. The physician also offered food and a drink, which the patient accepted. The patient revealed that he felt unsafe at his group home because his roommate sometimes became physically violent. Social work was ultimately consulted, and arrangements were made to find the patient a new group home.

24. Schneider LS, Dagerman KS, Insel P. Risk of death with atypical antipsychotic drug treatment for dementia: meta-analysis of randomized placebo-controlled trials. JAMA. 2005 Oct 19;294(15):1934-1943.
25. Khorassani F, Saad M. Intravenous olanzapine for the management of agitation: review of the literature. Ann Pharmacother. 2019 Aug;53(8):853-859.
26. Hunt NF, McLaughlin KC, Kovacevic MP, Lupi KE, Dube KM. Safety of intravenous olanzapine administration at a tertiary academic medical center. Ann Pharmacother. 2021 Sep;55(9):1127-1133.
27. Camm AJ, Karayal ON, Meltzer H, et al. Ziprasidone and the corrected QT interval: a comprehensive summary of clinical data. CNS Drugs. 2012 Apr 1;26(4):351-365.
28. Barbic D, Andolfatto G, Grunau B, et al. Rapid agitation control with ketamine in the emergency department: a blinded, randomized controlled trial. Ann Emerg Med. 2021 Dec;78(6):788-795.
29. Lin J, Figuerado Y, Montgomery A, et al. Efficacy of ketamine for initial control of acute agitation in the emergency department: a randomized study. Am J Emerg Med. 2021 Jun;44:306-311.
30. Mankowitz SL, Regenberg P, Kaldan J, Cole JB. Ketamine for rapid sedation of agitated patients in the prehospital and emergency department settings: a systematic review and proportional meta-analysis. J Emerg Med. 2018 Nov;55(5):670-681.
31. O'Connor L, Rebesco M, Robinson C, et al. Outcomes of prehospital chemical sedation with ketamine versus haloperidol and benzodiazepine or physical restraint only. Prehosp Emerg Care. 2019 Mar-Apr;23(2):201-209.
32. Preskorn SH, Zeller S, Citrome L, et al. Effect of sublingual dexmedetomidine vs placebo on acute agitation associated with bipolar disorder: a randomized clinical trial. JAMA. 2022 Feb;327(8):727-736.
33. Chan EW, Taylor DM, Knott JC, Phillips GA, Castle DJ, Kong DCM. Intravenous droperidol or olanzapine as an adjunct to midazolam for the acutely agitated patient: a multicenter, randomized, double-blind, placebo-controlled clinical trial. Ann Emerg Med. 2013 Jan;61(1):72-81.
34. Taylor DM, Yap CYL, Knott JC, et al. Midazolam-droperidol, droperidol, or olanzapine for acute agitation: a randomized clinical trial. Ann Emerg Med. 2017 Mar;69(3):318-326.e1.
35. Yap CYL, Taylor DM, Kong DCM, Knott JC, Taylor SE; Sedation for Acute Agitation in Emergency Department Patients: Targeting Adverse Events (SIESTA) Collaborative Study Group. Risk factors for sedation-related events during acute agitation management in the emergency department. Acad Emerg Med. 2019 Oct;26(10):1135-1143.
36. Marder SR, Sorsaburu S, Dunayevich E, et al. Case reports of postmarketing adverse event experiences with olanzapine intramuscular treatment in patients with agitation. J Clin Psychiatry. 2010 Apr;71(4):433-441.
37. Williams AM. Coadministration of intramuscular olanzapine and benzodiazepines in agitated patients with mental illness. Ment Health Clin. 2018 Aug 30;8(5):208-213.
38. Einarson A, Boskovic R. Use and safety of antipsychotic drugs during pregnancy. J Psychiatr Pract. 2009 May;15(3):183-192.
39. McKenna K, Koren G, Tetelbaum M, et al. Pregnancy outcome of women using atypical antipsychotic drugs: a prospective comparative study. J Clin Psychiatry. 2005 Apr;66(4):444-449.
40. Huybrechts KF, Hernández-Díaz S, Patorno E, et al. Antipsychotic use in pregnancy and the risk for congenital malformations. JAMA Psychiatry. 2016 Sep 1;73(9):938-946.
41. Wikner BN, Stiller CO, Bergman U, Asker C, Källén B. Use of benzodiazepines and benzodiazepine receptor agonists during pregnancy: neonatal outcome and congenital malformations. Pharmacoepidemiol Drug Saf. 2007 Nov;16(11):1203-1210.
42. Szpunar MJ, Freeman MP, Kobylski LA, et al. Risk of major malformations in infants after first-trimester exposure to benzodiazepines: results from the Massachusetts General Hospital National Pregnancy Registry for Psychiatric Medications. Depress Anxiety. 2022 Dec;39(12):751-759.
43. Gerson R, Malas N, Feuer V, Silver GH, Prasad R, Mroczkowski MM. Best practices for evaluation and treatment of agitated children and adolescents (BETA) in the emergency department: consensus statement of the American Association for Emergency Psychiatry. West J Emerg Med. 2019 Mar;20(2):409-418.
44. Shenvi C, Kennedy M, Austin CA, Wilson MP, Gerardi M, Schneider S. Managing delirium and agitation in the older emergency department patient: the ADEPT tool. Ann Emerg Med. 2020 Feb;75(2):136-145.
45. Tampi RR, Tampi DJ, Balachandran S, Srinivasan S. Antipsychotic use in dementia: a systematic review of benefits and risks from meta-analyses. Ther Adv Chronic Dis. 2016 Sep;7(5):229-245.
46. Meehan K, Zhang F, David S, et al. A double-blind, randomized comparison of the efficacy and safety of intramuscular injections of olanzapine, lorazepam, or placebo in treating acutely agitated patients diagnosed with bipolar mania. J Clin Psychopharmacol. 2001 Aug;21(4):389-397.
47. Peisah C, Chan DK, McKay R, Kurrle SE, Reutens SG. Practical guidelines for the acute emergency sedation of the severely agitated older patient. Intern Med J. 2011 Sep;41(9):651-657.
48. Reus VI, Fochtmann LJ, Eyler AE, et al. The American Psychiatric Association practice guideline on the use of antipsychotics to treat agitation or psychosis in patients with dementia. Am J Psychiatry. 2016 May;173(5):543-546.
49. Zarate CA Jr, Baldessarini RJ, Siegel AJ, et al. Risperidone in the elderly: a pharmacoepidemiologic study. J Clin Psychiatry. 1997 Jul;58(7):311-317.
50. McDermott CL, Gruenewald DA. Pharmacologic management of agitation in patients with dementia. Curr Geriatr Rep. 2019 Mar;8(1):1-11.
51. Schnitzer K, Merideth F, Macias-Konstantopoulos W, Hayden D, Shtasel D, Bird S. Disparities in care: the role of race on the utilization of physical restraints in the emergency setting. Acad Emerg Med. 2020 Oct;27(10):943-950.
52. Palmer BW, Harmell AL. Assessment of healthcare decision-making capacity. Arch Clin Neuropsychol. 2016 Sep;31(6):530-540.

The Critical ECG

Right Ventricular-Paced Myocardial Infarction, Failure to Sense, and Failure to Capture

By Jeremy Berberian, MD; William J. Brady, MD, FACEP; and Amal Mattu, MD, FACEP

Dr. Berberian is the associate director of emergency medicine residency education at ChristianaCare and assistant professor of emergency medicine at Sidney Kimmel Medical College, Thomas Jefferson University in Philadelphia, Pennsylvania. Dr. Brady is a professor of emergency medicine, medicine, and nursing, and vice chair for faculty affairs in the Department of Emergency Medicine at the University of Virginia School of Medicine in Charlottesville. Dr. Mattu is a professor, vice chair, and codirector of the Emergency Cardiology Fellowship in the Department of Emergency Medicine at the University of Maryland School of Medicine in Baltimore.

Objectives

On completion of this article, you should be able to:
- Describe the fundamentals of right ventricular pacing.
- Contrast the Sgarbossa criteria with the modified Sgarbossa criteria.
- Explain the role of the Sgarbossa criteria and modified Sgarbossa criteria in assessing for MI in the right ventricular-paced rhythm.

CASE PRESENTATION

An 89-year-old man with a history of dual-chamber permanent pacemaker placement presents with chest pain (*Figure 1*).

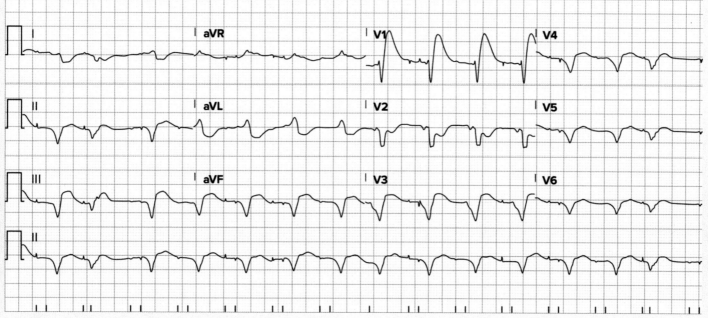

FIGURE 1. ECG of an 89-year-old man. *Credit:* EMRA.

ECG Findings

The patient's ECG shows an atrioventricular-paced (AV-paced) rhythm at 90 bpm, left axis deviation, prolonged QRS complex duration with left bundle branch block–like (LBBB-like) morphology, discordant ST elevation (STE) in lead V_1, ST depression (STD) in lead V_2, failure to capture, and intermittent failure to sense.

The fundamentals of right ventricular pacing include:
- Depolarization is initiated in the apex of the right ventricle.
- An abnormal but predictable pattern is produced that mimics an intrinsic LBBB except for leads V_1 through V_6, which will almost always have negatively oriented QRS complexes with a ventricular-paced rhythm.
  - These repolarization abnormalities confound the ECG's ability to detect an acute myocardial infarction (AMI) and other findings suggestive of acute coronary syndrome (ACS).

As with an intrinsic LBBB, the expected repolarization abnormalities in a paced rhythm follow the rule of appropriate discordance, which describes the relationship between the direction of the QRS complex and its ST segment. In other words, if the main vector of the QRS complex points up, there will be STD; if the QRS complex points down, there will be STE. Because of the repolarization abnormalities that confound the ECG's ability to detect AMI and other ACS findings

ACKNOWLEDGMENT

This case is reprinted from *Emergency ECGs: Case-Based Review and Interpretations*, available at www.emra.org/amazon or by scanning the QR code.

when a ventricular-paced rhythm occurs, the Sgarbossa criteria are required to diagnose MI. Importantly, a significant number of patients with AMI and a ventricular-paced rhythm will not have any abnormalities, Sgarbossa or otherwise, on their ECG.

The Sgarbossa criteria are based on the underlying principle that concordance and excessive discordance in LBBB are abnormal. The criteria assign a point value for any concordant STE (*Figures 2* and *3*) or excessively discordant STE (*Figure 4*). A score of 3 or greater is 98% specific for AMI, so the presence of criterion A or B is considered diagnostic of AMI. Criterion C is only assigned 2 points, so its presence alone is not diagnostic of AMI. However, with a right ventricular-paced rhythm, Sgarbossa criterion C has a 99% specificity for AMI.[1]

The modified Sgarbossa criteria includes Sgarbossa criteria A and B with a variation of criterion C. Instead of using a fixed cutoff of 5 mm for discordant STE, it uses a ratio of the STE height to the S-wave depth (*Figure 5*). An STE-S ratio ≥0.25 in 1 or more leads is considered diagnostic of AMI. This means that more than 5 mm of STE is permissible if there is a large S wave; less than 5 mm of STE may be diagnostic if the accompanying S wave is small.

The patient's ECG shows findings in leads V_1 and V_2 that meet modified Sgarbossa criterion C and Sgarbossa criterion B, respectively, both of which are diagnostic of an AMI. Identifying the J point in lead V_1 is difficult and best done by drawing a vertical line from lead V_2, where the J point is more obvious (*Figure 6*). The discordant STE ≥5 mm in lead V_1 is not diagnostic of AMI in the setting of an LBBB but has a 99% specificity for AMI in the setting of a right ventricular-paced rhythm (*Figure 7*).[1] The STD ≥1 mm in lead V_2 also meets Sgarbossa criterion B (*Figure 8*).

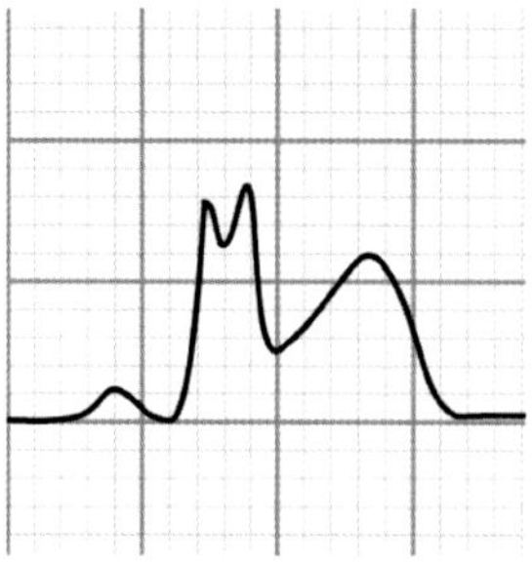

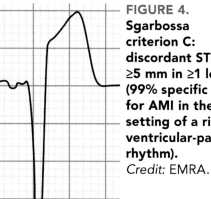

FIGURE 2. Sgarbossa criterion A: concordant STE ≥1 mm in ≥1 lead (5 points = diagnostic of AMI). *Credit:* EMRA.

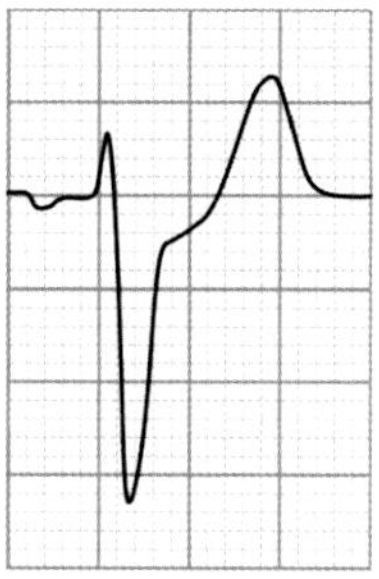

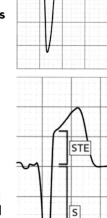

FIGURE 3. Sgarbossacriterion B: STD ≥1 mm in leads V_1, V_2, or V_3 (3 points = diagnostic of AMI). *Credit:* EMRA.

FIGURE 4. Sgarbossa criterion C: discordant STE ≥5 mm in ≥1 lead (99% specific for AMI in the setting of a right ventricular-paced rhythm). *Credit:* EMRA.

FIGURE 5. Modified Sgarbossa criterion C: STE-S ratio ≥0.25 in ≥1 lead (diagnostic of AMI). *Credit:* EMRA.

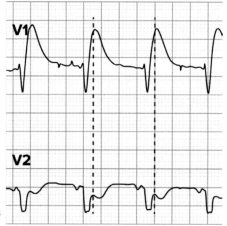

FIGURE 6. Using the J point in lead V_2, a vertical line can be extended up to help identify the J point in lead V_1. *Credit:* EMRA.

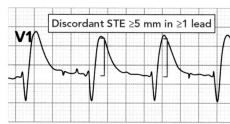

FIGURE 7. Discordant STE ≥5 mm in lead V_1 that meets Sgarbossa criterion C. *Credit:* EMRA.

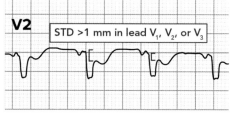

FIGURE 8. STD ≥1 mm in lead V_2 that meets Sgarbossa criterion B. *Credit:* EMRA.

Failure to Sense

The defining feature of failure to sense is asynchronous pacing — the pacemaker fails to sense the native cardiac activity. Failure to sense frequently presents as a pacer spike within a QRS complex, as seen on this patient's ECG. The second beat in the rhythm strip shows an atrial pacer spike followed by a premature ventricular contraction (PVC) with a ventricular pacer spike within the QRS complex (*Figure 9*). A retrograde P wave may be buried in the ascending limb of the PVC QRS complex, which is only possible because the atrium was not depolarized by the atrial pacing and, therefore, not refractory to retrograde conduction. In a normally functioning pacemaker, the pacer spike seen in the middle of the QRS complex would be inhibited by the pacer once it senses the native ventricular depolarization.

Common causes of failure to sense include a lead insulation break, a new intrinsic BBB, electrolyte abnormalities, and class IC antiarrhythmic drugs. Treatment is based on correcting the underlying etiology (eg, calcium for hyperkalemia).

Failure to Capture

The defining feature of failure to capture is the absence of depolarization after pacer spikes. The third beat in the rhythm strip shows an atrial pacer spike with no visible P wave on the ECG (see *Figure 9*). This is seen in all leads, including the leads

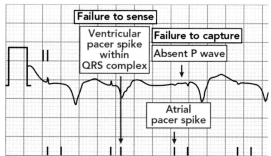

FIGURE 9. Failure to sense and failure to capture in the lead II rhythm strip. *Credit:* EMRA.

This patient went into cardiac arrest on his way to the cardiac catheterization laboratory and was unable to be resuscitated.

that typically show atrial activity the best (ie, II, III, aVF, and V$_1$), and is consistent with failure to capture. Note that this patient has a dual-chamber pacemaker (ie, AV-paced), and the presence of failure to capture with the atrial lead is far less concerning than it would be with the ventricular lead.

Common causes of failure to capture include electrode displacement, wire fracture, ischemia or infarct, and electrolyte abnormalities, especially hyperkalemia. Treatment is also based on correcting the underlying etiology (eg, calcium for hyperkalemia).

LEARNING POINTS

AMI in Right Ventricular-Paced Rhythms
Evaluate a paced ECG for ischemia, as would be done with an LBBB, using the Sgarbossa or modified Sgarbossa criteria:
- The presence of ≥1 of the following are diagnostic of AMI:
  - Concordant STE ≥1 mm in ≥1 lead
  - STD ≥1 mm in leads V$_1$, V$_2$, or V$_3$
  - Discordant STE ≥1 mm with a ratio of STE to S-wave depth ≥0.25 in ≥1 lead
- STD ≥1 mm in any of leads V$_4$ to V$_6$ increases sensitivity for AMI but has not been externally validated at the time of this publication and is not included in the most recent 2022 American College of Cardiology guidelines.[2]

Failure to Sense
- Pacemaker fails to sense native cardiac activity, leading to asynchronous pacing (*Figure 10*).
  - Sensing refers to the pacer's ability to recognize native cardiac beats.
- ECG shows pacer spikes before, after, or within P waves and QRS complexes.
- Causes include a lead insulation break, a new intrinsic BBB, electrolyte abnormalities, and class IC antiarrhythmic drugs (eg, flecainide).

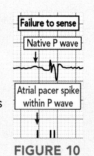

FIGURE 10

Failure to Capture
- Delivery of a pacing stimulus without subsequent myocardial depolarization (*Figure 11*)
- ECG shows absence of depolarization after pacer spikes.
- Causes are functional (eg, electrode displacement and wire fracture) and pathologic (eg, electrolyte disturbances and AMI).

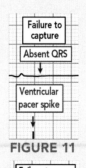

FIGURE 11

Failure to Pace
- A paced stimulus is not generated when expected (*Figure 12*).
- ECG shows decreased or absent pacemaker function.
- Causes include oversensing, a lead fracture, or an insulation defect.
  - Oversensing is pacing inhibited by noncardiac activity (eg, skeletal muscle activity) that is inappropriately recognized as native cardiac activity.

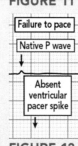

FIGURE 12

Pacemaker
- Pacer spikes are usually visible on the ECG, either at the bottom of the ECG or preceding the P wave or QRS complex.
  - Atrial pacing: spikes immediately precede P waves
  - Ventricular pacing: spikes immediately precede QRS complexes
  - Dual-chamber pacing: spikes immediately precede both P waves and QRS complexes
  - Biventricular pacing: two spikes immediately precede QRS complexes
- Atrial pacing
  - Pacemaker lead usually implanted in the right atrial appendage
  - Results in P waves with normal morphology
- Single ventricular pacing
  - Pacemaker lead usually implanted in the right ventricle apex
  - Results in an LBBB pattern in the limb leads and anteroseptal precordial leads
  - The major difference between an intrinsic LBBB and a single ventricular-paced rhythm is that the QRS complex will almost always be negatively oriented in leads V$_5$ and V$_6$ with a single ventricular-paced rhythm.
- Biventricular pacing
  - Two pacemaker leads usually implanted in the right ventricle apex and the surface of the posterior or lateral left ventricle
  - Typically results in a narrower QRS complex than with single ventricular pacing
  - Dominant R wave in lead V$_1$ +/– V$_2$ is common.
- An automatic implantable cardioverter-defibrillator will have a thick coil that differentiates it from a pacemaker.

REFERENCES

1. Kontos M, de Lemos J, Deitelzweig SB, et al. 2022 ACC expert consensus decision pathway on the evaluation and disposition of acute chest pain in the emergency department: a report of the American College of Cardiology Solution Set Oversight Committee. *J Am Coll Cardiol.* 2022 Nov 15;80(20):1925-1960.
2. Dodd KW, Zvosec DL, Hart MA, et al; PERFECT study investigators. Electrocardiographic diagnosis of acute coronary occlusion myocardial infarction in ventricular paced rhythm using the modified Sgarbossa criteria. *Ann Emerg Med.* 2021 Oct;78(4):517-529.

A Feared Complication of Cystic Fibrosis

By Fahad Uddin, DO; and
Erika Crawford, MD, FAAP, FACEP
Prisma Health Upstate in Greenville, South Carolina

Reviewed by Sharon E. Mace, MD, FACEP

Objective

On completion of this article, you should be able to:

■ Recognize, evaluate, and manage DIOS in patients with cystic fibrosis.

CASE PRESENTATION

A 13-year-old girl with cystic fibrosis presents with lower abdominal pain. She has a history of meconium ileus and is status post ostomy placement and takedown. Notably, shortly after she was born, she also had a prolonged meconium ileus that led to a bowel perforation, an exploratory laparotomy with bowel resection, and an ostomy and mucous fistula placement with subsequent reversal. She states that her current pain is constant and has been present for the past 3 days. Reported associated symptoms include nausea, nonbloody and nonbilious emesis, obstipation (her last bowel movement was 4 days ago), and no passage of flatus. The patient has had no recent fevers, dysuria, hematuria, or pulmonary-specific complaints such as coughing or dyspnea. She has a gastrostomy tube in place because of failure to thrive. Her mother states that the patient has decreased oral and enteral intake because she cannot tolerate either. When her symptoms started, the patient was evaluated at another facility, and CT of her abdomen was performed, which showed small bowel dilation concerning for distal intestinal obstruction syndrome (DIOS). However, she left that facility against medical advice and followed up with her primary care physician. Incidentally, a UTI was also found at that time and was treated prophylactically with ceftriaxone while awaiting culture results.

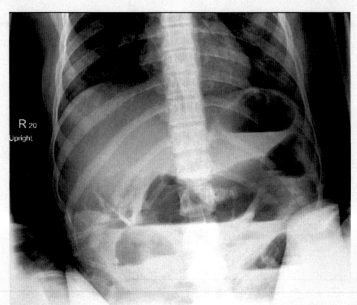

FIGURE 1. An upright anterior-posterior abdominal x-ray showing multiple dilated small bowel loops. *Credit: Fahad Uddin, DO; and Erika Crawford, MD, FAAP, FACEP.*

On examination, the patient appears pale and ill. She is tachycardic, with cool extremities and a delayed capillary refill time; she is also tachypneic, with a slight increased work of breathing and associated splinting. Her abdomen is mildly distended, and she has left and right lower quadrant tenderness; bowel sounds are normoactive in all quadrants. Her vital signs are BP 124/89, P 133, R 24, and T 36.8°C (98.2°F); SpO_2 is 100% on room air. Because of her presenting appearance and vital signs, the patient meets criteria for systemic inflammatory response syndrome (ie, SIRS), and the sepsis protocol is initiated. Screening laboratory tests, including blood cultures, a venous blood gas, and a urinalysis are obtained. The workup reveals respiratory alkalosis with an elevated lactate level of 3.2 mmol/L; a leukocytosis of 11.2×10^9/L; hemoconcentration with a hemoglobin level of 16.5 g/dL and a hematocrit measurement of 45.3%; an anion gap of 18 mmol/L; transaminitis with an AST level of 68 IU/L and an ALT level of 97 IU/L; and an elevated C-reactive protein level of 39.1 mg/L. Empiric cefepime and intravenous fluids are administered to treat sepsis and the patient's UTI. Two views of abdominal x-rays visualize multiple dilated loops of the small bowel with air-fluid levels (*Figures 1* and *2*). Pediatric surgery is urgently consulted and recommends nasogastric tube placement and a CT of the abdomen and pelvis with intravenous and enteral contrast. CT results support the x-ray findings and reveal a transition point within the left lower quadrant that involves the distal ileum (*Figures 3* and *4*). While sleeping in the emergency department, the patient has a few desaturation episodes, likely multifactorial due to her underlying history, acute illness, and decreased lung volumes from abdominal distension. A chest x-ray is ordered and demonstrates stable findings. She is given her home cystic fibrosis airway clearance regimen and oxygen supplementation.

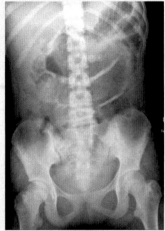

FIGURE 2. A supine anterior-posterior abdominal x-ray showing multiple dilated small bowel loops. *Credit: Fahad Uddin, DO; and Erika Crawford, MD, FAAP, FACEP.*

Discussion

Cystic fibrosis is a genetic disease that most commonly affects the respiratory system. However, the thick mucus secretions produced in the disease affect many other organ systems, including the GI, endocrine, and reproductive systems. Because of modern medicine, individuals with cystic fibrosis are living longer, and the incidence of these complications is rising. A feared GI complication of cystic fibrosis is DIOS, formerly known as meconium ileus equivalent. The syndrome was first described in 1945 and is an acute complete or incomplete obstruction of the ileocecal area of the small intestine secondary to inspissated intestinal contents.[1,2] It affects approximately 10% to 22% of individuals with cystic fibrosis but may affect many more because it is difficult to distinguish from other causes of obstruction.[3] The etiology of DIOS is unclear, but studies have shown that pancreatic enzyme deficiency plays a major role in its development, along with intestinal dysmotility and dehydration.[4] The patient in the case presentation has a history of pancreatic insufficiency for which she takes supplemental enzymes; her lack of oral and enteral intake and her nausea and vomiting are also likely risk factors for DIOS.

A case of DIOS can be hard to distinguish from a case of constipation. Both constipation and DIOS present with abdominal pain and distention and, potentially, with a palpable mass in the lower abdomen and decreased bowel movements.

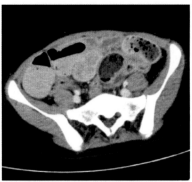

FIGURE 3. An axial view of the abdomen and pelvis CT showing multiple dilated small bowel loops with a transition point over the left lower quadrant of the abdomen. *Credit:* Fahad Uddin, DO; and Erika Crawford, MD, FAAP, FACEP.

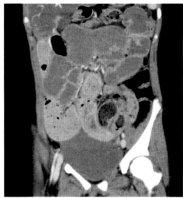

FIGURE 4. A coronal view of the abdomen and pelvis CT showing dilated small bowel loops with a transition point over the left lower quadrant of the abdomen. *Credit:* Fahad Uddin, DO; and Erika Crawford, MD, FAAP, FACEP.

In cases of constipation, however, symptoms are more gradual in onset, and the stool burden is more evenly distributed within the intestines. In cases of DIOS, the mass is almost always palpable in the right lower abdominal quadrant, where the ileocecal area is located. An abdominal x-ray can increase suspicion for DIOS by showing an accumulation of stool within only the distal ileum and right colon. An abdominal CT confirms DIOS by excluding other intestinal pathologies around this area of the abdomen, such as intussusception, bowel obstruction secondary to abdominal adhesions, volvulus, appendicitis, appendicular abscess, Crohn disease, fibrosing colonopathy, and malignancy.[2]

Treatment for DIOS depends on the severity of symptoms and whether the obstruction is complete or incomplete. Incomplete DIOS is managed nonsurgically through methods such as oral rehydration, stool softeners, osmotic laxatives, or enemas to alleviate the stool burden causing the obstruction. If the obstruction does not improve with these measures, osmotic contrasts can be used. Rarely, incomplete DIOS can lead to complete DIOS, in which case pediatric surgery should be consulted for laparotomy and manual decompression of the obstructed area.[4] Nasogastric tube decompression can also alleviate the obstruction and should be used on a case-by-case basis. If left untreated, DIOS can lead to intestinal ischemia and bowel perforation, both of which require surgical management.

CASE RESOLUTION

The patient was admitted to the pediatric ICU because of her clinical appearance and episodes of desaturation that required close monitoring. Pediatric pulmonology was consulted for her desaturation episodes and recommended close observation and administration of her home cystic fibrosis treatments (albuterol) and chest physiotherapy. The patient was subsequently weaned off supplemental oxygen without further desaturation episodes. She was also given piperacillin-tazobactam for broader antibiotic coverage. The pediatric surgery team elected to manage her bowel obstruction through nonoperative bowel decompression. She was also given an enteral contrast as both a diagnostic and therapeutic measure, which passed through the area of concern on repeat imaging 24 hours after admission. The patient subsequently had several bowel movements, and her diet was able to be advanced without any complications. The patient was discharged with a daily bowel regimen of lactulose and senna. She was advised to closely follow up with pediatric surgery and pulmonology as an outpatient.

REFERENCES

1. Houwen RH, van der Doef HP, Sermet I, et al. Defining DIOS and constipation in cystic fibrosis with a multicentre study on the incidence, characteristics, and treatment of DIOS. *J Pediatr Gastroenterol Nutr.* 2010 Jan;50(1):38-42.
2. Colombo C, Ellemunter H, Houwen R, Munck A, Taylor C, Wilschanski M; ECFS. Guidelines for the diagnosis and management of distal intestinal obstruction syndrome in cystic fibrosis patients. *J Cyst Fibros.* 2011 Jun;10(suppl 2):S24-S28.
3. Green J, Carroll W, Gilchrist FJ; Cochrane Cystic Fibrosis and Genetic Disorders Group. Interventions for treating distal intestinal obstruction syndrome (DIOS) in cystic fibrosis. *Cochrane Database Syst Rev.* 2018 Aug;2018(8):CD012798.
4. Sabharwal S, Schwarzenberg SJ. Cystic fibrosis: overview of gastrointestinal disease. UpToDate. Last updated July 26, 2023. https://www.uptodate.com/contents/cystic-fibrosis-overview-of-gastrointestinal-disease

Headache Presentations in the Emergency Department

By Paula N. Kreutzer, MD, MPH; and
Nicholas G. Maldonado, MD, FACEP
University of Florida College of Medicine, Gainesville

Reviewed by Andrew J. Eyre, MD, MS-HPEd

Objectives

On completion of this article, you should be able to:

■ Differentiate between primary and secondary headaches.

■ List the differential diagnosis of secondary headaches.

■ Explain how to diagnose the causes of secondary headaches.

Raam R, Tabatabai RR. Headache in the emergency department: avoiding misdiagnosis of dangerous secondary causes, an update. *Emerg Med Clin North Am.* 2021 Feb;39(1):67-85.

─ **KEY POINTS** ─────────────────────────

■ The likelihood of a secondary headache being from a dangerous cause can be gathered from a thorough history as well as neurologic and ophthalmologic examinations.

■ ACEP's clinical policy recommendations can be used to decide which patients with headaches can be diagnosed based on a bedside assessment and which need further testing.

■ In patients with headaches that peak in intensity within 1 hour, SAH can be safely ruled out by using the Ottawa SAH rule or noncontrast CT (within 6 hours of symptom onset). If results are negative and clinical suspicion persists, CT angiography or lumbar puncture can then be used to rule out SAH.

■ Nonopioid medications are the preferred treatment for acute primary headache. Specific secondary headache conditions require other interventions.

Headaches are a common reason that people present to the emergency department. Headaches can be classified as either primary or secondary. Primary headaches are more common, more benign, and include tension-type headaches, migraines, and cluster headaches. Secondary headaches are attributed to an underlying disorder that can be life-threatening: an aneurysm, a dissection, an infection or inflammation, or a space-occupying lesion; their presentations are variable and atypical. Fortunately, secondary headaches are relatively rare and often respond to the same analgesic agents used to treat more benign headaches. Emergency physicians can use diagnostic approaches and clinical policy recommendations to better differentiate a primary headache from the more dangerous secondary type.

Raam and Tabatabai describe an initial approach to the undifferentiated headache patient that includes assessing the patient's stability, addressing pain management, and ruling out secondary headache causes without overutilizing diagnostic testing. The authors also highlight the clinical features, diagnostic tests, interventions, and 14 conditions for emergency physicians to include in the differential diagnosis (*Table 1*).

Dangerous Causes of Secondary Headaches
AACG
Bacterial meningitis
CAD • ICAD • VAD
Cerebral infarction
CO poisoning
CVT
GCA
IIH
Occult trauma
Preeclampsia
Pituitary apoplexy
RCVS
SAH
Space-occupying lesion

TABLE 1. Differential diagnosis for secondary headaches

When gathering a patient's history, physicians should focus on the headache's characteristics (eg, time of onset, time-to-peak intensity, and quality), modifying factors, and associated symptoms. A sudden, severe headache with maximal intensity at onset (ie, a thunderclap headache) deserves special attention: It is a red flag symptom that indicates a subarachnoid hemorrhage (SAH). The classic thunderclap headache's peak time is usually within seconds to minutes but, according to the literature, can take up to 1 hour. Although a hallmark of SAH, thunderclap headaches are sometimes absent in SAH patients and can also be associated with other causes of secondary headaches (ie, cerebral venous thrombosis [CVT], cervical artery dissection [CAD], acute angle closure glaucoma [AACG], pituitary apoplexy, and reversible cerebral vasoconstriction syndrome [RCVS]). Dangerous headache etiologies can also be associated with headaches that are slow in onset (as with CVT) or recurrent (as with idiopathic intracranial hypertension [IIH]).

Headaches that have a positional quality, such as those that occur in supine position, or headaches that are worse in the morning or evening, may be associated with conditions that increase intracranial pressure, such as space-occupying lesions. Modifying factors can also provide clues to a specific cause. For example, giant cell arteritis (GCA) and AACG are associated with increasing age, especially patients aged 50 years and older. IIH is most likely to occur in obese women in their 20s and 30s. Pituitary apoplexy and preeclampsia should be high on the differential diagnosis for pregnant patients with headaches, especially when they are past 20 weeks' gestation. Space-occupying lesions should be suspected in any patient with a history of malignancy.

Medication use, specifically anticoagulants or oral contraceptives; immune status; and events that preceded headache onset are other important considerations in determining the cause. Bacterial meningitis and CVT can occur after head and neck infections. SAH or CAD can occur after physical exertion, coughing, or any activity that acutely elevates arterial pressure. CAD can also be preceded by blunt cervical trauma or chiropractic manipulation. Carbon monoxide (CO) poisoning should be suspected in headache patients who were recently exposed to smoke inhalation, engine exhaust, or inadequate ventilation of heating sources, especially when multiple household members are ill.

Associated symptoms also provide clues to the cause. Fever can be seen in bacterial meningitis and GCA; neck pain or stiffness in bacterial meningitis, CAD, and SAH; visual disturbances in GCA, CVT, IIH, AACG, preeclampsia, and pituitary apoplexy; and focal neurologic deficits in SAH, CVT, space-occupying lesions, and CAD (anterior circulation symptoms are seen with internal carotid artery dissection [ICAD], and posterior circulation symptoms are seen with vertebral artery dissection [VAD]). Some secondary headache causes have unique features: GCA is associated with jaw claudication and temporal artery abnormalities (eg, tenderness and swelling).

The physical examination should include detailed neurologic and ophthalmologic examinations that focus on mentation levels, new neurologic signs, and ocular abnormalities. Completely normal examination results are more common in benign conditions but can also be seen in headaches with dangerous etiologies. The presence of an altered mental status or focal neurologic deficits warrants further workup for secondary headache causes. Nuchal rigidity, jolt accentuation, and positive Kernig and Brudzinski signs suggest bacterial meningitis, but their absence does not rule out the condition. Ocular abnormalities include monocular vision loss in GCA and intracranial atherosclerotic disease, transient or persistent visual acuity changes or vision loss in IIH, papilledema in IIH and CVT, and associated cranial nerve palsies in CVT and pituitary apoplexy. In cases of AACG, patients can have isolated monocular pain, conjunctival injection, a mid-fixed dilated pupil, decreased visual acuity, and an intraocular pressure (IOP) greater than 21 mm Hg (but typically at least 30 mm Hg), which establishes the diagnosis.

After the history and physical examination, patients with acute headaches should be risk stratified. According to the American College of Emergency Physicians' (ACEP's) 2019 clinical policy, the Ottawa SAH rule is a highly sensitive decision rule that should be used to rule out SAH in headache patients with normal neurologic examinations and peak headache severity within 1 hour of pain onset (level B recommendation).

Serum laboratory workup has limited diagnostic utility in most cases of secondary headaches but can be useful for specific conditions. An elevated erythrocyte sedimentation rate ≥50 mm/hr is part of the diagnostic criteria for GCA; elevated C-reactive protein levels and platelet counts can also increase GCA's likelihood but may also be normal in positive cases. D-dimer testing has been studied in patients with CVT and has been found to have variable diagnostic accuracy that limits its usefulness. A diagnosis of preeclampsia can be established in pregnant patients with headaches through the presence of proteinuria, thrombocytopenia, renal insufficiency, or impaired liver function. Findings of hypoglycemia and hyponatremia can be signs of pituitary apoplexy. A diagnosis of CO poisoning can be established through co-oximetry that reveals an elevated CO level.

A 2008 ACEP clinical policy addresses which headache patients require neuroimaging. An emergent noncontrast head CT is required for headache patients with new sudden-onset severe headaches; with new abnormal findings on neurologic examination; or with HIV and a new type of headache (level B recommendations). An urgent noncontrast head CT, which can be arranged before discharge home, is recommended for headache patients older than 50 years who have a new headache but normal neurologic examination findings (level C recommendation).

ACEP's 2019 clinical policy recommends a normal noncontrast head CT (minimum third-generation scanner) within 6 hours of symptom onset in headache patients with normal neurologic examinations to rule out nontraumatic SAH. Importantly, however, a normal noncontrast head CT does not evaluate for most of the dangerous headache causes. For example, AACG is diagnosed based on an IOP assessment, and GCA and preeclampsia diagnoses do not require neuroimaging based on their specific diagnostic criteria from other specialty organizations. Other diagnoses require more advanced neuroimaging. CAD requires CT or MR angiography of the head and neck. CVT and IIH (to exclude alternative causes with IIH) require CT or MR venography of the head. Pituitary apoplexy and space-occupying lesions are diagnosed by MRI. Lastly, bacterial meningitis, IIH, and SAH require lumbar puncture to establish the diagnosis. CT angiography has an increasing role in the diagnostic workup for SAH, which is reflected in ACEP's clinical policy recommendation to perform lumbar puncture or CT angiography to safely rule out SAH in adult patients who are still at risk of SAH after a negative noncontrast head CT (level C recommendation).

Therapy should target treating the pain and the specific identified cause. ACEP recommends nonopioid medications to treat acute primary headaches (level A recommendation); it also recommends that physicians refrain from using the pain response to therapy as the sole diagnostic indicator of an acute headache's underlying etiology (level C recommendation). Raam and Tabatabai go into more detail on the therapies and interventions for specific dangerous causes of secondary headaches.

Critical Decisions in Emergency Medicine's LLSA literature reviews feature articles from ABEM's 2023 Lifelong Learning and Self-Assessment Reading List. Available online at acep.org/moc/llsa and on the ABEM website.

The Critical Procedure

Phimosis Treatment

By Steven J. Warrington, MD, MEd, MS
MercyOne Siouxland in Sioux City, Iowa

Objective

On completion of this article, you should be able to:

■ Discuss how to perform a foreskin dilation for patients with phimosis.

Introduction

Although most patients with phimosis (ie, stenosis of the distal aspect of the foreskin) do not require any intervention, the condition can lead to acute urinary obstruction that requires foreskin dilation to allow urine to pass. This uncommon procedure allows for follow-up on an outpatient basis.

Contraindications

■ None

Benefits and Risks

In addition to treating urinary obstructions, foreskin dilations can also be performed for catheter placement. Primary risks of dilation include damage to the glans of the penis or the urethral meatus. Trauma to the surrounding tissue can also occur. The procedure carries a risk of failure; in these cases, alternative therapy routes will need to be pursued, such as a dorsal slit.

Alternatives

The recommended initial attempt at treating phimosis is dilation alone, without a dorsal slit. However, dilation as a temporary treatment followed by circumcision or dorsal slit alone as the initial treatment are other alternatives. Suprapubic aspiration, suprapubic catheter placement, or referral to urology or other specialties who can perform these procedures are also alternatives to treating phimosis with dilation in the emergency department.

Reducing Side Effects

Manual attempts to retract the foreskin should be done gently; forced retraction is not only painful but can place the patient at risk of adhesion development. Additionally, care must be taken when readying for dilation to ensure that the urethral meatus is not included in the procedure so that inadvertent trauma is avoided. Also be aware of any signs of infection and prescribe antibiotics as appropriate.

Special Considerations

Pharmacologic therapy for pain and anxiety should be considered as part of phimosis treatment. Options include systemic medication, local anesthetics, regional anesthetics, or multiple routes of therapy.

TECHNIQUE

1. **Obtain** the patient's consent and the necessary equipment. Pretreat with pharmacologic agents if needed.

2. **Cleanse** and drape the area.

3. **Provide** local or regional anesthesia. Regional anesthesia can be obtained with a dorsal nerve block.

4. **Identify** the opening of the phimosis and insert the jaws of the hemostats between the glans and inner layer of foreskin. A fine metal probe can aid in initial insertion and identification of where to place the hemostats.

5. **Gently** use the hemostats to further separate the glans and inner foreskin, breaking adhesions when necessary.

6. **Determine** if the phimosis can be opened enough (depending on the purpose of the procedure).

7. **Consider** a dorsal slit if the opening is insufficient. If the hemostats can be inserted, consider a single clamp of dorsal foreskin to crush the tissue, but be careful to exclude the glans from this part of the procedure. Straight scissors can be used to incise the crushed tissue and open the phimosis.

8. **Consult** a specialist if no opening is identified. If no specialist is available and temporary therapy cannot be provided through the suprapubic route, consider the risky attempt of pushing the glans away from the distal phimosis and using the single clamp to crush the tissue; then create an incision with scissors. This route, however, can result in trauma to the glans and cosmetic issues.

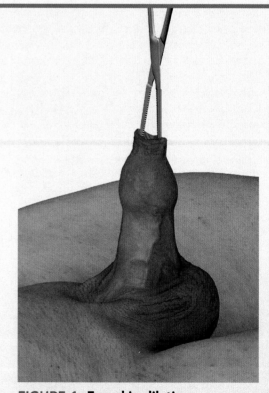

FIGURE 1. Foreskin dilation technique. *Credit:* ACEP.

Morel-Lavallée Lesion

By Steven Morrin, MD; Nick Copeli, MD; and
Victor Huang, MD, CAQSM
Northwell Health Orthopaedic Institute in New York

Reviewed by John Kiel, DO, MPH, FACEP, CAQSM

Objective

On completion of this article, you should be able to:
■ Explain the diagnostic and management methods for MLLs.

CASE PRESENTATION

A 20-year-old woman presents with progressively worsening right thigh pain after a motor vehicle collision that occurred 2 weeks ago. She was an unrestrained front passenger in a vehicle that crashed into a brick wall on the passenger's side, causing her to fall out of her seat and strike her right leg against the door.

Examination of the right lower extremity demonstrates a fluctuant collection that is tender to palpation along the lateral and posterior thigh. No erythema or warmth is noted, the compartments are soft, and neurovascular examination is normal. Plain x-rays of the femur and knee show no acute fractures or dislocations.

Background

A Morel-Lavallée lesion (MLL), named after the French physician who first identified it, is a closed internal degloving injury that leads to a hemolymphatic collection between the subcutaneous tissue and the underlying fascia. MLLs develop postoperatively or after trauma.[1,2] Although MLLs are commonly found in the proximal thigh overlying the greater trochanter, cases have also occurred in other locations including the trunk, low back, pelvis, knee, and scapula.[1-3] These lesions are often difficult to identify in the early phases of development because they grow insidiously. Various populations are at risk of MLLs including passengers in motor vehicle collisions, cyclists who experience road rash after a fall, and football players.[4] The mechanism of injury is typically high-energy blunt trauma that shears subcutaneous tissue off of the underlying fascia, leading to a disruption of lymphatic and blood vessels. The newly created space is then filled with liquefied fat, lymph, or blood. This process can occur in the initial hours after an injury, but some MLLs develop over days or months.[1,2] A chronic MLL occurs when the blood is reabsorbed and a fibrous capsule forms around the residual serosanguinous fluid.[1]

Physical Examination

A patient with an MLL typically presents with an enlarging painful lesion that usually occurs within hours to days after the initial injury.[1,5] When examining a patient for an MLL, emergency physicians should look for skin hypermobility, ecchymosis, tenderness to palpation, fluctuance, or soft tissue swelling.[1,6] Discoloration can take several days to fully develop. For this reason, up to one-third of MLL diagnoses are initially missed.[6] Complications of MLLs include progressive expansion of the lesion, skin breakdown and necrosis, recurrence, and infection.[1,3,5]

Imaging

Plain x-rays are used to assess for acute fractures or dislocations; however, x-rays have a limited ability to visualize MLLs and may reveal only a nonspecific, noncalcified soft tissue mass. Ultrasound and CT are more appropriate for initial emergency evaluation (*Figures 1* and *2*).[5]

Ultrasound findings of MLLs include a hypoechoic fluid collection that is deep to the hypodermis and superficial to the

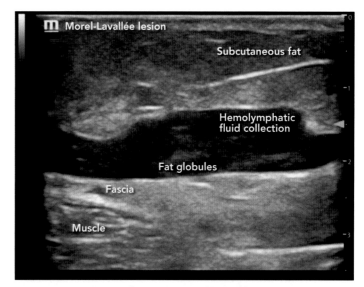

FIGURE 1. Point-of-care musculoskeletal ultrasound demonstrating a hypoechoic collection deep to the subcutaneous tissue and superficial to the fascia and musculature

muscle fascia, without internal flow with Doppler (see *Figure 1*).[1] The collection is usually compressible and can contain internal debris including fat globules.[1,5] MRI is the preferred imaging modality because its improved soft tissue contrast allows for the best characterization of the lesion.[1,5]

Mellado and Bencardino developed a classification system that categorizes lesions into six types based on MRI characteristics; however, this lesion classification does not correlate with treatment or clinical outcome.[1,3,7] Shen et al and Singh et al developed algorithmic approaches to determine the most appropriate management and likelihood of success.[1,3]

Management

The decision to manage these lesions conservatively or operatively is based on chronicity, lesion size, clinical presentation, imaging findings, and the lesion's proximity to concurrent soft tissue and bony injuries that may also require

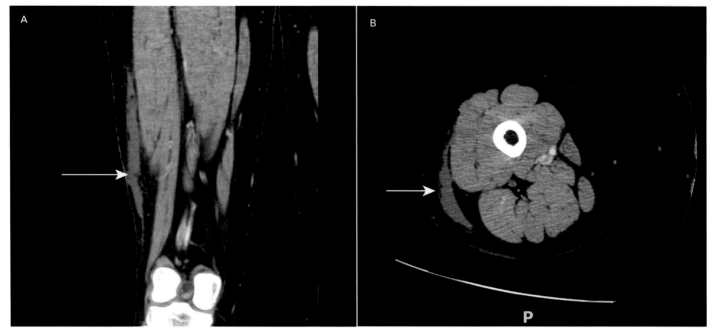

FIGURE 2. CT of the lower extremity with intravenous contrast demonstrating a subcutaneous perifascial collection of fluid that measures 7 cm × 2 cm × 15 cm, consistent with an MLL

operative management.[1,3,5] Management options include close observation without intervention, percutaneous drainage, sclerodesis, or surgical debridement.[1,6]

Adjunctive treatments such as serial aspiration, compression banding, and liposuction are sometimes performed to minimize additional soft tissue damage.[6] Compressive bandaging can be used for small, acute lesions without capsule formation that are located in the extremities.[1,3] Percutaneous drainage can be performed, but the likelihood of recurrence is high after this procedure, especially if the fluid volume is greater than 50 mL.[1,5] Sclerodesis involves aspirating fluid in the MLL, injecting a sclerosing agent, such as doxycycline, and then aspirating the solution. Sclerodesis induces fibrosis and can be performed in acute or chronic MLLs with less than 400 mL of fluid.[1]

Operative intervention with debridement is indicated if the overlying skin is necrotic or the fluid collection is large or difficult to aspirate percutaneously.[1] Open drainage or mass resection is indicated for chronic MLLs, especially with fibrous capsule formation. Quilting sutures, fibrin sealant, and low suction drains can be used to close the dead space, reducing recurrence and infection rates.[1,3]

Research on the success of close observation compared to surgical management is currently limited to smaller studies with subsequent meta-analyses. The data from orthopedic journals suggest that across the entire MLL patient population, nonoperative approaches such as compression wraps or percutaneous aspiration have limited efficacy compared to surgery.[1,3,6] However, emerging data show that less invasive techniques like sclerodesis have a high success rate, improved aesthetic outcomes, and less recurrence.[1-3]

CASE RESOLUTION

A surgical consult was requested to evaluate the patient's candidacy for operative intervention. The surgical team evaluated the patient in the emergency department and reviewed the imaging but did not feel that the patient's current clinical picture warranted immediate surgical intervention. A compressive wrap was placed over her leg, and she was scheduled for a follow-up appointment in 1 week. At the outpatient follow-up visit, the surgeon and patient decided to continue with conservative management with close observation, the compressive wrap, pain control, and warm compresses rather than operative management. She was cleared for all activity 3 months after her initial injury. At her 6-month follow-up visit, she reported that the collection had reduced in size, her pain had resolved, and she had no functional limitations with work or activity.

REFERENCES

1. Singh R, Rymer B, Youssef B, Lim J. The Morel-Lavallée lesion and its management: a review of the literature. *J Orthop.* 2018 Aug 28;15(4):917-921.
2. Jalota L, Ukaigwe A, Jain S. Diagnosis and management of closed internal degloving injuries: the Morel-Lavallée lesion. *J Emerg Med.* 2015 Jul;49(1):e1-e4.
3. Shen C, Peng JP, Chen XD. Efficacy of treatment in peri-pelvic Morel-Lavallee lesion: a systematic review of the literature. *Arch Orthop Trauma Surg.* 2013 May;133(5):635-640.
4. Tejwani SG, Cohen SB, Bradley JP. Management of Morel-Lavallee lesion of the knee: twenty-seven cases in the national football league. *Am J Sports Med.* 2007 Jul;35(7):1162-1167.
5. Amaravathi U, Singh S, Reddy AA, Mohammed M A, Ayyan SM. The Morel-Lavallée lesion. *J Emerg Med.* 2023 Jan;64(1):67-69.
6. Scolaro JA, Chao T, Zamorano DP. The Morel-Lavallee lesion: diagnosis and management. *J Am Acad Orthop Surg.* 2016 Oct;24(10):667-672.
7. Mellado JM, Bencardino JT. Morel-Lavallée lesion: review with emphasis on MR imaging. *Magn Reson Imaging Clin N Am.* 2005 Nov;13(4):775-782.

The Critical Image

A Cyanotic Infant

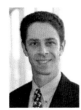

By Joshua S. Broder, MD, FACEP
Dr. Broder is a professor and the residency program director in the Department of Emergency Medicine at Duke University Medical Center in Durham, North Carolina.

Objectives

On completion of this article, you should be able to:

■ Recognize the classic chest x-ray findings of tetralogy of Fallot.

■ Explain the physiologic consequences of the anatomic defects of tetralogy of Fallot.

CASE PRESENTATION

A 2-month-old infant presents with intermittent cyanosis. His parents state that he has been having centrally distributed blue discoloration that lasts for approximately a minute, often when he is crying. They present a photograph taken during an episode that shows a pulse oximeter reading of 65%. The patient was born at 39 weeks' gestation by vaginal delivery; his mother lacked prenatal care. According to the parents, a heart problem was identified immediately after birth, and a procedure was performed, but they cannot describe the details.

The infant's vital signs are BP 116/83, P 147, R 42, and T 36.7°C (98.1°F); SpO_2 is 81% on room air. The patient appears in no acute distress. He does appear slightly cyanotic but has normal muscle tone and skin turgor and a capillary refill time of less than 2 seconds. He has a cleft upper lip but an otherwise normal head examination, including normal fontanelles. His cardiac examination demonstrates a continuous grade 3/6 murmur throughout the chest. He is tachypneic, with mild retractions and normal breath sounds. His abdomen is normal, and he has no pitting edema in his extremities. A chest x-ray is obtained (*Figure 1*).

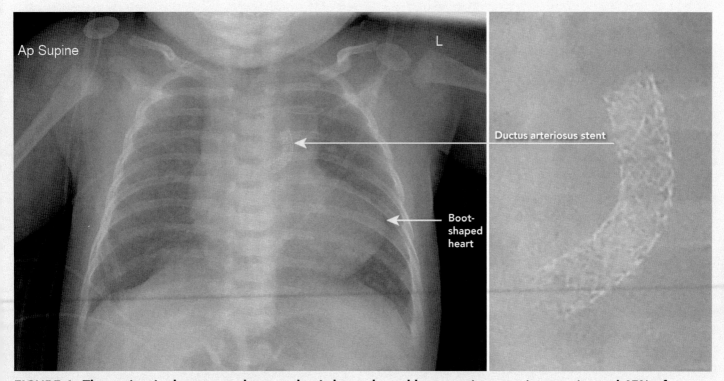

FIGURE 1. The patient's chest x-ray shows a classic boot-shaped heart, a sign seen in an estimated 65% of tetralogy of Fallot patients and attributed to the hypertrophied right ventricle.[1] A ductus arteriosus stent is visible.

Discussion

Tetrology of Fallot is a congenital heart defect that is characterized by a ventricular septal defect, pulmonic stenosis, right ventricular hypertrophy, and an abnormally positioned aorta that receives blood flow from both ventricles.[2] The right ventricular outflow tract is diminutive or absent, so blood does not flow from the right heart to the lungs. Instead, some blood is diverted from the aorta to the pulmonary arteries through the ductus arteriosus. Tetralogy of Fallot is, therefore, called a ductal-dependent lesion because infants rely on the ductus arteriosus' persistent patency for pulmonary blood flow and survival. The ductus arteriosus normally closes functionally by muscular contraction within 12 to 72 hours of birth unless kept open, initially, by the administration of prostaglandin E1 and,

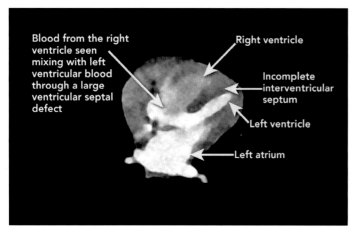

FIGURE 2. **An axial CT image obtained on the patient's third day of life (edited to remove surrounding structures).** Key abnormal anatomy and physiologic effects are seen. The interventricular septum is incomplete, resulting in a large ventricular septal defect. Deoxygenated blood from the right ventricle is seen mixing with oxygenated blood from the left ventricle — a right-to-left shunt. CT is not typically needed in acute management of tetralogy of Fallot, but images are included here to clarify anatomy and physiologic effects.

thereafter, by endovascular stenting.[3] In tetralogy of Fallot, some aortic blood flows through the ductus arteriosus to the lungs, takes up oxygen, and returns to the left atrium through the pulmonary veins. The oxygenated blood enters the left ventricle and mixes with deoxygenated blood entering from the right ventricle via the ventricular septal defect before being ejected into the aorta and on to the systemic circulation (*Figures 2* and *3*). Consequently, no matter how much oxygen is supplied to the lungs and absorbed into the blood, systemic blood does not achieve normal, high hemoglobin oxygen saturation levels. Pulse oximeter readings in the range of 80% may be "normal" and adequate for infants with tetralogy of Fallot.

During a hypercyanotic episode (also called a *tet spell*), which is often triggered by crying, infants become cyanotic because of an increase in shunting of deoxygenated blood from the right to the left ventricle; the increased fraction of deoxygenated blood decreases the hemoglobin oxygen saturation and

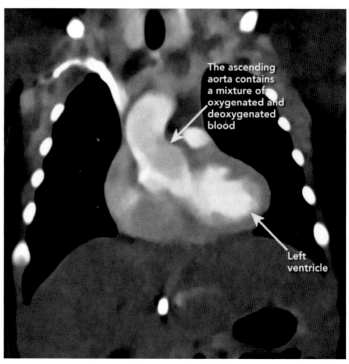

FIGURE 3. **A coronal CT image before placement of the ductus arteriosus stent.** The plume of blood in the ascending aorta contains a mixture of deoxygenated blood from the right ventricle and oxygenated blood from the left ventricle. This mixture results in the patient having a low arterial oxygen saturation, regardless of the FiO_2 supplied to the lungs.

increases the cyanotic appearance of the blood leaving the left ventricle for systemic circulation. Tet spells can be aborted by a knee-to-chest position of the infant, which increases systemic vascular resistance and left-sided heart pressures and reduces right-to-left shunting.[4] Worsening cyanosis and hypoxia that occur outside of a tet spell and are unresponsive to supplemental oxygen can indicate decreased pulmonary blood flow through the ductus arteriosus from etiologies such as anatomic closure of an unstented ductus or from stent occlusion. Other common causes of hypoxia, such as conditions that inhibit alveolar oxygen exchange (eg, pneumonia or pulmonary edema) would typically improve with increased FiO_2.

CASE RESOLUTION

The patient was admitted to the cardiology service and underwent echocardiography, which showed limited blood flow from the aorta through the ductus arteriosus to the pulmonary arteries. Cardiac catheterization was performed, and the ductus stent was dilated with a balloon to increase the diameter from 3.4 to 4.5 mm. The patient's oxygenation improved following this intervention.

REFERENCES

1. Haider EA. The boot-shaped heart sign. *Radiology*. 2008 Jan;246(1):328-329.
2. Facts about tetralogy of Fallot. CDC. Last reviewed February 3, 2023. https://www.cdc.gov/ncbddd/heartdefects/tetralogyoffallot.html
3. Iwashima S, Satake E, Uchiyama H, Seki K, Ishikawa T. Closure time of ductus arteriosus after birth based on survival analysis. *Early Hum Dev*. 2018 Jun;121:37-43.
4. Beerman LB. Tetralogy of Fallot. Merck Manual. Revised April 2023. https://www.merckmanuals.com/professional/pediatrics/congenital-cardiovascular-anomalies/tetralogy-of-fallot

Feature Editor: Joshua S. Broder, MD, FACEP. See also *Diagnostic Imaging for the Emergency Physician* (Winner of the 2011 Prose Award in Clinical Medicine, the American Publishers Award for Professional and Scholarly Excellence) and *Critical Images in Emergency Medicine* by Dr. Broder.

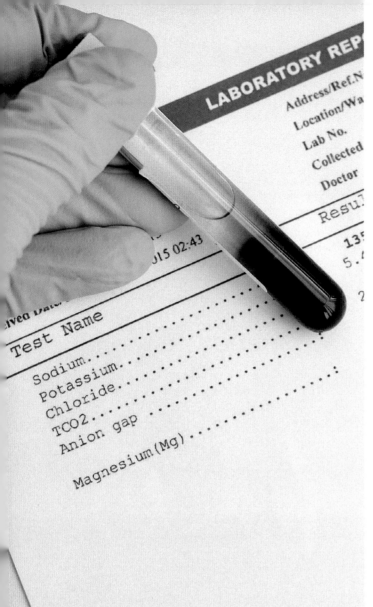

Balancing Act

Metabolic Acidosis

LESSON 18

By Ryan Yavorsky, DO; and Jonathan Glauser, MD, FACEP

Dr. Yavorsky is an assistant professor and Dr. Glauser is a professor of emergency medicine at Case Western Reserve School of Medicine, and both are faculty of the emergency medicine residency program at the Cleveland Clinic's MetroHealth Medical Center in Cleveland, Ohio.

Reviewed by Sharon E. Mace, MD, FACEP

Objectives

On completion of this lesson, you should be able to:

1. Recognize what constitutes metabolic acidosis.
2. Identify the underlying causes of an acidotic state.
3. Describe the process for evaluating mixed acid-base disturbances.
4. State the indications for and limitations of sodium bicarbonate therapy.
5. Discuss the management of toxic alcohol exposure.

From the EM Model

5.0 Endocrine, Metabolic, and Nutritional Disorders
    5.1   Acid-Base Disturbances
          5.1.1   Metabolic or Respiratory
                5.1.1.1   Acidosis

■ CRITICAL DECISIONS ■

- How is the primary acid-base disturbance determined?
- How is compensation for a primary acid-base disturbance evaluated?
- How are anion gap and delta gap used?
- What are the considerations in managing emergent acid-base disturbances?
- When should sodium bicarbonate be used to treat metabolic acidosis?
- How are toxic alcohol ingestions managed?
- What is propylene glycol, and what are its therapeutic implications?

Metabolic acidosis is common in acutely ill patients and has many potential causes. Treatment should be timely because the condition can lead to shock and respiratory failure. Further complicating matters, its potential presentations are numerous. Determining the cause of metabolic acidosis is the first priority since treatment depends on the etiology and is integral to the successful management of these critically ill patients.

■ CASE ONE

A 20-year-old woman presents with complaints of a flu-like illness. She states that for the past 2 days, she has been nauseated, vomiting, and short of breath. Her vital signs are BP 90/40, P 130, R 31, and T 36.7°C (98°F); SpO_2 is 98% on room air. Her lungs sound clear even though her respirations are deep and labored. Her physical examination reveals a nontender abdomen, dry mucous membranes, and poor skin turgor. She is alert but oriented to name only; no focal neurologic deficits are present. Intravenous access is obtained, and the emergency physician begins the patient's workup and treatment.

■ CASE TWO

A 50-year-old man presents via ambulance after he was found minimally responsive in a nearby parking lot. He cannot provide his history or any identification. He can nod his head to questions and intermittently follow commands. His speech is slurred, and his breath has a faint but distinctive smell. His vital signs are BP 80/40, P 120, R 22, and T 36.7°C (98°F); SpO_2 is 98% on room air. His Glasgow Coma Scale (GCS) score is 10. On neurologic examination, he has marked dysmetria with poor postural tone. His lungs are clear bilaterally, and his abdomen is nontender. Intravenous access is obtained, and workup and treatment are begun.

■ CASE THREE

A 5-year-old boy presents with an altered mental status. His parents report that the child was helping them clean the garage for an upcoming move. Shortly thereafter, the boy became somnolent and did not respond to verbal or physical stimuli. On arrival, his vital signs are BP 105/50, P 95, R 30, and T 36.7°C (98°F); SpO_2 is 85% on room air. He has a GCS score of 12; no focal neurologic deficits are noted. He has diffuse rhonchi bilaterally, and no abdominal tenderness is present. He is given a nonrebreather mask, and intravenous access is obtained.

Introduction

Emergency medicine is predicated on the ability to make critical decisions with limited time and information. Determining acid-base status is one of the most useful skills that an emergency physician has for guiding diagnosis and treatment. Acid-base status can be obtained from as few as two diagnostic serum blood draws and, when a disturbance is found, can substantially narrow the differential diagnosis by providing an etiology. After identifying the primary disturbance, emergency physicians must assess for compensatory effects and calculate relevant gaps to determine the proper management of metabolic acidosis.

CRITICAL DECISION

How is the primary acid-base disturbance determined?

Acid-base disturbances are categorized into one of four primary groups depending on a patient's blood pH level: metabolic acidosis, respiratory acidosis, metabolic alkalosis, or respiratory alkalosis (*Table 1*). A pH level below 7.35 indicates acidosis, and a pH level above 7.45 indicates alkalosis. After a patient's pH status is determined, the serum bicarbonate (ie, HCO_3^-) and carbon dioxide (ie, PCO_2) levels should be obtained. Normal ranges are 22 to 28 mEq/L for bicarbonate levels and 33 to 45 mm Hg for carbon dioxide levels. Metabolic acidosis is defined as acidosis with a decrease in the serum bicarbonate level; respiratory acidosis is an acidosis with an elevation in the carbon dioxide level. The reverse is true for metabolic and respiratory alkalosis: Metabolic alkalosis is marked by an elevated bicarbonate level, while respiratory alkalosis is marked by a decreased carbon dioxide level. A mixed primary disturbance can also occur when the blood pH level is normal but the carbon dioxide or bicarbonate level is abnormal.[1,2] In general, secondary compensation for a primary acid-base disturbance does not normalize pH blood levels.

These laboratory values are typically obtained from a basic metabolic panel and blood gas analysis. However, the bicarbonate level should be obtained from serum chemistry panels instead of blood gas samples when determining acid-base status because significant differences in levels can occur between the two measurement methods, and serum levels are more accurate.[3,4] The pH and carbon dioxide levels can be determined from either an arterial or venous sample. The pH levels from venous blood gas (VBG) and arterial blood gas (ABG) samples closely approximate each other (venous pH levels are approximately 0.03 less than arterial pH levels). Formulas have been derived to adjust venous carbon dioxide levels to the expected arterial levels.[5,6]

CRITICAL DECISION

How is compensation for a primary acid-base disturbance evaluated?

After the primary acid-base disturbance is determined, any acute compensation must be identified. Compensation refers to

	Metabolic Acidosis	Respiratory Acidosis	Metabolic Alkalosis	Respiratory Alkalosis
pH	Decreased	Decreased	Increased	Increased
Carbon dioxide	Normal	Increased	Normal	Decreased
Bicarbonate	Decreased	Normal	Increased	Normal
Compensation	Winters formula, delta gap	Increased 10 PCO_2 = increased 1 HCO_3^- and decreased 0.08 pH	Variable	Decreased 10 PCO_2 = decreased 2 HCO_3^- and increased 0.08 pH
Differential	Increased anion gap — methanol, uremia, DKA, propylene glycol, isoniazid, iron, lactic acid, ethylene glycol, salicylate toxicity (late toxicity stages)[7] Normal anion gap — hyperalimentation, Addison disease, RTA, diarrhea, normal saline infusion, acetazolamide, spironolactone	Lung disease, opioids, respiratory muscle fatigue	Loop diuretics, vomiting, antacids	Anxiety, high altitude (low PCO_2), pulmonary embolism, salicylate toxicity (early stages)[7]

TABLE 1. The four major categories of acid-base disturbances

the body's ability to use renal and respiratory systems to bring the pH level closer to the normal range, typically through the inverse process of the primary disturbance (eg, respiratory alkalosis would invoke metabolic acidosis as a compensatory mechanism).[2] In acute respiratory acidosis, every 10 mm Hg increase in the carbon dioxide level increases the bicarbonate level by 1 mEq/L and decreases the pH level by approximately 0.08. Over time, because of metabolic compensation, every 10 mm Hg increase in the carbon dioxide level depresses the pH level by only 0.03. However, the latter observation is more useful when evaluating carbon dioxide retention in patients with chronic obstructive pulmonary disease than when evaluating metabolic acidosis.

Respiratory alkalosis allows for a 2 mEq/L decrease in the bicarbonate level and a 0.08 increase in the pH level for every 10 mm Hg decrease in the carbon dioxide level. In metabolic alkalosis, compensation is minimal, if present at all, and is less helpful in an emergency department setting. Determining compensation in metabolic acidosis is done using Winters formula: $PCO_2 = ([1.5 \times serum\ HCO_3^-] + 8) \pm 2$. If the measured carbon dioxide value is lower than the carbon dioxide value calculated in Winters formula, there is an associated respiratory alkalosis. If the true carbon dioxide value is higher than the calculated carbon dioxide value, there is an associated respiratory acidosis.[2,6]

CRITICAL DECISION

How are anion gap and delta gap used?

If metabolic acidosis is the primary disturbance, determining the anion gap and delta gap can further elucidate the diagnosis. The anion gap is calculated with the formula $AG = Na^+ - (Cl^- + HCO_3^-)$. A normal anion gap value is between 10 and 14 mEq/L.[2] An abnormal anion gap value can be useful information in the critical care setting because only a limited number of processes cause an increased anion gap metabolic acidosis. When calculating the anion gap value, attention must be given to the albumin status. If hypoalbuminemia is present, expect the anion gap value to decrease by 2.5 mEq/L for every 1 g/dL decrease in the albumin level (assuming a normal albumin baseline of 4 g/dL).[2]

The delta gap should also be calculated in patients with metabolic acidosis. The formula used is $\Delta AG/\Delta HCO_3^-$, with an assumed anion gap baseline of 12 mEq/L and bicarbonate baseline of 24 mEq/L. In a simple case of increased anion gap metabolic acidosis, the delta gap value should be from 1 to 2. If the delta gap value is less than 1 (ie, a negative bicarbonate gap), an additional process is causing the bicarbonate level to decrease (eg, normal anion gap metabolic acidosis). If the delta gap value is greater than 2 (ie, positive bicarbonate gap), an associated metabolic alkalosis is likely contributing to the acid-base status.[2,6] A simple method of calculating for the presence of metabolic alkalosis is to add the delta gap value to the serum bicarbonate value. A value greater than 24 reveals an associated metabolic alkalosis; a value less than 24 reveals an associated normal anion gap metabolic acidosis.[2,6]

The osmolar gap can be calculated in patients with increased anion gap metabolic acidosis by using the formula plasma osmolality $(POsm) = 2(Na^+) + glucose\ level/18 + BUN\ level/2.8$ + the serum osmolality increase based on the type of alcohol ingested.[8] This value is then subtracted from the measured plasma osmolality. An osmolar gap greater than 10 mOsm/kg is considered elevated and can narrow the differential diagnosis.[2] This calculation is especially useful in differentiating between the types of toxic alcohol ingestions.

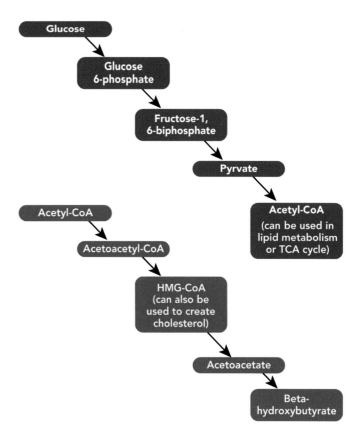

FIGURE 1. Glycolysis and ketogenesis overview. The process in *blue* depicts glycolysis, while the process in *green* depicts ketogenesis. This illustration focuses on substrates affected by insulin concentrations.

CRITICAL DECISION

What are the considerations in managing emergent acid-base disturbances?

DKA

Diabetic ketoacidosis (DKA) causes an increased anion gap metabolic acidosis. Insulin is integral for intracellular use of glucose and for glycolysis. A lack of insulin leads to a subsequent decrease in key enzymes that drive glycolysis (eg, fructose 1,6-bisphosphatase and pyruvate kinase), an increase in free fatty acid production and use, and an increase in ketone production through upregulation of HMG-CoA activity (*Figure 1*).[9-11] An oversimplified explanation of DKA is that the body uses the alternative sources of lipolysis and ketogenesis for energy because glycolysis and glucose transport are hindered. Management of DKA focuses on levels of potassium, insulin, and fluids (*Figure 2*). The potassium level should be checked prior to insulin administration to avoid unexpected intracellular shifts. If the potassium level is less than 3.3 mEq/L, insulin should be held, and 20 to 40 mEq of potassium should be administered per hour until the concentration rises above 3.3 mEq/L. If the potassium level is between 3.3 and 5.3 mEq/L, 20 mEq of potassium should be given with each liter of fluid for a goal concentration of 4 to 5 mEq/L. If the potassium concentration is greater than 5.3 mEq/L, no supplemental potassium should be given, and levels should be continuously monitored.[12]

Regular insulin can be administered using one of two regimens. The first is an intravenous bolus of 0.1 units/kg followed by a continuous infusion of 0.1 units/kg/hr. The second regimen is a

0.14-units/kg/hr infusion with no initial bolus. Within the first hour, the glucose level should decrease by 50 to 70 mg/dL. If the glucose level does not decrease, the insulin bolus should be doubled. Once glucose concentrations reach 200 mg/dL, the insulin infusion should be reduced to 0.05 units/kg/hr, with a goal glucose concentration of 150 to 200 mg/dL.[12]

Fluid administration is driven by volume status and the serum sodium level. The choice of fluids is determined by individual electrolyte concentrations, the pH level, and osmolarity (*Table 2*). After an initial evaluation, 1 L of 0.9% saline should be administered (if the patient is not in a decompensated hypervolemic state). If severe hypovolemia occurs, continue fluid resuscitation at a rate of 1 L of 0.9% saline/hr. If mild hypovolemia or euvolemia is present, calculate the corrected serum sodium level. If the sodium level is low, continue with the 0.9% saline infusion at 250 to 500 mL/hr. If the serum sodium level is high or normal, administer a 0.45% saline infusion at 250 to 500 mL/hr. Once the glucose concentration reaches 200 mg/dL, change the fluid infusion to 0.45% saline with 5% dextrose (D51/2NS) at 150 to 200 mL/hr.[6,12]

The efficacy of sodium bicarbonate therapy is widely debated.[6] Arguments for sodium bicarbonate administration cite that myocardial dysfunction, vasodilation, and a reduced catecholamine response are exacerbated by an acidotic state and are rapidly corrected by sodium bicarbonate administration. Arguments against sodium bicarbonate therapy state that its administration leads to hypervolemia and paradoxical CNS acidosis, which worsens electrolyte disturbances. It is generally accepted that sodium bicarbonate therapy is likely more useful in situations that are caused by a loss of bicarbonate than in situations that are caused by excess acid production.[6] The American Diabetes Association does recommend sodium bicarbonate therapy for DKA if the pH level is less than 6.9. Sodium bicarbonate therapy for DKA is provided by adding 100 mEq of sodium bicarbonate to 400 mL of water with 20 mEq of potassium supplementation and infusing over 2 hours for a goal pH level greater than 7.[6,13]

CRITICAL DECISION

When should sodium bicarbonate be used to treat metabolic acidosis?

Adverse effects of indiscriminate sodium bicarbonate use in metabolic acidosis include a decreased serum potassium level (potentially prolonging the QT interval and precipitating dysrhythmias) and a lowered serum calcium level (potentially decreasing left ventricular stroke volume, cardiac output, and blood

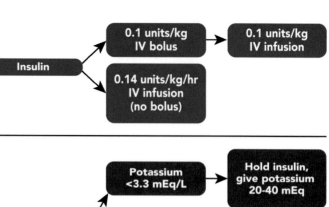

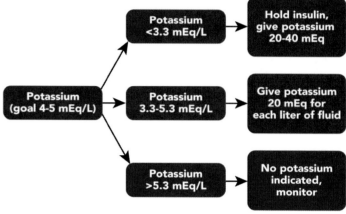

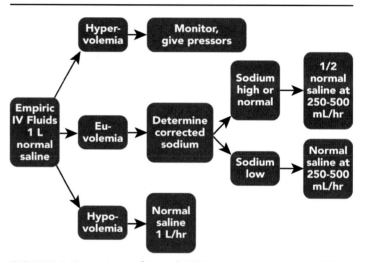

FIGURE 2. Overview of initial DKA management in adults

pressure). If respiratory insufficiency exists, the bicarbonate level can increase intracellular acidosis because the patient may be inadequately expiring carbon dioxide. If toxic alcohol poisoning is suspected, treatment may include fomepizole rather than sodium bicarbonate until methanol or ethylene glycol levels are determined. That said, sodium bicarbonate therapy is indicated for situations in which an ongoing loss of bicarbonate from diarrhea or renal tubular acidosis (RTA) occurs. Sodium bicarbonate can be given as an infusion for salicylate or tricyclic antidepressant poisoning, especially to enhance excretion of salicylates or to raise the pH level to 7 or above.[13]

CRITICAL DECISION

How are toxic alcohol ingestions managed?

Methanol, ethylene glycol, and isopropyl alcohol are common agents ingested for their intoxicating effects. Of the three, isopropyl alcohol is ingested the most, and all three types are often more potent than ethanol.[14] Given that each type of ingestion is associated with a unique treatment, emergency physicians must rapidly distinguish between each of the toxic alcohols (*Table 3*).

	Endogenous Plasma	0.9% Saline	Lactated Ringers
Sodium	135-145 mEq/L	154 mEq/L	130 mEq/L
Potassium	4.5-5 mEq/L	0 mEq/L	4 mEq/L
Chloride	94-111 mEq/L	154 mEq/L	109 mEq/L
Calcium	2.2-2.6 mEq/L	0 mEq/L	2.7 mEq/L
Magnesium	0.8-1 mEq/L	0 mEq/L	0 mEq/L
Bicarbonate	23-27 mEq/L	0 mEq/L	0 mEq/L
Lactate	1-2 mEq/L	0 mEq/L	28 mEq/L
Osmolarity	291 mOsm/L	308 mOsm/L	273 mOsm/L
pH	7.35-7.45	5	6.5

TABLE 2. Typical concentrations of crystalloid fluids

Methanol is commonly found in products such as wood alcohol, paint thinner, and certain cleaning supplies. Methanol's toxic effects are mediated through the metabolite formic acid. Clinical presentation of methanol intoxication usually includes ocular toxicity, but other effects such as parkinsonism or transverse myelitis can also occur. Methanol ingestion typically causes an elevated anion gap, osmolar gap, and lactic acid level. Importantly, however, as with any toxic alcohol ingestion in the early stages, the anion gap, osmolar gap, and lactic acid level can be normal. Treatment includes fomepizole or ethanol. Both fomepizole and ethanol inhibit alcohol dehydrogenase activity, thereby decreasing formic acid production.[11] Renal replacement therapy (RRT) is indicated if there are signs of end-organ dysfunction. If RRT is initiated, fomepizole is administered every 4 hours as opposed to every 12 hours.[15]

Ethylene glycol ingestion typically presents with altered mental status, renal failure, acute respiratory distress syndrome (ARDS), and occasionally, muscle spasms. Ethylene glycol is found in antifreeze, which is particularly dangerous to the pediatric population because of its bright color and sweet taste. Its toxic effects are mediated by its metabolism to oxalic acid and glycolic acid. Oxalic acid binds calcium to produce calcium oxalate crystals, leading to hypocalcemia and obstruction of the renal tubules. Ethylene glycol also elevates the anion gap, osmolar gap, and lactic acid level. The treatment is the same as it is for methanol ingestion.[11,14,16,17]

Isopropyl alcohol (isopropanol) is found in hand sanitizer and rubbing alcohol. It exhibits its toxic effects through its metabolism to acetone. Isopropyl alcohol is more potent than ethanol and can cause more severe intoxication, refractory hypotension, hemorrhagic gastritis, and sometimes, fruity-smelling breath.[16] Ingestion typically leads to an elevated osmolar gap but a normal anion gap and lactic acid level. Treatment is mainly supportive, with intubation sometimes required due to significant CNS depression. RRT can also be used in refractory cases.[11,16,17]

CRITICAL DECISION

What is propylene glycol, and what are its therapeutic implications?

Propylene glycol is a typically inactive substance in parenteral medications, namely intravenous medications (eg, nitroglycerin and phenobarbital). Continuous infusion of medications with propylene glycol as a solvent can lead to toxicity.[14,15] Because these medications are usually given in an inpatient setting, emergency physicians do not typically encounter this toxicity. Propylene glycol elevates the anion gap, osmolar gap, and lactic acid level. Presentations of its intoxication typically include renal failure or a sepsis-like syndrome. Treatment is largely based on RRT and limiting propylene glycol administration.[15]

Summary

Diagnosing and treating metabolic acidosis is a regular part of acute care. Diagnostic tools are available to aid in the evaluation of acid-base disorders and optimize the care of these acutely ill patients. Although metabolic acidosis has a broad differential, emergency physicians should be equipped to handle the specific associated endocrine, renal, and toxicology etiologies that are most likely to be encountered.

	Methanol	Ethylene Glycol	Isopropyl Alcohol
Location	Paint thinner, wood alcohol	Antifreeze	Rubbing alcohol, hand sanitizer
Metabolite	Formic acid	Oxalic acid, glycolic acid	Acetone
Presentation	Ocular disturbance	Altered mental status, renal failure, ARDS	Severe intoxication, gastritis, hypotension
Lactate	Elevated	Elevated	Normal
Anion gap	Elevated	Elevated	Normal
Osmolar gap	Elevated (serum osmolality increases 30.9 mmol/L for each 100 mg/dL)	Elevated (serum osmolality increases 16 mmol/L for each 100 mg/dL)	Elevated (serum osmolality increases 16.6 mmol/L for each 100 mg/dL)
Treatment	Fomepizole, ethanol, RRT	Fomepizole, ethanol, RRT	Supportive care, RRT

TABLE 3. Characteristics of toxic alcohols[8]

REFERENCES

1. Seigel TA. Deciphering acid-base disorders. ALiEM. Published September 16, 2013. https://www.aliem.com/deciphering-acid-base-disorders

2. Jones KM, Chiu WC. Acid-base disorders. In: Farcy DA, Chiu WC, Marshall JP, Osborn TM, eds. *Critical Care Emergency Medicine*. 2nd ed. McGraw-Hill Education; 2017:285-293.

3. Kim Y, Massie L, Murata GH, Tzamaloukas AH. Discrepancy between measured serum total carbon dioxide content and bicarbonate concentration calculated from arterial blood gases. *Cureus*. 2015 Dec 7;7(12):e398.

✔ Pearls

- Determine acid-base status from a serum bicarbonate level instead of from a blood gas analysis because the serum bicarbonate level is measured and, thus, more accurate than the calculated value from a blood gas analysis.

- Sodium bicarbonate therapy for metabolic acidosis is likely beneficial in cases associated with increased bicarbonate excretion but is less efficacious in cases from excess acid production.

- Levels of potassium, sodium, and glucose should be considered throughout the process of providing critical care to patients with DKA.

- Unlike methanol and ethylene glycol intoxications, isopropyl alcohol is associated with an elevated osmolar gap but a normal anion gap and lactic acid level.

- Methanol and ethylene glycol toxicity are treated with fomepizole or ethanol. Isopropyl alcohol toxicity is managed with supportive care. RRT is effective for all these toxic alcohol ingestions.

CASE RESOLUTIONS

CASE ONE

A fluid bolus of 0.9% saline was administered because of clinical concern for hypovolemia. Laboratory tests were obtained and were notable for a serum glucose level of 450 mg/dL, an increased anion gap, a pH level of 7, a serum bicarbonate level of 5 mEq/L, a potassium level of 5 mEq/L, a low corrected sodium level, and elevated serum concentrations of β-hydroxybutyrate. After diagnosing DKA, an additional 1 L of a 0.9% saline bolus was given, and the patient was placed on an infusion of 500 mL/hr. Potassium 20 mEq was given for every 1 L of fluid administered. A regular insulin infusion was started at 0.14 units/kg/hr. Serum levels of glucose, potassium, and sodium were measured every 2 hours. The patient's symptoms and laboratory results improved, and she was admitted to a step-down unit.

CASE TWO

A fluid bolus was immediately administered for hypotension after an examination revealed no signs of decompensated hypervolemia. A sepsis workup was initiated and included cultures and lactic acid measurements. The patient's blood pressure mildly improved with fluids. CT of the head was completed because of his decreased level of consciousness; it revealed no acute or emergent intracranial pathology. Laboratory results were notable for a normal lactic acid level, mild leukocytosis, mild hypoglycemia, a serum creatinine level of 15.8 mg/dL, a BUN level of 276 mg/dL, an elevated osmolar gap, a normal pH level, and an elevated anion gap. The patient was diagnosed with acute kidney injury with dehydration. His GCS score steadily worsened throughout his stay, and concern developed for his ability to protect his airway. The patient was intubated, and an orogastric tube was placed. Dark, coffee-ground gastric contents were observed in the tubing. Because of concern for hemorrhagic gastritis, the patient was started on a proton pump inhibitor; a blood type and screen was obtained; and his hemoglobin levels were trended. The patient was admitted to the ICU and was started on RRT.

CASE THREE

The patient's oxygen status was stabilized, and he was given a fluid bolus. Chest x-ray showed diffuse bilateral opacities. The initial concern was for pneumonia, so empiric broad-spectrum antibiotics were given after blood cultures were obtained. Laboratory results revealed an elevated lactic acid level, no leukocytosis, normal potassium and sodium levels, a low calcium level, and a creatinine level indicative of acute renal failure. Both the anion gap and osmolar gap were elevated. Examination of the patient's urine with a Wood lamp detected visible fluorescence. Fomepizole treatment was initiated, and nephrology was consulted because of concern for ethylene glycol ingestion complicated by ARDS. Nephrology recommended emergent RRT. Central access was obtained, and fomepizole dosing was increased. The patient's oxygen status remained low, so he was placed on a bilevel positive airway pressure machine for respiratory support and was then admitted to the pediatric ICU.

4. Yartsev A. Sources of error in blood gas analysis. Deranged Physiology. Updated March 29, 2023. https://derangedphysiology.com/main/required-reading/acid-base-disorders/Chapter%20112/sources-error-blood-gas-analysis

5. Chong WH, Saha BK, Medarov BI. Comparing central venous blood gas to arterial blood gas and determining its utility in critically ill patients: narrative review. Anesth Analg. 2021 Aug 1;133(2):374-378.

6. McCoin NS, Self WH. Acid-base disorders. In: Walls RM, Hockberger R, Gausche-Hill M, Erickson TB, Wilcox SR, eds. Rosen's Emergency Medicine: Concepts and Clinical Practice. Vol 2. 10th ed. Elsevier; 2022:1517-1524.

✖ Pitfalls

- Indiscriminately treating all cases of metabolic acidosis or DKA with sodium bicarbonate therapy. Sodium bicarbonate therapy should be reserved for severe or unique cases (eg, severe acidosis, tricyclic antidepressant ingestion, and RTA).

- Ruling out toxic alcohol ingestions based on a normal anion gap and osmolar gap. These measurements can be normal in the early stages of toxic alcohol ingestions.

- Neglecting to increase the frequency of fomepizole administration from every 12 hours to every 4 hours in patients on RRT.

- Initiating fomepizole alone for cases of methanol or ethylene glycol toxicity when end-organ dysfunction is present. Evidence of end-organ dysfunction warrants immediate RRT.

7. Barnett AK, Boyer EW. Salicylate (aspirin) poisoning: clinical manifestations and evaluation. UpToDate. Last updated May 10, 2023. https://www.uptodate.com/contents/salicylate-aspirin-poisoning-clinical-manifestations-and-evaluation

8. Kraut JA, Mullins ME. Toxic alcohols. N Engl J Med. 2018 Jan 18;378:270-280.

9. Dhillon KK, Gupta S. Biochemistry, ketogenesis. StatPearls [Internet]. StatPearls Publishing; 2023. Last updated February 6, 2023. https://www.ncbi.nlm.nih.gov/books/NBK493179/

10. Laffel L. Ketone bodies: a review of physiology, pathophysiology and application of monitoring to diabetes. Diabetes Metab Res Rev. 1999 Nov-Dec;15(6):412-426.

11. Gallagher N, Edwards FJ. The diagnosis and management of toxic alcohol poisoning in the emergency department: a review article. Adv J Emerg Med. 2019 May 22;3(3):e28.

12. Hirsch IB, Emmett M. Diabetic ketoacidosis and hyperosmolar hyperglycemic state in adults: treatment. UpToDate. Updated July 31, 2023. https://www.uptodate.com/contents/diabetic-ketoacidosis-and-hyperosmolar-hyperglycemic-state-in-adults-treatment

13. Judge BS. Metabolic acidosis: differentiating the causes in the poisoned patient. Emerg Med Clin North Am. 2022 May;40(2):251-264.

14. Bodford I. The unhappy drunk: toxic alcohols. emDOCs. Published September 16, 2015. http://www.emdocs.net/the-unhappy-drunk-toxic-alcohols/

15. Zar T, Graeber C, Perazella MA. Recognition, treatment, and prevention of propylene glycol toxicity. Semin Dial. 2007 May-Jun;20(3):217-219.

16. Bridwell R. EM@3AM: methanol toxicity. emDOCs. Published November 3, 2018. http://www.emdocs.net/em3am-methanol-toxicity

17. Beauchamp GA, Valento M. Toxic alcohol ingestion: prompt recognition and management in the emergency department. Emerg Med Pract. 2016 Sep 1;18(9):1-20.

CME Questions

Reviewed by Walter L. Green, MD, FACEP; and Sharon E. Mace, MD, FACEP

Qualified, paid subscribers to *Critical Decisions in Emergency Medicine* may receive CME certificates for up to 5 ACEP Category I credits, 5 *AMA PRA Category 1 Credits*™, and 5 AOA Category 2-B credits for completing this activity in its entirety. Submit your answers online at acep.org/cdem; a score of 75% or better is required. You may receive credit for completing the CME activity any time within 3 years of its publication date. Answers to this month's questions will be published in next month's issue.

1 A 17-year-old boy with a history of depression presents to the emergency department after being found acting abnormally by his grandmother. He is tachycardic, diaphoretic, and swinging his arms and legs aimlessly, but he calms when his grandmother talks to him. He is unable to answer any questions clearly and is moaning unintelligibly. What is the best next step?

A. Give intramuscular midazolam to get an improved examination
B. Obtain a blood glucose measurement
C. Obtain a urine drug screen
D. Restrain the patient to place an intravenous line

2 Which electrolyte derangement is least likely to cause agitation or altered mentation?

A. Hypercalcemia
B. Hypoglycemia
C. Hypokalemia
D. Hyponatremia

3 Which technique is a poor choice to de-escalate a situation with an agitated patient?

A. Addressing the patient by name and asking questions
B. Clearly and respectfully telling the patient that there will be consequences for unacceptable behavior
C. Having multiple physicians in the patient room to run the de-escalation
D. Offering a blanket or food to the patient

4 Which second-generation antipsychotic has the greatest risk of QT-interval prolongation?

A. Olanzapine
B. Quetiapine
C. Risperidone
D. Ziprasidone

5 Which medication is an appropriate choice for the given patient?

A. Haloperidol for a 22-year-old woman with a history of schizophrenia who is at 30 weeks' gestation
B. Lorazepam for an 80-year-old woman with fluctuating agitation
C. Midazolam for a 16-year-old boy with developmental delay
D. Olanzapine for a 44-year-old man with chronic stimulant use disorder

6 Which statement regarding a patient's capacity to make medical decisions is true?

A. Capacity can only be assessed by a psychiatrist
B. Capacity does not affect patient disposition
C. Capacity reflects a patient's understanding of their current situation
D. The patient must choose the intervention that is in their best interest

7 Which statement about physical restraint is correct?

A. A team of two people should be involved when implementing physical restraint
B. End-tidal CO_2 monitoring should only be considered for patients with suspected ingestions
C. If only two limbs can be restrained, ipsilateral arms and legs should be secured
D. The most common complication of physical restraint is skin breakdown

8 Which benzodiazepine can be safely given to patients with liver disease without an effect on its metabolism?

A. Alprazolam
B. Diazepam
C. Lorazepam
D. Midazolam

9 In which situation is discharge from the emergency department most appropriate?

A. 20-year-old man with no known medical history presents agitated and violent. He requires physical restraint and sedative medications to be worked up, but his workup is ultimately unrevealing. He remains agitated and altered on awakening.
B. 22-year-old man with a history of intravenous drug use presents with agitation. He is initially febrile and tachycardic and requires multiple doses of benzodiazepines to allow for safe care. He has been attempting to leave the emergency department but does not understand his current situation or the risks of leaving.
C. 35-year-old woman with schizophrenia, a history of medication nonadherence, and several recent psychiatric hospitalizations presents with agitation. She requires multiple doses of antipsychotics. No medical etiology of her agitation has been discovered.
D. 60-year-old man presents with agitation that is ultimately determined to be secondary to alcohol intoxication. After several hours of observation, he is clinically sober.

10 Which choice is most likely to cause agitation?

A. Benzodiazepine overdose
B. Depression
C. Opioid overdose
D. Sedative-hypnotic agent withdrawal

11 A patient is diagnosed with metabolic acidosis. The patient's carbon dioxide level is 12 mm Hg, and his serum bicarbonate level is 6 mEq/L. Is a concomitant process occurring with the metabolic acidosis?

A. No
B. Yes, the patient has an associated metabolic alkalosis
C. Yes, the patient has an associated respiratory acidosis
D. Yes, the patient has an associated respiratory alkalosis

12 **Which fluid should be given to a patient in diabetic ketoacidosis once the patient's serum glucose level reaches 200 mg/dL?**

A. 0.45% saline
B. 0.9% saline
C. 5% dextrose, 0.45% saline
D. 5% dextrose, lactated ringers

13 **Which laboratory values are most consistent with isopropyl alcohol toxicity?**

A. Elevated lactic acid levels, elevated anion gap, and normal osmolar gap
B. Elevated lactic acid levels, normal anion gap, and normal osmolar gap
C. Normal lactic acid levels, elevated anion gap, and elevated osmolar gap
D. Normal lactic acid levels, normal anion gap, and elevated osmolar gap

14 **What is the preferred treatment of ethylene glycol toxicity in a patient with acute renal failure and altered mental status?**

A. Fomepizole or ethanol
B. Renal replacement therapy, with fomepizole or ethanol used in conjunction
C. Sodium bicarbonate infusion
D. Supportive care and intravenous fluids

15 **A patient is diagnosed with metabolic acidosis. Her basic metabolic panel reveals a sodium level of 130 mEq/L, potassium level of 3.5 mEq/L, chloride level of 90 mEq/L, serum bicarbonate level of 5 mEq/L, BUN level of 35 mg/dL, and glucose level of 90 mg/dL. Further laboratory values show a bicarbonate value of 10 mEq/L on arterial blood gas analysis, a serum ethanol level of 0 g/dL, a serum osmolality of 350 mOsm/kg, and a lactic acid level of 4 mmol/L. What do these values indicate about the patient's anion gap and osmolar gap?**

A. Anion gap and osmolar gap are elevated
B. Anion gap and osmolar gap are normal
C. Anion gap is elevated and osmolar gap is normal
D. Anion gap is normal and osmolar gap is elevated

16 **What is a potential cause of metabolic acidosis?**

A. Early salicylate toxicity
B. High altitude
C. Late salicylate toxicity
D. Pulmonary embolism

17 **What is a common source of ethylene glycol?**

A. Antifreeze
B. Paint thinner
C. Rubbing alcohol
D. Wood alcohol

18 **What condition warrants the calculation of the anion gap and delta gap?**

A. Metabolic acidosis
B. Metabolic alkalosis
C. Respiratory acidosis
D. Respiratory alkalosis

19 **Which protein should be taken into consideration when calculating the anion gap?**

A. Alanine transaminase
B. Albumin
C. Alkaline phosphatase
D. Triglycerides

20 **Which laboratory test should be used to obtain a bicarbonate value?**

A. Arterial blood gas analysis
B. Basic metabolic panel
C. CBC
D. Venous blood gas analysis

ANSWER KEY FOR MONTH 2023, VOLUME 37, NUMBER 8

1	2	3	4	5	6	7	8	9	10	11	12	13	14	15	16	17	18	19	20
A	C	B	B	D	A	D	C	D	A	B	C	D	C	C	A	D	B	B	A

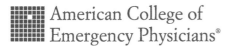
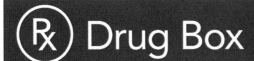

Drug Box

Intranasal Nalmefene

Frank LoVecchio, DO, MPH, FACEP
Valleywise Health Medical Center and ASU, Phoenix, Arizona

Objective
On completion of this column, you should be able to:
- Discuss the use of nalmefene for opioid overdose and compare it with naloxone.

Nalmefene is an opioid antagonist approved by the FDA in May 2023 as a nasal spray. It is the "first" nalmefene hydrochloride nasal spray for the emergency treatment of known or suspected opioid overdose in patients 12 years and older. Technically, intranasal naloxone is off-label.

Nalmefene is a 6-methylene analogue of naltrexone. It acts as an antagonist at the μ- and δ-opioid receptors and a partial agonist at the κ-opioid receptor. Intravenous nalmefene was approved in the United States in 1995 as an antidote for opioid overdose.

Nalmefene's major advantage is that it has a longer plasma half-life of about 11 hours compared to naloxone's 2-hour half-life. Nalmefene has been shown to reverse opioid intoxication for as long as 8 hours, reducing the need for continuous monitoring of intoxicated patients and repeated naloxone dosing. The American Heart Association recommends that naloxone or nalmefene be considered for the treatment of opioid-associated life-threatening emergencies.

Kinetics
Onset:
- IV: 2-5 min
- IM, SQ: 5-15 min
- IN: 2.5-5 min

Dosage:
- IV: 0.5 mg/70 kg; may administer a second dose of 1 mg/70 kg 2-3 min later, if necessary
- IN: 2.7 mg/0.1 mL; each unit dose of nasal spray delivers a single 2.7-mg dose

Time to peak:
- IM: 2.3 hr
- SQ: 1.5 hr
- IN: ~15 min (range: 10 min to 3 hr)

Bioavailability:
- IM, SQ: ~100%
- IN: ~80%

Half-life elimination:
- ~11 hr
- Slightly decreased clearance or longer duration may be noted in older adults and patients with kidney or liver disease.

Side Effects
The most common adverse reactions are nasal discomfort, headache, nausea, dizziness, hot flush, vomiting, anxiety, fatigue, nasal congestion, throat irritation, rhinalgia, decreased appetite, erythema, and hyperhidrosis. Nalmefene hydrochloride use in opioid-dependent patients may lead to opioid withdrawal.

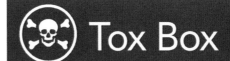

Tox Box

Poison Hemlock Ingestion

By Christian A. Tomaszewski, MD, MS, MBA, FACEP
University of California San Diego Health

Objective
On completion of this column, you should be able to:
- Explain the effects and treatment of poison hemlock ingestion.

Introduction
Poison hemlock (*Conium maculatum*) was used in ancient Athens to execute Socrates, who was condemned for corrupting the city's youth. Today, the plant is considered a non-native weed that grows throughout North America. It has a hollow stem and white flowers, grows up to 5 feet tall, and is occasionally mistaken for wild carrots or celery. All parts of the plant are toxic.

Mechanism of Action
- Nicotinic alkaloids including coniine
- *Early phase:* agonists at nicotinic acetylcholine receptors
- *Late phase:* inhibition of nicotinic acetylcholine receptors with paralysis

Kinetics
- Rapid coniine absorption after ingestion
- Toxic with ingestion of >150 mg of coniine (6-8 leaves)

Clinical Manifestations
(early stimulatory phase followed by a depressant phase)
- *Eyes:* mydriasis and blurred vision
- *GI:* salivation, nausea, and vomiting
- *Cardiac:* hypotension and tachycardia followed by bradycardia
- *Pulmonary:* bronchoconstriction and bronchorrhea followed by respiratory paralysis
- *Neuro:* ascending flaccid muscular paralysis, CNS depression, and seizures
- *Muscle:* pain and rhabdomyolysis

Diagnostics
- Basic metabolic panel; creatine phosphokinase test if severe symptoms
- Coniine isolated in blood and urine (not clinically useful)

Treatment
- Antiemetics
- Ventilatory support
- Benzodiazepines or barbiturates for seizures
- IV fluid bolus for hypotension
- Norepinephrine for fluid-unresponsive hypotension
- Fluids for rhabdomyolysis

Disposition
- Can discharge if improving or asymptomatic at 6 hours post ingestion

Critical decisions
in emergency medicine

Volume 37 Number 10: **October 2023**

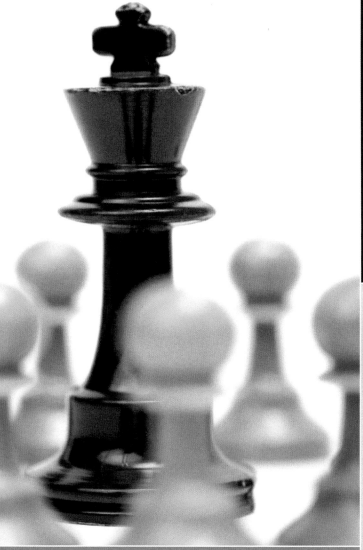

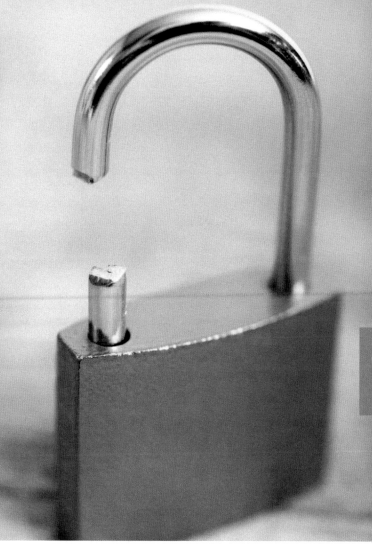

Caught Off Guard

Opportunistic infections have declined significantly in the era of highly active antiretroviral therapy for HIV, but these infections can still carry significant morbidity and mortality when they occur. To properly care for patients with HIV and AIDS, emergency physicians must know when to consider these infections, how to diagnose them, and when to initiate the appropriate treatment.

Security Breach

Pelvic inflammatory disease affects around 1 in 20 women during their lifetimes and, along with tubo-ovarian abscess, can lead to serious and life-altering consequences like infertility, ectopic pregnancy, peritonitis, and sepsis. Because early recognition and treatment can drastically improve patient outcomes, emergency physicians must promptly identify and appropriately manage these pelvic infections.

THE OFFICIAL CME PUBLICATION OF THE AMERICAN COLLEGE OF EMERGENCY PHYSICIANS

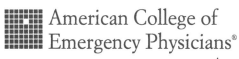
American College of Emergency Physicians®
ADVANCING EMERGENCY CARE

Critical decisions
in emergency medicine

Critical Decisions in Emergency Medicine is the official CME publication of the American College of Emergency Physicians. Additional volumes are available.

EDITOR-IN-CHIEF

Danya Khoujah, MBBS, MEHP, FACEP
University of Maryland, Baltimore, MD

SECTION EDITORS

Joshua S. Broder, MD, FACEP
Duke University, Durham, NC

Andrew J. Eyre, MD, MS-HPEd
Brigham and Women's Hospital/
Harvard Medical School, Boston, MA

John Kiel, DO, MPH, FACEP, CAQSM
University of South Florida Morsani College of Medicine, Tampa, FL

Frank LoVecchio, DO, MPH, FACEP
Valleywise, Arizona State University, University of Arizona, and Creighton University School of Medicine, Phoenix, AZ

Sharon E. Mace, MD, FACEP
Cleveland Clinic Lerner College of Medicine/
Case Western Reserve University, Cleveland, OH

Amal Mattu, MD, FACEP
University of Maryland, Baltimore, MD

Christian A. Tomaszewski, MD, MS, MBA, FACEP
University of California Health Sciences, San Diego, CA

Steven J. Warrington, MD, MEd, MS
MercyOne Siouxland, Sioux City, IA

ASSOCIATE EDITORS

Tareq Al-Salamah, MBBS, MPH, FACEP
King Saud University, Riyadh, Saudi Arabia/
University of Maryland, Baltimore, MD

Wan-Tsu Chang, MD
University of Maryland, Baltimore, MD

Ann M. Dietrich, MD, FAAP, FACEP
University of South Carolina School of Medicine, Greenville, SC

Kelsey Drake, MD, MPH, FACEP
St. Anthony Hospital, Lakewood, CO

Walter L. Green, MD, FACEP
UT Southwestern Medical Center, Dallas, TX

John C. Greenwood, MD
University of Pennsylvania, Philadelphia, PA

Nathaniel Mann, MD
University of South Carolina School of Medicine, Greenville, SC

George Sternbach, MD, FACEP
Stanford University Medical Center, Stanford, CA

EDITORIAL STAFF

Joy Carrico, JD, Managing Editor
jcarrico@acep.org

Alex Bass
Assistant Editor

Kel Morris
Assistant Editor

ISSN2325-0186 (Print)   ISSN2325-8365 (Online)

Contents

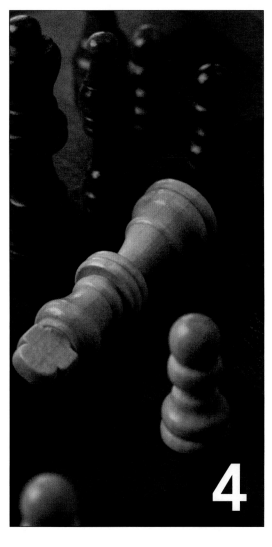

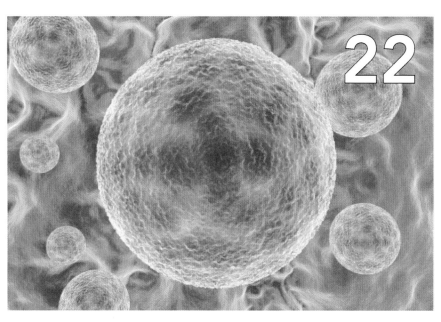
FEATURES

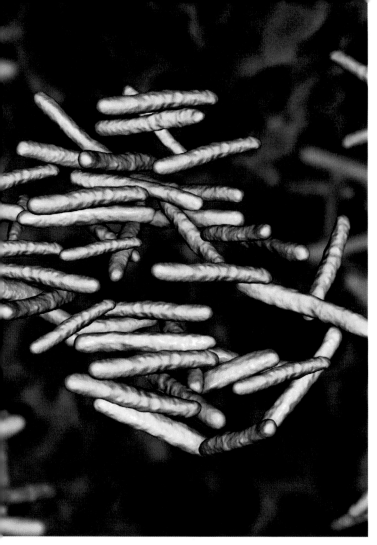

Caught Off Guard

Opportunistic Infections in Patients With HIV

LESSON 19

By Jordan Parker, MD; and Michael C. Bond, MD, FACEP
Dr. Parker is a resident in emergency and internal medicine at the University of Maryland Medical Center. Dr. Bond is a professor at the University of Maryland School of Medicine in Baltimore.

Reviewed by Frank LoVecchio, DO, MPH, FACEP

Objectives

On completion of this lesson, you should be able to:

1. Define AIDS-related OIs.
2. Recognize when OIs should be considered in HIV-positive patients.
3. Evaluate the safety of diagnostic and therapeutic lumbar puncture in patients with cryptococcal meningitis.
4. Compare preferred medications for prophylaxis against OIs.
5. Employ different diagnostic modalities for cryptococcal meningitis.
6. Recognize the importance of steroid therapy in patients with PCP.
7. Describe diagnostic and management strategies for oropharyngeal and esophageal candidiasis.

From the EM Model

10.0 Systemic Infectious Disorders
    10.6 Viral
        10.6.6 HIV/AIDS

■ CRITICAL DECISIONS ■

- When should there be concern for OIs in patients with HIV?

- Which infections should be considered and treated in patients with HIV who present with respiratory distress?

- How is PCP diagnosed and treated?

- How is cryptococcal meningitis diagnosed and treated?

- When should a lumbar puncture be performed in a patient with HIV and suspected cryptococcal meningitis?

- How are oropharyngeal and esophageal candidiasis diagnosed and treated?

Opportunistic infections (OIs) have declined significantly in the era of highly active antiretroviral therapy (HAART) for HIV, but these infections can still carry significant morbidity and mortality when they occur. To properly care for patients with HIV and AIDS, emergency physicians must know when to consider these infections, how to diagnose them, and when to initiate the appropriate treatment.

CASE PRESENTATIONS

CASE ONE

A 40-year-old man presents complaining of a headache that has been present for 3 weeks. He has a history of HIV and is taking antiretroviral therapy. His most recent CD4 lymphocyte count is 75 cells/μL. His symptoms now include fever, vomiting, and bilateral blurry vision. The physical examination shows bilateral papilledema with no focal neurologic deficits. A CT scan of the head and brain with contrast shows no space-occupying lesion.

CASE TWO

A 50-year-old woman presents with difficulty breathing. She is HIV positive; her most recent CD4 lymphocyte count is 150 cells/μL. She is on HAART but has been receiving no antibiotic prophylaxis. She has diffuse, bilateral crackles on pulmonary auscultation. She is tachypneic (R 36), with intercostal and supraclavicular retractions. She is also severely hypoxemic and requires a high-flow nasal cannula. A chest x-ray shows bilateral interstitial infiltrates (*Figure 1*).

CASE THREE

A 60-year-old man with no medical history presents with a sore throat, spots in his throat, and painful swallowing. He is sexually active with men and is not taking pre-exposure prophylaxis. On examination, he is found to be thin, with temporal muscle wasting. He has white plaques on his oropharynx that scrape off with a tongue depressor. Laboratory findings are notable for leukopenia, with a TLC of 800 cells/μL.

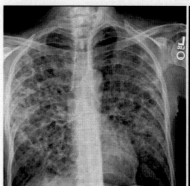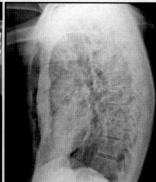

FIGURE 1. X-ray showing bilateral interstitial infiltrates. *Credit:* Copyright 2023 The Radswiki. Image courtesy of The Radswiki and Radiopaedia.org, rID: 11789. Used under license.

Introduction

An HIV infection causes destruction and dysfunction of the immune system. When left untreated, it can progress to AIDS. Patients with AIDS are susceptible to numerous infections and conditions.[1] CDC data show a decline in the number of new HIV infections between 2015 and 2019. Despite this improvement, as of 2019, an estimated 1.2 million people in the United States are HIV positive.[2] Although the use of antiretroviral therapy and antibiotic prophylaxis over the past several decades has caused a significant decline in the incidence of OIs, they still occur.[3,4] A significant number of people with HIV in the United States are undiagnosed, and many more are inadequately treated.[3] These patients remain at significant risk of developing OIs as their HIV infections progress. OIs typically occur when the CD4 lymphocyte count falls below 200 cells/μL. However, they can occur even in patients with higher CD4 lymphocyte levels.[4] Recent studies have shown the leading OIs in the United States include *Pneumocystis jirovecii* (formerly *Pneumocystis carinii*) pneumonia (PCP), disseminated *Mycobacterium avium* complex (MAC), and candidiasis.[4,5] Many other OIs, including tuberculosis, toxoplasmosis, and cryptococcal meningitis, can also cause significant morbidity and mortality. These infections must be considered when caring for patients with HIV.[4-6]

CRITICAL DECISION

When should there be concern for OIs in patients with HIV?

An increase in the risk of specific OIs is triggered as CD4 lymphocyte counts decline (*Table 1*). For example, the risk of PCP increases with a CD4 lymphocyte count less than 200 cells/μL. The risk of *Toxoplasma gondii* and *Cryptococcus neoformans* infections increases at a CD4 lymphocyte count less than 100 cells/μL. For MAC, the risk increases with a CD4 lymphocyte count less than 50 cells/μL.[5] This risk analysis is straightforward, but it becomes complicated when recent CD4 lymphocyte counts are unavailable because of inadequate access to care. Therefore, emergency physicians must sometimes use other tools to stratify risk.

Total lymphocyte count (TLC) can be obtained rapidly and has been well studied as a surrogate marker for a CD4 lymphocyte count. Numerous studies have been conducted to determine the optimal TLC cutoff to correlate to a CD4 lymphocyte count less than 200 cells/μL. Several have reported that a TLC range between 1,000 and 1,250 cells/μL or less correlate with a CD4 lymphocyte count less than 200 cells/μL.[7] However, many of these studies evaluated patients who were not taking antiretroviral therapy, a factor that must be considered. Although it is an imperfect tool, TLC can be used with caution to help risk stratify HIV-positive patients.

Another tool that can be used in the emergency department to assess the risk of OIs is a simple medication reconciliation. Taking certain antibiotics, such as trimethoprim-sulfamethoxazole (TMP-SMX), dapsone, pentamidine, or azithromycin, can suggest a CD4 lymphocyte count less than 200 cells/μL. Fluconazole 400 mg can be taken daily for prophylaxis against coccidioidomycosis and suggests a CD4 lymphocyte count less than 250 cells/μL. This

OI	CD4 Lymphocyte Count
Coccidioidomycosis	<250 cells/μL
PCP	<200 cells/μL
Candidiasis	<200 cells/μL
Histoplasmosis	<150 cells/μL
Toxoplasmosis	<100 cells/μL
Cryptococcal meningitis	<100 cells/μL
MAC	<50 cells/μL

TABLE 1. CD4 lymphocyte count risk threshold for OIs

regimen is typically seen in parts of the United States with a high incidence of coccidioidomycosis. Fluconazole is also used in 200-mg doses as suppressive therapy for cryptococcal meningitis.

Although regimens of TMP-SMX, dapsone, or atovaquone suggest prophylaxis against PCP and CD4 lymphocyte counts less than 200 cells/µL, TMP-SMX and atovaquone also provide prophylaxis against toxoplasmosis, which occurs at a CD4 lymphocyte count less than 100 cells/µL. Thus, patients on TMP-SMX or atovaquone may have CD4 lymphocyte counts between 50 and 200 cells/µL. Taking azithromycin suggests prophylaxis against MAC and correlates with a CD4 lymphocyte count less than 50 cells/µL.[7]

CRITICAL DECISION

Which infections should be considered and treated in patients with HIV who present with respiratory distress?

Respiratory infections are common in patients with HIV. They can occur at any CD4 lymphocyte count, but the risk of infection with specific pathogens increases as the CD4 lymphocyte count declines.[5,8] The most common pathogens that cause bacterial community-acquired pneumonia in patients with HIV (the same as in immunocompetent individuals) are *Streptococcus pneumoniae*, *Haemophilus influenzae*, and *Staphylococcus aureus*. Another pathogen that commonly causes community-acquired pneumonia in patients with HIV is *Pseudomonas aeruginosa*. Depending on specific geographic risk factors, patients with HIV are at greater risk of developing pulmonary infections from *Mycobacterium tuberculosis* (TB) and endemic fungi. It is especially important to ask patients with HIV about travel, recent hospital admissions, and homelessness.[5,8] Empiric antibiotic coverage is generally the same in patients with and without an HIV infection unless other concerns are present based on the history, CD4 lymphocyte count, examination, or diagnostic workup.[5]

Because of its associated morbidity and mortality, one of the most important OIs to consider is PCP. Mortality has been reported at 10% to 20% in patients with PCP, with higher rates for severe infections.[8,9] Fortunately, PCP has declined significantly over the past several decades because of prophylaxes and HAART.[3-5] The lifetime incidence of PCP was 70% to 80% in patients with AIDS in the pre-HAART era. Between 2008 and 2010, incidence declined to less than 0.5 cases per 100 person-years.[4] Despite the significant reduction in incidence, mortality remains high in those who become infected. *P. jirovecii* is still a relevant cause of pneumonia in patients whose HIV infections are undiagnosed, who are not treated with HAART, or whose illness has progressed to AIDS.[8] In HIV-positive patients with interstitial infiltrates and oropharyngeal candidiasis, the odds ratio for PCP has been reported at 11.81.[9] The specific clinical features that should raise suspicion of PCP include exertional dyspnea, diffuse interstitial infiltrates, inspiratory crackles, a subacute disease course, and oropharyngeal candidiasis (*Figure 2*).[8,9]

An HIV infection is also one of the greatest risk factors for the development of a TB infection. TB is a serious global concern. Its incidence is greater in people with HIV than without, but it is less common in the United States than elsewhere.[5,8,9] The clinical features that should increase suspicion of a pulmonary TB infection are cavitary infiltrates, fever for more than 7 days, and weight loss.[9,10] HIV-positive patients with histories of incarceration, homelessness, congregate housing, or

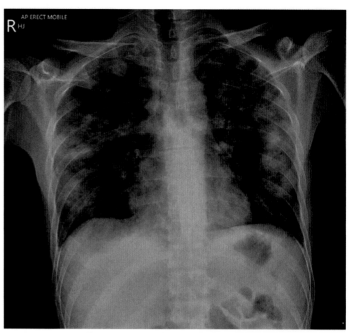

FIGURE 2.   Chest x-ray showing bilateral alveolar consolidations in a patient with a recent HIV diagnosis. *Credit:* Copyright 2023 Dr. Craig Hacking. Image courtesy of Dr. Craig Hacking and Radiopaedia.org, rID: 152246. Used under license.

travel to places with a high incidence of TB are at an increased risk of TB.[11] Empiric coverage is recommended for patients with HIV who have clinical and imaging findings consistent with TB. Diagnostic tests — including sputum smear, culture, and nucleic acid amplification — should be sent before empiric treatment is started. As a result, empiric coverage for TB is usually not initiated in the emergency department.[5]

Pulmonary infections from endemic fungi — coccidioidomycosis, histoplasmosis, and blastomycosis — are less common but must also be considered. The greatest risk factors for these infections are travel to and residence in endemic areas.[5,8,11] These infections are not typically diagnosed in the emergency department, and empiric coverage is not recommended.[5]

CRITICAL DECISION

How is PCP diagnosed and treated?

Diagnosis

The diagnosis of PCP can be challenging because immunofluorescent or cytochemical identification of the organism is required. Additionally, expectorated sputum samples have very low diagnostic sensitivity.[5] Induced sputum can be a viable option when paired with polymerase chain reaction testing. However, collecting sputum in the emergency department is challenging. Sensitivity ranges from 55% to 92% and likely depends on the sputum induction procedure used.[12,13]

There is another laboratory marker that can be used as a diagnostic tool. In patients with AIDS, a β-d-glucan level greater than 80 pg/mL has 92% sensitivity and 65% specificity for PCP.[14] In patients with AIDS and respiratory symptoms, a β-d-glucan level greater than 80 pg/mL has a sensitivity of 93%, specificity of 75%, and positive predictive value of 96%.[15] If this test is available in the emergency department, it can be a very helpful tool in the early diagnostic workup.

Lactate dehydrogenase (LDH) is another laboratory marker that is classically used. Studies have shown that an LDH level greater than 350 units/L in patients with PCP has a sensitivity of 78% to 100% and a specificity of 35.5% to 78%. The greatest challenge of using LDH is that it can be elevated because of several underlying conditions. In patients with HIV, LDH can also be elevated in the setting of pulmonary TB or bacterial pneumonias.[16] The low specificity and varying sensitivity across studies make LDH less helpful in isolation. However, the finding of a normal LDH level can reduce the concern for PCP in low-risk patients.

If these tests are readily available, it is reasonable to consider them early to guide management. Because of limited specificity, patients should still be covered with empiric antibiotics for other likely pathogens while awaiting a more definitive diagnosis. If clinical concern is high or the patient is critically ill, then empiric coverage for PCP prior to a confirmatory diagnosis is appropriate.

Treatment

Empiric coverage for PCP consists of TMP-SMX for 21 days. For moderate to severe disease, treatment is typically initiated with intravenous therapy and switched to oral therapy after the patient has improved. If a patient has contraindications to TMP-SMX therapy, alternative agents to consider are pentamidine or primaquine with clindamycin for moderate to severe disease. For mild to moderate disease, alternative therapy is dapsone or primaquine with clindamycin or atovaquone. Criteria for moderate to severe illness include a PaO_2 less than 70 mm Hg on room air or an alveolar-arterial DO_2 gradient greater than 35 mm Hg. In simpler terms, patients who require supplemental oxygen meet the criteria for moderate to severe disease. These patients benefit from corticosteroids. A common regimen is prednisone at a starting dose of 40 mg twice daily tapered over the course of 21 days.[5] Adjunctive corticosteroids in moderate to severe illness reduces mortality from PCP, with a number needed to treat (NNT) of 9 for patients not on HAART and an NNT of 23 for patients on HAART.[17]

CRITICAL DECISION

How is cryptococcal meningitis diagnosed and treated?

Cryptococcal meningitis typically presents as meningitis or encephalitis over approximately 2 weeks. Symptoms often include fever, headache, malaise, and sometimes, altered mental status.[5] Globally, cryptococcal meningitis accounts for 15% of AIDS-related deaths.[5,18] In high-income countries, 1-year mortality is reported to be as high as 20% to 30%. Delayed diagnosis has been identified as a major factor in the high morbidity and mortality associated with cryptococcal meningitis.[5,18-21] Prompt diagnosis and management to decrease intracranial pressure (ICP) and prevent long-term neurologic sequelae are essential.[20] Because they are often the first point of contact for patients who present for medical care, emergency physicians have a responsibility to consider this diagnosis.

The preferred diagnostic modality for cryptococcal meningitis is a lumbar puncture with opening pressure and a test for CSF cryptococcal antigen (CrAg). If CrAg testing is unavailable, then a CSF India ink test is recommended, but its sensitivity is only 60% to 80%. If a lumbar puncture cannot be performed, then a serum CrAg measurement can be obtained.[5,20,21] Serum CrAg testing is up to 99.7% sensitive and 94.1% specific, nearly equivalent to a CSF

CrAg test.[21] A lumbar puncture is still necessary to reduce ICP, but a serum CrAg measurement can guide empiric treatment.[5] If a serum CrAg test is positive, empiric coverage should be started with amphotericin B plus flucytosine.[22] While waiting for the results of a serum CrAg test, the physician should implement empiric coverage for bacterial and viral meningoencephalitis.

CRITICAL DECISION

When should a lumbar puncture be performed in a patient with HIV and suspected cryptococcal meningitis?

In patients with HIV who present with signs of a CNS infection, the differential diagnosis should include bacterial meningitis, cryptococcal meningitis, and toxoplasmosis. A *T. gondii* infection typically presents as focal encephalitis, which highlights the importance of a thorough neurologic examination.[5,23] Although serum CrAg testing has good sensitivity and specificity, a lumbar puncture should still be performed to evaluate for alternative pathologies, assess for elevated CSF pressure, and reduce elevated CSF pressure through therapeutic removal.[22] The longer the period of increased CSF pressure, the greater the risk of neurologic sequelae and mortality.[20,21] However, cryptococcal meningitis often causes symptoms that raise concern for lumbar puncture safety: papilledema, impaired mentation, and cranial neuropathies.[22]

The Infectious Diseases Society of America (IDSA) recommends a head CT scan in all HIV-positive patients with symptoms concerning for bacterial meningitis because immunocompromised patients are unable to mount an appropriate immune response to space-occupying lesions and can present without the usual neurologic findings.[24] Although MRI has better sensitivity than CT for cryptococcal lesions, it offers no advantage over CT for *Cryptococcus*-related masses.[25] Head CT is obtained not to evaluate for signs of

✔ Pearls

- TLC can be used as a surrogate for a CD4 lymphocyte count in patients with HIV; a TLC less than 1,000 to 1,250 cells/μL correlates to a CD4 lymphocyte count less than 200 cells/μL.

- *S. pneumoniae*, *H. influenzae*, and *S. aureus* are the most common pathogens responsible for bacterial community-acquired pneumonia in patients with HIV, the same as in the general population. Consideration should also be given to PCP, *P. aeruginosa*, and TB, which have greater incidences in patients with HIV than in those without.

- β-d-glucan is a useful laboratory test in the evaluation of patients with HIV and clinical features of PCP.

- For the management of PCP, adjunctive corticosteroids should be started in patients with moderate to severe disease (ie, those requiring supplemental oxygen).

- In patients with suspected cryptococcal meningitis and papilledema, lumbar puncture with an opening pressure and therapeutic CSF drainage is safe if the head CT shows no sign of a space-occupying lesion.

elevated ICP (which is common in cryptococcal meningitis), but rather to rule out brain shift as a cause. Elevated ICP can be caused by increased blood, brain, or CSF volume within the intracranial space. In the setting of elevated ICP due to increased CSF volume without brain shift, a lumbar puncture is considered safe.[26] If imaging does not show a space-occupying lesion, it is safe to perform large-volume therapeutic and diagnostic lumbar drainage in the setting of cryptococcal meningitis with an elevated (>30 mm Hg) opening pressure.[27,28]

No randomized controlled trial has specifically evaluated the safety of performing a lumbar puncture under these circumstances, but an overwhelming body of evidence shows that neurologic and clinical outcomes are better when elevated ICP is managed aggressively.[22,27-29] In patients with cryptococcal meningitis, the IDSA recommends prompt assessment of CSF pressure with a lumbar puncture and the reduction of elevated CSF pressure by 50% or to a normal pressure of less than 20 mm Hg.[24] Deviation from the IDSA guidelines on ICP management has been shown to increase neurologic sequelae.[29] Although a diagnostic lumbar puncture is important, emergency physicians must remember that a therapeutic lumbar puncture is essential in the setting of cryptococcal meningitis with elevated ICP.[20-22]

CRITICAL DECISION

How are oropharyngeal and esophageal candidiasis diagnosed and treated?

Esophageal and oropharyngeal candidiasis are common infections in patients with HIV, especially those with CD4 lymphocyte counts less than 200 cells/μL.[30] Oropharyngeal candidiasis is diagnosed clinically at the bedside when characteristic lesions are found on examination. Microscopic evaluation with potassium hydroxide can be used for diagnosis but is often not required if classic symptoms and examination findings are present.

Pseudomembranous candidiasis has lesions that are painless, white, and plaquelike. These lesions are found on the oral or pharyngeal mucosa and can be scraped off easily. The less common erythematous candidiasis presents with erythema, pain, and no plaques.[5,31,32] In esophageal candidiasis, typical symptoms include dysphagia, odynophagia, and pain behind the sternum. Upper endoscopic evaluation to confirm the diagnosis of esophageal candidiasis is unnecessary in patients whose condition improves with antifungal therapy.[5,30]

Patients who can tolerate oral intake can be safely discharged home with antifungal therapy. Treatment of oropharyngeal

candidiasis consists of oral fluconazole for 1 to 2 weeks. Topical agents can be used in patients who cannot take fluconazole because of drug interactions, adverse effects, or QTc prolongation. Topical agents to consider are miconazole buccal tablets, clotrimazole troches, nystatin suspension, itraconazole solution, and posaconazole suspension. Treatment for esophageal candidiasis consists of fluconazole or oral itraconazole solution. If a patient cannot tolerate oral intake because of their odynophagia, then intravenous fluconazole should be given. Alternatives include other azole agents, such as voriconazole or isavuconazole. The duration of therapy for esophageal candidiasis is 2 to 3 weeks.[31]

Oropharyngeal and esophageal candidiasis can occur together, but their treatment durations and alternative agents are different. Therefore, to determine whether there is esophageal involvement, physicians must ask patients about esophageal symptoms when concerned for oropharyngeal candidiasis.[30] If there is diagnostic uncertainty regarding esophageal involvement, a 2-week treatment course is a safe option because it falls within the recommended range for both conditions. Symptoms typically improve within the first 2 to 3 days of therapy.[5] If a patient returns to the emergency department because their condition is unimproved, consider alternative pathologies, such as drug-resistant *Candida albicans* and non–*C. albicans* species.[33] In patients with no history of HIV, oropharyngeal candidiasis without another clear risk factor or alternative explanation should raise suspicion for undiagnosed HIV.[34]

Summary

Patients with HIV are at risk of OIs that can cause significant morbidity and mortality. Emergency physicians evaluate undifferentiated patients in whom HIV status and CD4 lymphocyte count are often unknown. Therefore, all potential diagnoses must be considered, and appropriate diagnostic studies must be ordered. Laboratory findings must be thoroughly reviewed to assess the likelihood of undiagnosed HIV and the associated risk of OIs, which can drastically alter diagnosis and management. OIs have declined significantly since the advent of HAART, but it remains essential for emergency physicians to be fluent in the diagnostic workup and management of common OIs.

REFERENCES

1. Pantaleo G, Graziosi C, Fauci AS. The immunopathogenesis of human immunodeficiency virus infection. *N Engl J Med.* 1993 Feb 4;328(5):327-335.

2. U.S. Statistics. HIV.gov. Updated October 27, 2022. https://www.hiv.gov/hiv-basics/overview/data-and-trends/statistics

3. Buchacz K, Baker RK, Palella FJ Jr, et al; HOPS Investigators. AIDS-defining opportunistic illnesses in US patients, 1994-2007: a cohort study. *AIDS.* 2010 Jun 19;24(10):1549-1559.

4. Buchacz K, Lau B, Jing Y, et al; North American AIDS Cohorts Collaboration on Research and Design (NA-ACCORD) of IeDEA. Incidence of AIDS-defining opportunistic infections in a multicohort analysis of HIV-infected persons in the United States and Canada, 2000-2010. *J Infect Dis.* 2016 Sep 15;214(6):862-872.

5. Panel on Guidelines for the Prevention and Treatment of Opportunistic Infections in Adults and Adolescents with HIV. Guidelines for the prevention and treatment of opportunistic infections in adults and adolescents with HIV. National Institutes of Health. Updated July 24, 2023. https://clinicalinfo.hiv.gov/en/guidelines/hiv-clinical-guidelines-adult-and-adolescent-opportunistic-infections/whats-new

6. Palella FJ Jr, Delaney KM, Moorman AC, et al; HIV Outpatient Study investigators. Declining morbidity and mortality among patients with advanced human immunodeficiency virus infection. *N Engl J Med.* 1998 Mar 26;338(13):853-860.

━━━━━━━━━ ✖ **Pitfalls** ━━━━

■ Overlooking the possibility of a *P. jirovecii* infection in patients with HIV who present with bilateral pulmonary infiltrates and hypoxemic respiratory failure.

■ Forgetting to inquire about esophageal symptoms in patients with oropharyngeal candidiasis.

■ Neglecting to consider cryptococcal meningitis as the cause of a subacute headache in patients with HIV.

CASE RESOLUTIONS

CASE ONE
Empiric bacterial meningitis coverage was started. A lumbar puncture was performed, and the opening pressure was 40 mm Hg. Therapeutic lumbar drainage was completed with removal of 25 mL of CSF, and the closing pressure was 10 mm Hg. The patient had significant improvement in his headache and vision changes following the lumbar puncture. His CSF CrAg test was positive. He was started on amphotericin B and flucytosine and admitted to the hospital for further treatment.

CASE TWO
In the setting of this patient's HIV status, immunosuppression, clinical features, and chest x-ray, there was a high concern for PCP. A β-d-glucan test was ordered, and the levels were found to be elevated to 140 pg/mL, suggesting a diagnosis of PCP. A hypertonic saline nebulizer was given to obtain an induced sputum sample. The patient received TMP-SMX along with empiric community-acquired pneumonia coverage. Given her oxygen requirement and the high concern for PCP, adjunctive prednisone was also started at 40 mg twice daily. The patient was admitted to the hospital for further treatment. Her induced sputum sample stain and polymerase chain reaction tests were positive for PCP.

CASE THREE
Based on clinical features, the diagnosis of oropharyngeal candidiasis with likely esophageal involvement was made. A rapid HIV test was ordered, and the result was positive. The patient was able to tolerate oral intake without significant difficulty. He was informed of his diagnosis and provided with resources. He was scheduled for outpatient follow-up with an infectious disease specialist for further management of his newly diagnosed HIV and to initiate antiretroviral therapy. He was started on a 3-week course of oral fluconazole and discharged home.

7. Schreibman T, Friedland G. Use of total lymphocyte count for monitoring response to antiretroviral therapy. *Clin Infect Dis.* 2004 Jan 15;38(2):257-262.

8. Benito N, Moreno A, Miro JM, Torres A. Pulmonary infections in HIV-infected patients: an update in the 21st century. *Eur Respir J.* 2012 Mar;39(3):730-745.

9. Selwyn PA, Pumerantz AS, Durante A, et al. Clinical predictors of *Pneumocystis carinii* pneumonia, bacterial pneumonia and tuberculosis in HIV-infected patients. *AIDS.* 1998 May 28;12(8):885-893.

10. Lewinsohn DM, Leonard MK, LoBue PA, et al. Official American Thoracic Society/Infectious Diseases Society of America/Centers for Disease Control and Prevention clinical practice guidelines: diagnosis of tuberculosis in adults and children. *Clin Infect Dis.* 2017 Jan 15;64(2):111-115.

11. Lortholary O, Charlier C, Lebeaux D, Lecuit M, Consigny PH. Fungal infections in immunocompromised travelers. *Clin Infect Dis.* 2013 Mar;56(6):861-869.

12. Cruciani M, Marcati P, Malena M, Bosco O, Serpelloni G, Mengoli C. Meta-analysis of diagnostic procedures for *Pneumocystis carinii* pneumonia in HIV-1-infected patients. *Eur Respir J.* 2002 Oct;20(4):982-989.

13. Leigh TR, Parsons P, Hume C, Husain OA, Gazzard B, Collins JV. Sputum induction for diagnosis of *Pneumocystis carinii* pneumonia. *Lancet.* 1989 Jul 22;2(8656):205-206.

14. Sax PE, Komarow L, Finkelman MA, et al; AIDS Clinical Trials Gropu Study A5164 Team. Blood (1->3)-beta-D-glucan as a diagnostic test for HIV-related *Pneumocystis jirovecii* pneumonia. *Clin Infect Dis.* 2011 Jul 15;53(2):197-202.

15. Wood BR, Komarow L, Zolopa AR, Finkelman MA, Powderly WG, Sax PE. Test performance of blood beta-glucan for *Pneumocystis jirovecii* pneumonia in patients with AIDS and respiratory symptoms. *AIDS.* 2013 Mar 27;27(6):967-972.

16. Quist J, Hill AR. Serum lactate dehydrogenase (LDH) in *Pneumocystis carinii* pneumonia, tuberculosis, and bacterial pneumonia. *Chest.* 1995 Aug;108(2):415-418.

17. Ewald H, Raatz H, Boscacci R, Furrer H, Bucher HC, Briel M. Adjunctive corticosteroids for *Pneumocystis jiroveci* pneumonia in patients with HIV infection. *Cochrane Database Syst Rev.* 2015 Apr 2;2015(4):CD006150.

18. *Guidelines for Diagnosing, Preventing and Managing Cryptococcal Disease Among Adults, Adolescents and Children Living With HIV.* World Health Organization; 2022. http://www.ncbi.nlm.nih.gov/books/NBK581832

19. Salazar AS, Keller MR, Olsen MA, et al. Potential missed opportunities for diagnosis of cryptococcosis and the association with mortality: a cohort study. *EClinicalMedicine.* 2020 Oct 7;27:100563.

20. Aye C, Henderson A, Yu H, Norton R. Cryptococcosis—the impact of delay to diagnosis. *Clin Microbiol Infect.* 2016 Jul;22(7):632-635.

21. Temfack E, Rim JJB, Spijker R, et al. Cryptococcal antigen in serum and cerebrospinal fluid for detecting cryptococcal meningitis in adults living with human immunodeficiency virus: systematic review and meta-analysis of diagnostic test accuracy studies. *Clin Infect Dis.* 2021 Apr 8;72(7):1268-1278.

22. Perfect JR, Dismukes WE, Dromer F, et al. Clinical practice guidelines for the management of cryptococcal disease: 2010 update by the Infectious Diseases Society of America. *Clin Infect Dis.* 2010 Feb 1;50(3):291-322.

23. Luft BJ, Hafner R, Korzun AH, et al; ACTG 077p/ANRS 009 Study Team. Toxoplasmic encephalitis in patients with the acquired immunodeficiency syndrome. *N Engl J Med.* 1993 Sep 30;329(14):995-1000.

24. Tunkel AR, Hartman BJ, Kaplan SL, et al. Practice guidelines for the management of bacterial meningitis. *Clin Infect Dis.* 2004 Nov;39(9):1267-1284.

25. Charlier C, Dromer F, Lévêque C, et al. Cryptococcal neuroradiological lesions correlate with severity during cryptococcal meningoencephalitis in HIV-positive patients in the HAART era. *PLoS One.* 2008 Apr 16;3(4):e1950.

26. van Crevel H, Hijdra A, de Gans J. Lumbar puncture and the risk of herniation: when should we first perform CT? *J Neurol.* 2002 Feb;249(2):129-137.

27. Sun HY, Hung CC, Chang SC. Management of cryptococcal meningitis with extremely high intracranial pressure in HIV-infected patients. *Clin Infect Dis.* 2004 Jun 15;38(12):1790-1792.

28. Graybill JR, Sobel J, Saag M, et al; NIAID Mycoses Study Group; AIDS Cooperative Treatment Group. Diagnosis and management of increased intracranial pressure in patients with AIDS and cryptococcal meningitis. *Clin Infect Dis.* 2000 Jan;30(1):47-54.

29. Shoham S, Cover C, Donegan N, Fulnecky E, Kumar P. *Cryptococcus neoformans* meningitis at 2 hospitals in Washington, D.C.: adherence of health care providers to published practice guidelines for the management of cryptococcal disease. *Clin Infect Dis.* 2005 Feb;40(3):477-479.

30. Pappas PG, Kauffman CA, Andes DR, et al. Clinical practice guideline for the management of candidiasis: 2016 update by the Infectious Diseases Society of America. *Clin Infect Dis.* 2016 Feb 15;62(4):e1-e50.

31. Thompson GR III, Patel PK, Kirkpatrick WR, et al. Oropharyngeal candidiasis in the era of antiretroviral therapy. *Oral Surg Oral Med Oral Pathol Oral Radiol Endod.* 2010 Apr;109(4):488-495.

32. Vazquez JA. Optimal management of oropharyngeal and esophageal candidiasis in patients living with HIV infection. *HIV AIDS (Auckl).* 2010;2:89-101.

33. Patel PK, Erlandsen JE, Kirkpatrick WR, et al. The changing epidemiology of oropharyngeal candidiasis in patients with HIV/AIDS in the era of antiretroviral therapy. *AIDS Res Treat.* 2012;2012:262471.

34. Klein RS, Harris CA, Small CB, Moll B, Lesser M, Friedland GH. Oral candidiasis in high-risk patients as the initial manifestation of the acquired immunodeficiency syndrome. *N Engl J Med.* 1984 Aug 9;311(6):354-358.

Wellens Syndrome Type B

By Jeremy Berberian, MD; William J. Brady, MD, FACEP;
and Amal Mattu, MD, FACEP

Dr. Berberian is the associate director of emergency medicine residency
education at ChristianaCare and assistant professor of emergency medicine
at Sidney Kimmel Medical College, Thomas Jefferson University in
Philadelphia, Pennsylvania. Dr. Brady is a professor of emergency medicine,
medicine, and nursing, and vice chair for faculty affairs in the Department
of Emergency Medicine at the University of Virginia School of Medicine
in Charlottesville. Dr. Mattu is a professor, vice chair, and codirector of
the Emergency Cardiology Fellowship in the Department of Emergency
Medicine at the University of Maryland School of Medicine in Baltimore.

Objectives

On completion of this article, you should be able to:

■ Define the ECG diagnostic criteria and
   historical features of Wellens syndrome.

■ Explain the clinical significance of Wellens
   syndrome.

■ Describe the common ECG criteria for poor
   R-wave progression.

CASE PRESENTATION

A 63-year-old man presents due to an episode of chest pain with onset at rest that resolved a few hours prior to arrival (*Figure 1*).

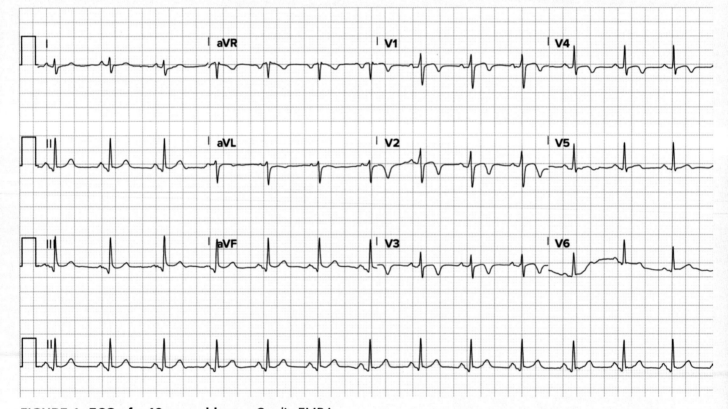

FIGURE 1. **ECG of a 63-year-old man.** *Credit:* EMRA.

ECG Findings

This ECG shows a normal sinus rhythm at 79 bpm, normal axis,
normal QRS complex duration, and T-wave inversion (TWI) in
leads V_1 to V_4. The J point in the inferior leads is isoelectric to the
TP segment but appears to be elevated relative to the PR segment;
however, this is confounded by a downsloping PR segment. There
appears to be ST depression in beats 1 and 3 of lead I, but this
is also confounded by a downsloping PR segment. Additionally,
there are Q waves in the inferior leads, but these are unlikely to be
clinically significant — pathologic Q waves are defined as having a
duration ≥40 msec and an amplitude ≥25% to 33% of accompanying
R-wave height.

The morphology of the precordial TWI is typically seen in
Wellens syndrome, also called left anterior descending (LAD)
coronary T-wave syndrome, which describes an abnormal T-wave
pattern seen in a pain-free state with a recent history of anginal
symptoms. These characteristic ECG findings were first described in
1982 by Dr. Hein J.J. Wellens, a Dutch cardiologist, who found that
75% of patients with this syndrome developed an anterior myocardial
infarction (MI) within a few weeks of hospital admission if no
intervention was performed.[1] The diagnostic criteria include:
- Biphasic (in Wellens type A) or deeply inverted (in Wellens
  type B, as seen in this example) T waves in precordial leads,
  typically V_2 to V_3 (*Figures 2* and *3*)

This patient was admitted for an urgent, but not emergent, cardiac catheterization. He was found to have a 99% occlusion of the proximal LAD, which was successfully treated with a stent.

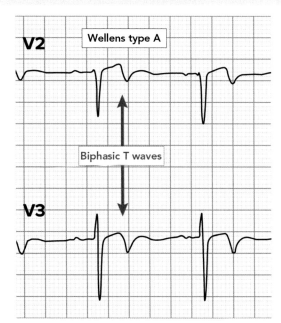

FIGURE 2. Biphasic T waves seen in Wellens type A (from a different ECG). *Credit:* EMRA.

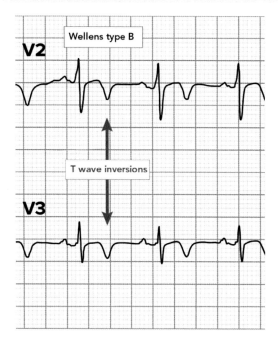

FIGURE 3. TWI seen in Wellens type B (from the case ECG). *Credit:* EMRA.

- Isoelectric or minimally elevated ST segment (<1 mm)
- No precordial Q waves
- Preserved precordial R-wave progression
- Normal or minimally elevated troponins

There is no universal definition for a preserved precordial R-wave progression, but common criteria include:

- R wave greater than 2 to 4 mm in lead V_3 or V_4
- R wave in lead V_4 greater than lead V_3 or lead V_3 greater than lead V_2
- R wave in lead V_3 greater than 3 mm

This ECG pattern is concerning for a critical stenosis or lesion of the proximal left LAD, and the T-wave abnormalities are thought to represent reperfusion after an ischemic event. Biphasic T waves, also called Wellens type A, are an early finding, and deeply inverted T waves, also called Wellens type B, are a later, more common finding (up to 75% of cases). Patients with these ECG findings in the appropriate clinical context have a high likelihood of developing an anterior MI within a short time frame and warrant admission for cardiac catheterization.[1] Coronary angiography is required to evaluate the need for early angioplasty or coronary bypass surgery, and provocative testing, especially exercise stress testing, should be avoided because it could precipitate an acute MI or cardiac arrest.[2-4]

It is important to recognize that these ECG findings were originally described in patients in a pain-free state. In fact, it is common to see these ECG changes persist from the painful presentation into the pain-free state because the ECG changes do not resolve until the LAD lesion is successfully managed with either percutaneous coronary intervention or a coronary artery bypass graft.

The term *Wellens waves* is sometimes used to describe these ECG findings in symptomatic patients. In these cases, the ECG changes are due to active ischemia. The term *pseudo-Wellens* is commonly used to describe these ECG findings when associated with causes other than LAD stenosis, such as left ventricular hypertrophy, pulmonary embolism, hypertrophic cardiomyopathy, intracranial hemorrhage, and right bundle branch block. In these cases, the ECG changes are due to repolarization abnormalities.

REFERENCES

1. de Zwaan C, Bär FW, Wellens HJJ. Characteristic electrocardiographic pattern indicating a critical stenosis high in left anterior descending coronary artery in patients admitted because of impending myocardial infarction. *Am Heart J.* 1982 Apr;103(4)(part 2):730-736.
2. de Zwaan C, FW Bär, Janssen JH, et al. Angiographic and clinical characteristics of patients with unstable angina showing an ECG pattern indicating critical narrowing of the proximal LAD coronary artery. *Am Heart J.* 1989 Mar;117(3):657-665.
3. Rhinehardt J, Brady WJ, Perron AD, Mattu A. Electrocardiographic manifestations of Wellens syndrome. *Am J Emerg Med.* 2002 Nov;20(7):638-643.
4. Patel K, Alattar F, Koneru J, Shamoon F. ST-Elevation myocardial infarction after pharmacologic persantine stress test in a patient with Wellens syndrome. *Case Rep Emerg Med.* 2014 Apr 2;2014:530451.

■ ACKNOWLEDGMENT ■

This case is reprinted from *Emergency ECGs: Case-Based Review and Interpretations,* available at emra.org/amazon or by using the QR code.

Winged Scapula: An Unusual Cause of Shoulder Dysfunction

By Evan Kuczynski, BA, EMT-B; and Sharon E. Mace, MD, FACEP
Emergency Department, Cleveland Clinic; and Cleveland Clinic
Lerner College of Medicine at Case Western Reserve University,
Cleveland, Ohio

Objective

On completion of this article, you should be able to:
■ Describe, identify, and treat a winged scapula.

CASE PRESENTATION

A 17-year-old boy presents with difficulty lifting his book bag and brushing his teeth for the past several days. He says that sitting in his chair at school and wearing his backpack are both uncomfortable. He has no history of illness and takes no medications. He denies smoking cigarettes or using other drugs. He reports landing on the right side of his upper back several days ago while wrestling. His vital signs are BP 110/80, P 86, R 14, and T 36.95°C (98.5°F); SpO$_2$ is 98% on room air. He has weakness when abducting his right arm. The examination reveals medial scapular winging (*Figure 1*). X-rays of the right scapula and the right shoulder do not show any fractures or dislocations.

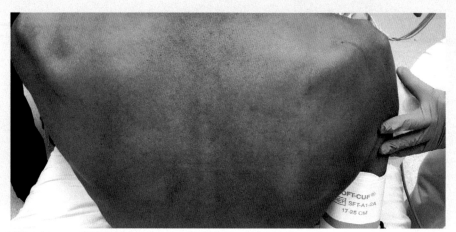

FIGURE 1. Photo of patient showing medial scapular winging at rest.
Credit: Sharon E. Mace, MD, FACEP, and the Cleveland Clinic Emergency Services Institute.

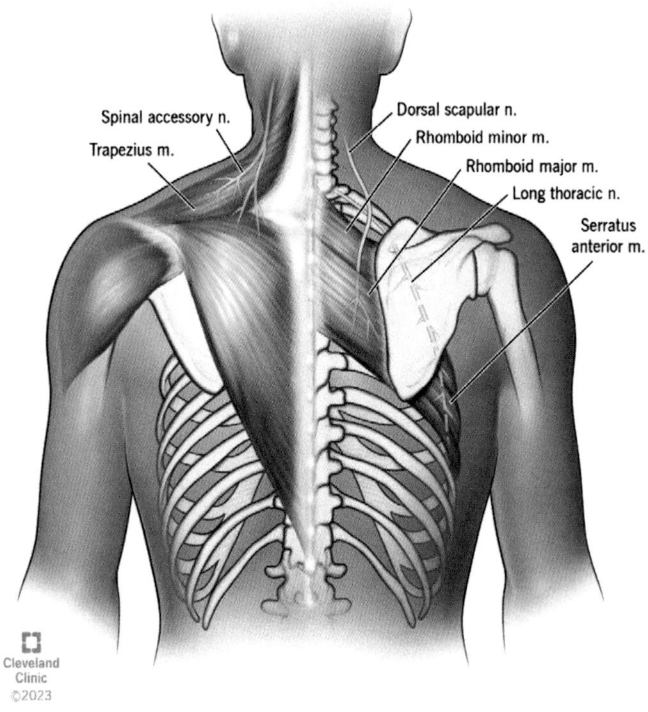

FIGURE 2. Muscles and nerves of the shoulder.
Credit: Reprinted with permission, Cleveland Clinic Foundation ©2023. All Rights Reserved.

Labels: Spinal accessory n.; Trapezius m.; Dorsal scapular n.; Rhomboid minor m.; Rhomboid major m.; Long thoracic n.; Serratus anterior m.; Cleveland Clinic ©2023

Discussion

Scapular winging, or winged scapula, is a rare condition in which palsy of the trapezius, rhomboids, or serratus anterior causes the scapula to detach (ie, wing) from the thoracic wall during movement. Most commonly, a lesion on the long thoracic nerve (LTN) causes palsy of the serratus anterior, resulting in medial scapular winging (*Table 1*).[1,2] LTN lesions that cause scapular winging can result from both traumatic and nontraumatic injuries.[2] Traumatic injury to the LTN is the most typical cause of scapular winging and results from overuse or acute trauma that stretches or compresses the LTN.[2-5] One study indicated that over 61% of LTN injuries were due to either acute trauma (whereby the arm was suddenly and forcefully moved forward or backward) or strenuous exertion.[4] Less commonly, scapular winging can occur laterally due to an injury to the spinal accessory (SAN) or dorsal scapular nerve (DSN). SAN injury is the most common cause of lateral winging, due to palsy of the trapezius (*Figure 2*).[3] Most often, injury to the SAN is iatrogenic, resulting from excision of lymph nodes or cervical masses (see *Table 1*).[1-3]

Clinical Findings

Patients who present with serratus anterior palsy can have weakness or posterior shoulder pain prior to or in conjunction with medial scapular winging.[1,5] If the patient is experiencing posterior shoulder pain or weakness without winging, obtaining a detailed history is important to differentiate serratus anterior palsy from other etiologies.[5] Winging due to serratus anterior palsy can be observed from behind the patient with arms resting at their sides and accentuated by having the patient press against the wall with

Nerve	Origination	Muscles Innervated	Muscle Function	Pertinent Examination Findings	Type of Winging	Common Etiology	Treatment
Long thoracic nerve	C5-C7	Serratus anterior	Upward rotation for abduction of the scapula	Medial winging during wall test, loss of final 30° of overhead abduction	Medial	Trauma, strenuous activities, or sports	Physical therapy for neurapraxic injury, surgery for severe cases
Dorsal scapular nerve	C4-C5	Levator scapulae (LS), rhomboid major (RM), and rhomboid minor (Rm)	Suspension (LS) and adduction (LS, RM, Rm) of the scapula	Lateral winging, weakness on scapular adduction on affected side	Lateral	Strenuous activity	(as above)
Spinal accessory nerve	Cranial nerve XI	Trapezius	Aids in elevation, adduction, and rotation of the scapula	Difficulty abducting affected shoulder past 90°, lateral winging on abduction, shoulder droop	Lateral	Iatrogenic injury	(as above)

TABLE 1. **Characteristics of winged scapula based on nerve involvement**

their arms in a push-up–like position (*Figure 3*).[2,3,5] Patients also commonly experience a loss in the end range of motion for arm abduction on the affected side.[1,3]

Patients who present with scapular winging due to trapezius or rhomboid palsy will have lateral winging and possibly pain in the affected shoulder.[2,3,6,7] Lateral winging can be observed from behind the patient. Although winging can be present at rest, it may be more obvious when patients abduct their arms.[3] Patients may also have difficulty abducting the arm on the affected side farther than 90°.[3] These patients may report having felt a sudden pain when lifting a heavy load overhead.[7] They may also experience pain due to muscle spasms from overcompensation of other muscles that insert on the scapula.[2]

Diagnostic Testing

X-rays of the shoulder and cervical spine are useful for ruling out other diagnoses.[3,5,8] If the diagnosis is uncertain or there are other concerns, an electromyogram can be used to definitively diagnose the affected nerves.[2,5,6] In some cases, MRI may be useful to detect winging due to a muscle tear.[7]

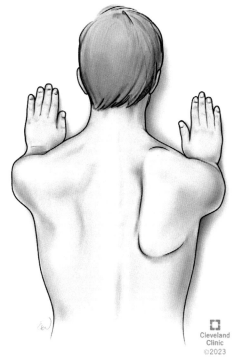

Cleveland
Clinic
©2023

FIGURE 3. Exacerbation of medial scapular winging while pushing on a wall. *Credit:* Reprinted with permission, Cleveland Clinic Foundation ©2023. All Rights Reserved.

Differential Diagnoses

Conditions that may cause shoulder pain, such as bony abnormalities of the cervical spine or shoulder, should be on the list of potential diagnoses for scapular winging.[5,8] Additionally, consider nerve lesions more proximal to the spinal cord that may be affecting the nerve roots where the LTN, DSN, or SAN originate (see *Table 1*).[8]

Treatment and Outcomes

Treatment for scapular winging typically includes pain management with NSAIDs and advising the patient to rest the affected shoulder.[6,8] Patients should also be given a referral for physical therapy. The majority of the literature agrees that conservative, nonoperative management through physical therapy is the best course within the first 2 years of injury.[1-3,6,7] Most patients experience a full recovery of function within that time.[1-3,7] When no recovery has been made after 2 years, operative management may be indicated.[1-3,6,7] Overall, the prognosis for patients with this type of injury is positive.

CASE RESOLUTION

Because the patient did not have a dislocation or fracture, no reduction or manipulation was necessary. The patient was discharged with NSAIDs and orders for a follow-up with physical therapy and orthopedics. In the orthopedic office several weeks later, the patient showed mild improvement. The decision was made to continue conservative treatment, including continuing with physical therapy. The patient experienced full resolution of his symptoms 2 years later.

REFERENCES

1. Gooding BWT, Geoghegan JM, Wallace WA, Manning PA. Scapular winging. *Shoulder Elbow.* 2014;6(1):4-11.
2. Martin RM, Fish DE. Scapular winging: anatomical review, diagnosis, and treatments. *Cur Rev Musculoskelet Med.* 2008;1(1):1-11.
3. Didesch JT, Tang P. Anatomy, etiology, and management of scapular winging. *J Hand Surg Am.* 2019 Apr;44(4):321-330.
4. Vastamäki M, Kauppila LI. Etiologic factors in isolated paralysis of the serratus anterior muscle: a report of 197 cases. *J Shoulder Elbow Surg.* 1993 Sep;2(5):240-243.
5. Wiater JM, Flatow EL. Long horacic nerve injury. *Clin Orthop Relate Res.* 1999 Nov;368:17-27.
6. Davis RL, Papachrisanthou ML. An unusual case of shoulder pain. *J Nurse Pract.* 2017 Jul 12;13(8):E403-E405.
7. Lafosse T, D'utruy A, El Hassan B, Grandjean A, Bouyer M, Masmejean E. Scapula alata: diagnosis and treatment by nerve surgery and tendon transfers. *Hand Surg Rehab.* 2022 Feb;41(suppl):S44-S53.
8. Waldman SD. Winged scapula syndrome. In: *Atlas of Uncommon Pain Syndromes.* 4th ed. Elsevier; 2020:245-247.

Early Anticoagulant Reversal After Trauma

By Kelechi Umoga, MD, MBA; and
Andrew J. Eyre, MD, MS-HPEd
Harvard Affiliated Emergency Medicine Residency; and
Brigham and Women's Hospital, Boston, Massachussetts

Objective

On completion of this article, you should be able to:

- Discuss the management of trauma patients who use anticoagulant medication.

Peck KA, Ley EJ, Brown CV, et al. Early anticoagulant reversal after trauma: a Western Trauma Association critical decisions algorithm. *J Trauma Acute Care Surg.* 2021 Feb 1;90(2):331-336.

KEY POINTS

- A combination of physical examination, imaging, and laboratory testing should be used to identify trauma patients with severe bleeding.

- Management of trauma patients on anticoagulants should include consideration of medication removal or reversal as well as surgical or procedural intervention.

- Each class of anticoagulants has unique mechanisms, reversal agents, and laboratory values that can be used for medication monitoring.

Introduction

Trauma evaluation, management, and outcomes in adult patients are often complicated by anticoagulation use, which primarily consists of vitamin K antagonists (VKAs), direct oral anticoagulation medications, and therapeutic low-molecular-weight heparins (LMWHs). This article summarizes the 2020 Western Trauma Association algorithm and guidelines for trauma patients who are — or may be — using anticoagulant medications.

Assess Degree of Injury and Bleeding

The extent of traumatic injury and bleeding should be rapidly assessed using the standard Advanced Trauma Life Support algorithm. Depending on patient-specific circumstances, this assessment often includes physical examination, imaging, and laboratory testing. Together, these tools are used to identify patients who have or may have severe bleeding, which the article defines as the "need for urgent/emergent operation or intervention, need for immediate transfusion, presence of hemorrhagic shock or hemorrhage into a critical organ or space including major intracranial, ocular, spine, cavitary, or extremity injuries."

Management of Anticoagulated Patients Without Severe Injury or Bleeding

These patients should be managed with simple hemostatic measures including direct pressure, pressure dressings, and suture control, when relevant, and should be monitored with serial physical examinations, laboratory tests, and imaging, as indicated.

Management of Anticoagulated Patients With Severe Injury or Bleeding

Management of severe bleeding in anticoagulated patients must involve removal or reversal of the anticoagulant in addition to the standard management of hemorrhagic shock (ie, appropriate surgical or procedural interventions and emergent resuscitation and transfusions). Care should be taken to avoid trauma-induced coagulopathy, and physicians should monitor for and address any hypothermia, thrombocytopenia, or acidosis.

Management of Specific Anticoagulant Medications

VKAs Such as Warfarin

VKAs disrupt the hepatic synthesis of factors II, VII, IX and X as well as proteins C and S, with the degree of anticoagulation measured by PT and INR. Anticoagulation by these agents is corrected through replacement of the deficient factors, typically with prothrombin complex concentrate (PCC) — four-factor PCC is the preferred agent. Other PCC options include three-factor PCC (factor IX complex) and activated PCC (anti-inhibitor coagulant complex). Fresh frozen plasma is a less expensive alternative, but it requires more time (for crossmatching and thawing) and large volumes for INR correction, which can lead to volume overload.

Direct Thrombin Inhibitors Such as Dabigatran

Dabigatran competitively binds the active site of thrombin, preventing thrombin-mediated conversion of fibrinogen to fibrin. Since dabigatran is heavily cleared by the kidneys, it can potentially be removed by hemodialysis. The only FDA-approved reversal agent for dabigatran is idarucizumab, a monoclonal antibody that binds dabigatran. It can be given as two successive doses of 2.5 g IV each for a total of 5 g. Although the most accurate tests to track dabigatran's effect — dilute thrombin time and ecarin clotting time — are not readily available, thrombin time and PTT can be used with some limitations. Thrombin time is extremely sensitive to dabigatran, and so a normal thrombin time reliably excludes clinically relevant dabigatran levels. By contrast, a prolonged PTT suggests the presence of dabigatran, but a normal value does not exclude it.

Factor Xa Inhibitors Such as Apixaban and Rivaroxaban

Factor Xa inhibitors directly inhibit factor Xa, resulting in decreased conversion of prothrombin to thrombin. The anti-Xa level is useful in determining the amount of clinically relevant anti-Xa drug present and is most reliable when calibrated to the specific drug. The only FDA-approved reversal agent for factor Xa inhibitors is andexanet alfa, a recombinant inactive protein with a structure similar to endogenous factor Xa that competitively binds and sequesters factor Xa inhibitors. It is administered in two different dosing levels depending on the specific factor Xa inhibitor taken, the dose taken, and the timing of the last dose. The lower dose is a bolus of 400 mg IV given at 30 mg/min followed by an infusion of 480 mg given at 4 mg/min for up to 120 minutes. The higher dose is a bolus of 800 mg given at 30 mg/min followed by an infusion of 960 mg given at 8 mg/min for up to 120 minutes. When the dose and timing of a factor Xa inhibitor are unknown, the higher-dose regimen is recommended. Four-factor PCC can also be used for management of severe bleeding in the setting of factor Xa–inhibitor use, although mortality with this option remains high.

LMWHs Such as Enoxaparin

LMWH (enoxaparin for the purposes of this guideline) binds and activates antithrombin, which inhibits factor Xa and, to a lesser extent, factor IIa. Like with factor Xa inhibitors, the anti-Xa level is useful for monitoring the amount of clinically relevant anti-Xa drug present. The recommended dose depends on the amount and timing of the enoxaparin administration. Protamine sulfate is recommended at 1 mg for every 1 mg of enoxaparin given within the prior 8 hours and at 0.5 mg for every 1 mg of enoxaparin given more than 8 hours ago. The intravenous doses should be given slowly, and the maximum recommended single dose is 50 mg in any 10-minute interval to avoid hypotension and anaphylaxis-like reactions.

Assessment for Ongoing Bleeding

Ongoing bleeding should be reassessed with repeated physical examinations, serial laboratory tests, and imaging, if indicated. If bleeding persists despite attempts with reversal agents and appropriate surgical intervention, reversal agents can be redosed or alternative agents considered.

Areas of Controversy and Existing Knowledge or Research Gaps

Additional research is needed to further refine the algorithm and study anticoagulation in acutely injured patients. The authors specifically note areas of controversy, such as the thrombotic risks associated with anticoagulation reversal, the timing of anticoagulation reinitiation, and the role of advanced testing such as thromboelastography and rotational thromboelastometry in anticoagulated patients.

Critical Decisions in Emergency Medicine's LLSA literature reviews feature articles from ABEM's 2023 Lifelong Learning and Self-Assessment Reading List. Available online at acep.org/moc/llsa and on the ABEM website.

Die-Punch Fracture of the Distal Radius

John Kiel DO, MPH, FACEP, CAQSM
University of South Florida Morsani College of Medicine, Tampa

Objective

On completion of this article, you should be able to:

- Describe the injury patterns of distal radius fractures and the uncommon pattern of a die-punch fracture.

CASE PRESENTATION

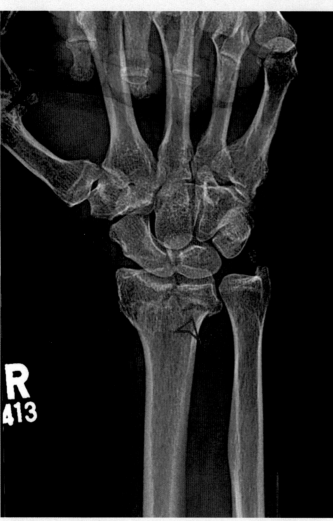

A 58-year-old man presents with right wrist and right shoulder pain after a fall 5 hours prior to arrival. The patient states he was at a bar when someone pushed him, causing him to fall and land on outreached arms. He denies any head injury or loss of consciousness. He states he took two ibuprofen pills when he got home. On physical examination, he has swelling and deformity of his wrist at the distal radius. He is grossly neurovascularly intact, and compartments are soft. The patient is given an oxycodone-acetaminophen pill and a tetanus booster. X-rays of the right shoulder are normal. X-rays of the wrist show comminuted, impacted fractures of the distal radius and ulna without displacement (*Figures 1* and *2*).

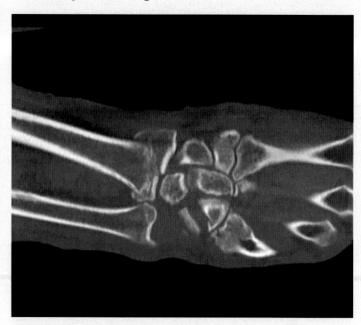

FIGURE 1. X-ray showing comminuted, impacted fracture of the distal radius with extension into the radiocarpal and distal radioulnar joint spaces. *Red arrow* indicates the die-punch fracture.

FIGURE 2. CT showing comminuted, impacted intra-articular fracture of the distal radius with extension into the radiocarpal and distal radioulnar joint spaces

Discussion

Distal radius fractures represent one of the most common fracture patterns in orthopedic trauma, constituting approximately 20% of fractures seen in the emergency department.[1] They represent a significant financial burden to the health care system and an economic burden due to lost productivity.[2] These injuries typically occur from a fall onto an outstretched hand with the forearm pronated and elbow extended. Patients often present with distal wrist pain, and an examination will reveal swelling, bruising, tenderness, and

frequently, deformity. X-rays are typically sufficient to make the diagnosis of a distal radius fracture; however, CT can be obtained to better clarify the injury pattern and to plan for surgical management.

The most common distal radius fracture is the Colles fracture, characterized by a fracture at the metaphysis with dorsal angulation. A Smith fracture, sometimes called a reverse Colles, is the same fracture but with volar angulation of the distal fragment. Other distal radius fractures include radial styloid fractures, which are typically nonsurgical when they occur in isolation; a chauffeur's fracture, which is a radial styloid fracture with intra-articular extension into the radiocarpal joint; and a Barton fracture, which is a distal radius fracture extending into the articular surface and associated with radiocarpal joint dislocation.

A die-punch fracture, which is one of the fractures in this case (along with a fracture of the radial half of the distal radius), is a fracture of the distal radius specifically at the lunate fossa of the articular surface of the distal radius. The lunate fossa represents nearly 50% of the articular surface of the radiocarpal joint.[3] The die-punch fracture is so called because the lunate punches into the distal radius like a die punches material. Die-punch fractures have intra-articular extension and typically require surgery due to their inherent instability. The mainstream treatment is open reduction and fixation with a volar locking plate.[4] Nonoperative management can be considered in uncomplicated, nondisplaced fractures.

CASE RESOLUTION

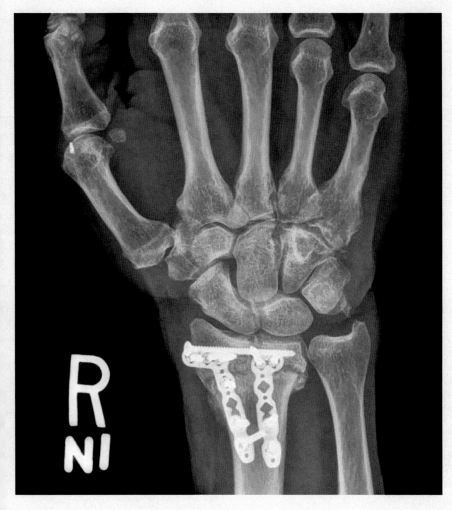

The patient was seen in the orthopedic clinic several days later. A CT scan was ordered, and the patient was screened for preoperative planning and surgical intervention. An open reduction and internal fixation was performed, and the patient was seen in the orthopedic clinic about 4 weeks later for a post-operation follow-up (*Figure 3*). At that time, the examination was reassuring, and he appeared to be healing appropriately. He was referred to physical therapy and subsequently lost to follow-up.

FIGURE 3. Postoperative x-ray showing dorsal plate and screw fixation of a distal radius fracture without change alignment or hardware complication. Mature bony bridging callus is noted.

REFERENCES

1. Meena S, Sharma P, Sambharia AK, Dawar A. Fractures of distal radius: an overview. *J Family Med Prim Care*. 2014 Oct-Dec;3(4):325-332.
2. Mauck BM, Swigler CW. Evidence-based review of distal radius fractures. *Orthop Clin North Am*. 2018 Apr;49(2):211-222.
3. Mekhail AO, Ebraheim NA, McCreath WA, Jackson WT, Yeasting RA. Anatomic and x-ray film studies of the distal articular surface of the radius. *J Hand Surg Am*. 1996 Jul;21(4):567-573.
4. Zhang X, Zhao Y, Hu C, et al. Comparative study of type B distal radius fractures with and without lunate facet involvement treated by volar locking plate, an observational study. *Int J Surg*. 2017 Aug;44:317-323.

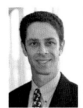

The Critical Image

A Critically Ill Patient

By Joshua S. Broder, MD, FACEP

Dr. Broder is a professor and the residency program director in the Department of Emergency Medicine at Duke University Medical Center in Durham, North Carolina.

Objectives

On completion of this article, you should be able to:

- Recognize common cognitive errors in image interpretation and employ strategies to avoid them.
- Describe targeted and systematic approaches to chest x-ray interpretation in critically ill patients.
- Identify medical devices on chest x-rays.
- Recall critical steps in addressing a retained intravascular wire.

CASE PRESENTATION

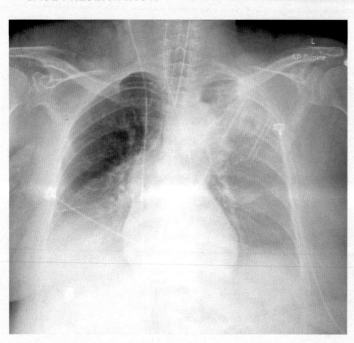

A 63-year-old woman presents with weakness, melena, and altered mental status. Her vital signs are BP 67/43, P 114, R 24, and T 35.7°C (96.3 °F); SpO_2 is 90% on room air. The patient is lethargic and ill appearing. Her mucous membranes are dry, and she has poor skin turgor. She is tachypneic with decreased breath sounds, and she has weak peripheral pulses and tachycardia. Her abdomen is nondistended, and she does not react to palpation. She has no focal neurologic deficits.

The patient is intubated, a central venous catheter is placed, and broad-spectrum antibiotics are initiated, along with blood products and a norepinephrine infusion. A chest x-ray is obtained (*Figure 1*).

FIGURE 1. Chest x-ray. The technique used is anteroposterior with the patient lying supine. With this technique, the heart appears larger than it would on a posteroanterior image. If present, free air beneath the diaphragm may be hidden. Pleural fluid spreads in the horizontal plane and may not be seen as a meniscus sign. In this position, a pneumothorax may be harder to detect.

Discussion

An important finding in this image may be unexpected to the viewer and thus less likely to be identified: a retained central venous catheter guidewire.

Using a database with information from over 40 US health care systems, a study of retained guidewires following central venous catheterization found that only one-third were recognized after completion of the procedure. The remainder were discovered with a delay of days to years — often on imaging obtained for other reasons. Retained guidewires can lead to serious complications, including dysrhythmia, vascular injury or thrombosis, cardiac injury and tamponade, and death.[1] Other studies have documented failures of emergency physicians, radiologists, and others to note retained guidewires on x-ray and CT.[2,3]

Many factors may contribute to the failure to recognize this important abnormality. The patient's clinical needs may limit the emergency physician's ability to devote time to systematic image interpretation. The patient may have multiple image findings and distractors for the physician interpreting the image. The viewer may be focused primarily on evaluating the image

for diagnostic information related to the patient's presentation and clinical condition (*Figure 2*). The image in this case is anteroposterior and supine, which is not ideal for the detection of some pathologies. Multiple procedures have been performed, and the viewer must consider findings related to the success, failure, or complications of those interventions (*Figure 3*). Multiple medical devices are present in the image, adding to its complexity and increasing the risk of a missed finding (see *Figure 3*). For a radiologist reviewing the image, the severity of the patient's illness and clinical priorities may not be evident.

Missed x-ray findings may also occur from multiple cognitive errors, including *satisfaction of search* and *inattentional blindness*. Satisfaction of search occurs when an evaluation process is ended prematurely following the identification of one finding — leading to a failure to recognize additional abnormalities.[2] Systematic strategies for image interpretation can reduce the risk of this error. Inattentional blindness is a phenomenon in which a finding is unrecognized, even if the viewer's gaze falls directly on the relevant portion of the image. In studies of inattentional blindness, radiologists tasked with identifying chest nodules failed to identify a gorilla embedded in the image in 83% of cases, despite their eyes scanning the portion of the image containing the gorilla.[4] Another contributor may include insufficient knowledge (ie, a finding is seen and registered but not recognized as abnormal or concerning).

In critical patients, the approach to chest x-ray interpretation can be modified to increase the likelihood of identifying all important findings. A redundant series of interpretations may be necessary to prevent a missed diagnosis related to satisfaction of search or inattentional blindness.

Targeted interpretation approaches have the advantage of prioritizing based on a patient's clinical presentation but risk missing other key findings and should be bolstered by systematic interpretations. Targeted approaches include:

- **Most-feared finding–based** (eg, tension pneumothorax). The image is reviewed first for the most ominous, life-threatening, or time-dependent problem. Other problems may be missed due to inattentional blindness and satisfaction of search.
- **Most-expected finding–based** (eg, pneumonia). The image is reviewed first for the most common or expected finding. Other findings may be missed, and findings indicative of other pathologies may be misconstrued as confirming the viewer's expectations.

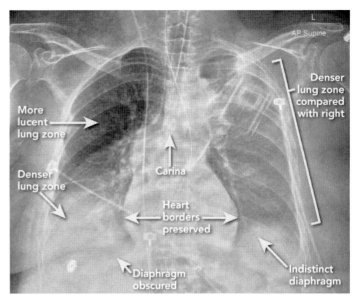

FIGURE 2. Chest x-ray with anatomic features labeled. The obscured diaphragms and densities in bilateral lung fields suggest pleural effusions or parenchymal infiltrates, or both.

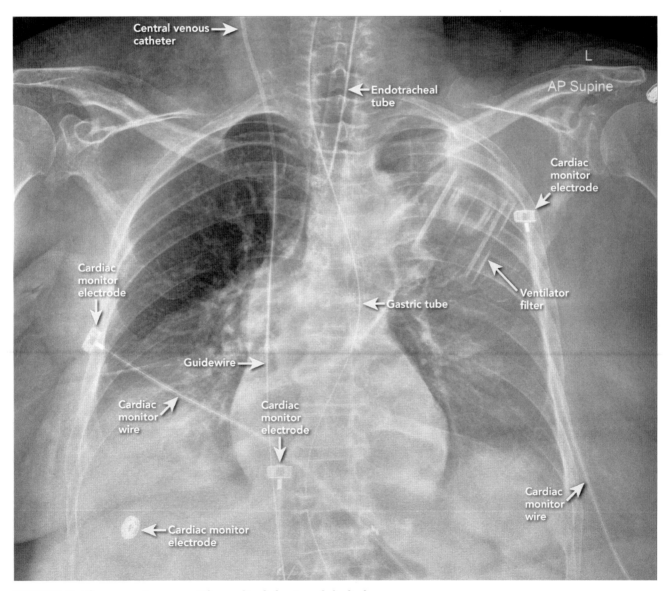

FIGURE 3. The same image with medical devices labeled.

- **Diagnosis-based.** The image is reviewed based on the differential diagnosis, with attention paid to finding signs of each condition. This approach combines targeted and systematic features but may lead to the viewer overlooking important findings of diagnoses not specifically considered or unrelated to the differential diagnosis.
- **Procedure- or complication-based.** This approach evaluates for expected findings and potential complications of a procedure. For example, the viewer may seek to answer questions such as: Is the device in the intended position, location, or configuration? Is a common complication of the procedure, such as pneumothorax, present or absent? This approach has the advantage of prioritizing the immediate intended and unintended consequences of a procedure but can miss unanticipated procedural complications or unrelated findings. Systematic approaches to interpretation include:
- **Anatomy-based.** The image is reviewed to identify and evaluate all anatomic structures within the field of view. Although systematic, this approach does not necessarily prioritize image review by probability, importance, time criticality, or other factors specific to an individual patient. It may overlook devices and findings not on the viewer's list of important anatomy.
- **Image-based.** This approach scans the image in a systemic fashion (eg, left to right, top to bottom, center to periphery) but does not prioritize factors related to the patient's condition, such as critical diagnoses or time-dependent abnormalities. It may also miss patterns that include findings in more than one region of the image.
- **Device-based.** This approach systematically reviews the image to identify all non-anatomic objects. It may distract from anatomic or pathologic findings not related to devices. Identifying a device does not guarantee the recognition of associated complications.

Once identified, intravascular wires require prompt removal. In most instances, removal under fluoroscopic guidance by an interventional radiologist is indicated. However, if the guidewire is still partially encased within the catheter, some authors have described a bedside technique for removal in which continuous negative pressure is exerted by aspirating the channel through which the wire is inserted while gradually withdrawing the catheter.[5] Sequentially clamping the catheter with forceps at the skin surface may be used with the suction technique.[6]

CASE RESOLUTION

The retained guidewire was not noted in the radiology report but was recognized by the emergency physician. The patient underwent wire retrieval with fluoroscopic guidance by an interventional radiologist (*Figure 4*).

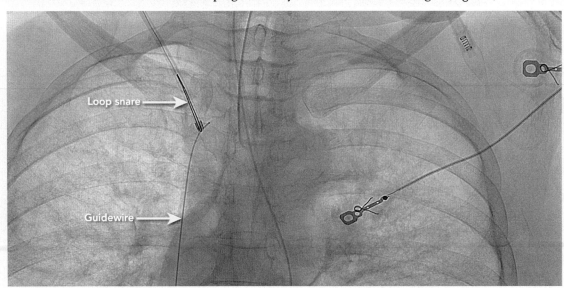

FIGURE 4. **An 8-French sheath has been inserted into the right internal jugular vein by an interventional radiologist.** A loop snare has been advanced to lasso the retained guidewire.

REFERENCES

1. Williams TL, Bowdle TA, Winters BD, Pavkovic SD, Szekendi MK. Guidewires unintentionally retained during central venous catheterization. *J Assoc Vasc Access.* 2014 Mar;19(1):29-34.
2. Lum TE, Fairbanks RJ, Pennington EC, Zwemer FL. Profiles in patient safety: misplaced femoral line guidewire and multiple failures to detect the foreign body on chest radiography. *Acad Emerg Med.* 2005 Jul;12(7):658-662.
3. Almehmi SE, Abaza M, Krishna VN, Almehmi A. Delayed diagnosis of a retained guidewire after bedside femoral venous catheter insertion: a preventable complication. *Radiol Case Rep.* 2022 Dec 22;17(3):647-649.
4. Drew T, Võ MLH, Wolfe JM. The invisible gorilla strikes again: sustained inattentional blindness in expert observers. *Psychol Sci.* 2013 Sep;24(9):1848-1853.
5. Mariyaselvam MZA, Patel V, Sawyer A, et al. A bedside rescue method for retrieving retained guidewires: the "suck out" technique. *J Vasc Access.* 2021 May;22(3):398-403.
6. Kannaujia AK, Bhargava T, Kumar A, Ambasta S. Retrieval of the lost guidewire immediately after central line insertion by the "clamp technique" — the preponderancy of a procedural checklist and prevention of catastrophe. *Indian J Anaesth.* 2022 May;66(suppl 3):S175-S176.

Feature Editor: Joshua S. Broder, MD, FACEP. See also *Diagnostic Imaging for the Emergency Physician* (Winner of the 2011 Prose Award in Clinical Medicine, the American Publishers Award for Professional and Scholarly Excellence) and *Critical Images in Emergency Medicine* by Dr. Broder.

Manual Reduction of Paraphimosis

Steven J. Warrington, MD, MEd, MS
MercyOne Siouxland, Sioux City, Iowa

Objective

On completion of this article, you should be able to:

- Explain the procedure for manual reduction of paraphimosis.

Paraphimosis occurs when the foreskin becomes stuck in a retracted position. Reduction helps with pain and prevents complications. Paraphimosis can occur naturally or as the result of failing to return the foreskin to its natural state of reduction; in either case, treatment is the same.

Contraindications

- None

Benefits and Risks

The primary benefit of reduction is to resolve the symptoms of paraphimosis, such as pain or urinary obstruction. Risks are relatively minimal and include discomfort, injury to the soft tissue, and failure to successfully reduce the foreskin.

Alternatives

The primary alternative to a manual reduction is a dorsal slit or a urologic or surgical consultation.

Minimizing Side Effects

There can be a significant amount of pain associated with this procedure, and the patient's inability to tolerate the pain may result in the reduction attempt failing. There are multiple potential approaches to alleviating the patient's pain, allowing for a successful manual reduction. The approach taken will depend on the available resources and the level of the patient's discomfort. In some cases, a topical anesthetic may be all that is required. However, oral or injectable medications may also be necessary, and some patients may require procedural sedation. Creating a treatment plan prior to attempting the procedure will help prevent the patient from experiencing unnecessary pain.

Special Considerations

There are multiple approaches to reducing edema, including using an ice pack (avoiding direct contact with the skin), sugar, or multiple small needle punctures.

TECHNIQUE

1. **Obtain** the patient's consent and necessary equipment. Consider pretreatment with pharmacologic agents or the need for adjunct therapies to reduce edema (ie, ice or sugar).

2. **Compress** the glans and foreskin gently but with continuously increased pressure applied to reduce the edema (*Figure 1*). Consider using gauze or drying the area if a topical anesthetic was applied.

3. **Focus** on compression of the glans. After a few minutes of compression and edema reduction, attempt to push the glans inward through the foreskin (*Figure 2*).

4. **Attempt,** if necessary, to reduce the paraphimosis by moving the foreskin distally while also pushing the glans inward through the paraphimotic ring.

5. **Use** additional adjuncts, such as ice, sugar, or small punctures if the procedure failed due to excess edema. If the patient was unable to tolerate complete compression, consider using procedural sedation. After addressing those issues, make another attempt.

6. **Consider** a dorsal slit if the procedure continues to fail despite edema-reducing measures and procedural sedation. A urologic consultation may be necessary.

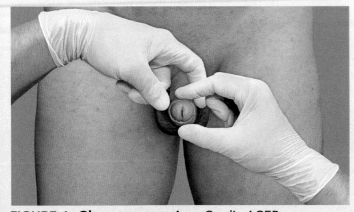

FIGURE 1. Glans compression. *Credit:* ACEP.

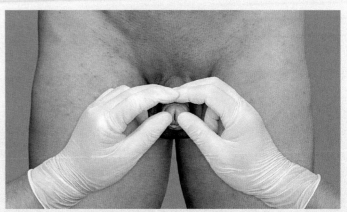

FIGURE 2. Foreskin reduction. *Credit:* ACEP.

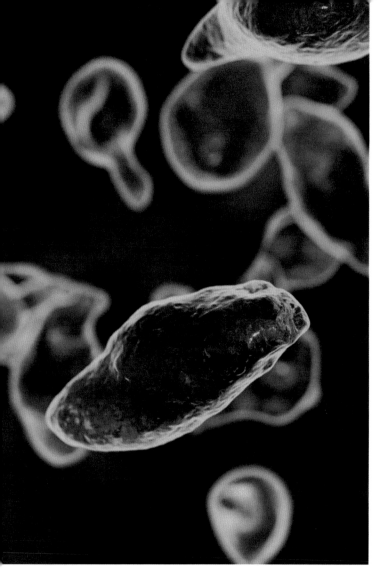

Security Breach

Presentations of Pelvic Inflammatory Disease

LESSON **20**

By Lucille Martin, MD; and Danya Khoujah, MBBS, MEHP, FACEP
Dr. Martin is an emergency medicine resident and Dr. Khoujah is a volunteer adjunct assistant professor of emergency medicine at the University of Maryland School of Medicine in Baltimore. Dr. Khoujah is also an attending physician with Tampa AdventHealth in Florida.

Reviewed by Ann M. Dietrich, MD, FAAP, FACEP

Objectives

On completion of this lesson, you should be able to:

1. Define PID and its common causes.
2. Differentiate PID from lower genital tract infections.
3. Evaluate patients with PID for TOA.
4. Treat PID and TOA, including in special populations.
5. Determine appropriate disposition and follow-up plans for patients with PID.
6. Counsel patients with PID on partner treatment, future sexual activity, and long-term complications.

From the EM Model

13.0 Obstetrics and Gynecology
    13.1 Female Genital Tract
        13.1.2 Infectious Disorders
            13.1.2.1 Pelvic Inflammatory Disease
                13.1.2.1.2 Tuboovarian Abscess

■ CRITICAL DECISIONS ■

- ■ How does PID present?

- ■ What clinical features should raise suspicion for TOA?

- ■ What laboratory testing and imaging should be obtained for patients with suspected PID?

- ■ How are PID and its complications treated?

- ■ When should patients with PID be admitted or discharged?

- ■ How should patients with PID be counseled when leaving the emergency department?

Pelvic inflammatory disease (PID) affects around 1 in 20 women during their lifetimes and, along with tubo-ovarian abscess (TOA), can lead to serious and life-altering consequences like infertility, ectopic pregnancy, peritonitis, and sepsis. Because early recognition and treatment can drastically improve patient outcomes, emergency physicians must promptly identify and appropriately manage these pelvic infections.

CASE ONE

A 20-year-old woman presents with worsening left-sided pelvic pain and subjective fevers for the past 3 days. She denies any vaginal discharge or discomfort. Her vital signs are BP 110/65, P 105, R 16, and T 38°C (100.4°F); SpO_2 is 100% on room air. She is well appearing but has a soft, tender abdomen in the left lower quadrant. During a pelvic examination, left-sided adnexal tenderness and a palpable mass are found. Because of these findings and her fever, the emergency physician suspects a gynecologic infection and inquires about the patient's sexual history. The patient insists that she has never been sexually active nor had any STIs.

CASE TWO

A 27-year-old woman who is G1P0 at 8 weeks' gestation by date of the last normal menstrual period presents with lower abdominal pain that has worsened over the past several days. She found out she was pregnant 2 weeks ago with a home pregnancy test and has not had her first obstetric appointment yet. Her gynecologic history includes chlamydia in her early 20s that was treated at the time of diagnosis. In addition to her lower abdominal pain, she has associated vaginal discharge and discomfort. Her vital signs are within normal limits; she is well appearing on examination but has moderate suprapubic tenderness. On pelvic examination, she has mucopurulent discharge, a friable cervix, cervical motion tenderness, and bilateral adnexal tenderness.

CASE THREE

A 22-year-old woman presents with worsening pelvic pain and vaginal discharge for the past several days. She was seen in the emergency department a month ago with similar symptoms and was treated for PID with a dose of intramuscular ceftriaxone and 2 weeks of doxycycline and metronidazole. She reports that her symptoms improved after treatment but returned a few days ago. She has had the same male sexual partner for the past 2 months and does not use barrier contraception. Her abdominal examination is benign, but her pelvic examination is significant for mucopurulent discharge, cervical motion tenderness, and uterine tenderness without an adnexal mass or tenderness.

Introduction

PID is a clinical syndrome characterized by inflammation of the upper genital tract, which consists of the uterus, fallopian tubes, ovaries, and pelvic peritoneum (*Figure 1*).[1] PID encompasses a range of inflammatory conditions including endometritis, salpingitis, TOAs, and pelvic peritonitis. PID most often occurs when a bacterial infection, like vaginitis or cervicitis, ascends from the lower genital tract, usually from sexual intercourse or retrograde menstruation.[2] These bacterial infections are most often caused by sexually transmitted infections (STIs) such as *Neisseria gonorrhoeae*, *Chlamydia trachomatis*, or *Mycoplasma genitalium*. Interestingly, however, 15% of PID cases are caused by respiratory or enteric organisms. The presence of bacterial vaginosis (BV) — a vaginal infection not caused by an STI but by an overgrowth of normal bacteria in the vagina — can impair the cervical barrier and allow infections to ascend and microorganisms to spread.[1] Untreated PID can become chronic if it lasts more than 30 days. The management of chronic PID, however, is not within the scope of emergency care.

PID is most common in young, sexually active women.[1] In the United States, PID accounts for approximately 30,000 emergency department visits yearly and is estimated to affect around 4% of women of reproductive age.[3,4] Because PID can be asymptomatic or cause vague, nonspecific symptoms, the condition is likely even more common than reported.[3] An estimated 15% of untreated chlamydial infections and even more gonococcal infections progress to PID. Diagnosing asymptomatic STIs and lower genital tract infections is of the utmost importance in PID prevention.[1] Notably, minors can consent to their own STI testing and treatment in all 50 states and the District of Columbia. The CDC lists the age of majority and the age of minor consent in all states on its website (cdc.gov/hiv/policies/law/states/minors.html).[5]

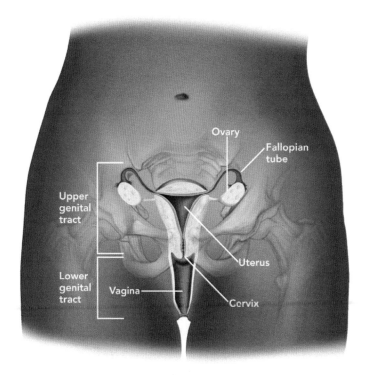

FIGURE 1. Diagram of the female reproductive system: upper versus lower genital tract. *Credit:* ACEP.

PID causes inflammatory changes along the upper genital tract, including the fallopian tubes. These changes may lead to long-term and serious complications such as ectopic pregnancy, infertility, and chronic pelvic pain in 10% to 20% of patients, even in those who have minimal or no symptoms.[4,6] Treatment delays are associated with higher complication rates, so recognition and timely treatment are critical.[7] PID can also be complicated by TOA, a pelvic abscess that can lead to serious infection, peritonitis, and sepsis.[8] Appropriate antibiotic treatment can prevent these complications. Historic data show that even when emergency department patients are diagnosed with PID, only 30% receive guideline-recommended antibiotic treatment.[9] As with STIs in general, effective infection control also includes counseling patients on getting their partners treated.[2]

CRITICAL DECISION

How does PID present?

PID should be suspected in sexually active women who present with acute pelvic pain that has no other clear etiology.[2] PID is most common in sexually active adolescents and young adults, particularly those who have a prior history of STIs.[4] Procedures such as intrauterine device (IUD) placements and surgical abortions are associated with an increased risk of PID — patients with recently placed IUDs are at an increased risk for 3 to 6 weeks after placement.[2,8,10,11] Other high-risk groups include people involved in commercial or survival sex; incarcerated individuals; and youths with substance misuse, mental health disorders, or disabilities. Patients with HIV are not at an increased risk of PID, but they are at a high risk of TOA when they have PID.[2]

Obtaining a thorough sexual history is essential for risk stratifying patients with suspected PID. Current and past sexual activities, medical treatment, and social history make up the sexual history. A basic framework for the sexual history can be remembered using the 5 Ps: partners, practice, protection, past history of STIs, and pregnancy) (*Table 1*). Assumptions about sexual orientation and practices should not be made based on patients' apparent or disclosed gender identity. The risk of STI transmission is present in women who have sex with women, both from sex with their female partners and from any male partners; up to 30% of women who have sex with women report having been with male partners within the past year.[12]

PID can be difficult to diagnose and, therefore, easily missed. Only around 40% of patients are symptomatic, and even then, the symptoms can be vague and nonspecific. No single clinical feature is sensitive or specific to the diagnosis of acute PID.[2] However, the most common presenting symptom of PID is acute-onset pelvic pain. The presence of mucopurulent cervical discharge or a known gonococcal or chlamydial infection is also highly predictive of PID.

PID must be differentiated from lower genital tract infections, namely vaginitis and cervicitis. Lower genital tract infections present similarly to PID with vaginal discomfort, mucopurulent discharge, dysuria, pruritus, and cervical friability, but they are not associated with pelvic pain or fever.[13] Cervical friability can be present by history (eg, intermenstrual or postcoital bleeding) or on physical examination; endocervical bleeding can be induced by gently passing a cotton swab through the cervical os.

Uterine, adnexal, or cervical motion tenderness are physical examination findings highly suggestive of PID; the presence of one or more of these findings should prompt the empiric diagnosis of PID in the absence of a different pelvic etiology. A classic PID finding is exquisite cervical motion

Sexual History

Partners
• Number of recent sexual partners
• Recent new sexual partners
• Genders of sexual partners

Practice
• Types of sexual activity and intercourse engaged in (and what body parts are involved)
• Involvement of substance use during sexual activity
• Sexual activity to meet needs (such as housing, money, food, or substances)

Protection
• Frequency of unprotected sexual activity
• Type of protection used

Past history of STIs
• Previous STI diagnoses (and if they were treated)
• Recency of latest STI testing and results
• Previous sexual partners diagnosed with STIs

Pregnancy
• Desire for pregnancy (and timing of desired pregnancy)
• Plan or method used to prevent pregnancy

TABLE 1. **The 5 Ps of a sexual history**[2]

tenderness — often known as the *chandelier sign* because the area is so tender that the patient reaches toward the ceiling (as if toward a chandelier) during a pelvic examination. The additional presence of fever (>38.3°C [100.9°F]) further supports the diagnosis of PID.

Laparoscopy is considered the gold standard for PID diagnosis but is, understandably, not often used, especially in patients with mild symptoms. Furthermore, laparoscopy may not detect early inflammation or endometritis and has high interobserver variability.[1,2]

An occasional complication of PID is Fitz-Hugh–Curtis syndrome, a perihepatitis caused by inflammation and adhesions in the liver capsule. This syndrome occurs in 4% to 14% of patients with PID (possibly more often in adolescents) and presents with right upper quadrant pain.[14]

PID can also occur during pregnancy, most often in the early stages of the first trimester before the cervical mucus plug and amniotic membrane can protect against ascending infection from the lower genital tract.[2,15,16] Rarely, PID can also present later in pregnancy.

Transgender and gender-nonconforming individuals are especially at risk of a missed PID diagnosis. Rates of gender-affirming genital surgery are low — many of these individuals transition socially without undergoing gender-affirming genital surgeries.[17] Physicians must not assume these surgeries have been completed. Instead, ask these patients about their previous surgeries and which organs are present so the risk of PID can be accurately assessed.[18] Transgender men (individuals assigned female at birth who identify as male) who have not had gender-affirming genital surgery (ie, a hysterectomy and oophorectomy, or bottom surgery) are still at risk of PID. Additionally, although rare,

PID has been diagnosed in transgender women (individuals assigned male at birth who identify as female) who have undergone gender-affirming genital surgery.[19]

CRITICAL DECISION

What clinical features should raise suspicion for TOA?

TOA is a serious and potentially life-threatening complication of PID. TOAs are intra-abdominal abscesses formed by the fusion of pelvic organs, most commonly the fallopian tubes and ovaries. Infections that cause TOA are often polymicrobial and contain mostly enteric or lower genital tract microbes whose invasion into the upper genital tract is commonly (but not exclusively) facilitated by STIs such as *N. gonorrhoeae*, *C. trachomatis*, or *M. genitalium*. TOA can also be caused by the spread of other intra-abdominal infections, appendicitis, inflammatory bowel disease, adnexal surgery, or malignancy.[8]

TOA should be suspected in patients with PID who present with unilateral pelvic pain, have an adnexal mass on examination, show no clinical improvement within 72 hours of appropriate antibiotics, or are ill appearing.[8] The diagnosis is not excluded by the lack of an adnexal mass because pelvic masses are frequently missed; one study reported that only 40% of masses from TOA were palpated on examination.[20,21] Patients with limited or challenging pelvic examinations may benefit from further imaging.

Patients with TOA are most likely to present with pelvic pain (>90%). Around 50% of patients with TOA have an associated fever. Approximately one-quarter of patients have nausea, a change in vaginal discharge, or vaginal bleeding. Leukocytosis is present in the blood work of around 77% of patients with TOA. A TOA diagnosis in a postmenopausal patient should raise concern for malignancy. The incidence of underlying malignancy in postmenopausal patients with TOA approaches 50% compared to a 1% incidence in premenopausal TOA patients.[8]

CRITICAL DECISION

What laboratory testing and imaging should be obtained for patients with suspected PID?

PID is a clinical diagnosis, so laboratory testing and imaging studies are not needed. However, several tests are helpful for confirming a PID diagnosis and, more importantly, for excluding other etiologies that cause similar symptoms.

Laboratory Testing

Because PID is often a complication of lower genital tract infections, testing for STIs is a prudent first step. STI testing should include testing for *C. trachomatis* and *N. gonorrhoeae* with nucleic acid amplification tests (NAATs) on vaginal or cervical samples. Self-obtained vaginal samples and first-void urine samples have become commonplace in clinical practice; they are more comfortable for patients and appear to have comparable sensitivity to endocervical swabs obtained by physicians during pelvic examinations.[22,23] However, when genital infections and PID are suspected, a pelvic examination offers important clinical information and should be conducted.

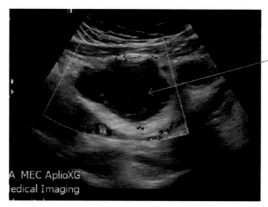

Right adnexa complex mas

FIGURE 2. Transvaginal ultrasound demonstrating a complex adnexal mass consistent with TOA.[33] *Credit: Jeh Wen Ho, Donald Angstetra, Richard Loong, and Tina Fleming (CC-BY [ncbi.nlm.nih.gov/pmc/articles/ PMC4009186/figure/fig2]).*

Testing for concomitant BV and trichomoniasis is usually done with saline microscopy of vaginal secretions (wet mount). However, microscopy has a sensitivity of only 50% for trichomoniasis so a negative wet mount should be followed by further testing with NAAT or culture testing. Testing for *M. genitalium* with NAAT (if available) should also be considered — it is present in 4% to 22% of patients with PID, and even to a higher degree in postabortal PID.[2] The presence of WBCs on the wet mount is concerning for cervicitis — they would be absent with BV alone.[1] Specifically, the presence of more than 10 WBCs/high power field is a finding sensitive for cervicitis, with a high negative predictive value. If cervical discharge appears normal and no WBCs are observed on the wet mount, a PID diagnosis is unlikely. Although testing for gonorrhea and chlamydia is important to obtain because positive results are highly associated with PID, negative results do not completely rule out PID. Patients whose results are negative for lower genital tract infections can still have PID.[2]

Pregnancy and its complications, such as ectopic pregnancy, should be ruled out through testing. A urinary tract infection as the source of symptoms should also be ruled out using a urinalysis with microscopy. Tests for

PID Findings
Fluid-filled fallopian tubes
Pelvic fat stranding with obscuration of fascial planes
Pelvic free fluid
Multicystic ovaries
Thickening of the uterosacral ligaments
Reactive lymphadenopathy
Adherence of ovary to surrounding structures on ultrasound (sliding organ sign)
Inflamed (hyperemic) fallopian tubes or ovaries on Doppler ultrasound

TABLE 2. Imaging findings suggestive of PID[1,20,25]

inflammatory markers, such as erythrocyte sedimentation rate and C-reactive protein level, and a WBC count can be helpful in confirming PID: Elevated levels increase the likelihood of PID and further differentiate PID from a lower genital tract infection.[1,2]

Imaging

Although imaging is not required to diagnose PID, it can be helpful in patients with vague clinical presentations. Imaging is necessary in patients suspected of having PID complications like TOA, or conditions that mimic PID, such as appendicitis, diverticulitis, ectopic pregnancy, or ovarian torsion. A highly specific imaging finding of PID is thickened, fluid-filled tubes, consistent with hydrosalpinx or pyosalpinx. TOA can appear as a complex, irregular adnexal mass or a tubo-ovarian complex, which is an inflammatory mass caused by fusion of pelvic structures like the ovaries and fallopian tubes (*Figure 2*).[20,24] Other imaging findings also raise suspicion for PID (*Table 2*).[25]

Imaging modalities for PID include pelvic ultrasound, CT, and MRI. Pelvic ultrasound, the first-line imaging modality, is accurate and relatively inexpensive.[20] CT and MRI are more accurate than ultrasound in diagnosing PID and TOA but are second line because they are more costly and because CT requires exposure to ionizing radiation.[8,20] However, CT or MRI may be preferred over ultrasound when there is concern for GI etiologies or malignancies.[8] A meta-analysis of the diagnostic accuracy of contrast-enhanced CT for acute PID showed a pooled sensitivity of 0.79 (95% confidence interval [CI], 0.52-0.93) and specificity of 0.99 (95% CI, 0.94-1.00).[26]

CRITICAL DECISION

How are PID and its complications treated?

Outpatient Treatment

Treatment of PID should include coverage of gonorrhea, chlamydia, and anaerobes (such as *Bacteroides fragilis*).[2] Regardless of the STI test results, the first-line treatment for uncomplicated PID is a single dose of intramuscular ceftriaxone and a 2-week course of doxycycline and metronidazole (*Table 3*). Metronidazole is a recent addition to the treatment guidelines, as is the ceftriaxone dose increase from 250 to 500 mg. Cefoxitin with concurrent probenecid or other parenteral third-generation cephalosporins can be used in place of ceftriaxone. Cross-reactivity to second- and third-

Intramuscular and Oral Antibiotic PID Treatment		
Ceftriaxone IM 500 mg once 1 g for >150 kg	Cefoxitin IM 2 g with probenecid PO 1 g once	Other third-generation parenteral cephalosporin (ceftizoxime, cefotaxime)

+

Doxycycline PO 100 mg twice daily for 14 days

+

Metronidazole 500 mg PO twice daily for 14 days

TABLE 3. **Outpatient antibiotic treatment for PID**[2]

generation cephalosporins in patients with reported penicillin allergies is negligible, so these regimens are likely appropriate for penicillin-allergic patients as well.[2,27] In the occasional patient who has a true IgE-mediated penicillin allergy or a known allergy to cephalosporins, ceftriaxone can be replaced by a single dose of gentamicin IM 240 mg. Levofloxacin can be used as an alternative to doxycycline.[2] Azithromycin is inadequate for the treatment of chlamydia because of high rates of failure.[2,28] Patients diagnosed with *M. genitalium* infections should also receive oral moxifloxacin 400 mg once daily for 14 days.

Inpatient Treatment

Some PID patients may need to be admitted for treatment with parenteral antibiotics — this includes patients who cannot tolerate oral medications, have failed treatment, are severely ill, have TOA, or are pregnant. PID patients who require intravenous antibiotics can receive ceftriaxone every 24 hours and doxycycline and metronidazole every 12 hours (*Table 4*). They can also receive intravenous cefotetan or cefoxitin every 12 hours instead of ceftriaxone. Other alternative parenteral treatments include ampicillin-sulbactam and doxycycline or clindamycin and gentamicin. The latter alternative regimen is ideal in pregnant patients because it does not contain doxycycline, which is contraindicated in the second and third trimesters. Other treatment considerations must also be made for pregnant patients with PID (*Table 5*).[2]

If PID is suspected in a patient with an IUD, the IUD can be left in place. However, if the patient does not improve after 72 hours of antibiotic therapy, the IUD should be removed.[2] These recommendations apply to hormonal and nonhormonal

Parenteral Antibiotic PID Treatment			Alternative Parenteral Treatment	
Ceftriaxone IV 1 g every 24 hr	Cefotetan IV 2 g every 12 hr	Cefoxitin IV 2 g every 6 hr	Ampicillin-sulbactam IV 3 g every 6 hr	Gentamicin 2-mg/kg loading dose, 1.5-mg/kg maintenance dose every 8 hr
+			+	+
Doxycycline PO or IV 100 mg every 12 hr			Doxycycline PO or IV 100 mg every 12 hr	Clindamycin IV 900 mg every 8 hr

+

Metronidazole PO or IV 500 mg every 12 hr

TABLE 4. **Inpatient antibiotic treatment for PID**[2]

Uncommon due to the mucus plug and amniotic membrane that protect from ascending infections

Most likely during early pregnancy

Increased risk of miscarriage, intrauterine fetal demise, preterm delivery, and neonatal death

Treatment:
- Clindamycin 900 mg every 8 hr
- Gentamicin 2-mg/kg loading dose and 1.5-mg/kg maintenance dose every 8 hr
- Doxycycline not recommended in second and third trimesters
- Admission for observation and treatment due to an associated high risk of complications

TABLE 5. **PID during pregnancy**[2,15,16]

IUDs based on extrapolations from nonhormonal IUD studies; no relevant studies are available for hormonal IUDs.

TOA

Unruptured TOAs should be treated with parenteral antibiotics until clinical improvement occurs. Ruptured TOAs, by contrast, require immediate surgical intervention.[29] The same parenteral antibiotic treatment for PID provides adequate coverage for TOA; patients can transition to an oral regimen as they improve clinically.[2,29] If patients are able to tolerate oral doxycycline and metronidazole, an oral regimen is preferred over intravenous formulations.[2] Clindamycin can also be used instead of metronidazole for anaerobic coverage.[7,27] *Escherichia coli* is among the most common organisms in TOA and can cause significant gram-negative sepsis, particularly in ruptured TOA cases.[8,30] *Actinomyces israelii* can cause TOA in patients with long-term IUDs and is usually also covered by the recommended antibiotic regimen.[8] If an unruptured TOA does not improve after parenteral treatment, surgical intervention is likely. TOAs between 4 and 6 cm require surgical intervention around 20% of the time; those larger than 10 cm require intervention more than 60% of the time. TOAs can be drained percutaneously under interventional radiologic guidance or through laparoscopy or laparotomy.[29]

Perihepatitis

PID patients with suspected perihepatitis (Fitz-Hugh–Curtis syndrome) do not typically require anything beyond the standard treatment.

CRITICAL DECISION

When should patients with PID be admitted or discharged?

For most patients, uncomplicated PID can be safely managed on an outpatient basis with oral antibiotics, but some patients should be admitted (*Table 6*). HIV status should not affect the disposition. The presence of HIV alone is not an indication for hospitalization or intravenous antibiotics. Outpatient management has been shown to be

Minimal to no improvement within 72 hours of initiating antibiotics

Pregnancy

TOA

Intractable nausea and vomiting

Inability to adhere to outpatient oral antibiotic treatment

Temperature >38.5°C (101.3°F) or ill appearing

Concern for other surgical emergencies, such as appendicitis, that cannot be ruled out

TABLE 6. **Indications for admitting patients with PID**[2]

just as effective as parenteral treatment in treating PID in patients with HIV.[2] Patients who are discharged should be given clear instructions to seek immediate medical attention if symptoms worsen or do not improve within 3 days — especially symptoms of fever, pain, and tenderness. In these cases, admission for further workup and parenteral antibiotics may be indicated.

Pregnant patients diagnosed with PID are at an increased risk of complications — including miscarriage, intrauterine fetal demise, preterm delivery, and neonatal death — and should be admitted for intravenous antibiotics and observation.[2,31] Patients with TOA should also be admitted. Patients with unruptured TOAs require treatment with intravenous antibiotics and observation for sepsis, leakage, or rupture.[7] Ruptured TOAs can lead to severe systemic infection and require immediate surgical management.[8]

CRITICAL DECISION

How should patients with PID be counseled when leaving the emergency department?

Effective treatment of PID also includes ensuring that patients' sexual partners from the past 60 days are treated to

✔ Pearls

- PID can lead to infertility, ectopic pregnancy, and chronic abdominal pain, even in patients with minimal or no symptoms.

- Treatment of uncomplicated PID should include gonococcal, chlamydial, and anaerobic coverage; the preferred regimen is ceftriaxone, doxycycline, and metronidazole.

- Partner treatment is an important part of effective STI treatment. If partners are unable to seek medical care, it is appropriate to consider offering antibiotics and educational information on STIs and prescribed medications to patients to give to their partners.

prevent reinfection. Patients should inform their partners of the need for medical evaluation and treatment. Physicians can notify a patient's sexual partners after obtaining permission from the patient. Sexual partners should be presumptively treated for chlamydia and gonorrhea, regardless of whether these pathogens were isolated in the patient.

Sometimes, partners with possible gonorrhea or chlamydia are unable or unwilling to seek medical treatment. In these cases, prescriptions and written information about the antibiotics and STIs can be given to patients to give to their partners. This practice is known as expedited partner therapy and is legal in most states. In partner therapy, physicians generally prescribe a single dose of oral cefixime 800 mg and oral doxycycline 100 mg twice daily for 7 days (or azithromycin 1 g if concerned about doxycycline adherence), recognizing that they are less effective than parenteral treatment with ceftriaxone.[32] Abstinence or consistent condom use is recommended until the antibiotic courses are completed for both partners. For single-dose regimens, precautions should be followed for 7 days. Patients can resume sexual activity once they and their partners complete their antibiotic courses and are asymptomatic.[2]

Patients must be made aware of the importance of adequate treatment for themselves and their partners to prevent persistent or worsening infection and long-term complications. Long-term complications occur in 10% to 20% of patients with PID. Their risk of infertility is 16% compared to 3% in patients without PID and 9% for ectopic pregnancy compared to 1% in patients without PID. PID patients may also develop chronic pelvic pain.[33]

Patients who test positive for any STI should be referred to the health department or primary care physician for testing for other STIs, including syphilis and HIV. Gonorrhea and chlamydia are reportable diseases in every state and can be reported by physicians, laboratories, or both. The CDC recommends retesting to detect treatment failures and reinfection for patients with chlamydia, gonorrhea, or trichomoniasis within 3 months of treatment completion for nonpregnant patients and within 4 weeks for pregnant patients. Testing before 4 weeks is not recommended because it can yield false-positive results.[2]

Summary

PID is a spectrum of inflammatory conditions of the female upper genital tract often caused by ascending infection from the lower genital tract, usually from gonorrhea and chlamydia but also numerous other microorganisms. Patients can present with a wide range of symptom severity, and even patients with minimal to no symptoms can suffer long-term consequences. Emergency physicians must be able to recognize PID in patients with pelvic pain, identify which patients need further workup for TOA, and treat them appropriately.

REFERENCES

1. Brunham RC, Gottlieb SL, Paavonen J. Pelvic inflammatory disease. *N Engl J Med.* 2015 May 21;372(21):2039-2048.

2. Workowski KA, Bachmann LH, Chan PA, et al. Sexually transmitted infections treatment guidelines, 2021. *MMWR Recomm Rep.* 2021 Jul 23;70(4):1-187.

3. Kreisel K, Flagg EW, Torrone E. Trends in pelvic inflammatory disease emergency department visits, United States, 2006-2013. *Am J Obstet and Gynecol.* 2018 Jan;218(1):117.e1-117.e10.

4. Kreisel K, Torrone E, Bernstein K, Hong J, Gorwitz R. Prevalence of pelvic inflammatory disease in sexually experienced women of reproductive age — United States, 2013–2014. *MMWR Morb Mortal Wkly Rep.* 2017 Jan 27;66(3):80-83.

5. State laws that enable a minor to provide informed consent to receive HIV and STD services. CDC. Last reviewed October 25, 2022. https://www.cdc.gov/hiv/policies/law/states/minors.html

6. Wiesenfeld HC, Sweet RL, Ness RB, Krohn MA, Amortegui AJ, Hillier SL. Comparison of acute and subclinical pelvic inflammatory disease. *Sex Transm Dis.* 2005 Jul;32(7):400-405.

7. Sweet RL. Treatment of acute pelvic inflammatory disease. *Infect Dis Obstet Gynecol.* 2011;2011:561909.

8. Chappell CA, Wiesenfeld HC. Pathogenesis, diagnosis, and management of severe pelvic inflammatory disease and tuboovarian abscess. *Clin Obstet Gynecol.* 2012 Dec;55(4):893-903.

9. Shih TY, Gaydos CA, Rothman RE, Hsieh YH. Poor provider adherence to the Centers for Disease Control and Prevention treatment guidelines in US emergency department visits with a diagnosis of pelvic inflammatory disease. *Sex Transm Dis.* 2011 Apr;38(4):299-305.

10. Savaris RF, Fuhrich DG, Maissiat J, Duarte RV, Ross J. Antibiotic therapy for pelvic inflammatory disease. *Cochrane Database of Syst Rev.* 2020 Aug 20;8(8):CD010285.

11. Russo JA, Achilles S, DePineres T, Gil L. Controversies in family planning: postabortal pelvic inflammatory disease. *Contraception.* 2013 Apr;87(4):497-503.

12. Xu F, Sternberg MR, Markowitz LE. Women who have sex with women in the United States: prevalence, sexual behavior and prevalence of herpes simplex virus type 2 infection — results from national health and nutrition examination survey 2001-2006. *Sex Transm Dis.* 2010 Jul;37(7):407-413.

13. Hainer BL, Gibson MV. Vaginitis. *Am Fam Physician.* 2011 Apr;83(7):807-815.

14. Peter NG, Clark LR, Jaeger JR. Fitz-Hugh-Curtis syndrome: a diagnosis to consider in women with right upper quadrant pain. *Cleve Clin J Med.* 2004 Mar;71(3):233-239.

15. Acquavella AP, Rubin A, D'Angelo LJ. The coincident diagnosis of pelvic inflammatory disease and pregnancy: are they compatible? *J Pediatr Adolesc Gynecol.* 1996 Aug;9(3):129-132.

✖ Pitfalls

- Assuming patients have certain sexual practices and social histories. Gather a thorough history without preconceived notions.

- Dismissing a TOA diagnosis in patients who do not appear to have an adnexal mass on physical examination.

- Excluding a PID diagnosis in patients with negative vaginal or endocervical STI results.

CASE ONE

A urine pregnancy test, vaginal swabs, and a transvaginal ultrasound were obtained to further evaluate the adnexal tenderness and mass. The patient's urine pregnancy test result was negative, and her urinalysis was normal. Her laboratory test results were significant for a leukocytosis of 14,000 WBC/mm^3 (14×10^9/L). Her transvaginal ultrasound showed hyperemia to the left adnexa, with a thickened, fluid-filled fallopian tube and a 4-cm adnexal mass that was concerning for TOA. STI results were pending, but the patient reported that she had not been sexually active.

The physician reassured the patient that although TOA is often associated with STIs like gonorrhea and chlamydia, it can also be caused by non-STI organisms such as *B. fragilis* or *Gardnerella vaginalis*. While her vaginal swab results were pending, the patient was started on antibiotics and admitted to the hospital for observation of signs of worsening infection and TOA rupture. The following day, she remained afebrile, and her pain improved. She was discharged home to follow up with her gynecologist.

CASE TWO

Because of the patient's pelvic tenderness, mucopurulent discharge, and friable cervix, PID was suspected. A pelvic ultrasound demonstrated an intrauterine pregnancy at 6 weeks' gestation and signs of adnexal adhesions concerning for PID. Because the patient was pregnant and had PID, she was admitted for intravenous antibiotics and close observation. The following day, her STI test results came back positive for chlamydia. She was treated with intravenous antibiotics and had no signs of miscarriage or other pregnancy complications during observation. She was discharged home after her inpatient stay.

CASE THREE

The patient's examination findings and history raised suspicion for PID recurrence. On further questioning, the patient revealed that she never told her partner about her PID diagnosis and that he was never evaluated or treated for STIs. The physician suspected that although the patient was appropriately treated, she was reinfected by her untreated partner. The patient was counseled on the importance of having her partner evaluated and treated for STIs and on the importance of abstaining from sexual activity until they both completed treatment and were asymptomatic. The patient was discharged home after being prescribed and starting another course of antibiotics for PID.

16. Marcinkowski KA, Mehta V, Mercier R, Berghella V. Pelvic inflammatory disease in pregnancy: a systematic review focusing on perinatal outcomes. *Am J of Obstet Gynecol MFM.* 2022 Jul;4(4):100643.

17. Weimer AK. Pelvic inflammatory disease in a male patient: the importance of understanding the transgender patient. *Proceedings of UCLA Healthcare.* 2017;21.

18. Kim H. Pelvic inflammatory disease in a male-to-female transsexual. *J Korean Soc Emerg Med.* 2015 Dec;26(6):609.

19. Reisner SL, Perkovich B, Mimiaga MJ. A mixed methods study of the sexual health needs of New England transmen who have sex with nontransgender men. *AIDS Patient Care STDS.* 2010 Aug;24(8):501-513.

20. Mynatt I. Gynecologic concepts. In: Ma OJ, Mateer JR, Reardon RF, Byars DV, Knapp BJ, Laudenbach AP, eds. *Ma and Mateer's Emergency Ultrasound.* 4th ed. McGraw-Hill; 2021:413-431.

21. Teisala K, Heinonen PK, Punnonen R. Transvaginal ultrasound in the diagnosis and treatment of tubo-ovarian abscess. *Br J Obstet and Gynaecol.* 1990 Feb;97(2):178-180.

22. Chinnock B, Yore M, Mason J, et al. Self-obtained vaginal swabs are not inferior to provider-performed endocervical sampling for emergency department diagnosis of *Neisseria gonorrhoeae* and *Chlamydia trachomatis. Acad Emerg Med.* 2021 Jun;28(6):612-620.

23. Centers for Disease Control and Prevention. Recommendations for the laboratory-based detection of *Chlamydia trachomatis* and *Neisseria gonorrhoeae* — 2014. *MMWR Recomm Rep.* 2014 Mar 14;63(RR-02):1-19.

24. Tougas DN, Brain P. 114. From IUD to PID: an uncommon cause of TOA. *J Pediatr Adolesc Gynecol.* 2023 Apr;36(2):221-222.

25. Revzin MV, Mathur M, Dave HB, Macer ML, Spektor M. Pelvic inflammatory disease: multimodality imaging approach with clinical-pathologic correlation. *Radiographics.* 2016 Sep-Oct;36(5):1579-1596.

26. Okazaki Y, Tsujimoto Y, Yamada K, et al. Diagnostic accuracy of pelvic imaging for acute pelvic inflammatory disease in an emergency care setting: a systematic review and meta-analysis. *Acute Med Surg.* 2022 Nov 9;9(1):e806.

27. Macy E, Blumenthal KG. Are cephalosporins safe for use in penicillin allergy without prior allergy evaluation? *J Allergy Clin Immunol Pract.* 2018 Jan-Feb;6(1):82-89.

28. Páez-Canro C, Alzate JP, González LM, Rubio-Romero JA, Lethaby A, Gaitán HG. Antibiotics for treating urogenital *Chlamydia trachomatis* infection in men and non-pregnant women. *Cochrane Database Syst Rev.* 2019 Jan 25;1(1):CD010871.

29. Kairys N, Roepke C. Tubo-ovarian abscess. *StatPearls [Internet].* StatPearls Publishing; 2023. Last updated June 12, 2023. https://www.ncbi.nlm.nih.gov/books/NBK448125

30. Landers DV, Sweet RL. Tubo-ovarian abscess: contemporary approach to management. *Rev Infect Dis.* 1983 Sep-Oct;5(5):876-884.

31. Guidance on the use of expedited partner therapy in the treatment of gonorrhea. CDC. Last reviewed August 18, 2021. https://www.cdc.gov/std/ept/gc-guidance.htm

32. Wiesenfeld HC, Hillier SL, Krohn MA, et al. Lower genital tract infection and endometritis: insight into subclinical pelvic inflammatory disease. *Obstet Gynecol.* 2002 Sep;100(3):456-463.

33. Ho JW, Angstetra D, Loong R, Fleming T. Tuboovarian abscess as primary presentation for imperforate hymen. *Case Rep Obstet Gynecol.* 2014;2014:142039.

CME Questions

Reviewed by Frank LoVecchio, DO, MPH, FACEP; and Ann M. Dietrich, MD, FAAP, FACEP

Qualified, paid subscribers to *Critical Decisions in Emergency Medicine* may receive CME certificates for up to 5 ACEP Category I credits, 5 *AMA PRA Category 1 Credits*™, and 5 AOA Category 2-B credits for completing this activity in its entirety. Submit your answers online at acep.org/cdem; a score of 75% or better is required. You may receive credit for completing the CME activity any time within 3 years of its publication date. Answers to this month's questions will be published in next month's issue.

1 **Below which CD4 lymphocyte count does the risk of opportunistic infections notably increase?**
   - A.   50 cells/μL
   - B.   200 cells/μL
   - C.   300 cells/μL
   - D.   500 cells/μL

2 **Which opportunistic infections are most common in the United States?**
   - A.   Candidiasis, *Cryptococcus*, and *Mycobacterium avium* complex
   - B.   Candidiasis, *M. avium* complex, and *Pneumocystis jirovecii* pneumonia
   - C.   *Cryptococcus*, *P. jirovecii* pneumonia, and tuberculosis
   - D.   *P. jirovecii* pneumonia, toxoplasmosis, and tuberculosis

3 **A man is seen in the emergency department for a cough and fever. He is taking highly active antiretroviral therapy and trimethoprim-sulfamethoxazole prophylaxis. Which pathogens could the trimethoprim-sulfamethoxazole be providing prophylaxis against, and what does this regimen suggest about his CD4 lymphocyte count?**
   - A.   *Cryptococcus*; CD4 lymphocyte count less than 100 cells/μL
   - B.   *Mycobacterium avium* complex; CD4 lymphocyte count less than 50 cells/μL
   - C.   *Pneumocystis jirovecii* and *Toxoplasma gondii*; CD4 lymphocyte count between 50 and 200 cells/μL
   - D.   *P. jirovecii*; CD4 lymphocyte count less than 200 cells/μL

4 **Below what total lymphocyte count should the concern for opportunistic infections be elevated?**
   - A.   1,000 cells/μL
   - B.   1,500 cells/μL
   - C.   1,750 cells/μL
   - D.   2,000 cells/μL

5 **Which elevated laboratory marker can suggest *Pneumocystis jirovecii* pneumonia in patients with HIV, and what is the positivity threshold?**
   - A.   β-d-glucan; 80 pg/mL
   - B.   β-d-glucan; 150 pg/mL
   - C.   Lactate dehydrogenase; 300 units/L
   - D.   Lactate dehydrogenase; 400 units/L

6 **Which adjunctive therapy has been shown to decrease mortality in patients with moderate to severe *Pneumocystis jirovecii* pneumonia?**
   - A.   Antifungal therapy
   - B.   Corticosteroids
   - C.   Trimethoprim-sulfamethoxazole
   - D.   Vitamin C

7 **Which diagnostic study is recommended if a lumbar puncture cannot be performed when there is concern for cryptococcal meningitis?**
   - A.   β-d-glucan
   - B.   Blood India ink stain
   - C.   Fungal blood culture
   - D.   Serum cryptococcal antigen

8 **In the setting of cryptococcal meningitis with elevated CSF pressure, therapeutic lumbar drainage should reduce CSF pressure by how much?**
   - A.   10%
   - B.   25%
   - C.   40%
   - D.   50%

9 **A woman presents with cough, fever, and shortness of breath. Her examination is notable for findings consistent with oropharyngeal candidiasis. Her chest x-ray shows interstitial infiltrates. The odds ratio for which pulmonary infection is increased by the presence of oropharyngeal candidiasis and interstitial infiltrates?**
   - A.   Endemic fungi
   - B.   *Pneumocystis jirovecii* pneumonia
   - C.   *Pseudomonas aeruginosa*
   - D.   Tuberculosis

10 **How are oropharyngeal and esophageal candidiasis typically diagnosed?**
   - A.   Clinically based on symptoms and examination findings
   - B.   Through a culture
   - C.   Via microscopic evaluation of oropharyngeal or esophageal lesions with potassium hydroxide
   - D.   Via upper endoscopy

11 **In a well-appearing and otherwise healthy patient diagnosed with a genital tract infection, which pelvic examination findings most strongly indicate the need for further imaging to rule out tubo-ovarian abscess?**
   - A.   Bilateral adnexal tenderness without a palpated mass
   - B.   Friable cervix with cervical motion tenderness and uterine tenderness
   - C.   Mucopurulent discharge with cervical motion tenderness
   - D.   Unilateral adnexal tenderness without a palpated mass

12 **What is the appropriate antibiotic treatment regimen for pelvic inflammatory disease?**

A. 250 mg of ceftriaxone IM and 1 g of azithromycin PO once

B. 250 mg of ceftriaxone IM once; 100 mg of doxycycline PO and 500 mg of metronidazole PO twice a day for 2 weeks

C. 500 mg of ceftriaxone IM and 100 mg of doxycycline PO twice a day for 2 weeks

D. 500 mg of ceftriaxone IM once; 100 mg of doxycycline PO and 500 mg of metronidazole PO twice a day for 2 weeks

13 **A 31-year-old woman presents with pelvic pain, dyspareunia, and increased vaginal discharge. She has a new sexual partner and does not use barrier protection. On pelvic examination, she has mucopurulent discharge and left adnexal fullness and tenderness. Her urine pregnancy test result is negative. What is the best first-line imaging test for this patient?**

A. CT of the pelvis with intravenous contrast

B. MRI of the pelvis

C. No imaging

D. Pelvic ultrasound

14 **A healthy 24-year-old woman presents with pelvic pain. Her last normal menstrual cycle was 5 weeks ago, and her urine pregnancy test result is positive. On examination, she has mucopurulent discharge, cervical motion, and bilateral adnexal tenderness. Transvaginal ultrasound shows an intrauterine pregnancy and inflammatory changes suggestive of pelvic inflammatory disease. How should this patient's condition be managed?**

A. Give azithromycin, ceftriaxone, and a 2-week course of metronidazole; recommend a follow-up appointment with obstetrics and gynecology in the next 3 days

B. Recommend pregnancy termination because of a high risk of maternal and fetal complications

C. Start ceftriaxone, doxycycline, and metronidazole; admit for antibiotics and observation

D. Start clindamycin and gentamicin and admit for antibiotics and observation

15 **Which patient with pelvic inflammatory disease can safely be discharged home?**

A. An otherwise healthy patient with a fever of 39°C (102.2°F), nausea, and vomiting

B. A patient diagnosed with pelvic inflammatory disease 3 days ago who returned for persistent pelvic pain

C. A well-appearing patient with HIV

D. A well-appearing patient with normal vital signs who was diagnosed with a 6-cm tubo-ovarian abscess

16 **What is an appropriate treatment regimen for a patient with pelvic inflammatory disease and a known anaphylactic allergy to penicillin?**

A. Admission for clindamycin and gentamicin administration

B. Outpatient treatment with ceftriaxone, doxycycline, and metronidazole

C. Outpatient treatment with a single dose of gentamicin followed by 2 weeks of doxycycline and metronidazole

D. Testing for gonorrhea and, if negative, treatment with doxycycline and metronidazole

17 **An otherwise healthy 20-year-old woman presents with right-sided pelvic pain for the past few days. She has a 5-cm complex fluid collection that is concerning for tubo-ovarian abscess. She has normal vital signs and is well appearing. What is the most appropriate management for this patient?**

A. Emergency surgery

B. Inpatient observation and intravenous antibiotics

C. Outpatient antibiotic treatment and close obstetrics and gynecology follow-up for repeat imaging in 48 to 72 hours

D. Percutaneous drainage with interventional radiology immediately after admission

18 **After being diagnosed with pelvic inflammatory disease, when can patients resume sexual activity without barrier protection?**

A. After the patient and their partner(s) have been asymptomatic for 48 hours

B. After the patient has negative repeat endocervical testing by their physician

C. Once the patient and their partner(s) have completed antibiotic treatment and are asymptomatic

D. Once the patient has been treated for at least 72 hours and their symptoms are improving

19 **A 59-year-old woman presents with right lower abdominal pain for the past several days. She has right lower quadrant tenderness without any nausea, vomiting, or diarrhea. Laboratory studies demonstrate leukocytosis. Further imaging is obtained and shows a possible tubo-ovarian abscess. Which condition should the physician be most concerned about in this patient?**

A. Concurrent urinary tract infection

B. GI tract infection

C. Malignancy

D. Ovarian torsion

20 **Which patient is most at risk of pelvic inflammatory disease?**

A. A patient who had an intrauterine device placed 3 months ago

B. A patient who had a surgical abortion in the past month

C. A patient who is 6 months pregnant

D. A patient with HIV who adheres to her antiretroviral therapy

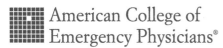
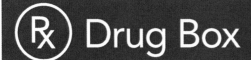

Drug Box

MgSO₄ IV in Severe COPD Exacerbation

Frank LoVecchio, DO, MPH, FACEP
Valleywise Health Medical Center and ASU, Phoenix, Arizona

Objective
On completion of this column, you should be able to:
■ Discuss the use of MgSO₄ IV in patients with severe COPD exacerbation.

The utilization of magnesium sulfate (MgSO₄) IV as an adjunct in severe chronic obstructive pulmonary disease (COPD) exacerbation remains controversial. In general, it has short-acting bronchodilator activity that is helpful for severe asthma attacks but was not previously recommended for COPD. Intravenous MgSO₄ has bronchodilator activity thought to arise from the inhibition of calcium influx into smooth muscle cells of the airway. A new systematic review and meta-analysis reported a decrease in hospitalization rates with emergency department utilization of MgSO₄ compared with a placebo (2C recommendation).[1]

For patients who presented with a severe COPD exacerbation that did not promptly respond to short-acting inhaled bronchodilators, an infusion of 2 g over 20 minutes of either MgSO₄ or a placebo was administered. The study found that MgSO₄ reduced hospital admissions compared with placebo (odds ratio [OR] 0.75; 95% confidence interval [CI], 0.60-0.92; I^2 = 28%, P = 0.18; n = 972; high-quality evidence). This translates to a reduction of 7 hospital admissions for every 100 adults treated with MgSO₄ (95% CI, 2-13 fewer). MgSO₄ may reduce the length of a hospital stay by a mean difference of 2.7 days (95% CI, 4.73-0.66 days) and improve dyspnea scores by a standardized mean difference of –1.40 (95% CI, –1.83 to –0.96).

The effect size of avoiding hospital admission, length of stay, and dyspnea scores is comparable to or better than that seen in the setting of acute asthma exacerbations.

In summary, assuming no contraindications, IV MgSO₄ should be encouraged for patients with severe COPD exacerbations that fail to improve with inhaled bronchodilator therapy.

The authors were unable to draw conclusions about the effects of nebulized MgSO₄ in COPD exacerbations for most of the outcomes.

Caution or Relative Contraindications
Intravenous MgSO₄ has an excellent safety profile. However, it is contraindicated in the presence of renal insufficiency, and hypermagnesemia can result in muscle weakness.

Adverse Events
Adverse events were uncommon. The most cited adverse events in the MgSO₄ groups were flushing, fatigue, nausea and headache, and hypotension.

Dosage
2 g infused over 20 min

REFERENCE
1. Ni H, Aye SZ, Naing C. Magnesium sulfate for acute exacerbations of chronic obstructive pulmonary disease. *Cochrane Database Syst Rev.* 2022 May 26;5(5):CD013506.

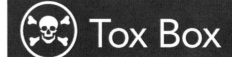

Tox Box

Acute Styrene Poisoning

By Christian A. Tomaszewski, MD, MS, MBA, FACEP
University of California San Diego Health

Objective
On completion of this column, you should be able to:
■ Describe the characteristics of acute styrene poisoning.

Introduction
Styrene monomer is a colorless, volatile, oily liquid with a sweet odor. The monomer is widely used for producing plastics, rubbers, and resins (eg, polystyrene). Exposure can occur at chemical worksites or from rail transportation accidents. Acute exposures are usually dermal or inhaled ("styrene sickness").

Mechanism of Action
■ Direct irritation and defatting of skin
■ Metabolite styrene oxide can cause hepatic damage

Kinetics
■ Hepatic metabolism to styrene epoxide
■ Half-life: 8 to 9 hr in blood, but up to days in adipose tissue

Range of Toxicity
■ 8-hr exposure limit (total weight average) is 100 ppm.
■ Neurologic symptoms start at ~300 ppm.
■ Danger to life starts at 2,500 ppm.

Clinical Manifestations
(usually in massive ingestions)
■ *Eyes and mucous membranes:* irritant
■ *GI:* nausea and vomiting
■ *Dermal:* skin irritation and erythema
■ *Pulmonary:* edema and bronchospasm
■ *Neurologic:* headache, ataxia, CNS depression, and peripheral neuropathy

Diagnostics
■ Comprehensive metabolic panel can be helpful in symptomatic cases.
■ Chest x-ray for pulmonary symptoms

Treatment
■ **Decontaminate**
  ● Remove contaminated clothing.
  ● Wash skin with soap and water.
■ Administer activated charcoal, if ingested.
■ Respiratory support with oxygen and β-agonists, as needed

Critical decisions
in emergency medicine

Volume 37 Number 11: **November 2023**

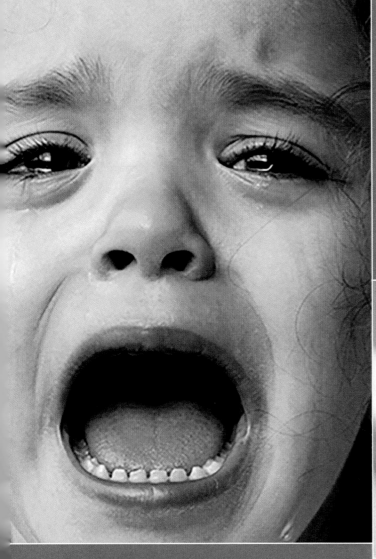

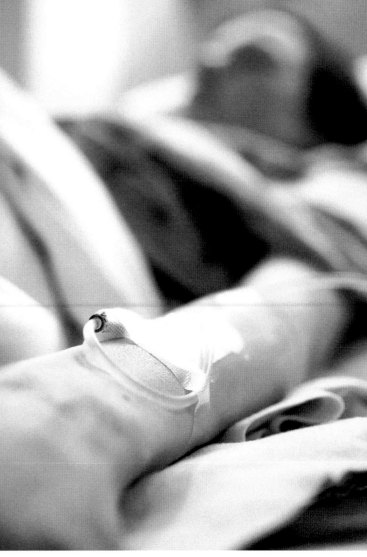

Brainstorm

Most pediatric head injuries seen in the emergency department are considered mild. Knowing how to classify head injury severity and when to order imaging in this patient population can be difficult, but it is important because certain tests carry with them the risks of radiation exposure. Emergency physicians must know the history and physical examination findings and decision-making rules that help identify which children with head injuries will benefit from imaging.

Stronger Than Ever

Frighteningly, some bacterial infections have become difficult or even impossible to treat with available antibiotics because the causative organisms have become resistant to historically effective therapies. To protect current and future patients from these so-called *superbugs*, emergency physicians must not only understand the current treatment options for antibiotic-resistant bacteria but also combat further resistance through judicious antibiotic stewardship.

Individuals in Control of Content

1. Jeremy Berberian, MD – Faculty
2. William J. Brady, MD, FACEP – Faculty
3. Matthew Carvey, MD – Faculty
4. Wade DeAustin, MD – Faculty
5. Jonathan Glauser, MD, FACEP, MBA – Faculty
6. Hunter Hoopes, DO – Faculty
7. Adeola A. Kosoko, MD, FACEP, FAAP – Faculty
8. Nicholas G. Maldonado, MD, FACEP – Faculty
9. Calliope Murphy, MD – Faculty
10. Megan J. Rivera, MD – Faculty
11. Stephen Sandelich, MD – Faculty
12. Mary Spring, DO – Faculty
13. Joshua S. Broder, MD, FACEP – Faculty/Planner
14. Ann M. Dietrich, MD, FACEP, FAAP – Faculty/Planner
15. Andrew J. Eyre, MD, MS-HPEd – Faculty/Planner
16. John C. Greenwood, MD, MS – Faculty/Planner
17. John Kiel, DO, MPH, FACEP, CAQSM – Faculty/Planner
18. Frank LoVecchio, DO, MPH, FACEP – Faculty/Planner
19. Amal Mattu, MD, FACEP – Faculty/Planner
20. Christian A. Tomaszewski, MD, MS, MBA, FACEP – Faculty/Planner
21. Steven J. Warrington, MD, MEd, MS – Faculty/Planner
22. Tareq Al-Salamah, MBBS, MPH, FACEP – Planner
23. Wan-Tsu Chang, MD – Planner
24. Kelsey Drake, MD, MPH, FACEP – Planner
25. Walter L. Green, MD, FACEP – Planner
26. Danya Khoujah, MBBS, MEHP, FACEP – Planner
27. Sharon E. Mace, MD, FACEP –Planner
28. Nathaniel Mann, MD – Planner
29. George Sternbach, MD, FACEP – Planner
30. Joy Carrico, JD – Planner/Reviewer

Contributor Disclosures. In accordance with the ACCME Standards for Integrity and Independence in Accredited Continuing Education, all relevant financial relationships, and the absence of relevant financial relationships, must be disclosed to learners for all individuals in control of content 1) before learners engage with the accredited education, and 2) in a format that can be verified at the time of accreditation. The following individuals have reported relationships with ineligible companies, as defined by the ACCME. These relationships, in the context of their involvement in the CME activity, could be perceived by some as a real or apparent conflict of interest. All relevant financial relationships have been mitigated to ensure that no commercial bias has been inserted into the educational content. William J. Brady, MD, FACEP holds an ownership interest in Medical Decisions. Joshua S. Broder, MD, FACEP, is a founder and president of OmniSono Inc, an ultrasound technology company, and a consultant on the Bayer USA Cardiac Imaging Advisory Board. Frank LoVecchio, DO, MPH, FACEP, receives speaking fees from ABBVIE for antibiotics. Sharon E. Mace, MD, FACEP, performs contracted research funded by Biofire Corporation, Genetesis, Quidel, and IBSA Pharma. Christian A. Tomaszewski, MD, MS, MBA, FACEP, performs contracted research for Roche, Pfizer, and AstraZeneca (site PI with financial support provided to institution). Andrew J. Eyre, MD, MS-HPEd is on the advisory board for MedVR Education. All remaining individuals with control over content have no relevant financial relationships to disclose.

This educational activity consists of two lessons, eight feature articles, a post-test, and evaluation questions; as designed, the activity should take approximately 5 hours to complete. The participant should, in order, review the learning objectives for the lesson or article, read the lesson or article as published in the print or online version until all have been reviewed, and then complete the online post-test (a minimum score of 75% is required) and evaluation questions. Release date: November 1, 2023. Expiration date: October 31, 2026.

Accreditation Statement. The American College of Emergency Physicians is accredited by the Accreditation Council for Continuing Medical Education to provide continuing medical education for physicians.

The American College of Emergency Physicians designates this enduring material for a maximum of 5 *AMA PRA Category 1 Credits*™. Physicians should claim only the credit commensurate with the extent of their participation in the activity.

Each issue of *Critical Decisions in Emergency Medicine* is approved by ACEP for 5 ACEP Category I credits. Approved by the AOA for 5 Category 2-B credits.

Commercial Support. There was no commercial support for this CME activity.

Target Audience. This educational activity has been developed for emergency physicians.

Critical Decisions in Emergency Medicine is a trademark owned and published monthly by the American College of Emergency Physicians, PO Box 619911, Dallas, TX 75261-9911. Send address changes and comments to Critical Decisions in Emergency Medicine, PO Box 619911, Dallas, TX 75261-9911, or to cdem@acep.org; call or text 888-817-2237.

The American College of Emergency Physicians (ACEP) makes every effort to ensure that contributors to its publications are knowledgeable subject matter experts. Readers are nevertheless advised that the statements and opinions expressed in this publication are provided as the contributors' recommendations at the time of publication and should not be construed as official College policy. ACEP recognizes the complexity of emergency medicine and makes no representation that this publication serves as an authoritative resource for the prevention, diagnosis, treatment, or intervention for any medical condition, nor should it be the basis for the definition of or standard of care that should be practiced by all health care providers at any particular time or place. Drugs are generally referred to by generic names. In some instances, brand names are added for easier recognition. Device manufacturer information is provided according to style conventions of the American Medical Association. ACEP received no commercial support for this publication.

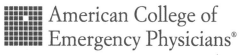

American College of Emergency Physicians®

ADVANCING EMERGENCY CARE

To the fullest extent permitted by law, and without limitation, ACEP expressly disclaims all liability for errors or omissions contained within this publication, and for damages of any kind or nature, arising out of use, reference to, reliance on, or performance of such information.

Critical decisions
in emergency medicine

Critical Decisions in Emergency Medicine is the official CME publication of the American College of Emergency Physicians. Additional volumes are available.

EDITOR-IN-CHIEF
Danya Khoujah, MBBS, MEHP, FACEP
University of Maryland, Baltimore, MD

SECTION EDITORS
Joshua S. Broder, MD, FACEP
Duke University, Durham, NC

Andrew J. Eyre, MD, MS-HPEd
Brigham and Women's Hospital/
Harvard Medical School, Boston, MA

John Kiel, DO, MPH, FACEP, CAQSM
University of South Florida Morsani College of Medicine, Tampa, FL

Frank LoVecchio, DO, MPH, FACEP
Valleywise, Arizona State University, University of Arizona, and Creighton University School of Medicine, Phoenix, AZ

Sharon E. Mace, MD, FACEP
Cleveland Clinic Lerner College of Medicine/
Case Western Reserve University, Cleveland, OH

Amal Mattu, MD, FACEP
University of Maryland, Baltimore, MD

Christian A. Tomaszewski, MD, MS, MBA, FACEP
University of California Health Sciences, San Diego, CA

Steven J. Warrington, MD, MEd, MS
MercyOne Siouxland, Sioux City, IA

ASSOCIATE EDITORS
Tareq Al-Salamah, MBBS, MPH, FACEP
King Saud University, Riyadh, Saudi Arabia/
University of Maryland, Baltimore, MD

Wan-Tsu Chang, MD
University of Maryland, Baltimore, MD

Ann M. Dietrich, MD, FAAP, FACEP
University of South Carolina School of Medicine, Greenville, SC

Kelsey Drake, MD, MPH, FACEP
St. Anthony Hospital, Lakewood, CO

Walter L. Green, MD, FACEP
UT Southwestern Medical Center, Dallas, TX

John C. Greenwood, MD
University of Pennsylvania, Philadelphia, PA

Nathaniel Mann, MD
University of South Carolina School of Medicine, Greenville, SC

George Sternbach, MD, FACEP
Stanford University Medical Center, Stanford, CA

EDITORIAL STAFF
Joy Carrico, JD, Managing Editor
jcarrico@acep.org

Alex Bass
Assistant Editor

Kel Morris
Assistant Editor

ISSN2325-0186 (Print)   ISSN2325-8365 (Online)

Contents

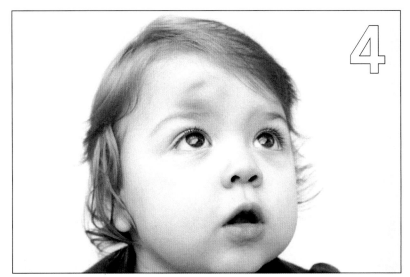

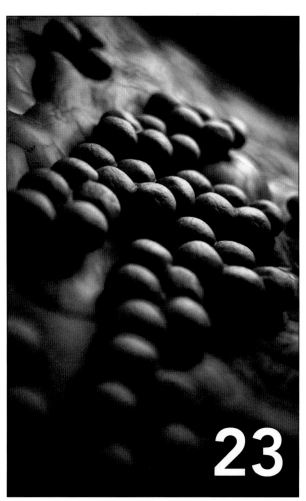

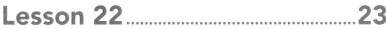

FEATURES

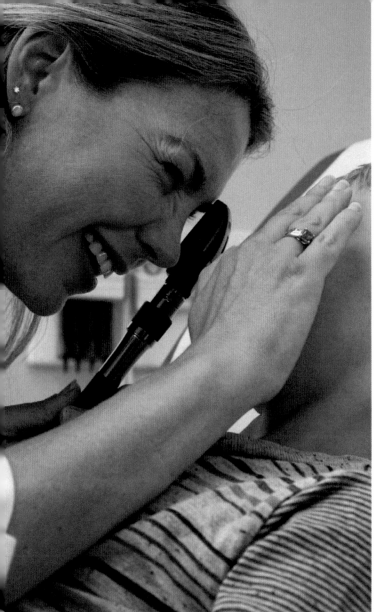

Brainstorm

Pediatric Head Injuries

LESSON **21**

By Adeola A. Kosoko, MD, FACEP, FAAP;
Calliope Murphy, MD; and Mary Spring, DO
Dr. Kosoko is an emergency physician and pediatric emergency
physician, and Dr. Murphy and Dr. Spring are residents in
emergency medicine at McGovern Medical School, University of
Texas Health Sciences Center at Houston.

Reviewed by Ann M. Dietrich, MD, FACEP, FAAP

Objectives

On completion of this lesson, you should be able to:

1. Identify and categorize pediatric head trauma.

2. Describe appropriate emergency medical evaluations for children with head injuries.

3. Diagnose and manage pediatric concussions.

4. Determine the appropriate disposition for children with TBIs.

From the EM Model

18.0 Traumatic Disorders
    18.1 Trauma
        18.1.6 Head Trauma
            18.1.6.1 Intracranial Injury

▬ CRITICAL DECISIONS ▬

- How are pediatric TBIs classified?

- What history and physical examination features indicate the need for imaging in children with head injuries?

- What pediatric head injury decision tools can suggest the need for advanced imaging?

- What are concussions, and how are they diagnosed?

- What are the criteria for a safe discharge home after an mTBI?

- What are appropriate discharge care instructions for pediatric patients with mTBIs?

Most pediatric head injuries seen in the emergency department are considered mild. Knowing how to classify head injury severity and when to order imaging in this patient population can be difficult but is important because certain tests carry the risks of radiation exposure. Emergency physicians must know the history and physical examination findings and decision-making rules that help identify which children with head injuries will benefit from imaging.

■ CASE ONE

A 2-month-old boy is brought in by his mother and grandmother after he fell from his mother's arms. The mother reports that she dropped the child after she fell asleep while breastfeeding him. The boy cried immediately after he fell onto the wooden floor. On arrival, the baby is well appearing. His examination reveals a small, soft area on his right parietal region; when palpated, he cries. Swaddling appears to calm him, and he has been eating well.

■ CASE TWO

A 14-year-old girl presents after another dancer at dance practice accidentally kicked the front of her head. She arrives on a backboard and wearing a cervical collar. When asked if she lost consciousness from the event, the girl is unsure. Onlookers report that the girl fell to the ground after being kicked and then started crying. She complains of a mild headache and states that she feels a little nauseated and confused about the events that transpired.

■ CASE THREE

A 12-year-old boy presents by ambulance after an all-terrain vehicle (ATV) accident. The boy was tossed from his ATV after it flipped on its side. He was not wearing a helmet. The boy is brought in on a backboard and is wearing a cervical collar. He has multiple abrasions to his face and body. Soon after being transferred to a bed, he becomes unresponsive.

Introduction

When children hit their heads, they are usually brought to the emergency department by their loved ones or caretakers who are seeking guidance. Emergency physicians have the important job of determining the severity of traumatic brain injuries (TBIs) and appropriately evaluating patients without overusing imaging that would expose pediatric patients to unnecessary radiation. Fortunately, most head injuries seen in the emergency department are minor and allow for recovery with minimal consequences. In these cases, emergency physicians have the responsibility of instructing pediatric patients and their caregivers on how to manage these head injuries to ensure the best possible outcome.

CRITICAL DECISION

How are pediatric TBIs classified?

Accurate classification of pediatric TBIs is important because it affects management and patient outcomes. Head injuries can be classified by severity as mild, moderate, or severe. Moderate and severe TBIs are frequently grouped together as clinically important TBIs (ciTBIs). Mild, or minor, TBIs (mTBIs) are the most common and, with appropriate symptomatology, may meet the criteria for a concussion. On the Glasgow Coma Scale (GCS), an mTBI includes scores 13 to 15, a moderate TBI includes scores 9 to 12, and a severe TBI includes scores 8 and lower (*Table 1*).[1] Furthermore, mTBIs are often uncomplicated, without any overt CT findings, while moderate and severe TBIs usually have associated abnormalities on imaging.

Clinically significant outcomes (eg, prolonged hospitalization, intubation, neurosurgical intervention, or death) are rarely associated with mTBIs. However, even when children have low-risk features for a significant head injury, emergency physicians must complete a thorough history and physical examination to identify the risk of poor outcomes.

CRITICAL DECISION

What history and physical examination features indicate the need for imaging in children with head injuries?

History

When gathering a patient's history, physicians should obtain collateral information from EMS, the patient's family, or bystanders whenever possible. In children younger than 2 years, keep in mind the developmental stages and the possibility of abuse. Physicians should also keep in mind that older children with TBIs may be under the influence of alcohol or drugs, which will affect assessment results and make them unreliable historians.

Behavior	Response	Score
Eye opening response	Opens spontaneously	+4
	Opens to verbal stimuli	+3
	Opens to pain only	+2
	No response	+1
Verbal response	Oriented	+5
	Confused	+4
	Inappropriate words	+3
	Incomprehensible sounds	+2
	No response	+1
Motor response	Obeys commands	+6
	Localizes to pain	+5
	Withdraws to pain	+4
	Abnormal flexion posturing	+3
	Abnormal extensor posturing	+2
	No response	+1

13-15 point = minor brain injury
9-12 points = moderate brain injury
3-8 points = severe brain injury

TABLE 1. GCS for adults and older children

Symptoms that suggest intracranial injury include a severe headache, vision changes, confusion (or irritability in a preverbal child), and mood disturbances. TBIs should be more readily suspected in children with a severe mechanism of injury, such as a motor vehicle collision that involved a vehicle rollover, the patient's ejection from the vehicle, or death of another passenger in the vehicle; a fall of more than 5 feet; a head strike by a high-impact object, or a bicycle accident without a helmet.

An isolated episode of vomiting without other high-risk symptoms is rarely associated with ciTBI. However, persistent episodes of vomiting can highly suggest ciTBIs in children. According to the CATCH2 study, four or more episodes of vomiting increase the symptom's sensitivity for TBI to 99.5%.[2]

Physical Examination

Any pediatric patient who presents with suspected head trauma should undergo a systematic physical examination to avoid missing any injuries. During the initial evaluation, a patient's general appearance, signs of trauma, and GCS score should be noted. The method to determine the GCS score for a pediatric patient is slightly different from that for adults. Specifically, the verbal response score depends on the child's age (*Table 2*).[1] GCS scores less than or equal to 14 are concerning for ciTBIs and may indicate that imaging is appropriate.

Physical examination findings that suggest underlying skull fractures can be signs of a severe TBI. Signs of a basilar skull fracture include CSF rhinorrhea or otorrhea, hemotympanum, periorbital ecchymosis (raccoon eyes),

and postauricular ecchymosis (Battle sign) (*Figure 1*). A boggy, nonfrontal hematoma greater than 2 cm suggests a skull fracture and an associated intracranial injury. Any depressions, step-offs, or crepitus at the scalp are also concerning for skull fractures. Additionally, a full fontanel or papilledema suggests increased intracranial pressure and a ciTBI. Outside of the head examination, any focal weakness, neurologic deficit, or bruit on auscultation of the carotid arteries are potential TBI red flags.

CRITICAL DECISION

What pediatric head injury decision tools can suggest the need for advanced imaging?

Excessive radiation exposure can be detrimental to children over time. However, head CT is the test of choice to evaluate for ciTBI in the emergency department. Pediatric head injury decision tools help determine when the benefits of CT for identifying TBIs outweigh the risks posed by radiation exposure. The Pediatric Emergency Care Applied Research Network (PECARN) pediatric head injury prediction rule, the Canadian assessment of tomography for childhood head injury (CATCH) rule, and the children's head injury algorithm for the prediction of important clinical events (CHALICE) rule are the most popular decision-making rules for determining which children with head injuries are likely to benefit from a CT scan. These three decision rules differ by the

Behavior	Response <2 Years Old	Response ≥2 Years Old	Score
Eye opening	Opens spontaneously	Opens spontaneously	+4
	Opens to verbal stimuli	Opens to verbal stimuli	+3
	Opens to pain only	Opens to pain only	+2
	No response	No response	+1
Verbal response	Coos, babbles	Oriented	+5
	Cries irritably	Confused	+4
	Cries in response to pain	Inappropriate words	+3
	Moans in response to pain	Incomprehensible sounds	+2
	No response	No response	+1
Motor response	Moves spontaneously	Obeys commands	+6
	Withdraws to touch	Localizes to pain	+5
	Withdraws to pain	Withdraws to pain	+4
	Flexor posturing to pain	Flexor posturing to pain	+3
	Extensor posturing to pain	Extensor posturing to pain	+2
	No response	No response	+1

TABLE 2. GCS for young children

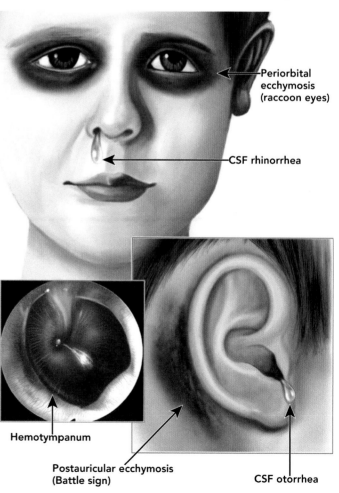

FIGURE 1. **Signs of a skull fracture.** *Credit: ACEP.*

Periorbital ecchymosis (raccoon eyes)

CSF rhinorrhea

Hemotympanum

Postauricular ecchymosis (Battle sign)

CSF otorrhea

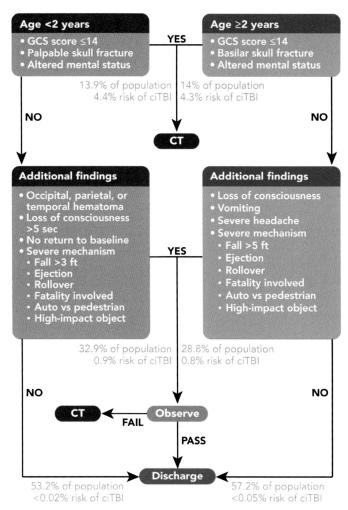

Age <2 years	Age ≥2 years
• GCS score ≤14	• GCS score ≤14
• Palpable skull fracture	• Basilar skull fracture
• Altered mental status	• Altered mental status

YES

13.9% of population 14% of population
4.4% risk of ciTBI 4.3% risk of ciTBI

NO → **CT** ← **NO**

Additional findings	Additional findings
• Occipital, parietal, or temporal hematoma	• Loss of consciousness
• Loss of consciousness >5 sec	• Vomiting
• No return to baseline	• Severe headache
• Severe mechanism	• Severe mechanism
▪ Fall >3 ft	▪ Fall >5 ft
▪ Ejection	▪ Ejection
▪ Rollover	▪ Rollover
▪ Fatality involved	▪ Fatality involved
▪ Auto vs pedestrian	▪ Auto vs pedestrian
▪ High-impact object	▪ High-impact object

YES

32.9% of population 28.8% of population
0.9% risk of ciTBI 0.8% risk of ciTBI

NO **NO**

CT ← **FAIL** ← **Observe**

PASS

Discharge

53.2% of population 57.2% of population
<0.02% risk of ciTBI <0.05% risk of ciTBI

FIGURE 2. PECARN pediatric head trauma algorithm.[3] *Credit: ACEP.*

questions asked, targeted age groups and injury severity, and presentation of results.[3] One prospective cohort study compared the three decision rules in children at a tertiary emergency department and found that the PECARN rule is the only decision rule to correctly identify all ciTBIs, making it likely the most sensitive decision rule for determining which children should undergo a CT scan, which should be observed, and which should be discharged home (*Figure 2*).[4] In 2021 PECARN published a study on the risk of TBIs in children younger than 3 months old who had sustained minor blunt head trauma. The authors concluded that although the PECARN criteria identified infants younger than 3 months old at low risk of ciTBI, there were infants at low risk whose CT scan indicated a TBI, suggesting the need for caution in this age group.[5]

CRITICAL DECISION

What are concussions, and how are they diagnosed?

Concussions are diagnosed clinically based on the history and physical examination. The diagnosis can be difficult to make because symptoms can be vague and elusive — it is possible that some symptoms will develop only after the initial evaluation. The history of patients with concussions suggests a physiologic disruption to the brain from a traumatic event such as a direct blow to the head, neck,

or face. Forces from a blow can damage axons and open electrolyte channels in the brain, leading to symptoms of headaches, confusion or disorientation, altered mental status, amnesia (for memories before or after the event), loss of balance, or changes in vision. Headaches are the most common symptom. Occasionally loss of consciousness occurs but only in about 10% of concussions. In preverbal children, concussions are more likely to present with intractable fussiness or somnolence.

Random accidental injuries can cause concussions in children of any age. However, concussions in older children are most often caused by sports. Consequences of sports-related concussions include migraine headaches, depression, anxiety, and cognitive issues at school or during daily activities. A feared complication of repeated concussions is chronic neurodegenerative disease. Second impact syndrome may result from a second head injury that occurs while a patient is recovering from an initial concussion. Even a minor second head injury can cause increased brain edema in a patient with second impact syndrome.[6,7] Because of these serious long-term consequences, properly diagnosing athletes with concussions and counseling them on the recovery process are important.

No imaging or laboratory tests are used to diagnose a concussion. Recently, the FDA approved a panel of two biomarkers, glial fibrillary acidic protein and ubiquitin C-terminal hydrolase-L1, for detecting intracranial abnormalities. However, their use is not yet approved for children, and it is unclear if they are useful in helping diagnose a concussion, especially in the emergency department.[6]

CRITICAL DECISION

What are the criteria for a safe discharge home after an mTBI?

When CT is not recommended, the next step is often observation in the emergency department. For lower-risk patients, however, the observation should take place at home if their caretakers are reliable and willing. For patients who undergo observation in the emergency department, an escalation in care is in order if new high-risk symptoms develop; if these symptoms do not develop, discharge home is appropriate. There is no optimal length of the observation period, but most observations do not last past 6 hours after injury onset — a diagnosis of a significant intracranial injury more than 6 hours after injury in a well-appearing child is rare. After the observation period, another neurologic examination should be performed to demonstrate that the child is not deteriorating. During this repeat neurologic examination, the child's ambulation should be observed, their GCS score should be 15, and they should have no vision changes or focal neurologic deficits.[8] If a patient suffered polytrauma, any extracranial injuries should also be addressed and stabilized.[7]

If a patient receives a CT in the emergency department, the physician should ensure that the scan is negative for any intracranial abnormalities prior to discharge. Physicians should also consider their personal proficiency with reading CTs before basing the disposition decision on their interpretation of the scan. A GCS score of 15 combined with a normal CT is generally a good indicator that a patient can be safely discharged.

Admission should be considered for patients who ingested drugs or alcohol and for patients with additional traumatic injuries. Children who are unable to tolerate oral intake despite antiemetics; who are having severe, refractory pain; or who are having difficulty with coordination, vision, or ambulation may need further observation in the hospital prior to being discharged home. Referral to a concussion specialist or neurologist should be considered for children with a history of multiple concussions or persistent migraines, both of which can increase their risk of a complicated recovery.

If nonaccidental trauma is suspected, admission may be needed to ensure the child's safety. Nonaccidental pediatric trauma (ie, child abuse) should be considered, especially in preverbal children and children who rely solely on adults to describe their mechanism of injury. Abusive head trauma occurs with blunt injury to the head or aggressive shaking. Shaken baby syndrome includes the triad of subdural hematoma, retinal hemorrhage, and encephalopathy. An emergency department evaluation for nonaccidental trauma in a preverbal child typically includes x-rays (a skeletal survey), serum and urine testing, and a head CT scan, if they present with a head injury. Retinal hemorrhages can be identified on fundoscopy; emergency physicians may not be as adept at performing this examination on young children, so an ophthalmology consultation can be useful in these cases. Also, a social worker or a physician who specializes in child abuse can help determine a safe disposition for suspected victims of nonaccidental trauma.

CRITICAL DECISION

What are appropriate discharge care instructions for pediatric patients with mTBIs?

The decision to discharge home should be based on a normal mental status, improved symptoms, the absence of risk factors that warrant a CT scan (or a normal CT scan, if performed), and the absence of other indications for hospital observation (eg, other injuries, bleeding disorder, and worsening symptoms). A child should only be discharged home if there is a dependable parent or guardian who can care for them and identify a worsening course (*Table 3*).

Physicians should instruct caretakers that the child may initially be tired and should be allowed to nap or rest more often than usual. However, if the child becomes lethargic or difficult to arouse, they should immediately return to the emergency department for further evaluation. Other return precautions include increased vomiting, worsening headaches, increased alteration of consciousness, or new-onset focal neurologic deficit (eg, vision loss or extremity weakness). Caretakers do not necessarily need to wake the child from sleep outside of their regular schedule to check for these symptoms. Caretakers should also be instructed to follow up with the child's primary care physician for an evaluation after a concussion to determine when it is safe to return to sports and to address any concerns regarding symptom resolution. Additionally, there are concussion clinics and specialists in pediatric neurology and sports

Things to Check Before Recommending Discharge
Patient tolerates oral intake
Caregiver understands return precautions
Normal repeat neurologic examination
Absence of focal neurologic deficits
Negative head CT imaging (if applicable)
GCS score of 15
No other unaddressed extracranial injuries

TABLE 3. **Head injury discharge checklist**

medicine that can assist with determining when it is appropriate for the child to return to activities.

No specific medications are prescribed for concussion management. Antiemetics such as ondansetron can be helpful for postconcussive vomiting. Postconcussive headaches can be treated with NSAIDs or acetaminophen, as needed. Most children with mTBIs recover completely within 2 weeks. Symptoms may be prolonged, however, in patients who have had previous concussions.

Cognitive Rest

Most children benefit from up to 2 days of cognitive rest and a gradual return to normal activities. To temper symptoms, children should initially avoid bright lights and loud noises. As part of their gradual recovery, children should use electronic entertainment and communication devices with conservative limits on screen time.

Physical Rest

Children should rest up to 2 days before gradually returning to physical activity. Returning to school and a full cognitive load should occur before fully returning to sports activities. Prior to returning to physical activity, pediatric patients' neurocognitive function should be reevaluated by their pediatrician or a physician at a concussion specialty clinic (eg, neurology, neurosurgery, trauma, or sports medicine). The follow-up physician should explain to the patient and caregivers how physical activity will gradually be reintroduced. For example, after the first follow-up visit with a physician, the patient can expect to be cleared for moderate aerobic activity; after completing moderate aerobic activity without symptoms for 24 hours, the patient can expect to advance to the next phase of activity, such as a sport-specific activity.[8,9]

✔ Pearls

- The PECARN rule has great sensitivity to determine which patients can forgo CT scans.

- Patients with concussions should gradually return to their normal levels of activity.

- A significant intracranial hemorrhage is rarely diagnosed more than 6 hours after injury onset.

CASE RESOLUTIONS

CASE ONE

The child's parietal region was boggy, and his behavior had not returned to normal — he continued to display fussiness and irritability. The concerned physician obtained a CT scan of the patient's head; it revealed a linear, nondisplaced parietal skull fracture with an overlying scalp hematoma and a 2-mm subdural hematoma. The patient had a neurosurgical consultation and was observed overnight in an inpatient unit, where he received frequent neurologic checks.

During his evaluation the next day, no changes were noted in the child's neurologic status. Acetaminophen was ordered for pain. The child tolerated breastfeeding well. A fundoscopic evaluation by ophthalmology did not reveal any retinal hemorrhages. A social worker was consulted because of the child's young age and the nature of his injury; however, no evidence of abuse was found. The mother and grandmother reported corroborating histories that matched the baby's injury, and they were timely and demonstrated appropriate concern with bringing the child to the emergency department. The child was discharged home to his mother the next day.

CASE TWO

Per the PECARN rule, CT was not recommended for the dancer with the head injury. The patient did not have any pain, tenderness, or focal neurologic findings, so her backboard was removed, and she was cleared from her cervical collar.

The girl was observed in the emergency department for 2 hours. Her parents reported that she was behaving normally and that they would feel comfortable monitoring her at home. She was able to drink juice, eat crackers, and walk normally. She was discharged home in the care of her parents, who understood the return precautions.

CASE THREE

Because of his deteriorating mental status, the boy was intubated using rapid sequence intubation. A CT scan demonstrated an epidural hematoma with a midline shift. The patient was given hypertonic saline intravenously and was expeditiously transferred to another facility for pediatric neurosurgery. On arrival at the other facility, the patient was rushed to the operating room for an emergency craniotomy.

Summary

When children with head injuries present to the emergency department, the injury severity must be determined to differentiate cases that need emergency intervention from cases that simply need supportive care. Proper classification of head injuries allows for appropriate evaluation and management. Clinical decision rules such as the PECARN rule help prevent unnecessary CT use and radiation exposure. Fortunately, most pediatric patients with head injuries have an uncomplicated course and can be discharged home. Before these patients are discharged home, however, their caretakers must be thoroughly educated on the type of care to provide to prevent poor outcomes.

✖ Pitfalls

- Forgetting that a boggy, nonfrontal scalp hematoma (>2 cm) is highly suggestive of a skull fracture and TBI.

- Overlooking the importance of worsening nausea or vomiting or changes in mental status during observation. These symptoms warrant increased concern for a ciTBI.

- Discharging children with head injuries home for continued observation without considering their caretakers' reliability in providing care and understanding of return precautions.

- Failing to educate athletes with concussions on second impact syndrome and the importance of rest and recovery before returning to sports-related activities.

MDCALC REFERENCES

PECARN Pediatric Head Injury/Trauma Algorithm. https://www.mdcalc.com/calc/589/pecarn-pediatric-head-injury-trauma-algorithm

CATCH Rule. https://www.mdcalc.com/calc/3954/catch-canadian-assessment-tomography-childhood-head-injury-rule

CHALICE Rule. https://www.mdcalc.com/calc/3953/chalice-childrens-head-injury-algorithm-prediction-important-clinical-events-rule

REFERENCES

1. Haydel MJ, Weisbrod LJ, Saeed W. Pediatric head trauma. In: *StatPearls [Internet]*. StatPearls Publishing; 2023. https://www.ncbi.nlm.nih.gov/books/NBK537029/
2. Harper JA, Klassen TP, Balshaw R, Dyck J, Osmond MH; Pediatric Emergency Research Canada Head Injury Study Group. Characteristics of vomiting as a predictor of intracranial injury in pediatric minor head injury. *CJEM*. 2020 Nov;22(6):793-801.
3. Kuppermann N, Holmes JF, Dayan PS, et al; Pediatric Emergency Care Applied Research Network (PECARN). Identification of children at very low risk of clinically-important brain injuries after head trauma: a prospective cohort study. *Lancet*. 2009 Oct 3;374(9696):1160-1170.
4. Easter JS, Bakes K, Dhaliwal J, Miller M, Caruso E, Haukoos JS. Comparison of PECARN, CATCH, and CHALICE rules for children with minor head injury: a prospective cohort study. *Ann Emerg Med*. 2014 Aug;64(2):145-152.e5.
5. Abid Z, Kupperman N, Tancredi DJ, Dayan PS. Risk of traumatic brain injuries in infants younger than 3 months with minor blunt head trauma. *Ann Emerg Med*. 2021 Sep;78(3):321-330.e1.
6. Mannix R, Bazarian JJ. Managing pediatric concussion in the emergency department. *Ann Emerg Med*. 2020 Jun;75(6):762-766.
7. Stillman A, Alexander M, Mannix R, Madigan N, Pascual-Leone A, Meehan WP. Concussion: evaluation and management. *Cleve Clin J Med*. 2017 Aug;84(8):623-630.
8. Wing R, James C. Pediatric head injury and concussion. *Emerg Med Clin North Am*. 2013 Aug;31(3):653-675.
9. Schunk JE, Schutzman SA; Pediatric head injury. *Pediatr Rev*. 2012 Sep;33(9):398-411.

Atrial-Sensed, Ventricular-Paced Rhythm With Failure to Capture

By Jeremy Berberian, MD; William J. Brady, MD, FACEP; and Amal Mattu, MD, FACEP

Dr. Berberian is the associate director of emergency medicine residency education at ChristianaCare and assistant professor of emergency medicine at Sidney Kimmel Medical College, Thomas Jefferson University in Philadelphia, Pennsylvania. Dr. Brady is a professor of emergency medicine, medicine, and nursing, and vice chair for faculty affairs in the Department of Emergency Medicine at the University of Virginia School of Medicine in Charlottesville. Dr. Mattu is a professor, vice chair, and codirector of the Emergency Cardiology Fellowship in the Department of Emergency Medicine at the University of Maryland School of Medicine in Baltimore.

Objectives

On completion of this article, you should be able to:

■ Identify an atrial-sensed, ventricular-paced rhythm on a 12-lead ECG.

■ Describe the ECG findings seen with failure to capture.

■ Differentiate between an intrinsic LBBB and the LBBB-like morphology seen with RV pacing.

■ **CASE PRESENTATION** ■

An 82-year-old man presents with near syncope (*Figure 1*).

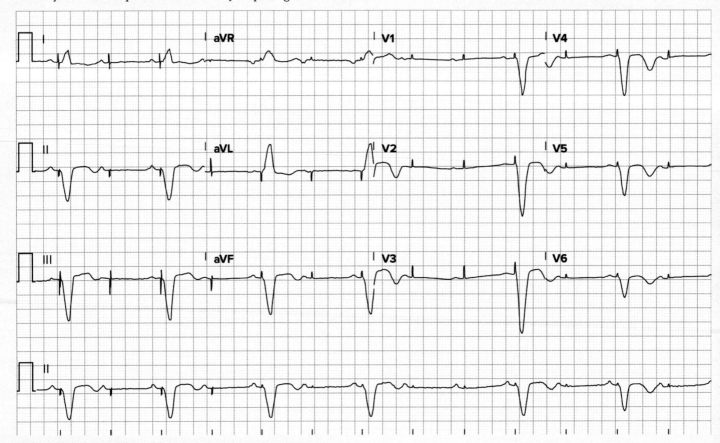

FIGURE 1. ECG of an 82-year-old man. *Credit:* EMRA.

ECG Findings

This ECG shows an atrial-sensed, ventricular-paced rhythm with an average ventricular rate of 36 bpm, left axis deviation, a prolonged QRS complex duration with a left bundle branch block–like (LBBB-like) morphology, and frequent failure to capture (*Figure 2*). The QRS complex in lead V_6 is negatively oriented, which is normal for right ventricular (RV) pacing.

The P-QRS-T complexes associated with the 1st, 3rd, 5th, 7th, 10th, and 12th pacer spikes show a normal atrial-sensed, ventricular-paced rhythm. A native P wave is sensed by the pacemaker, which then triggers a paced ventricular beat (*Figure 3*).

This patient's workup was notable for hyperkalemia due to acute renal failure. He was aggressively treated for hyperkalemia, after which his ECG normalized.

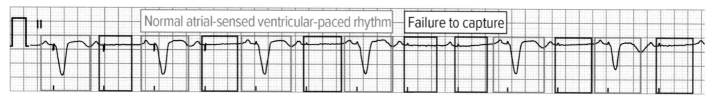

FIGURE 2. **The lead II rhythm strip shows an atrial-sensed, ventricular-paced rhythm (*green boxes*) with frequent failure to capture (*red boxes*).** *Credit:* EMRA.

The 2nd, 4th, 6th, 8th, 9th, 11th, and 13th pacer spikes show failure to capture. The defining feature of failure to capture is the absence of depolarization after a pacer spike (*Figure 4*). Common causes of failure to capture include electrode displacement, wire fracture, ischemia or infarct, and electrolyte abnormalities (especially hyperkalemia). Treatment is based on correcting the underlying etiology (eg, calcium for hyperkalemia).

LEARNING POINTS

Pacemaker
- Pacer spikes are usually visible on the ECG, either at the bottom of the ECG or preceding the P wave or QRS complex.
- Atrial pacing
  - Pacemaker lead usually implanted in the right atrial appendage
  - Results in P waves with normal morphology
- Single ventricular pacing
  - Pacemaker lead usually implanted in the right ventricle apex
  - Results in an LBBB pattern in the limb leads and anteroseptal precordial leads
  - The major difference between an intrinsic LBBB and a single ventricular-paced rhythm is that the QRS complex will almost always be negatively oriented in leads V_5 and V_6 with a single ventricular-paced rhythm.
- Biventricular pacing
  - Two pacemaker leads usually implanted in the right ventricle apex and the surface of the posterior or lateral left ventricle
  - Typically results in a narrower QRS complex than with single ventricular pacing
  - Dominant R wave in lead V_1 +/− V_2 is common.
- An automatic implantable cardioverter-defibrillator will have a thick coil that differentiates it from a pacemaker.

Failure to Capture
- Delivery of a pacing stimulus without subsequent myocardial depolarization
- ECG shows absence of depolarization after pacer spikes.
- Causes include functional (eg, electrode displacement and wire fracture) and pathologic (eg, electrolyte disturbances and AMI).

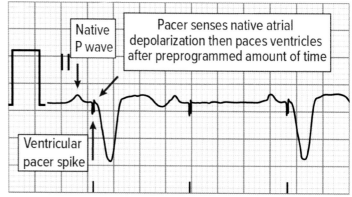

FIGURE 3. **The initial P-QRS-T complex of the lead II rhythm strip shows an atrial-sensed, ventricular-paced rhythm.** *Credit:* EMRA.

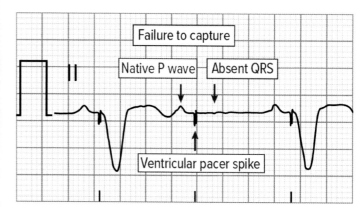

FIGURE 4. **The second P wave of the lead II rhythm strip is sensed by the pacemaker, which then triggers a pacer spike.** The absence of subsequent ventricular depolarization is called failure to capture. *Credit:* EMRA.

ACKNOWLEDGMENT

This case is reprinted from *Emergency ECGs: Case-Based Review and Interpretations,* available at emra.org/amazon or by using the QR code.

Clinical Pediatrics

Lung Injuries From Vaping

By Wade DeAustin, MD; and Stephen Sandelich, MD

Milton S. Hershey Medical Center, Hershey, Pennsylvania

Reviewed by Ann Dietrich, MD, FACEP, FAAP

Objective

On completion of this article, you should be able to:

■ Recognize EVALI and manage it appropriately.

CASE PRESENTATION

A 16-year-old boy without a significant medical history presents with a dry cough, a sore throat, nausea, vomiting, and fever for 2 days. Although the patient tested positive for COVID-19 2 weeks ago, he says that his viral symptoms resolved before his current symptoms started. He also reports unintentional weight loss over the past few months and that he had been smoking and vaping marijuana daily but has recently cut back.

The patient's initial vital signs are BP 101/70, P 130, R 24, and T 38.9°C (102°F); his SpO_2 is 98% on room air. On evaluation, he appears nontoxic but is slightly pale and dehydrated, which is evident from dry mucous membranes. His capillary refill time is normal. He is tachycardic, has mildly increased work of breathing, and has sounds of mild crackling near the bases of his lungs. His initial laboratory analysis reveals hyponatremia (134 mEq/L); an anion gap of 15 mEq/L; leukocytosis (19 × 10^9/L, with neutrophil predominance); slight anemia (12.5 g/dL); a negative D-dimer level; and an elevated INR (1.4), PTT (37 sec), and total bilirubin level (2.7 mg/dL); additionally, his C-reactive protein level is 20.75 mg/dL, and his erythrocyte sedimentation rate is 101 mm/hr. A blood culture is also obtained. His chest x-ray reveals no cardiopulmonary abnormality (*Figure 1*). Except for sinus tachycardia, his ECG is otherwise normal (*Figure 2*). Because of his appearance, examination findings, and initial workup, he is treated empirically for sepsis with fluid resuscitation (2 L of normal saline) and antibiotics (1 g of ceftriaxone). After the initial resuscitation, his vital signs stabilize, and he is admitted.

On admission, further workup reveals a negative respiratory viral panel, normal troponin level, and elevated BNP level (433 pg/mL). An echocardiogram shows normal biventricular function. CT of the abdomen and pelvis detects bilateral ground-glass opacities in the lower lungs and trace pleural effusions that are concerning for multifocal pneumonia (this finding is also seen in COVID-19 infections); hepatomegaly; a small volume of free fluid in the abdomen, likely reactive; soft tissue edema; and no appendicitis. Hepatitis laboratory tests are negative.

On hospital day 2, the patient's oxygen needs increase, and he is upgraded to the pediatric ICU. High-flow nasal cannula therapy is initiated to maintain an SpO_2 above 90%. A repeat chest x-ray shows diffuse pulmonary edema, and a chest CT shows confluent ground-glass opacities with bilateral trace pleural effusions that are concerning for diffuse alveolar hemorrhage (*Figures 3* and *4*). High-dose corticosteroids are initiated. Lung injury from e-cigarette use is suspected.

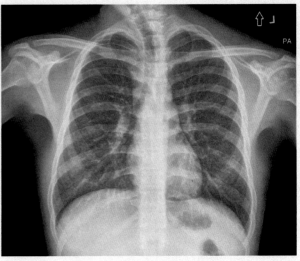

FIGURE 1. Chest x-ray revealing no cardiopulmonary abnormality. *Credit:* Wade DeAustin, MD; and Stephen Sandelich, MD.

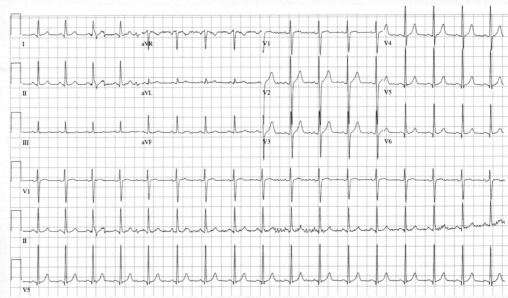

FIGURE 2. ECG showing sinus tachycardia. *Credit:* Wade DeAustin, MD; and Stephen Sandelich, MD

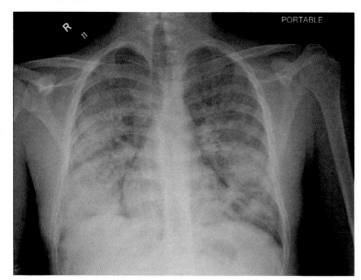

FIGURE 3. Chest x-ray showing confluent ground-glass opacities with bilateral trace pleural effusions.
Credit: Wade DeAustin, MD; and Stephen Sandelich, MD.

Discussion

E-cigarette use, or vaping, was initially intended for tobacco cessation. E-cigarettes were first approved for use in Europe in 2006 and in the United States in 2007.[1] Vaping, however, has become a significant public health concern, especially for adolescents because of increased use since 2017.[2] Vaping has substantial consequences separate from the risks of traditional cigarette smoking.[3] According to the National Survey on Drug Use and Health, in 2021 8.1% of people (31.1 million people) between the ages of 12 and 20 years have vaped nicotine products.[4] Of those 12 years and older who vape, 71% use nicotine, 40% use marijuana, and 19% use flavoring.

E-cigarettes contain a battery, heat source, and reservoir for the substance to be vaped.[5] Vaping solutions usually contain nicotine mixed with other ingredients, such as propylene glycol, glycerol, and concentrated flavoring compounds. Up to 100 different chemicals have been identified in vaping solutions, including tobacco-specific nitrosamines, aldehydes, metals, volatile organic compounds, phenolic compounds, polycyclic aromatic hydrocarbons, flavorings, and tobacco alkaloids.[6-9]

E-cigarette– or vaping-associated lung injury (EVALI) became a new diagnosis in 2019.[10-12] Its incidence appears to be dropping somewhat, possibly because of a law passed in December 2019 that raised the federal minimum age for the purchase of tobacco products, including e-cigarettes, from 18 to 21 years.[13]

The pathophysiology of EVALI is multifactorial and not completely understood. Exposure to chemicals in vaping solutions can damage any lung tissue and potentially lead to acute lung injury or diffuse lung inflammation. When these chemicals are inhaled, the body and lung tissue treat them like microscopic foreign bodies, leading to local inflammation and an immune-driven response that further damages tissue.[14-19]

Most patients with EVALI are young and previously healthy. Symptoms are usually nonspecific and mimic a viral illness; they present gradually over days to weeks.[18,19] CDC data reveal that 95% of patients initially present with respiratory symptoms, including coughing, chest pain, and shortness of breath; 77% have GI symptoms of vomiting, abdominal pain, and diarrhea; and 85% have constitutional symptoms, such as fever, chills, and weight loss. Physical examination generally reveals tachycardia (55%), tachypnea (45%), and hypoxia (57%). Pulmonary examination may reveal decreased or adventitious breath sounds (crackles or wheezes) or may be normal.[12]

Laboratory testing commonly reveals leukocytosis and an elevated erythrocyte sedimentation rate and C-reactive protein level; transaminitis may also be present. An infectious disease workup — including respiratory viral panels and testing for *Streptococcus pneumoniae*, *Legionella pneumophila*, *Mycoplasma pneumoniae*, endemic mycoses, and opportunistic infections — should be considered to rule out alternative diagnoses.[12] A chest x-ray should be obtained for all patients, and a chest CT should be considered for patients who appear to have severe or

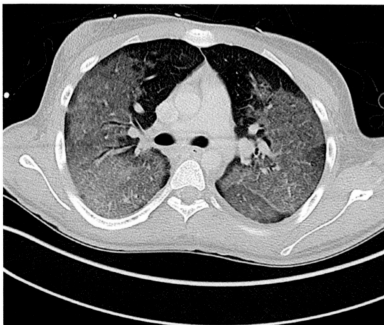
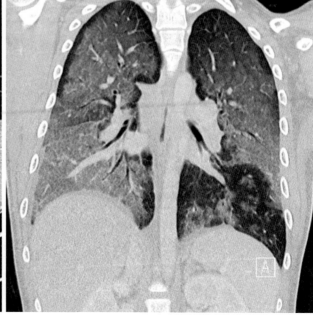

FIGURE 4. Chest CT showing confluent ground-glass opacities with bilateral trace pleural effusions.
Credit: Wade DeAustin, MD; and Stephen Sandelich, MD.

worsening disease. Imaging findings associated with EVALI include pulmonary infiltrates on chest x-ray and ground-glass opacities on chest CT. EVALI is a diagnosis of exclusion; once other potential causes have been excluded, physicians should use the CDC diagnostic criteria to diagnose EVALI (*Table 1*).

Most patients with EVALI require hospital admission. Admission criteria include respiratory distress, hypoxia, ill appearance, or significant comorbidities. Treatment for EVALI is predominantly supportive, ensuring the stability of the patient's respiratory status. The degree of respiratory distress and failure varies, so respiratory interventions must be tailored to each patient. Some patients require only minimal oxygen supplementation via nasal cannula, while others (up to one-third) require endotracheal intubation and mechanical ventilation. Extracorporeal membrane oxygenation may be necessary for severe cases.[20]

Systemic corticosteroids may help blunt the inflammatory response, but evidence is limited.[12,20-22] Ranges for corticosteroid dosages, durations, and tapers vary in the literature. Emergency

EVALI Diagnostic Criteria
Use of an e-cigarette within 90 days before symptom onset
Presence of a pulmonary infiltrate, such as opacities on chest x-ray or ground-glass opacities on chest CT scan
No evidence of an infection or an infection has been ruled out
No plausible alternative diagnosis

TABLE 1. The CDC's definition of EVALI

physicians should tailor corticosteroid treatment to each patient, ideally after consulting a pulmonary specialist. Many patients with EVALI receive antibiotics for concurrent infections. An important part of EVALI treatment and prevention is encouraging patients to avoid e-cigarette use entirely. Education on EVALI and the risks of vaping for the general population, especially for adolescents, is also crucial.

CASE RESOLUTION

On hospital day 5, the patient required continuous positive airway pressure because of worsening hypoxic respiratory failure. After slow improvement of his respiratory status, the patient was diagnosed with acute hypoxemic respiratory failure from EVALI. On hospital day 11, he was weaned from supplemental oxygen therapy. He was discharged on hospital day 13 with instructions to take 30 mg of prednisone twice daily and 2 puffs of budesonide-formoterol twice daily. He was also educated on vaping and smoking cessation.

REFERENCES

1. Salzman GA, Alqawasma M, Asad H. Vaping associated lung injury (EVALI): an explosive United States epidemic. *Mo Med*. 2019 Nov-Dec;116(6):492-496.
2. Cullen KA, Gentzke AS, Sawdey MD, et al. E-cigarette use among youth in the United States, 2019. *JAMA*. 2019 Dec 3;322(21):2095-2103.
3. Hamberger ES, Halpern-Felsher B. Vaping in adolescents: epidemiology and respiratory harm. *Curr Opin Pediatr*. 2020 Jun;32(3):378-383.
4. Key substance use and mental health indicators in the United States: results from the 2020 National Survey on Drug Use and Health. Substance Abuse and Mental Health Services Administration. Published October 2021. https://www.samhsa.gov/data/sites/default/files/reports/rpt35325/NSDUHFFRPDFWHTMLFiles2020/2020NSDUHFFR1PDFW102121.pdf
5. Vaping devices (electronic cigarettes) drug facts. National Institute on Drug Abuse. Published January 8, 2020. https://nida.nih.gov/publications/drugfacts/vaping-devices-electronic-cigarettes
6. Herrington JS, Myers C. Electronic cigarette solutions and resultant aerosol profiles. *J Chromatogr A*. 2015 Oct 30;1418:192-199.
7. Kucharska M, Wesołowski W, Czerczak S, Soko R. Testing of the composition of e-cigarette liquids — manufacturer-declared vs true contents in a selected series of products. *Med Pr*. 2016;67(2):239-253.
8. Park JA, Crotty Alexander LE, Christiani DC. Vaping and lung inflammation and injury. *Annu Rev Physiol*. 2022 Feb 10;84:611-629.
9. St Helen G, Eaton DL. Public health consequences of e-cigarette use. *JAMA Intern Med*. 2018 Jul 1;178(7):984-986.
10. Pray IW, Atti SK, Tomasallo C, Meiman JG. E-cigarette, or vaping, product use–associated lung injury among clusters of patients reporting shared product use — Wisconsin, 2019. *MMWR Morb Mortal Wkly Rep*. 2020 Mar 6;69(9):236-240.
11. Kalininskiy A, Bach CT, Nacca NE, et al. E-cigarette, or vaping, product use associated lung injury (EVALI): case series and diagnostic approach. *Lancet Respir Med*. 2019 Dec;7(12):1017-1026.
12. Siegel DA, Jatlaoui TC, Koumans EH, et al; Lung Injury Response Clinical Working Group; Lung Injury Response Epidemiology/Surveillance Group. Update: interim guidance for health care providers evaluating and caring for patients with suspected e-cigarette, or vaping, product use associated lung injury — United States, October 2019. *MMWR Morb Mortal Wkly Rep*. 2019 Oct 18;68(41):919-927.
13. Rules, regulations and guidance: the Historic Tobacco Control Act. US Food and Drug Administration. Updated December 21, 2019. https://www.fda.gov/tobacco-products/products-guidance-regulations/rules-regulations-and-guidance
14. Fuoco FC, Buonanno G, Stabile L, Vigo P. Influential parameters on particle concentration and size distribution in the mainstream of e-cigarettes. *Environ Pollut*. 2014 Jan;184:523-529.
15. Geiss O, Bianchi I, Barahona F, Barrero-Moreno J. Characterisation of mainstream and passive vapours emitted by selected electronic cigarettes. *Int J Hyg Environ Health*. 2015 Jan;218(1):169-180.
16. Goel R, Durand E, Trushin N, et al. Highly reactive free radicals in electronic cigarette aerosols. *Chem Res Toxicol*. 2015 Sep 21;28(9):1675-1677.
17. Sussan TE, Gajghate S, Thimmulappa RK, et al. Exposure to electronic cigarettes impairs pulmonary anti-bacterial and anti-viral defenses in a mouse model. *PLoS One*. 2015 Feb 4;10(2):e0116861.
18. Kligerman S, Raptis C, Larsen B, et al. Radiologic, pathologic, clinical, and physiologic findings of electronic cigarette or vaping product use-associated lung injury (EVALI): evolving knowledge and remaining questions. *Radiology*. 2020 Mar;294(3):491-505.
19. Shinbashi M, Rubin BK. Electronic cigarettes and e-cigarette/vaping product use associated lung injury (EVALI). *Paediatr Respir Rev*. 2020 Nov;36:87-91.
20. Layden JE, Ghinai I, Pray I, et al. Pulmonary illness related to e-cigarette use in Illinois and Wisconsin — final report. *N Engl J Med*. 2020 Mar 5;382(10):903-916.
21. Davidson K, Brancato A, Heetderks P, et al. Outbreak of electronic-cigarette–associated acute lipoid pneumonia — North Carolina, July-August 2019. *MMWR Morb Mortal Wkly Rep*. 2019 Sep 13;68(36):784-786.
22. Maddock SD, Cirulis MM, Callahan SJ, et al. Pulmonary lipid-laden macrophages and vaping. *N Engl J Med*. 2019 Oct 10;381(15):1488-1489.

The Critical Procedure

Anoscopy

By Steven J. Warrington, MD, PhD
MercyOne Siouxland in Sioux City, Iowa

Objective

On completion of this article, you should be able to:

■ Recall the indications for an anoscopy and how to perform one.

Introduction

Anoscopy is an adjunct for rectal examination that can be useful in certain situations. For instance, anoscopy can provide additional information on the source of bleeding in patients with a distal lower GI bleed. Additionally, it can aid in rectal foreign body removal by visualizing the foreign body and guiding physicians with instrument insertion.

Contraindications

■ Imperforate anus

Benefits and Risks

The primary benefit of anoscopy is better visualization of potential anal pathology such as masses, foreign bodies, and sources of bleeding. Few risks are associated with the procedure. Anoscopy can be painful and can cause bleeding from minor trauma to the mucosa. Anal pathology may not be identified on anoscopy; in such cases, patients will require further evaluation with procedures like sigmoidoscopy or colonoscopy. Reusable anoscopes pose the risk of infectious disease transmission if not well sterilized; disposable anoscopes limit this risk.

Alternatives

The appropriate alternative to anoscopy depends to some degree on the indication for an anoscopy. Some emergency departments may offer a rigid sigmoidoscopy that may be able to visualize anal pathology. For foreign bodies, operative examination for removal may be more appropriate than anoscopy. For patients with suspected slow lower GI bleeds, a colonoscopy or stool evaluation for blood may be better alternatives.

Reducing Side Effects

Although an anoscopy carries few risks, the procedure can be anxiety provoking and uncomfortable. Attention to adjunctive medications is important to improve patients' tolerability of the examination. Depending on the situation, procedural sedation may be appropriate. However, other factors should also be taken into account when considering procedural sedation, like whether the patient will require further care and whether operative examination or colonoscopy would be better alternatives.

Special Considerations

Involuntary rectal spasms and reflexes may make initial insertion of the anoscope difficult; slow, gentle pressure during insertion helps make the process smoother. During anoscope withdrawal, these involuntary rectal responses can push the anoscope out quicker than intended; pressure should be kept on the anoscope while withdrawing it to prevent this reaction.

TECHNIQUE

1. **Discuss** the procedure with the patient and ensure they understand it.

2. **Obtain** consent if required by the state or institution.

3. **Perform** a digital rectal examination first to identify any masses, bleeding, or sources of pain.

4. **Lubricate** the anoscope and obturator, with the obturator completely inserted into the anoscope.

5. **Use** gentle, constant pressure on the back of the obturator to insert the anoscope into the anus.

6. **Advance** the anoscope while asking the patient to lightly bear down. Continue to hold the obturator in place to ensure it is not dislodged during anoscope insertion.

7. **Continue** advancing the anoscope until its flange reaches the edge of the rectum.

8. **Remove** the obturator. If the anoscope does not have a light source, use a portable light source. Visualize the field; then slowly withdraw the anoscope while visualizing more of the area. Swabs may be needed to visualize the mucosa directly.

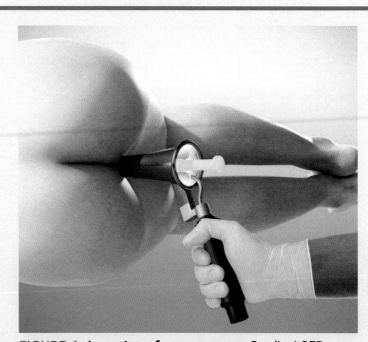

FIGURE 1. Insertion of an anoscope. *Credit:* ACEP.

The LLSA Literature Review
Shoulder Dislocations

By Megan J. Rivera, MD; and
Nicholas G. Maldonado, MD, FACEP
Duke University School of Medicine in Durham,
North Carolina; and the University of Florida
College of Medicine in Gainesville

Reviewed by Andrew J. Eyre, MD, MS-HPEd

Objectives

On completion of this article, you should be able to:

■ Explain how appropriate shoulder reduction techniques are selected.

■ Name the most successful shoulder reduction techniques for each type of shoulder dislocation.

Gottlieb M. Shoulder dislocations in the emergency department: a comprehensive review of reduction techniques. *J Emerg Med.* 2020 Apr;58(4):647-666.

KEY POINTS

■ Shoulder dislocations are a common presentation in the emergency department. Physicians should be familiar with the different reduction techniques for this condition.

■ There are multiple shoulder reduction techniques. Each has advantages, disadvantages, and varying success rates.

■ The reduction technique chosen will depend on the type of shoulder dislocation, the patient, the physician, and factors specific to the health care system.

■ Slow and guided movements should be pursued over rapid or forceful movements. If the first attempt fails, physicians should consider an alternative maneuver.

Joint dislocations are common orthopedic emergencies; shoulder dislocations, in particular, are among the most often seen presentations. Shoulder dislocations are classified as anterior, posterior, or inferior based on the position of the humeral head relative to the glenoid fossa. There are multiple reduction techniques available to achieve anatomic alignment, and the choice depends on the type of shoulder dislocation being reduced. Gottlieb provides a comprehensive review of the 26 major shoulder reduction techniques, describing each technique and its modifications in detail with pictorial representations; the review also highlights the success rates, advantages, and disadvantages of each technique.

Factors related to the patient, physician, and health system also influence which shoulder reduction technique is chosen. Patient factors to consider include body habitus, pain tolerance, comorbidities, and sedation risk factors. Other factors related to the patient include the body positions they can tolerate during the reduction; whether this is a first-time or recurrent dislocation; and where the reduction will be performed (eg, in the field or a hallway bed of the emergency department). Physician factors include the physician's experience with reductions and how many people are available to assist with the reduction. Health system factors include the emergency department's census, available resources, and time constraints.

Two variables associated with higher rates of failed reduction are (1) delays in emergency department presentation and reduction attempts and (2) repeated reduction attempts. Repeated reduction attempts also increase the risk of neurovascular injuries. Thus, important aspects to emergency care include performing shoulder reductions as soon as possible and striving for a successful reduction on the first attempt. Emergency physicians must also know multiple shoulder reduction techniques in case the first attempt is unsuccessful; however, data that compare specific techniques are limited.

Based on Gottlieb's review, *Table 1* summarizes the major shoulder reduction techniques and their reported success rates. The table also references each technique's targeted anatomic location, the positioning the technique requires, and the number of operators needed to perform each technique. For example, a patient with an anterior shoulder dislocation is able to sit upright but is unable to lie in bed. Only one physician is available to perform the shoulder reduction. An appropriate technique for this scenario is the Bokor-Billman technique, which has been reported to have no complications and a 100% success rate. In another example, a patient with an anterior shoulder dislocation is able to lie prone, and one physician is available but has strict time constraints. According to the table, the Stimson maneuver would be an appropriate reduction technique.

Some techniques — the Cunningham, Davos/Aronen, FARES, and GONAIS — have the advantage of requiring no sedation in selected patients. Techniques such as the Davos/Aronen, GONAIS, and the modified Milch can be taught as self-reduction techniques, which is especially useful for patients with recurrent shoulder dislocations or patients who require reduction in places outside of the emergency department. Scapular manipulation has several modifications to its original prone technique, making it flexible in terms of patient positions and the number of operators needed.

Gottlieb cautions that several reduction techniques have been associated with higher risks of injury. For example, the Hippocratic method for reduction is no longer recommended because the axillary pressure exerted during this technique increases the risks of a humerus fracture and neurovascular injury. The modified Kocher technique that uses axial humeral traction, the Nicola method, and the traction-countertraction technique have also been associated with injuries. Although expertise in all shoulder reduction techniques is not realistic, emergency physicians should know how to perform the most successful shoulder reductions for each type of shoulder dislocation and should avoid techniques with the highest risk of complications. Additionally, they should know how to select an appropriate reduction technique based on a patient's presentation and should tailor their approach to patient, physician, and health system limiting factors.

16 *Critical Decisions in Emergency Medicine*

Anatomic Location (% Dislocations)	Patient Position or Position of Comfort	Operators Required	Technique	Reported Success Rates
Anterior dislocation (96.4%)	Sitting upright	One operator	Bokor-Billmann technique	100%
			Cunningham technique	100%
			Chair method	96.6%-100%
			Nicola method	88.6%-100%
			Davos method/Aronen technique	60%-86%
			Modified seated Spaso method	79.4%, Matsumoto et al modification
		Two operators	Legg reduction maneuver	Data lacking
	Supine	One operator	Elbow technique	100%
			Janecki forward elevation maneuver	92.6%-100%
			FARES method	85.7%-100%
			Milch technique	69.2%-100%
			Kocher technique	68%-100%
			Spaso method	66.7%-100%
			Zahiri technique	84.6%
			Hippocratic method	72.5%-100%, no longer recommended
		Two operators	Traction-countertraction method	91.5%-100%
		Three operators	Double traction method	90%-100%
	Prone	One operator	Modified prone Milch techniques	100%, Lacey and Crawford modification; 90%, McNair modification
			Scapular manipulation	78.4%-100%
		No operator	Stimson technique	28% first attempt, 91.3% overall
	Lateral decubitus (affected side facing ceiling)	One operator	Modified Nicola method	100%, Bhan and Mehara modification
		Two operators	Pendel method (also called Eskimo technique)	77.3%
	Standing	One operator	GONAIS method	Data lacking
	Any position	One operator	Axial traction with acromial fixation	100%
			External rotation maneuver (ERM)	78%-100%
		One or two operators	Modified scapular manipulation techniques	Data lacking for modified techniques
Posterior dislocation (3%)	Supine or sitting upright	One operator	DePalma "lever" method	Data lacking
			Caudal traction	Data lacking
	Sitting upright	Two operators	Wilson technique	100%, data limited
Inferior dislocation (0.6%)	Supine	One operator	Two-step maneuver	Data lacking
		Two operators	Traction-countertraction method	Data lacking

TABLE 1. Shoulder reduction techniques based on anatomic location, patient position, and number of operators required

Critical Decisions in Emergency Medicine's LLSA literature reviews feature articles from ABEM's 2023 Lifelong Learning and Self-Assessment Reading List. Available online at acep.org/moc/llsa and on the ABEM website.

Critical Cases in Orthopedics and Trauma
High-Pressure Injection Injury

By John Kiel DO, MPH, FACEP, CAQSM
University of South Florida Morsani College of Medicine — Tampa

Objective

On completion of this article, you should be able to:

■ Recognize and appropriately manage a high-pressure injection injury.

CASE PRESENTATION

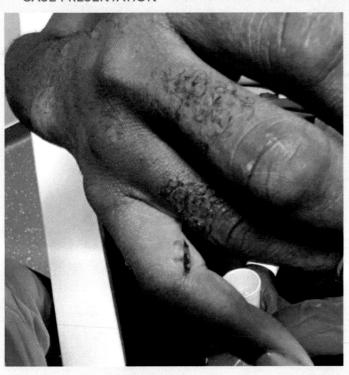

A 57-year-old man presents with a laceration to his right little finger after using a pressure washer at a car wash just prior to arrival. He describes the pain in his finger as aching and throbbing and says he cannot move his hand or finger without significant pain. On examination, a small laceration is noted on the radial side of his fifth digit, which is relatively hemostatic (*Figure 1*). Tenderness and crepitus extend along the dorsal and ulnar sides of the finger and hand. X-rays are obtained; they show subcutaneous emphysema in the ulnar aspect of the hand and wrist (*Figures 2* and *3*).

FIGURE 1. A small laceration on the radial side of the pinky finger

Discussion

A high-pressure injection injury is a traumatic condition characterized by extensive soft tissue damage and a benign high-pressure entry wound. The condition is a surgical emergency, with amputation rates as high as 30%.[1] The incidence is relatively rare and estimated to be approximately 1/600 hand traumas. The most common demographic is young male laborers who use paint, automotive grease, solvents, or diesel oil.[2] The nondominant hand is typically affected, and the index finger is the most-injured digit.[3] The patient in the case presentation injured the fifth digit of his nondominant right hand.

The mechanism of injury for this type of injury is an injection force of up to 10,000 psi delivered at a speed of up to 400 mph; a force as low as 100 psi is enough to break the skin. The pathophysiologic process involves the initial injury, chemical irritation, inflammation, and subsequent secondary infection. The anatomical injury usually involves dissection along planes of least resistance, such as neurovascular bundles. Vascular occlusion can lead to local soft tissue necrosis.

On initial evaluation, the time since the event must be determined. The average time from the event to evaluation by a physician is usually around 9 hours. The type of injected material is another critical piece of information to determine. Injection of clean water or air is generally considered low risk. Paint produces a large, early inflammatory response with a high rate of amputation. Grease guns cause a more blunted inflammatory response with a lower risk of amputation.

The most common location of high-pressure injection injuries is the hands and fingers. Paradoxically, the injury typically appears benign on first evaluation because immediately after the injection, only a small injection site or laceration appears, with minimal or no pain. Eventually, pain and paresthesia occur. In toxic cases, the injured site becomes edematous, pale, and severely tender to palpation over time. The diagnosis is primarily a clinical one based on a thorough history and physical examination. Depending on the injectate, x-rays may show radiopaque material and subcutaneous emphysema.

Treatment generally involves an early emergent consultation with a hand surgeon. The patient should be splinted and immobilized. Nonoperative management can be considered for injections of air, water, or chicken vaccine. However, more than half of these injuries will ultimately require an operation.

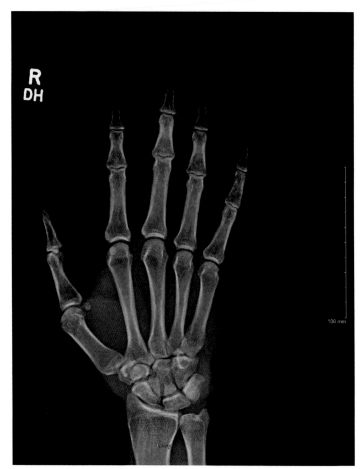

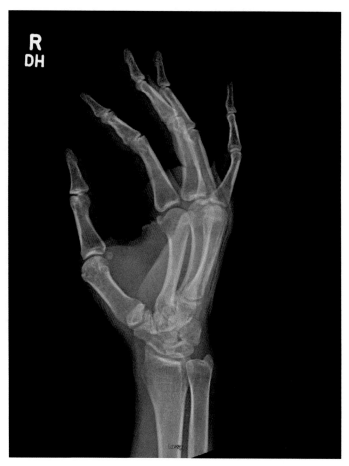

FIGURE 2. Posteroanterior x-ray showing subcutaneous emphysema along the ulnar aspect of the hand and wrist

FIGURE 3. Lateral x-ray demonstrating subcutaneous emphysema along the ulnar aspect of the hand and wrist

Early surgical decompression and debridement is often indicated for any caustic substances. Delays in treatment after 10 hours increase the risk of amputation. Tetanus vaccinations should be updated and broad-spectrum antibiotics should be initiated. Digital blocks are contraindicated because the wound is already under high pressure.

In general, the complications and prognosis of high-pressure injection injuries depend on the type of injectate.

The amputation rate approaches 50% for injuries from organic solvents (paint, paint thinner, diesel fuel, jet fuel, oil).[4] Delays in treatment increase the risk of infection. Variables that can be used prognostically to help predict outcomes include the time from injury to treatment, force of injection, volume injected, and composition of material. Rare late complications include oleogranulomas, fibrohistiocytic tumors, and squamous cell carcinomas.[5]

CASE RESOLUTION

The patient was evaluated by orthopedic surgery. During this assessment, the patient reported a significant decrease in swelling and denied any neurologic symptoms. Compartments were soft and compressible. The patient's tetanus vaccination was updated. He was also initiated on cephalexin for prophylaxis, and his laceration was repaired. After serial examinations to ensure compartments remained soft and symptoms continued to improve, the patient was discharged with an order for outpatient follow-up.

REFERENCES

1. Collins M, McGauvran A, Elhassan B. High-pressure injection injury of the hand: peculiar MRI features and treatment implications. *Skeletal Radiol.* 2019 Feb;48(2):295-299.
2. Hart RG, Smith GD, Haq A. Prevention of high-pressure injection injuries to the hand. *Am J Emerg Med.* 2006 Jan;24(1):73-76.
3. Saadat P, Turla S, Vadmal M. Fibrohistiocytic tumor of the hand after high-pressure paintgun injury: 2 case reports. *J Hand Surg Am.* 2005 Mar;30(2):404-408.
4. Hogan CJ, Ruland RT. High-pressure injection injuries to the upper extremity: a review of the literature. *J Orthop Trauma.* 2006 Jul;20(7):503-511.
5. Eells AC, McRae M, Buntic RF, et al. High-pressure injection injury: a case report and systematic review. *Case Reports Plast Surg Hand Surg.* 2019 Dec 18;6(1):153-158.

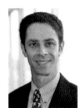
By Joshua S. Broder, MD, FACEP
Dr. Broder is a professor and the residency program director in the Department of Emergency Medicine at Duke University Medical Center in Durham, North Carolina.

The Critical Image

A Child With Periorbital Swelling

Objectives

On completion of this article, you should be able to:

- Risk stratify pediatric patients with suspected orbital cellulitis and determine the need for imaging.
- Select appropriate imaging for suspected orbital cellulitis in children.
- Identify CT findings of orbital cellulitis.

CASE PRESENTATION

A 5-year-old boy presents with a day-long headache and right periorbital edema. He completed a 10-day amoxicillin treatment for otitis media a week ago. Three days ago, his rhinorrhea recurred. He has no other medical history, and his immunizations are up to date. His vital signs are BP 126/69, P 112, R 28, and T 38.5°C (101.3°F); SpO_2 is 97% on room air. The patient is alert and in no acute distress. He has right periorbital swelling with mild erythema (*Figure 1*). His extraocular movements are intact, although he complains of pain with eye motion. His pupillary and conjunctival examinations and visual acuity are normal. He has no focal neurologic deficits, and his neck is supple.

His WBC count is $16.9 \times 10^9/L$ (normal $3.8\text{-}14 \times 10^9/L$), with 75% neutrophils. His erythrocyte sedimentation rate is 35 mm/hr (normal 0-13 mm/hr) and C-reactive protein level is 2.49 mg/dL (normal ≤0.85 mg/dL). Ampicillin-sulbactam and clindamycin are administered, and a CT scan with intravenous contrast is obtained.

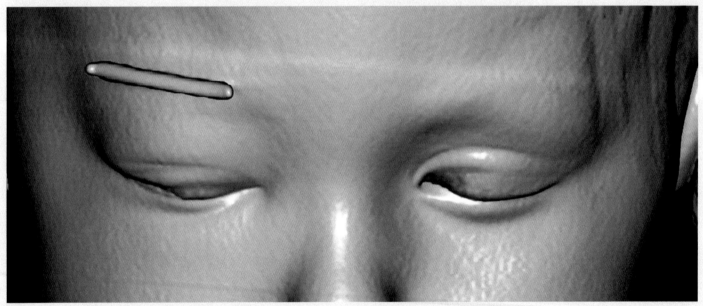

FIGURE 1. A skin surface reconstruction of the patient's periorbital region from CT images demonstrating the extent of swelling. The bar above the right eye is a CT skin marker. The CT reconstruction does not reflect skin color.

Discussion

Periorbital (preseptal) cellulitis and orbital (postseptal) cellulitis have similar clinical presentations in children, although the natural histories are likely different.[1] Periorbital cellulitis is a soft tissue infection anterior to the thin fibrous orbital septum. Orbital cellulitis is an infection of the orbital contents that typically arises from an adjacent sinus infection. A retrospective review found that 91% of orbital cellulitis cases in children were associated with sinus infections, compared with just 9% of periorbital cellulitis cases.[2] The thin medial wall of the orbit allows easy penetration of infection from the adjacent ethmoid sinus; ethmoid sinusitis was found in 86% of orbital cellulitis

cases in one study.[2] Extension of infection from the maxillary sinuses, which neighbor the orbits inferiorly, was identified in 60% of orbital cellulitis cases; a minority of cases were associated with frontal and sphenoid sinus infections.[2] Orbital cellulitis rarely arises without one of these associated conditions. Thus the common belief among physicians that periorbital cellulitis progresses to orbital cellulitis is probably a misconception. Preceding or concurrent sinusitis can suggest orbital cellulitis.

Although periorbital and orbital cellulitis share the features of periorbital edema, erythema, and fever, the two conditions can be distinguished by other signs and symptoms. Orbital cellulitis inflames and can even entrap muscles of the orbit, causing pain

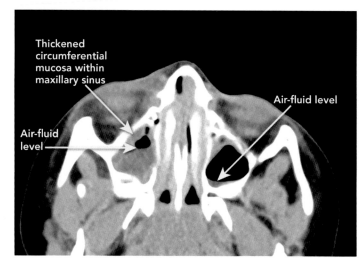

FIGURE 2. **An axial CT slice with intravenous contrast, viewed with a soft tissue window, demonstrating bilateral maxillary sinus fluid, greater in the right than in the left.** In the context of fever and nasal discharge, these findings are diagnostic of maxillary sinusitis.

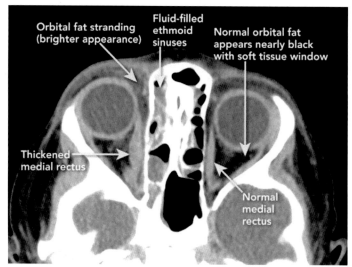

FIGURE 3. **An axial CT slice with intravenous contrast demonstrating bilateral ethmoid sinus fluid.** Given the patient's clinical symptoms, this finding is diagnostic of ethmoid sinusitis. The right orbit has abnormal inflammatory findings, including fat stranding and thickening of the right medial rectus muscle, compared to structures of the left orbit. These findings are diagnostic of orbital cellulitis.

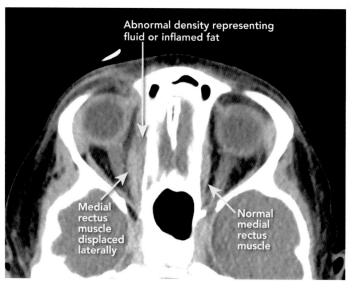

FIGURE 4. **A fluid collection medial to the right medial rectus muscle**

with eye movements and, sometimes, limitation of eye motion (leading to disconjugate gaze and diplopia from one mobile and one entrapped eye). More extreme cases of orbital cellulitis can lead to proptosis and visual impairment from pressure on the optic nerve or globe — this type of visual impairment is sometimes difficult to distinguish from complaints of visual impairment related to eyelid edema. When orbital edema increases pressure on the optic nerve or globe, the pupil of the affected eye can be sluggish, be unreactive, or demonstrate an afferent pupillary defect. These features are generally absent in periorbital cellulitis and, therefore, can aid in risk stratifying patients. Laboratory testing plays a supportive role but cannot rule out orbital cellulitis.[1]

Imaging is appropriate when orbital cellulitis is suspected, and CT of the orbits with intravenous contrast is the most appropriate and readily available test in most emergency departments. Intravenous contrast enhances structures with high blood flow and may reveal rim enhancement of an abscess. CT both without and with contrast is unnecessary and increases costs and radiation exposure without diagnostic benefit.[3] CT without intravenous contrast may be appropriate for patients with contraindications to contrast; some findings of orbital cellulitis (eg, proptosis, orbital fat stranding, and thickening or asymmetry of the orbital muscles) are still identifiable on CT without intravenous contrast.[3] Brain CT may also be indicated if the differential diagnosis includes brain abscess and complications of orbital cellulitis such as cavernous sinus thrombosis. X-rays are not indicated for suspected orbital cellulitis.[3] MRI of the orbits without and with intravenous contrast is considered equally appropriate to orbital CT with contrast by the American College of Radiology.

Normal sinus spaces are air filled and appear black on CT (using either bone or soft tissue windows), and the mucosa lining the sinuses is normally thin and barely apparent. Fluid is normally absent within healthy sinuses. Findings of orbital cellulitis are fluid and mucosal thickening of the ethmoid or maxillary sinuses, which are nearly always abnormal in cases of orbital cellulitis (*Figures 2, 3,* and *4*).[4] In fact, the absence of adjacent sinusitis on CT makes orbital cellulitis highly unlikely.[2]

When examination findings are equivocal (ie, lacking highly suggestive abnormalities such as proptosis, visual abnormalities or abnormal pupillary response, or restriction of eye movements and diplopia), empiric therapy without imaging may be appropriate. The antibiotic coverage recommended for pediatric orbital cellulitis and periorbital cellulitis is similar: agents such as amoxicillin-clavulanic acid or ampicillin-sulbactam. Methicillin-sensitive *Staphylococcus aureus* was isolated in 26% of cases, followed by *Streptococcus intermedius* (21%), *Cutibacterium* (formerly *Proprionibacterium*) *acnes* (15%), *Streptococcus pyogenes* (13%), *Streptococcus pneumoniae* (7%), and methicillin resistant *S. aureus* (5%). One-third of cases grew more than one organism.[5]

A retrospective review found that oral therapy may be as effective as intravenous therapy, but no well-controlled trials have addressed this question.[6,7] In one series, most cases of orbital cellulitis resolved without surgical intervention.[8] In another study, surgery (including sinus surgery) was performed in almost 40% of cases, perhaps reflecting practice preferences in different centers.[5]

CASE RESOLUTION

The patient was admitted and improved with intravenous antibiotics. He was discharged with a 14-day course of amoxicillin-clavulanic acid.

REFERENCES

1. Pelletier J, Koyfman A, Long B. High risk and low prevalence diseases: orbital cellulitis. *Am J Emerg Med.* 2023 Jun;68:1-9.
2. Botting AM, McIntosh D, Mahadevan M. Paediatric pre- and post-septal peri-orbital infections are different diseases. A retrospective review of 262 cases. *Int J Pediatr Otorhinolaryngol.* 2008 Mar;72(3):377-383.
3. Kennedy TA, Corey AS, Policeni B; Expert Panel on Neurologic Imaging. ACR Appropriateness Criteria® orbits vision and visual loss. *J Am Coll Radiol.* 2018 May;15(5)(supp):S116-S131.
4. Dankbaar JW, van Bemmel AJ, Pameijer FA. Imaging findings of the orbital and intracranial complications of acute bacterial rhinosinusitis. *Insights Imaging.* 2015 Oct;6(5):509-518.
5. Anosike BI, Ganapahty V, Nakamura MM. Epidemiology and management of orbital cellulitis in children. *J Pediatric Infect Dis Soc.* 2022 May 30;11(5):214-220.
6. Cannon PS, Mc Keag D, Radford R, Ataullah S, Leatherbarrow B. Our experience using primary oral antibiotics in the management of orbital cellulitis in a tertiary referral centre. *Eye (Lond).* 2009 Mar;23(3):612-615.
7. Al-Nammari S, Roberton B, Ferguson C. Towards evidence based emergency medicine: best BETs from the Manchester Royal Infirmary. Should a child with preseptal periorbital cellulitis be treated with intravenous or oral antibiotics? *Emerg Med J.* 2007 Feb;24(2):128-129.
8. Gonçalves R, Menezes C, Machado R, Ribeiro I, Lemos JA. Periorbital cellulitis in children: analysis of outcome of intravenous antibiotic therapy. *Orbit.* 2016 Aug;35(4):175-180.

Feature Editor: Joshua S. Broder, MD, FACEP. See also *Diagnostic Imaging for the Emergency Physician* (Winner of the 2011 Prose Award in Clinical Medicine, the American Publishers Award for Professional and Scholarly Excellence) and *Critical Images in Emergency Medicine* by Dr. Broder.

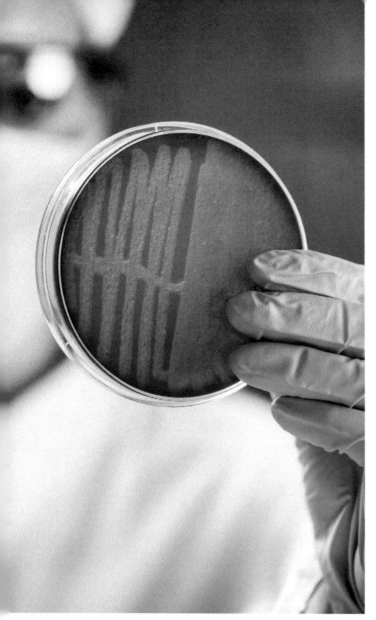

Stronger Than Ever

Organisms Resistant to Antibiotics: An Update

LESSON **22**

By Matthew Carvey, MD; and
Jonathan Glauser, MD, FACEP, MBA
Dr. Carvey is a resident at MetroHealth Medical Center and the
Cleveland Clinic. Dr. Glauser is a professor at Case Western
Reserve University School of Medicine in Cleveland, Ohio.

Reviewed by John C. Greenwood, MD, MS

Objectives

On completion of this lesson, you should be able to:

1. Describe factors that enable the development of bacterial resistance.
2. Prescribe effective therapies for MRSA infections.
3. Appraise current therapies for treating infections caused by CRE.
4. Manage the spread of VRE.
5. Compare treatment options for *N. gonorrhoeae*.
6. Practice antibiotic stewardship.

From the EM Model

10.0   Systemic Infectious Disorders
      10.8   Drug Resistance

■ CRITICAL DECISIONS ■

- When should MRSA be considered, and which strategies are effective against it?

- How can the spread of CRE be managed or prevented?

- How have VRE evolved, and how can emergency physicians contain and prevent their spread?

- How has resistant *N. gonorrhoeae* developed, and how should it be managed?

Frighteningly, some bacterial infections have become difficult or even impossible to treat with available antibiotics because the causative organisms have become resistant to historically effective therapies. To protect current and future patients from these so-called *superbugs*, emergency physicians must not only understand the current treatment options for antibiotic-resistant bacteria but also combat further resistance through judicious antibiotic stewardship.

■ CASE ONE

An 8-year-old girl without any reported immunodeficiency presents with a febrile illness, left ankle swelling, and an inability to walk. She was recently discharged 2 days after a left distal tibial fracture, with a small break in the skin that was treated with local wound care and plaster fixation. No vascular catheters are in place. Her vital signs are BP 107/66, P 164, R 38, and T 38.5°C (101.3°F); SpO$_2$ is 98% on room air. A physical examination reveals that she is tired but arousable and consolable by family. Her lungs are clear on auscultation, and she has a nontender abdomen. The cast is bivalved to expose the fracture site. She has significant pain and yellow discharge from the left distal tibia, which now appears to be open at the prior injury site. A CBC shows a leukocytosis of 27 × 10⁹/L. Her urinalysis results are negative, and her blood glucose level is 87 mg/dL on a point-of-care test.

■ CASE TWO

A 61-year-old man with a medical history of myelodysplastic syndrome was recently admitted for a stem cell transplant. On hospital day 9 after the transplant, he developed nonodorous and nonbloody diarrhea. On post-transplant day 13, the patient presents with neutropenic fever. He has no other significant medical history. He has no indwelling urinary or fecal catheter or implanted port. His vital signs include BP 105/65, P 89, R 20, and T 38.6°C (101.5°F). Physical examination findings show an arousable older man who appears unwell. His lungs are clear on auscultation, and his abdomen is nontender. He has no skin breakdown or pressure ulcers.

■ CASE THREE

A 21-year-old woman presents with dysuria and vaginal discharge of 2 days' duration. The patient states that her male partner also developed dysuria and urethral discharge. She wants to be treated for a sexually transmitted infection. She states that she and her partner usually use barrier protection but did not do so 1 week ago. The patient denies any joint pain. She has no rash or sores. A urinalysis shows no WBCs.

Introduction

Antibiotic management is essential to the practice of emergency medicine. Unfortunately, organisms are evolving and developing resistance to the antibiotics that physicians prescribe. As a result, some infections can no longer be treated with available antimicrobials. This lesson provides an update on treatment options, focusing on four organisms that have generated considerable concern in the health care community: methicillin-resistant *Staphylococcus aureus* (MRSA), carbapenem-resistant Enterobacterales (CRE), vancomycin-resistant enterococci (VRE), and resistant *Neisseria gonorrhoeae*.

CRITICAL DECISION

When should MRSA be considered, and which strategies are effective against it?

MRSA infections have been widespread for years. Resistance initially occurred among very ill hospitalized patients and then within the community. MRSA is now a major pathogen implicated in orthopedic infections and can cause an infection in nearly every other organ system.[1] It is the predominant source of skin and soft tissue infections, and it represents a significant burden to the health care system.[2] Outbreaks are especially common in certain groups of patients. Patients who were recently hospitalized or confined to nursing facilities are at high risk. Other patients at risk include those who received antibiotics during a hospital stay, were on recent steroid therapy, have a history of injection drug use, are HIV positive (especially with CD4 counts <500 cells/μL), are on hemodialysis, have diabetes mellitus, have pressure ulcers, or had prior MRSA infections.[3,4]

Rapid assays have shortened laboratory turnaround times for the diagnosis of MRSA from the traditional 48 to 96 hours. Some rapid MRSA assays use bacteriophage technology, and others use polymerase chain reaction (PCR) techniques. Nasal PCR swab results can be returned within hours. Extranasal

Oral	Parenteral
• Clindamycin	• Ceftaroline
• Doxycycline	• Daptomycin
• Linezolid	• Linezolid
• Rifampin	• Quinupristin-dalfopristin
• Trimethoprim-sulfamethoxazole	• Tigecycline
	• Vancomycin
	• Ceftobiprole*

*Currently unavailable in the United States

TABLE 1. Antibiotics with activity against MRSA

screening includes testing for MRSA in wounds, the rectum, and the axilla, with PCR results returned within as few as 2 hours.[3] For emergency departments that do not have access to rapid assays for MRSA, physical examination findings may include a wound that fails to heal over time despite treatment or a large, diffuse area of cellulitis on the skin. A history of MRSA skin infections can also increase suspicion for a current infection.

Unlike some resistant organisms, MRSA responds to multiple treatments (*Table 1*). Clindamycin, trimethoprim-sulfamethoxazole, and tetracyclines are usually effective oral treatments. MRSA is generally also susceptible to rifampin; however, because resistance to rifampin can develop rapidly, this antibiotic should be used in conjunction with another agent — rifampin monotherapy is generally not recommended. *S. aureus* species that are resistant to methicillin tend to also be resistant to other β-lactam agents. Ceftaroline, a cephalosporin that the FDA approved in 2010 for the treatment of MRSA, and ceftobiprole, which is currently not FDA approved, are exceptions.[5]

Intravenous antibiotics that are generally effective for MRSA include clindamycin, vancomycin, and ceftaroline. Vancomycin can be given at 0.5 to 2 g every 6 to 8 hours, but the dosage varies by patient and clinical status (eg, renal function). Culture data will often include antibiotic sensitivities and effectiveness (minimum inhibitory concentration [MIC]). When the vancomycin MIC is greater than 1 µg/mL, other agents such as daptomycin may be more effective.[6] However, daptomycin is not effective for pulmonary infections; alternative therapy should be considered in these cases. Other agents effective against MRSA include tigecycline and linezolid. Limitations to linezolid include thrombocytopenia, serotonin syndrome, lactic acidosis, and peripheral neuropathy. Rifampin has been evaluated as an adjunct treatment for MRSA infections. The ARREST trial demonstrated that adjunctive rifampin provides no overall benefit over standard antibiotic therapy in adults with MRSA bacteremia.[7] However, it currently remains an acceptable alternative therapy.

Most skin abscesses — including those caused by MRSA — can be cured with adequate surgical drainage alone. For simple, drainable abscesses less than 5 cm in diameter in nontoxic, afebrile patients, antibiotic therapy is not required to meet the standard of care.[8]

Health care professionals should take precautions when interacting with patients infected with MRSA. Standard precautions against MRSA include gowns and gloves during all contact with infected patients and their environment — and certainly for wound drainage.

CRITICAL DECISION

How can the spread of CRE be managed or prevented?

Pathogens in the order Enterobacterales are among the most common in humans. They have been implicated in meningitis, peritonitis, pneumonia, cystitis, and bacteremia.[9] A variety of Enterobacterales pathogens have developed antibiotic resistance, including *Enterobacter* species, *Escherichia coli*, and *Klebsiella pneumoniae*. Carbapenemases are enzymes that destroy all β-lactam antibiotics, including carbapenems, which have a broad antimicrobial spectrum. *K. pneumoniae* carbapenemase (KPC) is the most frequently encountered carbapenemase, but there are other CRE organisms that carry a carbapenemase. Carbapenem-resistant *K. pneumoniae* (CRKP) was first reported in the northeast United States in the early 2000s and has since spread across the country.[10]

KPC is the most prevalent extended-spectrum β-lactamase, at a 47% to 90% prevalence in the United States.[11] Newer enzymes that confer resistance are the metallo-β lactamases, named for the presence of zinc at their active site to facilitate hydrolysis. Exposure to a health care setting, mechanical ventilation, and antimicrobials are among the prominent risk factors for infections with CRE.[12] Recent exposure to carbapenems, cephalosporins, fluoroquinolones, and vancomycin also increase the risk of CRE infections.

CRE were uncommon in the United States before 1992. Imipenem resistance was first reported in 2004 and reached a 4.3% prevalence by 2010. Despite combination antibiotic therapy, the mortality rate of infections with CRE is 23.5%, representing significantly high clinical failure rates.[11] One review of CRKP studied 40 patients from acute and long-term care hospitals. Patients were generally older adults with multiple comorbidities. Among this group, 11 patients died during the

Antibiotics
• Aminoglycosides: gentamicin and amikacin
• Colistin
• Doxycycline
• Tigecycline
• Ceftazidime-avibactam
• Meropenem-vaborbactam
• Plazomicin
• Eravacycline

TABLE 2. **Antibiotics with potential use against CRE**

index hospitalization, 23 were discharged to nursing homes, and only 4 were discharged home. Patients with CRE genitourinary or bloodstream infections were often incontinent and exposed to multiple medical devices.[13]

The potential to spread CRE via orofecal contact means that all individuals, including healthy community members, are potential carriers of CRE — possibly for years. So far, CRE have mainly infected the chronically ill. Risk factors for CRE acquisition include recent exposure to a health care setting, admission to a long-term care facility, an immunocompromised status, recent urinary catheterization, recent mechanical ventilation, dialysis, and previous antibiotic use. Some patients are clearly more at risk, such as solid-organ transplant recipients and those receiving bone marrow transplantation or chemotherapy.

Treatment options for CRE include aminoglycosides, such as amikacin or polymyxin, which are potentially nephrotoxic. Moreover, reports of polymyxin-resistant strains of *Klebsiella* have emerged. Doxycycline can be effective for mild CRKP infections, such as urinary tract infections (UTIs) in well-appearing patients. The most common antimicrobials for treating CRE are a polymyxin backbone coupled with targeted antibiotic therapy or in a triple combination with a carbapenem, rifampin, or tigecycline.[14-17] As of 2023, Enterobacterales remain susceptible to colistin and tigecycline. However, resistance to tigecycline monotherapy is emerging.[18] Since 2015, the FDA has approved four new CRE-directed antimicrobials: ceftazidime-avibactam (2015), meropenem-vaborbactam (2017), plazomicin (2018), and eravacycline (2018) (*Table 2*).[19]

✔ Pearls

- Antibiotic use collectively contributes to the development of antibiotic-resistant microbes.

- Shortening the duration of antimicrobial therapy can help decrease bacterial resistance without affecting treatment efficacy.

- Removal of intravascular or urinary catheters can cure UTIs in some cases.

- Using antibiotics with a narrow spectrum and that target a specific organism can prevent the emergence of bacterial resistance.

CDC guidelines for monitoring and controlling the spread of CRE are[20]:
- Follow good hand hygiene. Wash hands with soap and water or use a waterless, alcohol-based hand rub before and after patient contact.
- Use contact precautions. Wear a gown and gloves when in contact with colonized or infected sites or body fluids. Predictors of future rectal CRE carriage include exposure to antimicrobials (especially fluoroquinolones), admission from another health care facility, and a span of less than 3 months from the first positive CRE test.
- Implement health care personnel education. Contaminated equipment can spread CRE.
- Minimize devices used during routine patient care. Central venous catheters, endotracheal intubation, and urinary catheters can spread CRE.
- Form patient and staff cohorts. Infected patients should be placed in the same area away from noninfected patients. Noninfected patients should each have their own room.
- Notify the laboratory and infection prevention staff immediately when CRE are detected.
- Practice antimicrobial stewardship. Use antibiotics only for appropriate indications and durations. Use the narrowest antibiotic spectrum that can effectively treat the target organism.
- Ensure the duration of antimicrobial therapy is appropriate, which can also help decrease bacterial resistance without affecting treatment efficacy.
- Screen for CRE. Screen patient contacts and epidemiologically linked patients.

Clinical care facilities should review culture results from the preceding 6 to 12 months to determine whether previously unrecognized CRE have been present. High-risk units such as ICUs may be the initial source. Surveillance cultures taken from the perianal or rectal site are usually the most productive. Antimicrobial stewardship should be directed at decreasing the use of antimicrobials and medical devices such as indwelling urinary catheters.

CRITICAL DECISION

How have VRE evolved, and how can emergency physicians contain and prevent their spread?

Hospital-acquired infections with VRE are increasingly common. VRE are among the major nosocomial antimicrobial-resistant pathogens globally. VRE were first reported in the 1980s in Europe and have been found in medical, pediatric, and ICU settings in the United States for many years since.[21] VRE have been associated with bacteremia, endocarditis, meningitis, UTIs, wound infections, and infected central venous lines. These bacteria can spread from hands or gloves of health care workers and from environmental surfaces. Tympanic thermometers, rectal thermometers, bed rails, bedside tables, and ECG leads are all at risk of colonization.

Resistance varies by the isolate. Most VRE isolates are *Enterococcus faecium*. More than 60% of *E. faecium* isolates have shown vancomycin resistance; lower rates of resistance have been found for *Enterococcus faecalis* isolates. Although *E. faecalis* is less common and, apparently, less lethal in patients with enterococcal bacteremia, it appears to have a much greater inclination to

Antibiotics
• Ceftriaxone
• Daptomycin
• Gentamicin (high resistance has been reported)
• Imipenem (*E. faecalis*)
• Lefamulin
• Linezolid
• Nitrofurantoin, fosfomycin, ampicillin, or amoxicillin (each given as monotherapy to treat UTIs)
• Quinupristin-dalfopristin
• Rifampin
• Streptomycin
• Teicoplanin*
• Telavancin (skin infections)
• Tigecycline

*Currently unavailable in the United States

TABLE 3. Antibiotics that may be active against VRE

transfer the determinant for vancomycin resistance to *S. aureus*. Surveillance cultures are usually obtained from rectal or perirectal swabs or stool samples. Cultures can also be obtained from draining wounds and areas of skin breakdown.

Risk factors for VRE colonization and infection include prior antimicrobial therapy, exposure to contaminated surfaces, residence in long-term care facilities, and decubitus ulcers. Cephalosporin, antianaerobic, and vancomycin exposure increase the risk of a later VRE infection. Underlying medical conditions such as cancer, end-stage renal disease and dialysis, organ transplantation, and conditions that require ICU care also pose a risk of VRE infection. The risk of colonization and infection increases with greater levels of daily exposure to VRE, including the number of colonized patients within the same unit.

Prevention, control, and eradication strategies for VRE include:
- Practice good hand hygiene. Use antimicrobial soaps with chlorhexidine and alcohol-based hand rubs.
- Use contact precautions, including wearing a gown and gloves.
- Practice antimicrobial stewardship.
- Isolate or cohort VRE carriers.
- Improve environmental cleaning and decontamination of equipment.
- If all other measures fail, temporarily close affected units.

Appropriate treatment of an antibiotic-resistant enterococcal infection depends on the site of the infection. Antibiotic therapy for VRE may be institution dependent. Treatment decisions generally vary according to local resistance patterns and occur in concert with an infectious disease service (*Table 3*). VRE-associated UTIs may still respond to ampicillin, nitrofurantoin, fosfomycin, amoxicillin, or simply removal of the infective indwelling foley catheter, when feasible. Treatment for endocarditis may require combination therapy (eg, daptomycin, gentamicin, or ampicillin) or necessitate valve replacement. Linezolid, daptomycin, and tigecycline are also active against many strains of *E. faecium* and *E. faecalis*. Tigecycline can be given instead of daptomycin if the patient has renal insufficiency. Quinupristin-dalfopristin remains active against most strains of vancomycin-resistant *E. faecium*, but resistance patterns

Antibiotic	Dosage	Organisms	Adverse Effects	Notes
Aztreonam	UTI: 500-1,000 mg every 8-12 hr Severe infections: up to 2 g every 6-8 hr; lower dosage for decreased renal function	Gram-negative aerobic bacteria, such as *P. aeruginosa*	Cough, neutropenia, *Clostridioides difficile*–associated diarrhea, and toxic epidermal necrolysis	Pregnancy category B
Ceftaroline	Parenteral cephalosporin with half-life of 2-3 hr 600 mg IV every 12 hr Lower range for renal insufficiency	*S. aureus*, including MRSA and vancomycin-intermediate and vancomycin-resistant *S. aureus* *E. faecalis*, but not *E. faecium*	Positive Coombs test, *C. difficile*–associated diarrhea, renal failure, and hyperkalemia	Pregnancy category B Caution with history of penicillin/cephalosporin/carbapenem allergy (angioedema, urticarial, or anaphylaxis reaction with β-lactams) May enhance warfarin's anticoagulant effect
Colistin/colistimethate	2.5-5 mg/kg per day in 2-4 divided doses Lower doses for renal insufficiency	Resistant gram-negative infections (eg, *Pseudomonas aeruginosa* and *Acinetobacter*)	Bronchospasm, nephrotoxicity, slurred speech, and vertigo	Pregnancy category C
Daptomycin	Half-life of 8 hr Skin and soft tissue infections: 4 mg/kg IV once daily for 7-14 days Bacteremia, osteomyelitis: 6 mg/kg daily	Enterococci including VRE Staphylococci (MRSA or methicillin sensitive *S. aureus*)	Anemia, neutropenia (reversible on discontinuation), edema, chest pain, hypokalemia, nausea, abdominal pain, *C. difficile*–associated diarrhea, eosinophilic pneumonia, and myopathy/elevated creatine phosphokinase	Pregnancy category B
Fosfomycin	Uncomplicated UTI: 3 g, once Complicated UTI, prostatitis: 3 g every 3 days for 21 days	*E. coli* and *E. faecalis*	*C. difficile*–associated diarrhea, angioedema, hepatic necrosis, headache, vaginitis, optic neuritis, and aplastic anemia	Pregnancy category B
Linezolid	Half-life of 5-7 hr Adult: 600 mg PO or IV every 12 hr No renal dose adjustment	MRSA Enterococci including VRE Multidrug-resistant *S. pneumoniae*	Thrombocytopenia, pancreatitis, decreased hemoglobin, *C. difficile*–associated diarrhea, rhabdomyolysis, serotonin syndrome, lactic acidosis, myelosuppression, and optic neuropathy	Pregnancy category C
Polymyxin B	15,000 to 25,000 units/kg per day, divided every 12 hr Reduce for renal impairment	*P. aeruginosa* CRE	Facial flushing, weakness/neuromuscular blockade, nephrotoxicity, ataxia, and respiratory paralysis	
Quinupristin-dalfopristin	7.5 mg/kg IV every 12 hr Central catheter required due to phlebitis	MRSA, including vancomycin failure *E. faecium*, not *E. faecalis*	Hyperbilirubinemia, pain at infusion site, mesenteric artery occlusion, pancreatitis, pancytopenia, paraplegia, and *C. difficile*–associated diarrhea	Pregnancy category B
Tigecycline	100 mg IV initially, then 50 mg every 12 hr	MRSA and methicillin-susceptible isolates CRE Other gram-positive and gram-negative infections	Phlebitis, hyponatremia, pancreatitis, *C. difficile*–associated diarrhea, and hepatic failure Increases concentration of warfarin Structurally similar to tetracyclines (photosensitivity)	Pregnancy category D Use in patients older than 8 yr

Only the side effects of greatest concern in emergency medicine are listed. Dosages are within the suggested range only and can be modified based on individual patient characteristics in consultation with infectious disease specialists.

TABLE 4. Antibiotics effective against resistant infections

are emerging. Imipenem has some activity against *E. faecalis*. Telavancin is approved for the treatment of some skin infections caused by susceptible gram-positive bacteria and has activity against enterococci.[22] Lefamulin is an emerging FDA-approved pleuromutilin that binds the 50S ribosomal subunit and has activity against VRE (*Table 4*).[23]

CRITICAL DECISION

How has resistant *N. gonorrhoeae* developed, and how should it be managed?

The global incidence of gonorrhea in 2016 was 20/1000 women and 26/1000 men, translating to 86.9 million new cases that year.[24] In 2017, an estimated 5,548 cases of gonorrhea per 100,000 men who have sex with men (MSM) were reported, according to a survey of 16 major US metropolitan areas.[25] *N. gonorrhoeae* has historically developed resistance to antibiotics rather quickly (*Table 5*). Treatment options for gonorrhea are now limited to dual therapy with third-generation cephalosporins in combination with azithromycin. Combination therapy remains the standard of treatment. In the United States, *N. gonorrhoeae* isolates with intermediate resistance and infections that fail to respond to CDC-recommended therapies must be reported. Decreasing cephalosporin susceptibility has been observed.

As of 2023, the CDC has not received reports of verified clinical treatment failures for gonococcal infections treated with a cephalosporin in the United States. Previous reports of treatment failures were ultimately determined to be reinfections. One case of dual therapy failure was reported in 2016. Gentamicin 240 mg IV or IM in combination with azithromycin is an emerging alternative to the combination of ceftriaxone and azithromycin. However, gentamicin with azithromycin remains inferior to the standard treatment of ceftriaxone with azithromycin.[26] Cefixime 800 mg PO remains an option for uncomplicated gonorrhea.[27] Current guidelines recommend 250 to 500 mg of ceftriaxone IM, along with azithromycin 1 g PO to cover other pathogens such as chlamydia. Doxycycline and cefixime can be used in uncomplicated cases of gonorrhea. Zoliflodacin is another emerging antimicrobial option.[28] In cases of cephalosporin allergy, azithromycin 2 g PO can be used. However, cases of gonorrhea with high levels of resistance to azithromycin have been identified.

Antibiotics
• Cefixime
• Ciprofloxacin
• Other fluoroquinolones
• Penicillins
• Sulfanilamide
• Tetracyclines
• Spectinomycin*

*Currently unavailable in the United States

TABLE 5. Antibiotics that are ineffective against *N. gonorrhoeae*

Current nucleic acid amplification tests do not detect genetic markers of cephalosporin-resistant gonorrhea. In cases of treatment failure, culture-based methods are needed for antimicrobial susceptibility testing. Therefore, patients who return with persistent or recurrent symptoms after being tested with non–culture-based methods should be retested for gonorrhea by culture. Treatment failure can represent reinfection. However, emergency physicians must maintain a high level of suspicion for gonococcal resistance, especially in MSM, cases from the West Coast or Hawaii, and patients who were recently treated with cefixime. Because of its developing resistance, other treatment options for gonococcal infection have been investigated. Spectinomycin showed similar cure rates to that of ceftriaxone in one report, but this drug is unavailable in the United States.[29] If new treatment strategies, drugs, or possibly vaccines for gonorrhea are not developed, the infection may become untreatable.

Summary

Development of microbial resistance to antibiotics has been well-documented for years. Addressing this problem likely requires several strategies, only some of which are under the control of emergency physicians. The strategies that can be controlled include curbing unnecessary antibiotic use and more closely targeting specific bacterial agents. Unlike CRE, VRE, and resistant gonorrhea, MRSA infection can be treated with available agents. Public policy changes on patent life and market exclusivity may be needed to encourage the development of new antibiotics.

✖ Pitfalls

- Prescribing antibiotics for nonbacterial infections.

- Selecting antibiotics with a broader spectrum than needed for a given infection.

- Failing to practice standard hand hygiene.

- Prescribing antibiotics after drainage of an uncomplicated abscess smaller than 5 cm.

- Using invasive devices (eg, urinary catheters) too broadly.

- Delaying removal of invasive devices.

REFERENCES

1. Ribau AI, Collins JE, Chen AF, Sousa RJ. Is preoperative *Staphylococcus aureus* screening and decolonization effective at reducing surgical site infection in patients undergoing orthopedic surgery? A systematic review and meta-analysis with a special focus on elective total joint arthroplasty. *J Arthroplasty*. 2021 Feb;36(2):752-766.e6.

2. Hindy JR, Haddad SF, Kanj SS. New drugs for methicillin-resistant *Staphylococcus aureus* skin and soft tissue infections. *Curr Opin Infect Dis*. 2022 Apr 1;35(2):112-119.

3. Rebmann T, Aureden K; Association for Professionals in Infection Control and Epidemiology. Preventing methicillin-resistant *Staphylococcus aureus* transmission in long-term care facilities: an executive summary of the APIC Elimination Guide. *Am J Infect Control*. 2011 Apr;39(3):235-238.

4. Torres K, Sampathkumar P. Predictors of methicillin-resistant *Staphylococcus aureus* colonization at hospital admission. *Am J Infect Control*. 2013 Nov;41(11):1043-1047.

■ CASE ONE

The girl underwent blood and wound culture testing for a suspected MRSA infection. Results of the initial blood cultures came back positive for MRSA bacteremia, with the wound culture growing the same organism. The initial treatment with vancomycin failed; the organism was found to be resistant on culture sensitivities. However, combination therapy with linezolid and rifampicin exhibited a good response. The orthopedic team completed surgical debridement of the left distal tibia and regularly changed the dressings. The patient was discharged after 1 week of hospitalization, when she was able to walk with assistance. At a follow-up visit 1 week later, she had no discharge from the left tibial surgical site, her fever had cleared, and her mental status had returned to baseline.

■ CASE TWO

The man had a workup for febrile neutropenia secondary to a stem cell transplant, including blood and urine cultures. He was started on cefepime and vancomycin for presumed febrile neutropenia. Blood cultures were positive for VRE. Vancomycin was discontinued, and daptomycin was started. On hospital day 15, the patient developed progressive septic shock. His antibiotics were broadened further from cefepime to meropenem. On hospital day 17, he developed progressive multi-organ failure, and after discussion with the family, his goals of care were changed to comfort care only. The patient later died.

■ CASE THREE

The woman underwent nucleic acid amplification testing for gonorrhea and chlamydia by urine specimen. An endocervical specimen was also collected. Results of these tests came back positive for gonorrhea and negative for chlamydia on day 2. She returned to the emergency department and was treated with 250 mg of ceftriaxone and 1 g of oral azithromycin. The patient was discharged with instructions to use barrier protection during sex. On day 3, the endocervical specimen returned positive for azithromycin-resistant gonococci. At a scheduled followed-up visit with her primary care physician on day 5, she reported decreased vaginal discharge and dysuria. No further treatment was discussed, and the patient was educated on dual antibiotic therapy for azithromycin-resistant gonococci.

5. Watkins RR, Holubar M, David MZ. Antimicrobial resistance in methicillin-resistant *Staphylococcus aureus* to newer antimicrobial agents. *Antimicrob Agents Chemother.* 2019 Sep 9;63(12):e01216-19.

6. Murray KP, Zhao JJ, Davis SL, et al. Early use of daptomycin versus vancomycin for methicillin-resistant *Staphylococcus aureus* bacteremia with vancomycin minimum inhibitory concentration >1 mg/L: a matched cohort study. *Clin Infect Dis.* 2013 Jun;56(11):1562-1569.

7. Thwaites GE, Scarborough M, Szubert A, et al; United Kingdom Clinical Infection Research Group. Adjunctive rifampicin for *Staphylococcus aureus* bacteraemia (ARREST): a multicentre, randomised, double-blind, placebo-controlled trial. *Lancet.* 2018 Feb 17;391(10121):668-678.

8. Talan DA. Lack of antibiotic efficacy for simple abscesses: have matters come to a head? *Ann Emerg Med.* 2010 May;55(5):412-414.

9. Schwaber MJ, Carmeli Y. Carbapenem-resistant Enterobacteriaceae: a potential threat. *JAMA.* 2008 Dec 24;300(24):2911-2913.

10. Park SO, Liu J, Furuya EY, Larson EL. Carbapenem-resistant *Klebsiella pneumoniae* infection in three New York City hospitals trended downwards from 2006 to 2014. *Open Forum Infect Dis.* 2016 Dec 2;3(4):ofw222.

11. Cury AP, Girardello R, Duarte AJDS, Rossi F. KPC-producing Enterobacterales with uncommon carbapenem susceptibility profile in Vitek 2 system. *Int J Infect Dis.* 2020 Apr;93:118-120.

12. Gupta N, Limbago BM, Patel JB, Kallen AJ. Carbapenem-resistant Enterobacteriaceae: epidemiology and prevention. *Clin Infect Dis.* 2011 Jul 1;53(1):60-67.

13. Kontopidou F, Giamarellou H, Katerelos P, et al; Group for the Study of KPC-producing *Klebsiella pneumoniae* infections in intensive care units. Infections caused by carbapenem-resistant *Klebsiella pneumoniae* among patients in intensive care units in Greece: a multi-centre study on clinical outcome and therapeutic options. *Clin Microbiol Infect.* 2014 Feb;20(2):O117-O123.

14. Smith HZ, Kendall B. Carbapenem resistant Enterobacteriaceae. In: *StatPearls [Internet].* StatPearls Publishing; 2023. https://www.ncbi.nlm.nih.gov/books/NBK551704/

15. Lee J, Patel G, Huprikar S, Calfee DP, Jenkins SG. Decreased susceptibility to polymyxin B during treatment for carbapenem-resistant *Klebsiella pneumoniae* infection. *J Clin Microbiol.* 2009 May;47(5):1611-1612.

16. Gomez-Simmonds A, Nelson B, Eiras DP, et al. Combination regimens for treatment of carbapenem-resistant *Klebsiella pneumoniae* bloodstream infections. *Antimicrob Agents Chemother.* 2016 May 23;60(6):3601-3607.

17. Lee GC, Burgess DS. Treatment of *Klebsiella pneumoniae* carbapenemase (KPC) infections: a review of published case series and case reports. *Ann Clin Microbiol Antimicrob.* 2012 Dec 13;11:32.

18. Morrill HJ, Pogue JM, Kaye KS, LaPlante KL. Treatment options for carbapenem-resistant Enterobacteriaceae infections. *Open Forum Infect Dis.* 2015 May 5;2(2):ofv050.

19. Lutgring JD. Carbapenem-resistant Enterobacteriaceae: an emerging bacterial threat. *Semin Diagn Pathol.* 2019 May;36(3):182-186.

20. National Center for Emerging and Zoonotic Infectious Diseases, Division of Healthcare Quality Promotion. Facility guidance for control of carbapenem-resistant Enterobacteriaceae (CRE). November 2015 update — CRE toolkit. CDC. Published November 2015. https://stacks.cdc.gov/view/cdc/79104

21. Karanfil LV, Murphy M, Josephson A, et al. A cluster of vancomycin-resistant *Enterococcus faecium* in an intensive care unit. *Infect Control Hosp Epidemiol.* 1992 Apr;13(4):195-200.

22. Krause KM, Renelli M, Difuntorum S, Wu TX, Debabov DV, Benton BM. In vitro activity of telavancin against resistant gram-positive bacteria. *Antimicrob Agents Chemother.* 2008 Jul;52(7):2647-2652.

23. Gould IM, Gunasekera C, Khan A. Antibacterials in the pipeline and perspectives for the near future. *Curr Opin Pharmacol.* 2019 Oct;48:69-75.

24. Kirkcaldy RD, Weston E, Segurado AC, Hughes G. Epidemiology of gonorrhea: a global perspective. *Sex Health.* 2019 Sep;16(5):401-411.

25. Yaesoubi R, Cohen T, Hsu K, et al. Evaluating spatially adaptive guidelines for the treatment of gonorrhea to reduce the incidence of gonococcal infection and increase the effective lifespan of antibiotics. *PLoS Comput Biol.* 2022 Feb;18(2):e1009842.

26. Hazra A, Collison MW, Davis AM. CDC sexually transmitted infections treatment guidelines, 2021. *JAMA.* 2022 Mar 1;327(9):870-871.

27. Yang F, Yan J. Antibiotic resistance and treatment options for multidrug-resistant gonorrhea. *Infect Microbes Dis.* 2020 Jun;2(2):67-76.

28. Bai ZG, Bao XJ, Cheng WD, Yang KH, Li YP. Efficacy and safety of ceftriaxone for uncomplicated gonorrhoea: a meta-analysis of randomized controlled trials. *Int J STD AIDS.* 2012 Feb;23(2):126-132.

29. Unemo M, Shafer WM. Antimicrobial resistance in *Neisseria gonorrhoeae* in the 21st century: past, evolution, and future. *Clin Microbiol Rev.* 2014 Jul;27(3):587-613.

CME Questions

Reviewed by **Ann M. Dietrich, MD, FACEP, FAAP; and John C. Greenwood, MD, MS**

Qualified, paid subscribers to *Critical Decisions in Emergency Medicine* may receive CME certificates for up to 5 ACEP Category I credits, 5 *AMA PRA Category 1 Credits™*, and 5 AOA Category 2-B credits for completing this activity in its entirety. Submit your answers online at acep.org/cdem; a score of 75% or better is required. You may receive credit for completing the CME activity any time within 3 years of its publication date. Answers to this month's questions will be published in next month's issue.

1 A 1-year-old boy presents after a motor vehicle collision. The child was improperly restrained, sitting in his parent's lap in the back passenger seat. In response to pain, the patient is opening his eyes, crying, and withdrawing. What is his Glasgow Coma Scale score?

   A.   7
   B.   8
   C.   9
   D.   10

2 A 4-year-old girl presents after falling off a 2-foot-tall stool. Her mother states that the child appears to feel well, has not lost consciousness, and is at her neurologic baseline. Other than a frontal scalp hematoma, the patient's physical examination is reassuring. What is the next step for managing this patient?

   A.   Discharge home
   B.   Head CT scan
   C.   Nonaccidental trauma workup
   D.   Observation

3 A 14-month-old boy presents after a rollover motor vehicle collision. The patient was restrained in a weight-appropriate car seat in the back seat. His eyes are open, and he is looking around the room. He is inconsolably crying and moving all extremities spontaneously. His vital signs are stable. What is the next step in his management?

   A.   Discharge home with parents
   B.   Head CT scan
   C.   Observation
   D.   Skull x-ray

4 Which finding is concerning for a basilar skull fracture?

   A.   Epistaxis
   B.   Hematemesis
   C.   Postauricular ecchymosis
   D.   Proptosis

5 A 6-week-old boy presents after rolling and falling out of his cradle, according to his caregiver. The patient has a Glasgow Coma Scale score of 15. On examination, he has a soft, flat fontanel and pupils that are reactive and equal in size. He is moving all extremities spontaneously. On fundoscopy, bleeding in the retina is found. What is the best next step?

   A.   Discharge home with strict return precautions
   B.   Nonaccidental trauma workup
   C.   Observation
   D.   Ophthalmology consultation

6 A 6-year-old girl with no medical history presents after a fall from a second-story balcony. On arrival, the patient is alert and oriented. Her eyes open spontaneously, and she can follow commands. The decision is made to observe the patient in the emergency department. One hour into the patient's stay, she begins to have multiple episodes of vomiting and displays behavioral changes. What is the best next course of action?

   A.   Administer 2 mg ondansetron, orally dissolving tablet
   B.   Consult neurosurgery
   C.   Order a head CT scan
   D.   Restart the observation period

7 A 2-year-old boy presents after crawling out of his crib and falling a height of 3 feet. The fall was unwitnessed, but his mother thinks he hit his head. She reports that the child started crying immediately and never lost consciousness. He is well appearing, without an altered mental status. On examination, the patient has a small abrasion on his left arm but no focal neurologic deficits. No hematoma or points of tenderness are found on his head. He is observed in the emergency room for 4 hours. When the physician returns to the room, the boy is smiling and continues to be well appearing. What is the best next step?

   A.   Administer an oral challenge
   B.   Discharge the patient
   C.   Order a head CT scan
   D.   Repeat the neurologic examination

8 A 14-year-old girl presents after her head was hit by an opponent's elbow in a basketball game. The patient was hit during a jump for a rebound play. She did not lose consciousness. The patient reports initially having only a headache, later followed by one vomiting episode while she was sitting on the bench. On physical examination, she has no focal neurologic deficits, is sensitive to light, and reports she is nauseated. She is observed for several hours in the emergency department, where she tolerates crackers. Her repeat neurologic examination is normal. The physician decides to discharge the patient home. Which symptom would warrant a prompt return to the emergency department?

   A.   Anxiety
   B.   Difficulty concentrating at school the next day
   C.   Headache the next day
   D.   Left lower-extremity weakness

9 A 16-year-old girl arrives after colliding with her teammate during a volleyball game 3 hours ago. The patient reports confusion, a posterior headache, and one episode of vomiting. She remembers the event. The physician suspects a concussion. Which imaging study can confirm a concussion?

- A. Brain MRI scan
- B. Head CT scan
- C. No imaging study
- D. Skull x-ray

10 When should a neurology consultation be considered for a child with a concussion?

- A. When the child also has a history of seizures
- B. When the child has a Glasgow Coma Scale score of 14
- C. When the child has had multiple concussions
- D. When the child loses consciousness after the traumatic event

11 Which antibiotic is most likely to be effective against a methicillin-resistant Staphylococcus aureus infection?

- A. Cephalexin
- B. Clindamycin
- C. Nafcillin
- D. Oxacillin

12 Which choice indicates the greatest risk of infection with carbapenem-resistant Enterobacterales?

- A. Decubitus ulcer
- B. Exposure to contaminated surfaces
- C. Pyelonephritis in a previously healthy young patient
- D. Treatment with meropenem in the past 3 months

13 Which antibiotic is most likely to be effective for treating carbapenem-resistant Enterobacterales?

- A. Azithromycin
- B. Colistin
- C. Mupirocin
- D. Vancomycin

14 What is a vancomycin-resistant enterococcal infection most likely to be associated with?

- A. Infected central venous line
- B. Pharyngitis
- C. Pneumonia
- D. Sexually transmitted infection

15 Which choice is a risk factor for a vancomycin-resistant enterococcal infection?

- A. End-stage renal disease
- B. Isolating colonized patients in a separate ward
- C. No antibiotic therapy in the past 12 months
- D. Use of alcohol-based hand rubs

16 Which abscess is most likely to heal without antibiotic therapy if surgically drained?

- A. Abscess in an infant younger than 3 months
- B. Abscess larger than 5 cm in a febrile patient
- C. Abscess smaller than 5 cm in a patient who is nontoxic and afebrile
- D. Abscess with significant surrounding cellulitis

17 Which strategy is recommended for preventing vancomycin-resistant enterococcal infections?

- A. Hand hygiene with antimicrobial soaps with chlorhexidine and alcohol-based hand rubs
- B. Immunization against Enterococcus
- C. Routine stool cultures of emergency department patients
- D. Widespread use of N95 respirators

18 Which treatment is included in the treatment guidelines for Neisseria gonorrhoeae infection?

- A. Ceftriaxone and azithromycin
- B. Ciprofloxacin
- C. Intramuscular penicillin with probenecid
- D. Sulfa drugs such as sulfamethoxazole

19 Which strategy constitutes appropriate antimicrobial stewardship?

- A. Broad use of germ-resistant bed rails and IV poles
- B. Incentivizing pharmaceutical companies to develop new and effective antibiotics
- C. Withholding antibiotics from febrile toxic patients pending culture and sensitivity results
- D. Withholding antibiotics if a disease is not thought to be caused by a bacterial infection; limiting antibiotics to the narrowest spectrum needed to treat a specific infection

20 Which antibiotic is a novel treatment option for resistant Neisseria gonorrhoeae infection?

- A. Daptomycin
- B. Fosfomycin
- C. Linezolid
- D. Zoliflodacin

ANSWER KEY FOR OCTOBER 2023, VOLUME 37, NUMBER 10

1	2	3	4	5	6	7	8	9	10	11	12	13	14	15	16	17	18	19	20
B	B	C	A	A	B	D	D	B	A	D	D	D	D	C	C	B	C	C	B

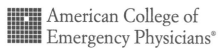
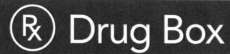

Drug Box

Methylnaltrexone for OIC

Hunter Hoopes, DO; and Frank LoVecchio, DO, MPH, FACEP
Valleywise Health Medical Center and ASU, Phoenix, Arizona

Objective
On completion of this column, you should be able to:
- Discuss the benefits of methylnaltrexone for OIC.

Methylnaltrexone, a quaternary derivative of naltrexone, is an FDA-approved medication for the treatment of chronic opioid-induced constipation (OIC). Methylnaltrexone's efficacy has been documented in patients with cancer and terminal illness. Although documentation of its use in the emergency department is sparse, its relatively rapid onset (~2 hr) makes it a useful adjunct for patients with refractory OIC who have failed conventional treatments, such as laxatives, enemas, and disimpaction. The literature suggests that patients experience significant relief from OIC after a single dose compared with placebo.[1]

Methylnaltrexone cannot cross the blood-brain barrier and, thus, counteracts the undesired effects of itching and constipation without affecting the pain relief that opioids provide.[2] Cost can be a barrier. The subcutaneous solution (12 mg/0.6 mL) is around $172, and a 90-day supply of 150-mg tablets costs more than $2,000.

Mechanism of Action
Methylnaltrexone binds to receptors in the gut, blocking the peripheral effects of opioids on the GI tract while sparing their central analgesic effects.

Pharmacokinetics (Metabolism)
- Conjugation in the liver by sulfotransferase isoforms and aldo-keto reductase into methylnaltrexone sulfate and methyl-6-naltrexol
- Majority excreted unchanged through the kidneys and GI tract
- Half-life elimination: 15 hr
- Time to peak in serum:
  - Tablets: 3.5 hr (1.5 hr fasting);
  - Parenteral: 0.5 hr, SQ or IV (off label)

Side Effects
Abdominal pain (4%), diarrhea (3%), hyperhidrosis (2%), headache (1%), and vomiting (1%) are most commonly reported. Use should be avoided in patients with known or suspected obstruction because of the risk of perforation. Symptoms of opioid withdrawal, including chills, anxiety, and yawning, can occur but are uncommon.

Dosage (in Adults)
- 450-mg tablet once daily
- 12 mg SQ once daily

Pediatric and Pregnancy Categories
Methylnaltrexone has not been studied in pediatric or pregnant populations, but animal studies suggest that it has no effect on organogenesis in rats and rabbits.

REFERENCES
1. Peacock WF, Slatkin NE, Israel RJ, Stambler N. First-dose efficacy of methylnaltrexone in patients with severe medical illness and opioid-induced constipation: a pooled analysis. *J Emerg Med.* 2022 Feb;62(2):231-239.
2. Methylnaltrexone prescribing information. Salix Pharmaceuticals. Revised April 2020. https://shared.salix.com/shared/pi/relistor-pi.pdf?id=811664a

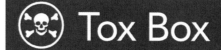

Tox Box

Colchicine Toxicity

By Christian A. Tomaszewski, MD, MS, MBA, FACEP
University of California San Diego Health

Objective
On completion of this column, you should be able to:
- List treatment recommendations for colchicine overdose.

Introduction
Colchicine, commonly prescribed for gout and pericarditis, has a narrow therapeutic index. Repeated or excessive oral dosing can progress to multisystem organ failure and death days after exposure.

Mechanism of Action
- Binds to tubulin, inhibiting microtubule formation (mitosis)
- GI and blood cells affected first because of rapid division

Dosage
- >0.5 mg/kg associated with systemic toxicity
- >0.8 mg/kg associated with death

Kinetics
- *Absorption (rapid):*
  - High oral bioavailability, 25%-40%
  - Volume of distribution >2 L/kg (up to 21 L/kg in overdose)
- *Excretion:*
  - Half-life is 10-30 hr
  - Hepatic metabolized
  - 20%-30% renally cleared

Clinical Manifestations
- *GI:* nausea, vomiting, and diarrhea (early)
- *Cardiac:* cardiogenic shock, bradycardia, and heart block
- *Pulmonary:* acute respiratory distress syndrome
- *Renal:* kidney injury
- *Hepatic:* centrilobular necrosis
- *Blood:* pancytopenia
- *Neuro:* confusion, decreased reflexes, and delayed neuropathy

Diagnostics
- Screening for glucose and acetaminophen levels
- CBC and comprehensive metabolic panel if symptomatic
- ECG if symptomatic

Treatment
- Activated charcoal (oral) if <2 hr post ingestion and airway can be protected (multidose may have a limited role)
- Hypotension
  - IV fluid bolus
  - Vasopressors (norepinephrine, milrinone) for inotropic support
  - Venoarterial extracorporeal membrane oxygenation has been used.
- Continuous renal replacement therapy for anuric renal failure
- Enhanced elimination unlikely to be useful (high volume of distribution)
- Multiple unproven therapies (eg, multidose activated charcoal, whole blood exchange transfusion, and colony-stimulating factor for pancytopenia)
- Anticolchicine antibodies (only experimental)

Disposition
- If asymptomatic, monitor serious overdoses for 6-8 hr
- If symptomatic, admit

Critical decisions
in emergency medicine

Volume 37 Number 12: **December 2023**

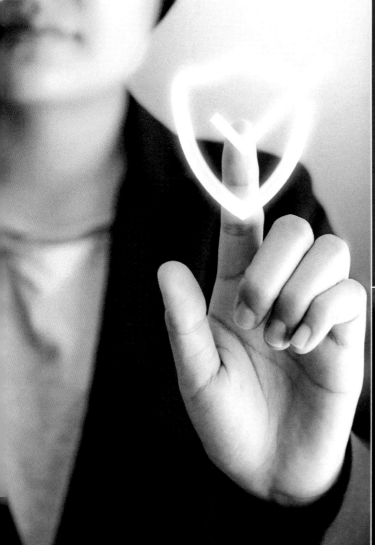

Lifelong Learner

The American Board of Emergency Medicine's mission is to ensure the highest standards in the specialty of emergency medicine. It does so through its voluntary continuing certification process that emergency physicians complete if they want to be ABEM certified. Participation in continuing certification ensures that physicians are engaged in a program of continuous professional development that conforms to the national standards for their specialty.

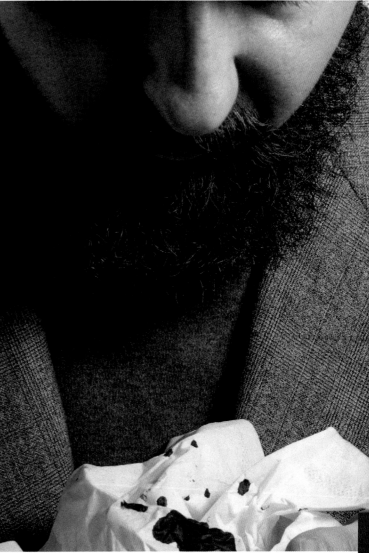

Red Alert

Hemoptysis is a common complaint that exists on a spectrum of disease — ranging from benign and self-limited to critical and life-threatening. The challenge for emergency physicians is to accurately classify the severity of the disease causing the hemoptysis and apply the appropriate critical interventions to patients who present with life-threatening hemorrhage.

THE OFFICIAL CME PUBLICATION OF THE AMERICAN COLLEGE OF EMERGENCY PHYSICIANS

Individuals in Control of Content

1. Melissa A. Barton, MD – Faculty
2. Jeremy Berberian, MD – Faculty
3. William J. Brady, MD, FACEP – Faculty
4. Florian Capobianco III, DO – Faculty
5. Aaron D'Amore, MD – Faculty
6. Alan John, MD – Faculty
7. Samuel M. Keim, MD, MS – Faculty
8. Ryan Long, MD – Faculty
9. Sean Lynch, DO – Faculty
10. Jonathan Reeder, MD – Faculty
11. Christopher T. Stem, MD – Faculty
12. Kyle Thomas, MD – Faculty
13. Emilee Young-Rizk, DO – Faculty
14. Elizabeth Zivick, MD – Faculty
15. Joshua S. Broder, MD, FACEP – Faculty/Planner
16. Ann M. Dietrich, MD, FAAP, FACEP – Faculty/Planner
17. Andrew J. Eyre, MD, MS-HPEd – Faculty/Planner
18. Walter L. Green, MD, FACEP – Faculty/Planner
19. Danya Khoujah, MBBS, MEHP, FACEP – Faculty/Planner
20. John Kiel, DO, MPH, FACEP, CAQSM – Faculty/Planner
21. Frank LoVecchio, DO, MPH, FACEP – Faculty/Planner
22. Amal Mattu, MD, FACEP – Faculty/Planner
23. Christian A. Tomaszewski, MD, MS, MBA, FACEP – Faculty/Planner
24. Steven J. Warrington, MD, PhD – Faculty/Planner
25. Tareq Al-Salamah, MBBS, MPH, FACEP – Planner
26. Wan-Tsu Chang, MD – Planner
27. Kelsey Drake, MD, MPH, FACEP – Planner
28. John C. Greenwood, MD, MS –Planner
29. Sharon E. Mace, MD, FACEP –Planner
30. Nathaniel Mann, MD – Planner
31. George Sternbach, MD, FACEP – Planner
32. Joy Carrico, JD – Planner/Reviewer

Contributor Disclosures. In accordance with the ACCME Standards for Integrity and Independence in Accredited Continuing Education, all relevant financial relationships, and the absence of relevant financial relationships, must be disclosed to learners for all individuals in control of content 1) before learners engage with the accredited education, and 2) in a format that can be verified at the time of accreditation. The following individuals have reported relationships with ineligible companies, as defined by the ACCME. These relationships, in the context of their involvement in the CME activity, could be perceived by some as a real or apparent conflict of interest. All relevant financial relationships have been mitigated to ensure that no commercial bias has been inserted into the educational content. William J. Brady, MD, FACEP holds an ownership interest in Medical Decisions. Joshua S. Broder, MD, FACEP, is a founder and president of OmniSono Inc, an ultrasound technology company. Andrew J. Eyre, MD, MS-HPEd is on the advisory board of Med VR Education. Frank LoVecchio, DO, MPH, FACEP, receives speaking fees from ABBVIE for antibiotics. Christian A. Tomaszewski, MD, MS, MBA, FACEP, performs contracted research for Roche, Pfizer, and AstraZeneca (site PI with financial support provided to institution). All remaining individuals with control over content have no relevant financial relationships to disclose.

This educational activity consists of two lessons, eight feature articles, a post-test, and evaluation questions; as designed, the activity should take approximately 5 hours to complete. The participant should, in order, review the learning objectives for the lesson or article, read the lesson or article as published in the print or online version until all have been reviewed, and then complete the online post-test (a minimum score of 75% is required) and evaluation questions. Release date: December 1, 2023. Expiration date: November 30, 2026.

Accreditation Statement. The American College of Emergency Physicians is accredited by the Accreditation Council for Continuing Medical Education to provide continuing medical education for physicians.

The American College of Emergency Physicians designates this enduring material for a maximum of 5 *AMA PRA Category 1 Credits™*. Physicians should claim only the credit commensurate with the extent of their participation in the activity.

Each issue of *Critical Decisions in Emergency Medicine* is approved by ACEP for 5 ACEP Category I credits. Approved by the AOA for 5 Category 2-B credits.

Commercial Support. There was no commercial support for this CME activity.

Target Audience. This educational activity has been developed for emergency physicians.

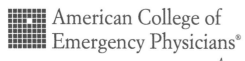

American College of Emergency Physicians®

ADVANCING EMERGENCY CARE

Critical decisions in emergency medicine

Critical Decisions in Emergency Medicine is the official CME publication of the American College of Emergency Physicians. Additional volumes are available.

EDITOR-IN-CHIEF

Danya Khoujah, MBBS, MEHP, FACEP
University of Maryland, Baltimore, MD

SECTION EDITORS

Joshua S. Broder, MD, FACEP
Duke University, Durham, NC

Andrew J. Eyre, MD, MS-HPEd
Brigham and Women's Hospital/
Harvard Medical School, Boston, MA

John Kiel, DO, MPH, FACEP, CAQSM
University of South Florida Morsani College of Medicine, Tampa, FL

Frank LoVecchio, DO, MPH, FACEP
Valleywise, Arizona State University, University of Arizona, and Creighton University School of Medicine, Phoenix, AZ

Sharon E. Mace, MD, FACEP
Cleveland Clinic Lerner College of Medicine/
Case Western Reserve University, Cleveland, OH

Amal Mattu, MD, FACEP
University of Maryland, Baltimore, MD

Christian A. Tomaszewski, MD, MS, MBA, FACEP
University of California Health Sciences,
San Diego, CA

Steven J. Warrington, MD, MEd, MS
MercyOne Siouxland, Sioux City, IA

ASSOCIATE EDITORS

Tareq Al-Salamah, MBBS, MPH, FACEP
King Saud University, Riyadh, Saudi Arabia/
University of Maryland, Baltimore, MD

Wan-Tsu Chang, MD
University of Maryland, Baltimore, MD

Ann M. Dietrich, MD, FAAP, FACEP
University of South Carolina School of Medicine, Greenville, SC

Kelsey Drake, MD, MPH, FACEP
St. Anthony Hospital, Lakewood, CO

Walter L. Green, MD, FACEP
UT Southwestern Medical Center, Dallas, TX

John C. Greenwood, MD
University of Pennsylvania, Philadelphia, PA

Nathaniel Mann, MD
University of South Carolina School of Medicine, Greenville, SC

George Sternbach, MD, FACEP
Stanford University Medical Center, Stanford, CA

EDITORIAL STAFF

Joy Carrico, JD, Managing Editor
jcarrico@acep.org

Alex Bass
Assistant Editor

Kel Morris
Assistant Editor

ISSN2325-0186 (Print)   ISSN2325-8365 (Online)

Contents

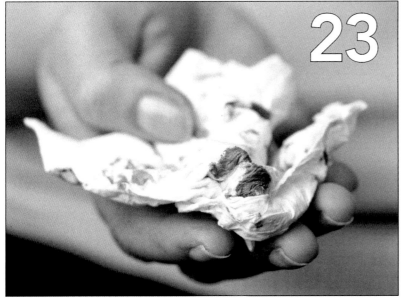

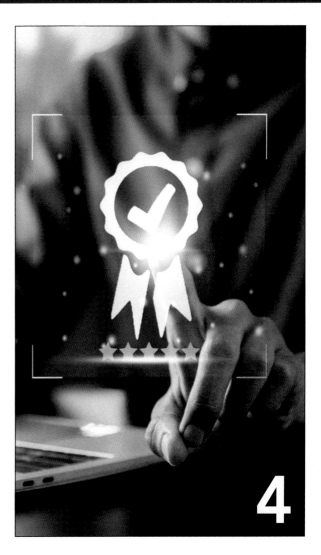

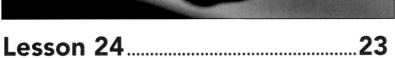

FEATURES

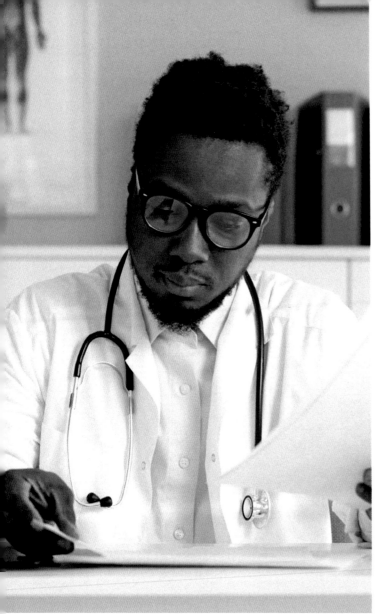

Lifelong Learner

ABEM Continuing Certification

LESSON 23

By Samuel M. Keim, MD, MS; and Melissa A. Barton, MD
Dr. Keim is a professor and chair of the Department of Emergency Medicine and a professor in the Division of Epidemiology and Biostatistics at the Mel and Enid Zuckerman College of Public Health and the University of Arizona College of Medicine in Tucson. Dr. Barton is the director of medical affairs for the American Board of Emergency Medicine.

Reviewed by Danya Khoujah, MBBS, MEHP, FACEP

Objectives

On completion of this lesson, you should be able to:

1. Explain the evolution of ABEM's continuing certification process.
2. Recognize the most recent changes to the ABEM continuing certification process.
3. Identify continuing certification requirements.
4. Discuss methods to meet the IMP requirement.
5. Explain the benefits of the optional modules that do not count toward continuing certification requirements.

From the EM Model

20.0 Other Core Competencies of the Practice of Emergency Medicine
    20.2 Practice-Based Learning and Improvement

▬ CRITICAL DECISIONS ▬

- What are ABEM's requirements for continuing certification, and how are they met?

- How is the IMP requirement met?

- Why should ABEM certification be maintained?

- What are the best ways to prepare for taking MyEMCert modules?

- Why take the optional modules that do not count toward continuing certification requirements?

The American Board of Emergency Medicine (ABEM) has a mission to ensure the highest standards in the specialty of emergency medicine. It does so through its voluntary continuing certification process that emergency physicians complete if they want to be ABEM certified. Participation in continuing certification ensures that physicians are engaged in a program of continuous professional development that conforms to the national standards for their specialty.

■ CASE ONE

KG is a 42-year-old ABEM-certified physician with 21 years of experience and ABEM certification. She has read about ABEM's revised continuing certification process and wonders how this new format differs from the traditional high-stakes recertification examination.

■ CASE TWO

JK is a 59-year-old ABEM-certified physician who took the ConCert Exam one last time in 2022 before retirement. He was informed that his next ABEM certification period is only for 5 years and that he must pay an annual fee. He does not understand why his continuing certification requirements have changed when he is nearing retirement. He had planned on taking the ConCert Exam and not having to do anything else.

■ CASE THREE

JM is a 35-year-old diplomate who became ABEM certified 2 years ago. She works in a critical access emergency department and is unclear about how to satisfy the IMP requirement.

Introduction

The American Board of Medical Specialties (ABMS) requires that all medical specialty member boards have a continuing certification process to provide ongoing learning and a periodic external assessment of each board-certified physician's cognitive expertise. The primary aim of continuing certification is to help maintain the highest standards for safe and quality patient care. An assessment helps to assure patients, physicians, and other stakeholders that ABEM-certified physicians (also known as diplomates) are continually working to improve the emergency care that they provide.

History of Continuing Certification

When the ABMS was founded in the 1930s, physicians who achieved board certification were issued lifetime certificates; they were never required to take another examination to remain certified. Beginning in the 1970s, some ABMS member boards began to require continuing certification by issuing time-limited certificates to ensure higher quality standards for their certified physicians. Two ABMS member boards, the American Board of Family Medicine and ABEM, always had a continuing certification requirement and never offered lifetime certificates.

Because of rapid medical advances and patient safety concerns described in the Quality of Health Care in America Committee of the Institute of Medicine report issued in 1999, lifetime certification offered by some of the ABMS member boards was felt to be insufficient.[1] Career-long performance standards were no longer ensured by initial certification and annual continuing medical education (CME) activities, which may not address gaps in competency.[2] State medical licensing board interventions existed, but there were no national standards to evaluate physician engagement in a career-long program of ongoing professional development. As a result, in 2000 the ABMS outlined a set of standards for ongoing professional development known as *maintenance of certification* (MOC), now called continuing certification, that all ABMS member boards are required to follow.

Initial certification and continuing certification activities have been shown to enhance patient safety, improve the quality of patient care, and reduce health care costs.[3-6] ABEM continually reassesses the continuing certification experience for certified physicians and works to make continuing certification relevant and user-friendly while adhering to ABMS standards.

Keeping ABEM's Continuing Certification Process Relevant

ABEM convened a continuing certification summit of stakeholder organizations in emergency medicine in October 2014. Participants critically reviewed ABEM's continuing certification process and the 2015 ABMS Continuing Certification Standards. Roundtable discussions included strengths of the current program, opportunities for improvement, assessing professionalism, identifying and addressing competency gaps, and enhancing relevancy.

ABEM surveyed its over 36,000 certified physicians in 2017 about continuing certification. Physicians (93%) responded that they preferred an at-home examination with shorter, more frequent open-book tests instead of the existing high-stakes recertification examination (ConCert Exam).[7] Physicians agreed that medical knowledge should be tested to maintain certification.

Informed by the stakeholder summit, the ABEM diplomate survey, and emerging research on knowledge translation, ABEM redesigned its continuing certification process to align with the ABMS revised Standards for Continuing Certification.[8] In 2021, the ABMS approved their new Standards for Continuing Certification, effective in 2024. These standards require a certification period of 5 years or less, something that physicians agreed with during the discovery phase leading up to its implementation.

Additional Changes to Continuing Certification

In 2021, ABEM enacted a Code of Professionalism and implemented a 5-year certification period along with an annual fee requirement for all newly certified or recertified physicians. Annual fees are a standard practice within the certification community; ABEM was nearly the last ABMS member board to implement one.

The ABEM Board of Directors designed a new fee structure in response to physician feedback. Physicians indicated in a survey that they would prefer an annual fee over large, episodic fees. One of the rationales was that an annual fee would more easily align with CME funding through employers. Beginning in 2021, physicians who certify or recertify receive a 5-year certificate and must pay an annual fee. The fee is an annual requirement and not an additional fee; it takes the place of paying for individual activities. Physicians have the option of paying the annual fee for all 5 years of certification in one lump sum during the first year of their 5-year certification or making annual payments. The fee can be paid at any time during the year but must be paid to access continuing certification activities. Nonpayment of the annual fee could eventually result in decertification.

Several factors contributed to the decision to change the certification cycle to 5 years:

- The ABMS Continuing Certification Standards require all member boards to change their certification cycles from 10 years to 5 years or less. Physicians will move to a 5-year certificate when their current certificates expire.
- Five-year certification cycles create a more continuous approach to keeping up with medical knowledge and key advances in the specialty.

The public and patient groups view the 10-year certification process as too long for keeping up with changes. A recent ABEM/Harris Poll found that when emergency physicians were asked how frequently they should be tested to maintain certification, 54% responded that testing should take place at least once per year.[9]

The Professionalism and Professional Standing component of continuing certification serves as a screening mechanism to ensure that board-certified physicians maintain professional behavior and that there are no sanctions against their medical licenses by any state medical licensing boards. Participants in the continuing certification process must continuously hold a current, active, valid, full, unrestricted, and unqualified license to practice medicine in at least one jurisdiction in the United States, its territories, or Canada and in each jurisdiction where they practice. Participants in the continuing certification process must report to ABEM all currently and previously held licenses.[10] This requirement is especially important for physicians who work in multiple states, such as emergency physicians doing locum tenens.

Any license that is conditional, under probation, or limits the physician to a specific practice setting does not meet this continuing certification requirement, including licenses in states where the physician may not be practicing. If even one of a physician's licenses does not meet these standards, ABEM may revoke certification. Because state medical boards report to one another through the Federation of State Medical Boards, a sanction against a physician in one state can result in another state revoking the physician's medical license, even when the physician has not acted out of accordance in the second state. Physicians should also be mindful that states can choose to suspend medical licenses due to civil or criminal matters unrelated to the clinical practice of medicine, such as being charged with driving under the influence, domestic violence, or failure to pay child support. ABEM maintains an appeal process for physicians who do not fulfill the requirements of the ABEM Policy on Medical Licensure.

ABEM-certified physicians must also comply with the ABEM Code of Professionalism.[11] ABEM's Code of Professionalism requires that physicians "refrain from conduct that the Board determines, in its sole judgement, to be sufficiently egregious that it is inconsistent with ethical behavior by a physician." If physicians do not comply with this code, they can be subject to review under ABEM's disciplinary action process that can result in decertification. ABEM also maintains an appeal process for physicians who do not fulfill the requirements described in the Code of Professionalism.

ABEM intentionally aligns continuing certification requirements with work that clinically active emergency physicians routinely perform. Accordingly, ABEM has developed ways to help physicians meet reporting requirements in as seamless a way as possible. For example, ABEM worked with the American College of Emergency Physicians (ACEP) to provide automatic Improvement in Medical Practice (IMP) requirement credit for physicians who participate in the Clinical Emergency Data Registry (CEDR). CEDR houses data used to comply with federal quality measure reporting, enabling participating emergency physicians to monitor and assess their adherence to nationally established quality measures.

ABEM diplomates want a clear description of their pending continuing certification requirements. ABEM provides this information through the "✓ ABEM Reqs" tool on their public website (abem.org/checkreqs). A diplomate can see specific certification requirements by entering the year that their certificate expires and the length of their certification (5 or 10 years). Physicians can also view which requirements are complete and which are outstanding through their profile on the secure portal (accessible at abem.org). Physicians are encouraged to contact ABEM directly (abem@abem.org) should any questions arise about their continuing certification requirements.

CRITICAL DECISION

What are ABEM's requirements for continuing certification, and how are they met?

For physicians who currently hold a *10-year certificate* (that is, those who certified or last recertified between 2012-2021), there are four parts to continuing certification:

- Professionalism and Professional Standing;
- Lifelong Learning and Self-Assessment (LLSA);
- Assessment of Knowledge, Judgement, and Skills; and
- IMP.

These physicians pay activity fees for LLSAs, the ConCert Exam, and MyEMCert modules.

✔ Pearls

- Ideas for fulfilling the IMP component of continuing certification are in a drop-down menu on ABEM's secure portal. Most clinically active emergency physicians will be able to select one of the available options based on performance measures already being tracked by their hospitals.

- Diplomates can take MyEMCert modules by themselves at any time in any location. Taking one module each year provides diplomates with knowledge of the most current advances in emergency medicine and spreads out certification requirements to make the modules more manageable.

- CME credit can be earned for every LLSA activity and MyEMCert module. Diplomates are encouraged to take advantage of this relatively low- or no-cost CME option.

Physicians whose *certifications are for 5 years* (ie, those who certified or recertified in 2021 or later) have three components for continuing certification:

- Professionalism and Professional Standing;
- IMP; and
- MyEMCert modules (which combine the LLSA and Assessment of Knowledge, Judgement, and Skills requirements).

These physicians pay an annual fee.

LLSA

ABEM's requirement for meeting the LLSA component is completion of four LLSA activities within the first 5 years of a 10-year certification period. *LLSAs are required only for physicians with a 10-year certification.* LLSAs will no longer be available in 2026. MyEMCert modules incorporate aspects of LLSAs that physicians have historically found favorable, such as relevancy and currency. Physicians who are uncertain if they must complete LLSAs should consult the ✓ ABEM Reqs tool or contact ABEM for guidance.

The LLSA component is a list of 10 to 15 emergency medicine–relevant articles that is released annually until 2026. The activity is designed to be self-study, but many emergency physicians find it useful to discuss the LLSA readings in a group setting to enhance learning. After reviewing the articles, each diplomate then takes an open-book test (20-30 questions) based on the readings, with three attempts per registration to pass; a score of 85% or higher is considered passing. ABEM-certified physicians can also take the LLSA tests for EMS, medical toxicology, and pediatric emergency medicine, even if not certified in these areas. These subspecialty LLSA activities count toward meeting emergency medicine continuing certification requirements.

To enhance the value of LLSAs, ABEM provides the option to obtain CME credit for completed LLSA activities and MyEMCert modules from external providers. Physicians can obtain 7 to 15 *AMA PRA Category 1 Credits*™ for each LLSA activity or 9 *AMA PRA Category 1 Credits*™ for the successful completion of a MyEMCert module; physicians can choose to receive these credits from ACEP. Of the over 27,200 LLSA tests and MyEMCert modules taken in 2022, the CME activity was selected by 80% of test takers.

✖ Pitfalls

- Participating in unethical activities, even when unrelated to the practice of medicine, can lead to sanctions against a physician's medical license and, potentially, a loss of board certification.

- Forgetting to register for relatively inexpensive CME activities before taking LLSA tests or MyEMCert modules.

- Falling behind on annual LLSA tests or MyEMCert modules can lead to time-consuming cramming in the last 5 years of certification; keeping up with these requirements annually is best.

Assessment of Knowledge, Judgement, and Skills

Physicians whose certifications expire in 2026 or earlier had the option of taking the ConCert Exam in their last 5 years of certification as part of the renewal process. This option became unavailable after 2022, when the ConCert Exam was discontinued. Taken at a proctored computer-testing center, the ConCert Exam used to be ABEM's only external assessment of diplomates' cognitive skills.

A common misunderstanding some physicians had was that if they took the ConCert Exam, their certification would renew for 10 years. Taking the ConCert Exam to renew ABEM certification is just one of several requirements for maintaining certification — the ConCert Exam alone does not renew certification.

In 2021, ABEM launched MyEMCert, an online, open-book, module-based assessment. MyEMCert became available as the alternative to the ConCert Exam. Physicians who hold a 10-year certificate are required to complete four MyEMCert modules in the second 5 years of certification. Physicians who hold a 5-year certificate are required to complete four MyEMCert modules during their certification period.

The modules are organized by content area, allowing physicians to select and retain information related to specific clinical topics. Each module contains about 50 questions, with approximately 70% on presentation-based knowledge and 30% on key advances. Key advance questions are based on practice advances, clinical policy alerts, and suggestions from the literature but are not necessarily related to a module's topic. Physicians can complete the modules in whatever order they choose but must complete them without assistance from others. Physicians have 4 hours to complete each module (although they can pause the examination and stop the clock from running) and have three attempts in the calendar year to pass each one. Diplomates also receive immediate feedback on the accuracy of their responses and the rationale for the correct answers.

Content for all ABEM assessments is derived from *The Model of Clinical Practice of Emergency Medicine*, an outline of the knowledge, skills, and abilities required of ABEM-certified emergency physicians. This outline is routinely updated through a collaboration of leaders of emergency medicine organizations to reflect clinical emergency medicine. MyEMCert modules cover eight topics:

- Abdominopelvic;
- Abnormal vital signs and shock;
- Head and neck;
- Neurology;
- Nontraumatic musculoskeletal;
- Social and behavioral health;
- Thoracorespiratory; and
- Trauma and bleeding.

Writing test questions that are relevant, important, and fair is a priority in developing MyEMCert questions. Questions are written by a team of trained, volunteer item writers who are board-certified, clinically active emergency physicians and are edited by ABEM directors who are also clinically active in emergency medicine. Content for key advance items is developed by emergency physicians and a clinical pharmacist who are experts in evidence-based medicine.

CRITICAL DECISION

How is the IMP requirement met?

The IMP certification component emphasizes practice-based learning related to patient care and professionalism. The vast majority of clinically practicing emergency physicians can get credit for the IMP portion of certification through process improvement work that their department is already doing. ABEM may be contacted directly with any questions about IMP requirements.

The four required steps for the IMP component include (1) measure 10 or more patients with a specific condition or clinical situation; (2) compare this metric to a national standard of care; (3) implement an improvement; and (4) reassess performance in achieving the practice performance metric. For physicians with a 10-year certification, the practice improvement activity must be completed once during the first 5 years and once during the second 5 years of each 10-year certification period. Physicians with a 5-year certification are required to complete one practice improvement activity during their certification.

The IMP requirement is usually considered the easiest component of the continuing certification process to meet. Every emergency department has performance metrics that are tracked to guide practice changes to improve patient care. Emergency physicians can meet the IMP requirement by using their practice's group data if physician-specific data is available. However, sometimes emergency physicians are unaware of the metrics that are monitored and could be used to fulfill the IMP component. Examples of emergency department measures that meet this requirement span the entire spectrum of care, from tracking door-to-thrombolytic therapy for acute stroke patients to screening patients for the risk of opioid use disorder prior to prescribing medications (*Table 1*). For physicians who work in lower-acuity settings like urgent care centers, meeting the IMP portion can be more challenging.

ABEM has a menu of options for IMP attestation. Additionally, ABEM allows physicians to submit individualized practice improvement attestations that must include pre- and postintervention data. Externally developed practice improvement activities are also available for physicians who cannot identify an option from ABEM's list on its website (*Table 2*).

CRITICAL DECISION

Why should ABEM certification be maintained?

Although ABEM board certification is voluntary and not required to be a licensed physician, the reality is that many hospitals, medical staff organizations, and third-party payors require board certification. Because patients do not choose their emergency physician, ABEM certification demonstrates to the public that an emergency physician is adhering to a career-long program of continuous professional development. ABEM certification is also associated with higher reimbursement — on average, an additional $43,000 in annual compensation per physician.[12]

Certification is important for professional self-regulation and serves as a social contract with the public. Historically, physicians did not adequately address health care costs and quality, and as a result, federal statutes and regulations were imposed. To remain a field with high levels of professional self-regulation, medicine must demonstrate to the public that physicians undergo regular assessment of their skills and knowledge through specialty certification boards like ABEM.

ABEM certification promotes lifelong learning. MyEMCert is an assessment *for* learning rather than an assessment *of* learning. An assessment of learning tests medical knowledge and diagnostic skills. The Qualifying (written) Exam is an assessment of learning. It ensures that physicians who want to become board-certified meet the minimum standard set by the board. MyEMCert is an assessment for learning because it covers current practices in emergency medicine and provides immediate feedback about whether questions have been correctly answered, as well as rationales for correct answers. It also provides additional resources in case physicians need to fill specific knowledge gaps. The overall goal is for physicians to integrate what they learn from MyEMCert modules into their clinical practice.

If ABEM certification lapses, it can be regained in different ways.[13] If the certificate expired less than 5 years ago and four or fewer LLSA tests or two MyEMCert modules were missed while certified, certification can be regained by making up missed requirements. If certification expired more than 5 years ago or if more than four LLSA test requirements were missed while certified, a physician must pass four MyEMCert modules and then the Oral Certification Exam to regain certification. Physicians in these situations are encouraged to contact ABEM directly for assistance.

CRITICAL DECISION

What are the best ways to prepare for taking MyEMCert modules?

MyEMCert is open book, so study requirements are minimal. However, resources are available for review before or while taking a module. ABEM recommends reviewing all available key advance synopses prior to taking any module because questions about any key advance can be included in any module. Written synopses are available for each key advance, and some have video reviews.

Study points are another resource that diplomates have indicated are useful in preparing for modules; each module topic has study points. Study points do not provide examples of module questions but rather focus on areas of study and preparation. Other resources include a no-cost demo module, sample questions, a quick start guide, and a number of frequently asked questions. All available resources can be found at abem.org/myemcert-resources.

CRITICAL DECISION

Why take the optional modules that do not count toward continuing certification requirements?

ABEM offers several modules that provide additional learning opportunities. They do not count toward continuing certification requirements but are available at no cost, offer associated CME activities, and provide clinical practice updates that help emergency physicians acquire knowledge important to their specialty.

Area	IMP
Time-related	• Door-to-doctor time • Emergency department length of stay for discharged psychiatric and transferred patients • Throughput time improvement • Time to disposition decision
Infectious disease–related	• Sepsis guidelines, use of DART toolkit • Septic shock: repeat lactate level measurement and lactate clearance rate of ≥10% • Antibiotic stewardship • Appropriate testing for children with pharyngitis • Appropriate treatment for children with upper respiratory infection • Antibiotic treatment for adults with acute bronchitis: avoidance of inappropriate use • Antibiotics within a specific time • Blood culture before antibiotics • Immunization status • COVID-19 patient management
Stroke-related	• Head CT within 45 min of arrival • Thrombolytic consideration or use in eligible patients • Door-to-puncture time for endovascular stroke treatment • Stroke activations and care pathways
Cardiac-related	• Door-to-balloon time for acute myocardial infarction (AMI) • Transfer time to another facility for AMI intervention • Aspirin at arrival for AMI or chest pain • Assessment for chest pain • Median time to ECG for AMI or chest pain • Improving care for patients with chest pain • Cardiac resuscitation and postresuscitation care • Screening for high blood pressure and follow-up documented
Appropriate imaging	• Appropriate CT use for: minor blunt head trauma (adult or pediatric population), suspected pulmonary embolus, and abdominal pain in adults • Appropriate imaging for renal and ureteral colic • Appropriate imaging for trauma patients • Imaging for low-back pain • Ultrasound for diagnosing abdominal pain (pediatric population) • Ultrasound determination of pregnancy location in pregnant patients with abdominal pain • Appropriate use of neuroimaging for patients with primary headache, a normal neurologic examination, and no trauma • Avoidance of head CT for patients with uncomplicated syncope
Advancing health equity	• Increasing collection and data integrity of race, ethnicity, language preference, and health-related social needs • Use of data to identify a health equity focus • Access to linguistically and culturally appropriate care • Securing pregnancy-related care for Black, American Indian, and Alaskan native women • Consultation to social work to improve health insurance and prescription access • Consultation to mental health and substance use disorder specialists for at-risk populations • Auxiliary aids for patients with communication disabilities

Area	IMP
Pain management and sedation	• Time to pain management • Reassessment of pain after analgesia • Procedural sedation safety
Patient safety, error reduction, and complication avoidance	• Prevention of central venous catheter bloodstream infections • Ultrasound use for central line insertion • Appropriate Foley catheter use • Medication error reduction • Appropriate use of restraints and seclusion • Management of the intoxicated or alcohol withdrawal patient • Reassessment of vital signs at discharge • Planning safer and more effective aftercare • Reducing discrepancies between emergency physician and radiologist x-ray interpretation • Notification of regional poison control center for poisoned patients • Safe ventilator management • Adherence to indications for blood transfusions
Substance use disorder and mental health	• Initiate medication for opioid use disorder (MOUD) • Assure outpatient follow-up for MOUD • Evaluation for risk of OUD • Use of statewide electronic pain medication prescribing system • Opioid overdose management • Adherence to opioid prescribing recommendations for chronic pain • Implementing an alcohol withdrawal management guideline • Screening for substance use disorder • Referral to outpatient community mental health • Depression screening • Integration of behavioral health
Palliative care	• Use of palliative care consultation • Discussion of end-of-life care goals • Integration of hospice into emergency care • Adherence to POLST registry according to state standards
Additional common measures and activities	• Left without being seen • Unscheduled return visits • Ongoing Professional Practice Evaluation • Focused Professional Practice Evaluation • Improvement of difficult airway management • Asthma pathways • EMA Clinical Performance Improvement Program • Pregnancy test for female abdominal pain patients • Appropriate use of urine culture

TABLE 1. Patient care practice improvement activities approved by ABEM

The Resuscitation module is open book and was developed to enhance physician knowledge, skills, and abilities in evaluating and resuscitating newborns, children, and adults. ABEM is working to promote it as a way to fulfill state CME requirements and hospital credentialing requirements. It provides six *AMA PRA Category 1 Credits*™ from ACEP. Diplomates have three opportunities per calendar year to take and pass the Resuscitation module.

Two other new modules from ABEM, the Substance Use Disorder and Opioid Use Disorder modules, are also open book and available at no cost to ABEM-certified physicians. Article summaries and video synopses are available with these two modules. Physicians can claim a total of six CME credits between the two modules. These credits can be applied toward the new DEA requirement. Those who take the MyEMCert Social and Behavioral Health module and opt for the CME activity can apply two credits toward the DEA requirement as well.

Summary

Continuing certification for ABEM-certified physicians helps ensure the highest standards for the specialty of emergency medicine. Developed as a response to patient safety concerns, ABEM's continuing certification process assesses varied aspects of physician performance beyond licensure and traditional CME activities.

Unrestricted state licensure and adherence to the ABEM Policy on Medical Licensure and Code of Professionalism

Available to All ABEM and Former ABEM-Certified Physicians
ACEP CEDR
ACEP E-QUAL initiatives: substance abuse disorder
ACEP E-QUAL initiatives: acute stroke and venous thromboembolism
ACEP E-QUAL initiatives: acute infections
American Academy of Pediatrics Revise II: reducing excessive variability in infant sepsis evaluation
Available to Specific Groups
Multispecialty Portfolio Approval Program

TABLE 2. Externally developed practice improvement activities approved by ABEM

remain the foundation of the professionalism component. The LLSA activity features articles relevant to the day-to-day clinical practice of emergency medicine and allows ABEM-certified physicians to concentrate on areas of interest such as EMS, medical toxicology, or pediatric emergency medicine. MyEMCert modules keep physicians up to date on the most current advances in the clinical practice of emergency medicine. Completing the IMP component allows diplomates to document the many quality improvement activities that emergency physicians contribute to. ABEM continues to incorporate feedback to improve the certification process and make it easier for emergency physicians to complete.

CASE RESOLUTIONS

CASE ONE

The current certification has been shortened from 10 to 5 years, and MyEMCert modules have replaced the traditional high-stakes ConCert Exam. MyEMCert was designed to be less burdensome and more relevant to physicians' clinical practice than the ConCert Exam. Instead of taking an 8-hour, closed-book examination at a testing center (like with the ConCert Exam), physicians can choose when to take the MyEMCert modules, which are open book and provide immediate responses on correct answers and answer rationales. Testing on key advances in emergency medicine is also incorporated into MyEMCert modules. This new process of testing incorporates learning and can identify gaps in each physician's knowledge. LLSA articles and ideas for MyEMCert Key Advances can be submitted to ABEM by any diplomate for consideration.

CASE TWO

The ConCert Exam has been only one of several requirements for ABEM continued certification. Passing the ConCert Exam alone has not been enough to renew certification in the past.

The 5-year certification cycle was put into effect to align with the new ABMS Standards for Continuing Certification (effective in 2024) that require a certification period of 5 years or less, something that diplomates indicated they agreed with during the discovery phase leading up to the implementation of shorter certification periods. Becoming and staying certified now requires that activities are completed on a more frequent basis. This allows physicians to stay up to date in the current practice of emergency medicine and aligns with public opinion that emergency physicians should be tested more frequently to maintain certification.

Annual fees are a standard practice within the certification community. ABEM was one of the last ABMS member boards to implement an annual fee. Additionally, diplomates indicated in a survey that they would prefer an annual fee over large, episodic fees because an annual fee more easily aligns with CME funding through employers. The fee is an annual requirement and not an additional fee; it takes the place of paying for individual activities.

CASE THREE

Satisfying the IMP activity for continuing certification should be relatively easy for emergency physicians. Tracking physician performance is common in different settings for emergency care. Any hospital that accepts Medicare and Medicaid has performance metrics that it tracks for its emergency department. Measurements can include, for example, The Joint Commission's Core Measure, an improvement in documentation, a doctor-patient communication measurement, or patient safety event reporting. Emergency physicians can meet the IMP requirement by using their practice's group data if physician-specific data are available. ABEM has a menu of options for IMP attestation. Additionally, ABEM allows physicians to submit individualized practice improvement attestations that must include pre- and postintervention data. Externally developed practice improvement activities are also available for physicians who cannot identify an option from ABEM's list on its website.

REFERENCES

1. Institute of Medicine (US) Committee on Quality of Health Care in America. *Crossing the Quality Chasm: A New Health System for the 21st Century.* National Academy Press; 2001.

2. Davis D, O'Brien MA, Freemantle N, Wolf FM, Mazmanian P, Taylor-Vaisey A. Impact of formal continuing medical education: do conferences, workshops, rounds, and other traditional continuing education activities change physician behavior or health care outcomes? *JAMA.* 1999 Sep 1;282(9):867-874.

3. Holmboe ES, Wang Y, Meehan TP, et al. Association between maintenance of certification examination scores and quality of care for Medicare beneficiaries. *Arch Intern Med.* 2008 Jul 14;168(13):1396-1403.

4. Galliher JM, Manning BK, Petterson SM, et al. Do professional development programs for maintenance of certification (continuing certification) affect quality of patient care? *J Am Board Fam Med.* 2014 Jan-Feb;27(1):19-25.

5. Gray BM, Vandergrift JL, Johnston MM, et al. Association between imposition of a maintenance of certification requirement and ambulatory care-sensitive hospitalizations and health care costs. *JAMA.* 2014 Dec 10;312(22):2348-2357.

6. Brennan TA, Horwitz RI, Duffy FD, et al. The role of physician specialty board certification status in the quality movement. *JAMA.* 2004 Sep 1;292(9):1038-1043.

7. 2017-2018 annual report. American Board of Emergency Medicine. https://www.abem.org/public/docs/default-source/publications/2017-2018-annual-report.pdf?sfvrsn=4e06cef4_8

8. American Board of Medical Specialties. Standards for continuing certification. Published October 29, 2021. https://www.abms.org/board-certification/board-certification-standards/standards-for-continuing-certification/

9. American Board of Emergency Medicine. The American public supports board certification and continuous learning for emergency physicians. Published May 16, 2023. https://www.abem.org/public/news-events/abem-news/2023/05/16/the-american-public-supports-board-certification-and-continuous-learning-for-emergency-physicians

10. American Board of Emergency Medicine. Policy on medical licensure. Published February 2023. https://www.abem.org/public/docs/default-source/policies-faqs/policy-on-medical-licensure.pdf?sfvrsn=1d17ccf4_10

11. American Board of Emergency Medicine. Policy on Professionalism and Professional Standing. https://www.abem.org/public/docs/default-source/policies-faqs/abem-code-of-professionalism.pdf?sfvrsn=17b1c3f4_8.

12. Reisdorff EJ, Masselink LE, Gallahue FE, et al. Factors associated with emergency physician income. *J Am Coll Emerg Physicians Open.* 2023 Apr;4(2):e12949.

13. American Board of Emergency Medicine. Policy on regaining certification. Published July 2023. https://www.abem.org/public/docs/default-source/policies-faqs/policy-on-regaining-certification.pdf?sfvrsn=1bb6c9f4_12

Acknowledgement: The authors would like to acknowledge Mary Nan S. Mallory, MD, MBA and Catherine A. Marco, MD, who authored a version of this article published in 2018.

The Critical ECG
Left Arm–Left Leg Lead Reversal

By Jeremy Berberian, MD; William J. Brady, MD, FACEP;
and Amal Mattu, MD, FACEP

Dr. Berberian is the associate director of emergency medicine residency
education at ChristianaCare and assistant professor of emergency medicine
at Sidney Kimmel Medical College, Thomas Jefferson University in
Philadelphia, Pennsylvania. Dr. Brady is a professor of emergency medicine,
medicine, and nursing, and vice chair for faculty affairs in the Department
of Emergency Medicine at the University of Virginia School of Medicine
in Charlottesville. Dr. Mattu is a professor, vice chair, and codirector of
the Emergency Cardiology Fellowship in the Department of Emergency
Medicine at the University of Maryland School of Medicine in Baltimore.

Objectives

On completion of this article, you should be
able to:

■ Identify the ECG abnormalities that suggest
lead reversal.

■ Describe the ECG findings seen with LA-LL
lead reversal.

CASE PRESENTATION

A 79-year-old woman is being admitted for a hip fracture and undergoes a preoperative ECG (*Figure 1*).

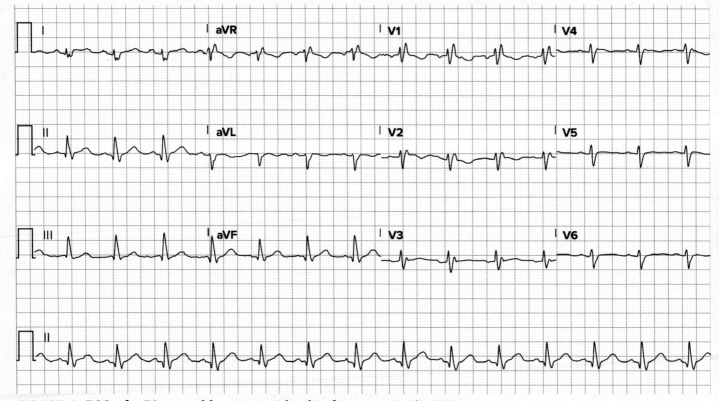

FIGURE 1. ECG of a 79-year-old woman with a hip fracture. *Credit:* EMRA.

ECG Findings

This ECG shows left arm–left leg (LA-LL) lead reversal.
A notable finding in this ECG that should prompt concern for
LA-LL lead reversal is the prominent P wave in lead I compared
to lead II. In general, the P wave should be more prominent in lead
II than lead I in normal sinus rhythm with correct lead placement.
Figure 2 shows a repeat ECG with correct lead placement.

ECG findings seen with LA-LL lead reversal include (*Figure 3*
and *Table 1*):

• In comparison to normal P-QRS-T complexes (ie, normal
sinus rhythm with normal lead placement), leads I and II
switch places, meaning that the normal findings in lead I are
noted in lead II and vice versa.

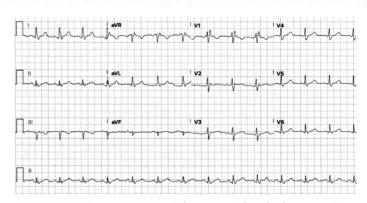

FIGURE 2. Repeat ECG with correct lead placement.
Credit: EMRA.

CASE RESOLUTION

A repeat ECG with correct lead placement was obtained and was unremarkable.

ACKNOWLEDGMENT

This case is reprinted from *Emergency ECGs: Case-Based Review and Interpretations*, available at www.emra.org/amazon or by scanning the QR code.

- In comparison to normal P-QRS-T complexes (ie, normal sinus rhythm with normal lead placement), leads aVL and aVF switch places, so the normal findings in lead aVL are noted in lead aVF and vice versa.

- Lead III is inverted, meaning that the P-QRS-T complexes are all oriented in the opposite direction from the normal P-QRS-T complexes (ie, normal sinus rhythm with normal lead placement).
- Lead aVR is unchanged.

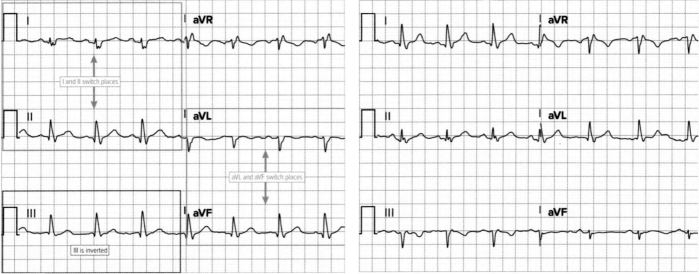

FIGURE 3. Comparison of the limb leads from the case ECG that shows LA-LL lead reversal with the repeat ECG that shows correct lead placement. *Credit:* EMRA.

	I	II	III	aVR	aVL	aVF	V1-V6
LA-RA	Inverted	Switches with III	Switches with II	Switches with aVL	Switches with aVR	No change	No change
LA-LL	Switches with II	Switches with I	Inverted	No change	Switches with aVF	Switches with aVL	No change
LA-RL	Looks like II	Unchanged	Flatline	Looks like inverted II	Looks identical to aVF	Looks identical to aVL	No change
RA-LL	Switches with inverted III	Inverted	Switches with inverted I	Switches with aVF	No change	Switches with aVR	No change
RA-RL	Looks like inverted III	Flatline	Unchanged	Looks identical to aVF	Looks like inverted III	Looks identical to aVR	No change
LA-LL + RA-RL	Flatline	Looks like inverted III	Inverted	Looks identical to aVL	Looks identical to aVR	Looks like inverted III	No change
Dextrocardia	Inverted	Switches with III	Switches with II	Switches with aVL	Switches with aVR	No change	Dominant S wave and poor R-wave progression

Note: RL is a ground lead, so RL-LL reversal does not result in any significant changes

TABLE 1. A summary of lead reversal. *Credit:* EMRA.

Baking Soda Intoxication

By Florian Capobianco III, DO;
Emilee Young-Rizk, DO; Christopher T. Stem, MD;
and Elizabeth Zivick, MD
Medical University of South Carolina, Charleston

Reviewed by Ann M. Dietrich, MD, FAAP, FACEP

Objectives

On completion of this article, you should be able to:

- Educate parents and caregivers about baking soda intoxication in infants.
- Explain how to properly monitor and titrate intravenous fluids for infants with hypernatremia.

CASE PRESENTATION

A 6-week-old, previously healthy, late preterm female infant presents with respiratory distress. Two days prior, she had a cough, congestion, and decreased activity and oral intake. Over the past 12 hours, these symptoms worsened. The infant typically consumes 2 to 4 ounces of formula every 2 to 3 hours, but her intake has decreased to about 1 ounce every 2 to 3 hours. Her parents report that they added a half teaspoon of baking soda and a half teaspoon of corn syrup to each of her feeds over the past 4 weeks to decrease the infant's fussiness and colic. Her mother says that adding a pinch of baking soda to infant formula is a family home remedy. She has not discussed its use with her daughter's pediatrician.

The patient's physical examination reveals significant dehydration, a sunken fontanel, and a prolonged capillary refill time of 3 seconds. Additionally, the infant has marked bradypnea. Laboratory tests are remarkable for significant hypernatremic metabolic alkalosis with compensatory hypercapnic respiratory acidosis (*Table 1*). The hypernatremia is so profound (>200 mEq) that it is unreadable. After a pediatric nephrology consultation, the patient is given three 10-mL/kg normal saline boluses and is started on 5% dextrose plus normal saline at 2.75 times the maintenance rate. Her head ultrasound shows no obvious signs of cerebral edema or venous sinus thrombosis, and her chest x-ray is unremarkable. Her respiratory panel is positive for rhinovirus and enterovirus. She is placed on a 2-L/min nasal cannula because of her increased work of breathing and is admitted to the pediatric critical care unit for management of severe hypernatremic metabolic alkalosis.

Comprehensive Metabolic Panel	
Sodium	>200 mmol/L
Potassium	4.3 mmol/L
Chloride	129 mmol/L
Bicarbonate	50 mmol/L
BUN	41 mg/dL
Creatinine	1.3 mg/dL
Glucose	267 mg/dL
Calcium	8.8 mg/dL
Total bilirubin	1 mg/dL
AST	42 units/L
ALT	20 units/L
Alkaline phosphatase	418 units/L
Albumin	3.4 g/dL
Total protein	5.6 g/dL
CBC	
WBC	15.8 × 10⁹/L
Hemoglobin	10 g/dL
Hematocrit	38.5%
Platelets	250 × 10⁹/L

Urinalysis	
pH	8.5
Blood	Trace
Nitrite	Negative
Specific gravity	1.02
Ketones	Negative
RBC	2/high power field
WBC	1/high power field
Leukocyte esterase	Negative
Bilirubin	Negative
Mucus	Few
Urobilinogen	<2 mg/dL
Venous Blood Gas	
pH	7.61
PCO_2	73 mm Hg
PO_2	95 mm Hg
Bicarbonate	73.5 mmol/L
Miscellaneous	
Magnesium	3.1 mg/dL
Phosphorus	7.1 mg/dL
Procalcitonin	0.38 ng/mL

TABLE 1. The patient's initial laboratory test results after presenting to the emergency department

Discussion

Baking soda (sodium bicarbonate) is an easily obtainable agent used in many products, such as deodorant, household cleaner, and mouthwash. In medical applications, it is marketed as an antacid for adults and is recommended at dosages of 1 to 2.5 teaspoons (not exceeding 5 teaspoons) a day. It is not recommended for antacid use in children younger than 6 years.[1] A teaspoon of baking soda contains approximately 42 mEq each of sodium and bicarbonate, which can potentially lead to lethal hypernatremia and metabolic alkalosis.[2] Although warning labels about intoxication in children are required on all baking soda products, this patient's case presentation reveals a lack of preventive guidance from physicians.[3] Physicians should be

inquiring about how much children are consuming *and* the specifics of what they are consuming. The patient in this case consumed a half teaspoon of sodium bicarbonate in 4 ounces of formula with each feed, totaling approximately 170 mEq/L/day. This value is 3.5 times the amount of sodium and 4.5 times the amount of bicarbonate found in standard oral electrolyte repletion beverages.[2] Increased sodium bicarbonate intake in infants combined with their decreased ability to concentrate urine (compared with adults) makes electrolyte and acid-base imbalance likely.

An appropriate serum sodium level is 135 to 145 mmol/L; once this level exceeds 160 mmol/L, CNS abnormalities can occur. CNS symptoms in infants and children range from agitation, irritability, and increased thirst to more severe CNS depression.[3,4] The infant in this case had symptoms of respiratory distress, decreased oral intake, and increased fatigue that could have been attributed to her viral infections; however, these symptoms are also consistent with hypernatremia. Only a few cases of baking soda intoxication in children have been described in the literature, all between the years 1987 and 2001.[2,3,5] In these reports, sodium levels ranged from 160 to 193 mmol/L, lower than in the case presentation. Given the severity of the patient's hypernatremia, she was at significant risk of severe complications such as seizures or demyelination. However, she did not experience these more severe complications, perhaps because her sodium ingestion was gradual rather than acute, allowing for appropriate compensatory respiratory acidosis.

Rapid correction of hypernatremia can lead to seizures and cerebral edema.[6] Therefore, correction should be done slowly, at a rate of approximately 0.5 mEq/L/hr.[7,8] Multiple fluids of different tonicities should be given in the pediatric critical care unit, where the critical care team can closely regulate and titrate sodium levels (*Figure 1*).

Despite the potential lethal side effects of baking soda, multiple websites and community chat boards endorse using baking soda for child-rearing purposes — for instance, as a cleaning agent for bottles and sleeping equipment, as a bathing solution for rashes, and as a treatment for colic. Although the vast majority of websites do not recommended baking soda for colic in infants because of the risk of electrolyte abnormalities, families can still find information on the internet that supports its use.

The American Academy of Pediatrics and Bright Futures guidelines recognize that well-child visits with outpatient

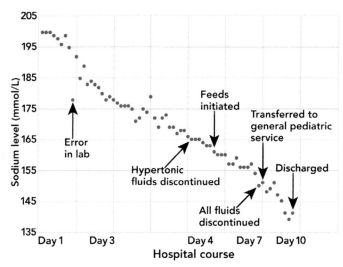

FIGURE 1. **Sodium level trend throughout the patient's hospital stay.** Specific milestones are indicated. *Credit:* ACEP.

pediatricians are the foundation of preventive pediatrics.[9] These office visits allow for educational opportunities on topics like normal growth and development throughout childhood, injury prevention, appropriate discipline, and socialization. Pediatricians should also discuss how much milk infants are consuming and should specifically instruct parents to not mix any harmful substances into the bottle the milk is served in. In the acute setting, careful history taking can reveal if the infant has been exposed to harmful substances and can facilitate a timely diagnosis to prevent lethal complications.

CASE RESOLUTION

During the first 24 hours of admission, the patient required two boluses of 5 mL/kg 3% hypertonic saline to avoid an overly rapid sodium correction. Several rates of normal saline fluids were administered over the first 2 hospital days to maintain a sodium correction rate of 0.5 mmol/L/hr. Intravenous fluids were ultimately transitioned to two different types of fluids that were administered simultaneously: a hypertonic solution (10% dextrose plus 1.1% saline) with an isotonic solution (10% dextrose plus 0.45% saline plus 75 mEq/L sodium bicarbonate). Sodium bicarbonate was added to fluids on hospital day 3 to address the relatively rapid correction of metabolic alkalosis and the resultant hyperchloremia. The two fluid bags were titrated to the maintenance rate to slowly correct sodium levels.

The patient was monitored on an EEG for 3 days; her EEG was unremarkable and showed no seizure activity. A brain MRI without contrast was performed on day 3 of hospitalization; no intracranial abnormalities or edema was noted. On day 4, once the patient's sodium level was approximately 160 mmol/L, oral feeds were initiated and hypertonic saline fluids were discontinued while isotonic fluids were continued. Her sodium levels decreased over the course of 7 days to 152 mmol/L, and she was transferred to the pediatric hospital unit. All fluids were discontinued shortly after, when her sodium level was 150 mmol/L and stable. The patient was discharged 10 days after admission with a sodium level of 141 mmol/L and bicarbonate level of 23 mmol/L (see *Figure 1*). At her 2-week follow-up visit, her sodium level remained stable at 140 mmol/L, and she had no neurologic abnormalities or deficits.

REFERENCES

1. Sodium bicarbonate (oral route, intravenous route, subcutaneous route) side effects. Mayo Clinic. Updated November 1, 2023. https://www.mayoclinic.org/drugs-supplements/sodium-bicarbonate-oral-route-intravenous-route-subcutaneous-route/side-effects/drg-20065950
2. Fuchs S, Listernick R. Hypernatremia and metabolic alkalosis as a consequence of the therapeutic misuse of baking soda. *Pediatr Emerg Care.* 1987 Dec;3(4):242-243.
3. Spandorfer P, Alessandrini E. Sugar and spice and everything nice. *Pediatr Ann.* 2001 Oct;30(10):603-606.
4. Finberg L, Kiley J, Luttrell CN. Mass accidental salt poisoning in infancy. A study of a hospital disaster. *JAMA.* 1963 Apr 20;184(3):187-190.
5. Nichols MH, Wason S, Gonzalez del Rey J, Benfield M. Baking soda: a potentially fatal home remedy. *Pediatri Emerg Care.* 1995 Apr;11(2):109-111.
6. Sterns R. Disorders of plasma sodium — causes, consequences, and correction. *N Engl J Med.* 2015 Jan 1;372(1):55-65.
7. Fang C, Mao J, Dai Y, et al. Fluid management of hypernatremic dehydration to prevent cerebral oedema: A retrospective case control study of 97 children in China. *J Paediatr Child Health.* 2010 Jun;46(6):301-303.
8. Kahn A, Blum D, Casimir G, Brachet E. Controlled fall in natremia in hypertonic dehydration: possible avoidance of rehydration seizures. *Eur J Pediatr.* 1981 Feb;135(3):293-296.
9. Hsu H, Lee SY, Lai CM, Tsai WL, Chiu HT. Effects of pediatric anticipatory guidance on mothers of young children. *West J Nurs Res.*2018 Mar;40(3):305-326.

Cerumen Removal

By Steven J. Warrington, MD, PhD
MercyOne Siouxland in Sioux City, Iowa

Objective

On completion of this lesson, you should be able to:
- Remove cerumen buildup using saline irrigation.

Introduction

Cerumen of the ear can cause symptoms, such as dizziness, hearing loss, and anxiety, that prompt its removal. Cerumen removal is a relatively safe procedure and can be done in the emergency department, sometimes by nursing or other ancillary staff.

Contraindications

- Recent ear surgery
- Tympanic membrane perforation
- Myringotomy tubes
- Middle-ear disease
- Radiation therapy to the ear area
- Severe otitis externa
- Sharp foreign bodies in the auditory canal
- Vertigo
- Uncooperativeness

Benefits and Risks

The primary benefit of cerumen removal depends on the reason for removal. For instance, removal may be needed to evaluate the tympanic membrane in a patient with suspected otitis media or to treat patients who are anxious about symptoms that cerumen impaction has caused.

General risks exist for cerumen removal, along with specific risks depending on the exact method used. General risks include injury to the ear canal or tympanic membrane and failure to remove the cerumen. More specific risks include reactions to agents used during the process, such as dermatitis or allergic reactions when agents like docusate or mineral oil are used. Other risks include vertigo, pain, and otitis externa.

Alternatives

Multiple methods for cerumen removal exist, some of which can be performed in the emergency department and others that require referral to a specialist. Some emergency departments have equipment like loops or spoons for manual cerumen removal. These tools can lead to quicker removal and fewer reactions and infections compared to methods that use water or other topical treatments. Specialists who remove cerumen may use these instruments for removal along with binocular microscopes.

Consideration must also be given to which topical agent to use during removal. The literature does not agree on which agent or time frame is most effective.

TECHNIQUE

1. **Decide** if cerumen removal should be performed in the emergency department. If so, obtain the patient's consent. Attempt manual removal initially, as appropriate.

2. **Pretreat** with a cerumenolytic, if warranted. Allow it to sit or otherwise use it as suggested.

3. **Obtain** materials and equipment for cerumen removal, including a 60-mL syringe, an irrigation basin, body temperature water or saline, and a disposable catheter tip for the syringe. A water-absorbent pad and suction device can reduce mess during the procedure. Some departments will have more formal tools and equipment to use.

4. **Set up** the equipment and position the patient in an upright or semi-upright position.

5. **Use** gentle traction to lift the ear superior and posterior to help straighten the auditory canal. Insert the catheter to the edge of the external auditory canal and direct the catheter upward, which will allow water to enter the ear and the cerumen-water mixture to flow out without obstruction.

6. **Gently** irrigate the canal while watching for cerumen.

7. **Intermittently** check the canal for any remaining cerumen and to determine when to end the procedure and whether it was successful.

8. **Consider** using a few drops of isopropanol to help evaporate residual moisture (if appropriate for the patient).

9. **Determine** if prophylactic antibiotic or antiseptic drops are indicated.

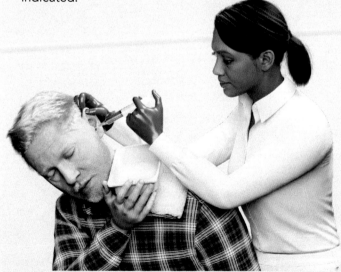

FIGURE 1. Cerumen removal technique using saline irrigation. *Credit:* ACEP.

Many agents are used. Examples of agents outside of water include peroxide, sodium bicarbonate, docusate, and mineral oil. Some agents focus on softening, while others focus on hydrating and breaking up cerumen. Applying a cerumenolytic before irrigation may increase the success rate of cerumen removal.

Reducing Side Effects

Some literature suggests antibiotic or antiseptic drops for a few days after cerumen removal to prevent otitis externa. The risk of otitis externa is higher for certain populations like diabetic patients. Additionally, mixtures with a steroid can provide some relief if the irrigation process is prolonged. The temperature of water during the irrigation process should be close to body temperature. Otherwise, caloric stimulation can occur, which can be an unpleasant experience for patients.

Special Considerations

Some of the literature suggests deferring treatment of patients with cerumen buildup because 25% to 30% will have at least moderate resolution of symptoms within a week of onset without intervention. Patients should be counseled to avoid ear candling, which has not been shown to be of significant benefit and, instead, may worsen the condition or cause other conditions such as burns. Isopropanol drops are sometimes given after irrigation to help with residual water but should not be used in patients with a perforated, or possibly perforated, tympanic membrane.

Critical Cases in Orthopedics and Trauma
Multiligamentous Knee Injury

By Ryan Long, MD; and Sean Lynch, DO
University of South Florida Morsani College of Medicine, Tampa

Reviewed by John Kiel, DO, MPH, FACEP, CAQSM

Objective

On completion of this lesson, you should be able to:

■ Identify and appropriately manage prehospital knee dislocations that reduced spontaneously.

CASE PRESENTATION

A 26-year-old woman presents with severe right knee pain and instability after slipping and falling while walking across a parking lot 2 days ago. She describes a sensation of her knee bending backward and being loose after the fall. She was seen at another emergency department and was discharged with a soft knee brace; she received no advanced imaging because her knee spontaneously reduced. Later that night, she felt her knee dislocate and reported to a different hospital, where imaging showed a posterior knee dislocation (*Figures 1* and *2*). Her knee was reduced; she was placed in a knee immobilizer and was transferred to a level I trauma center.

Her physical examination demonstrates a grossly effused, tender, and warm right knee without outward evidence of penetrating injury, ecchymosis, or epidermal violation. She is unable to bear weight on the affected limb. Dorsalis pedis and posterior tibial pulses are 2+ bilaterally. Ligamentous testing is limited by the degree of swelling. Sensation is decreased in the distribution of the lateral peroneal and saphenous nerves. Weakness is present with right lower-extremity plantar flexion and extension.

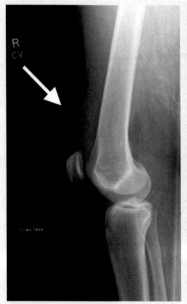

FIGURE 1. Lateral x-ray showing an effusion in the suprapatellar recess (*white arrow*)

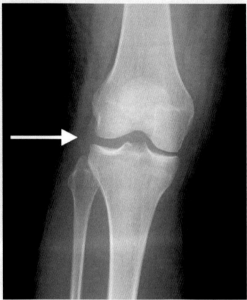

FIGURE 2. Posteroanterior x-ray showing varus widening of the joint space, which suggests ligament instability (*white arrow*)

Discussion

Knee dislocations are rare injuries. They are typically associated with multiligamentous injuries in which the tibia and femur dissociate, usually due to a high-energy mechanism of injury. Obesity alone, however, may predispose a patient to knee dislocations without high-energy mechanisms and can complicate the time to diagnosis if physical examination is limited.[1] Although subsequent knee deformity is an obvious indicator of knee dislocation, up to 50% of knee dislocations spontaneously reduce prior to the physical examination.[2] X-ray results are often normal because bony injuries are uncommon. Consequently, suspicion for knee dislocation should be high even after a thorough history and physical examination.

A multiligamentous injury should be considered equivalent to a knee dislocation and should be treated as such until proven otherwise, even when from a low-velocity mechanism (as with this patient). Knee dislocations frequently include concomitant meniscal, chondral, nerve, and vascular injuries.[3,4] The most-feared complication of knee dislocation is vascular injury with an anatomically susceptible popliteal artery from firm tethering both above and below the popliteal fossa.[3-5] Vascular injuries can lead to amputation in as many as 18% of cases with appropriate intervention and 86% of cases with delayed treatment.[3,5] Additionally, the incidence of nerve injury may be as high as

25% — the common peroneal nerve and its branches are at greatest risk.[5]

Patients with true knee dislocations will present on physical examination with global knee laxity with or without deformity.[3] This finding is an important distinction from a patellar dislocation, which does not result in lax intrinsic knee ligaments, even if the patient describes a sensation of instability. Specific ligament testing may further identify involved structures, and laxity of two or more major ligaments alone suggests a multiligamentous knee injury and warrants further workup. At a minimum, anterior and posterior drawer tests as well as varus and valgus stress tests should be performed and documented.[3] Careful and methodical assessment for instability should be done to avoid iatrogenic injury to neurovascular structures. Neurovascular status should be assessed with sensation, motor, and strength testing as well as assessment of distal pedal pulses. The ankle-brachial index (ABI) can be used to evaluate for vascular compromise — an ABI less than 0.9 is 100% sensitive for injury.[3,5] Notably, normal vascular examination findings do not exclude arterial injury. Clinical suspicion combined with the patient's history should drive the decision for further imaging when no abnormalities are found.[3]

Plain x-rays should initially be obtained to evaluate for fractures and dislocations. In patients with suspected knee dislocations, further imaging is indicated. Options include ABI ultrasound, arterial Doppler ultrasound, CT angiography, MR angiography, MRI, and possibly serial pulse examinations depending on the clinical context. CT angiography is the most time efficient and commonly used, but no consensus or evidence-based opinion has been made about its universal use for these injuries. Opinions vary from ubiquitous use, to a stepwise approach after an abnormal ABI, to skipping it altogether if it would delay surgical intervention (like in cases of a clinically ischemic extremity).[3,6] MR angiography is available but uncommonly used because it is rarely obtained in a timely manner. MRI is the imaging method of choice because it can specifically identify soft tissue injuries (eg, ligaments, menisci, and cartilage) to appropriately classify the injury and direct future intervention.[2,3,6] MRI may also further define occult fractures of the involved bony structures.

If a patient presents with an obvious knee deformity and compromised distal pulses, the first step is to reduce the knee with manipulation, preferably with the patient under procedural sedation. Then, the knee should be stabilized with a posterior long leg splint, which helps prevent repeat subluxation of the already unstable joint.[3] If a pulse is present, a stepwise evaluation can be started with a physical examination and plain x-rays, followed by advanced imaging as indicated.

The decision to manage multiligamentous knee injuries conservatively or operatively depends on the nature of the injured knee structures. If limb-threatening ischemia or vascular compromise is detected (on angiography or otherwise), surgical intervention is emergently indicated — rates of amputation can reach 86% if revascularization is not achieved within 6 to 8 hours of onset.[3,6] Physicians should not delay surgical intervention for additional imaging if limb ischemia is highly suspected.

Several studies have evaluated conservative versus operative management of soft tissue injuries associated with knee dislocation. The general consensus is that operative repair yields better long-term results.[3,6-8] Even if patients do not require emergent surgical repair and are discharged, they should be provided with orthopedic surgery follow-up. Specific surgical interventions are dictated by the injured structures, degree of injury, and injury chronicity. Surgery should occur within 3 weeks of injury: Delayed intervention can lead to excessive scarring that impairs operative techniques.[3] Nonoperative management alone can be considered in sedentary populations or an older adult who is not a good surgical candidate.[6]

Managing long-term sequelae of multiligamentous knee injuries is challenging but important, especially in otherwise healthy, active populations. Aside from neurovascular complications, patients can suffer long-term, debilitating chronic pain, arthrofibrosis, traumatic osteoarthritis, joint stiffness, or persistent joint instability. Such chronic effects can significantly impede athletic performance or even daily activities. Consequently, appropriate postoperative physical therapy is critical to improving patient outcomes.[3,6]

CASE RESOLUTION

CT angiography did not identify any vascular abnormalities; hemarthrosis was present. MRI of the affected knee demonstrated a medial tibial plateau fracture; a depressed subchondral fracture of the lateral femoral condyle; partial tears of the posterior and anterior cruciate ligament, along with the lateral collateral ligament; complete medial and lateral meniscus tears with extrusion; a complete tear of the distal biceps femoris; and a high-grade tear of the popliteus muscle (*Figure 3*). The patient was fitted with a posterior long leg splint with a U-splint of the right lower extremity. She was also provided a leg pillow for comfort and was discharged with outpatient orthopedic surgery follow-up.

Two weeks post injury, she underwent surgical intervention for right knee open peroneal nerve neurolysis and amniotic membrane wrapping, lateral collateral ligament repair with augmentation, and medial meniscal repair. The patient was subsequently discharged with physical therapy, pain control, and regular follow-up. Postoperative restrictions included range-of-motion restrictions of 0° to 90° degrees and non–weight-bearing status for 6 weeks to protect the meniscal repair. Her recovery was complicated by Achilles contracture, noted 10 days after her surgery. Her care was further complicated by her lack of health insurance; no records were available for subsequent follow-up.

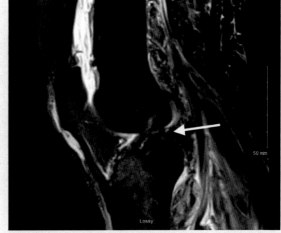

FIGURE 3. MRI (*sagittal view*) demonstrating a partial anterior cruciate ligament tear (*white arrow*)

REFERENCES

1. Marin EL, Bifulco SS, Fast A. Obesity. A risk factor for knee dislocation. *Am J Phys Med Rehabil*. 1990 Jun;69(3):132-134.
2. Figueroa F, Sandoval A, Figueroa D. Schenck's knee dislocation (KD) I injury: An uncommon pattern. *J Clin Orthop Trauma*. 2021 May;16:230-232.
3. Rihn JA, Groff YJ, Harner CD, Cha PS. The acutely dislocated knee: evaluation and management. *J Am Acad Orthop Surg*. 2004 Sep-Oct;12(5):334-346.
4. Yu JS, Goodwin D, Salonen D, et al. Complete dislocation of the knee: spectrum of associated soft-tissue injuries depicted by MR imaging. *AJR Am J Roentgenol*. 1995 Jan;164(1):135-139.
5. Medina O, Arom GA, Yeranosian MG, Petrigliano FA, McAllister DR. Vascular and nerve injury after knee dislocation: a systematic review. *Clin Orthop Relat Res*. 2014 Sep;472(9):2621-2629.
6. Fanelli GC, ed. *The Multiple Ligament Injured Knee: A Practical Guide to Management*. Springer; 2004.
7. Richter M, Bosch U, Wippermann B, Hofmann A, Krettek C. Comparison of surgical repair or reconstruction of the cruciate ligaments versus nonsurgical treatment in patients with traumatic knee dislocations. *Am J Sports Med*. 2002 Sep-Oct;30(5):718-727.
8. Levy BA, Dajani KA, Whelan DB, et al. Decision making in the multiligament-injured knee: an evidence-based systematic review. *Arthroscopy*. 2009 Apr;25(4):430-438.

Acute Flank Pain

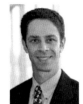

By Joshua S. Broder, MD, FACEP
Dr. Broder is a professor and the residency program director in the Department of Emergency Medicine at Duke University Medical Center in Durham, North Carolina.

Objectives

On completion of this article, you should be able to:

■ Recognize the similarities between presentations of renal colic and renal infarction.

■ Identify risk factors for renal infarction.

■ Select the appropriate CT technique when renal infarction is suspected.

CASE PRESENTATION

A 24-year-old man presents with sudden and severe left flank and abdominal pain that is associated with vomiting. The patient describes the pain as 10/10 in intensity. He denies hematuria and dysuria and has never had kidney stones. His medical history is significant for obesity (he weighs 140 kg [308 lb]), diabetes, and nonischemic cardiomyopathy with an ejection fraction less than 15%. His vital signs are BP 158/70, P 130, R 22, and T 37.7°C (99.9 °F); SpO$_2$ is 99% on room air.

The patient is lying on his right side and appears to be in severe pain. His cardiac rhythm is regular, with no audible abnormal heart sounds. His lungs are clear on auscultation. His abdomen is nontender, but the patient does complain of left costovertebral angle tenderness. He has moderate edema of both legs. His lipase level and liver and renal function tests are normal. His urinalysis is negative for RBCs. A CT scan with intravenous contrast is performed (*Figures 1-4*).

FIGURE 1. CT scan with intravenous contrast, axial image. Contrast is seen in the kidneys during the corticomedullary phase of enhancement. The normal renal cortex enhances brightly during this phase, while the normal renal pyramids do not yet enhance. A renal infarct extends through the cortex to the surface of the left kidney and can be distinguished from renal pyramids, which do not extend to the kidney surface.

Labels in Figure 1:
- Normal renal pyramids do not extend to renal surface
- Normal renal cortex brightly enhances with contrast
- Normal renal pyramids do not enhance with contrast
- Wedge-shaped hypodensity (a renal infarct) extends through renal cortex to renal surface

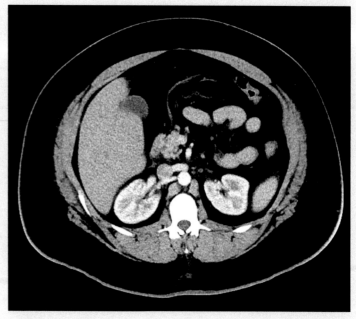

FIGURE 2. CT with intravenous contrast in the same patient 3 months prior. An axial image corresponding to Figure 1. The left kidney does not show signs of infarction.

Discussion

Renal infarction shares many signs and symptoms with renal colic, including sudden, severe flank pain that is often accompanied by nausea, vomiting, and macroscopic or microscopic hematuria (present in 82% of renal infarcts).[1] Risk factors for renal infarction include any reason for arterial embolism; one case series identified atrial fibrillation (65%), prior thromboembolic events (35%), hypertension (53%), mitral stenosis (35%), and ischemic heart disease (41%) in patients with renal infarction.[1] Because of their clinical similarity, renal infarct and its risk factors should be considered when renal colic is on the differential diagnosis. An important corollary is that if an unsuspected renal infarction is discovered with imaging, it should prompt further evaluation for causes and sources of arterial thromboembolism.

Although CT without intravenous contrast is the most appropriate initial imaging option for suspected urologic stone disease according to the American College of Radiology, this protocol can miss renal infarcts, which are best seen on a contrast-enhanced CT scan.[2] Without contrast, an infarcted region may be faintly visible as an area of lower density than the surrounding renal cortex. With intravenous contrast, the infarcted region does not enhance and stands out in distinct relief against the surrounding renal cortex, which enhances brightly during the corticomedullary phase of contrast injection (occurring between 25 and 70 sec after contrast injection and corresponding to the portal venous phase of the commonly performed general abdominal CT scan) (see *Figures 1* and *3*).[3,4] This diagnostic advantage of intravenous contrast must be weighed against the advantages of noncontrast CT, which include avoiding the risks and cost of contrast. Also, noncontrast renal CT often applies low-radiation dose techniques, of particular interest for patients younger than 40 years and patients who need repeat CT scans for follow-ups of known conditions.[5]

Identification of a renal infarction does not require an unenhanced CT scan before administration of intravenous contrast. Additionally, intravenous contrast is unlikely to disguise clinically relevant ureteral stones; one study found that very small stones were detected in the presence of intravenous contrast (sensitivity was 88%, 95%, 99%, and 98% for stones ≥2, ≥3, ≥4, and ≥5 mm, respectively).[6] For this reason, if both renal stones and renal infarction are suspected, a single CT scan with intravenous contrast is usually sufficient to answer both clinical questions, rather than a noncontrast scan followed by a contrast-enhanced CT scan. Emergency physicians should consider the differential diagnosis and choose the CT technique appropriate to the individual patient's diagnostic needs.

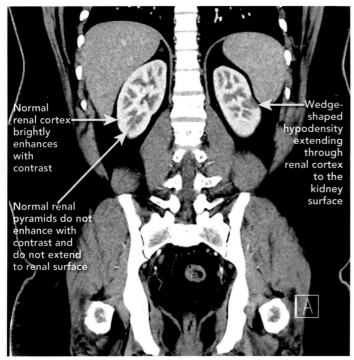

FIGURE 3. CT with intravenous contrast, coronal image, again demonstrating a left renal infarct

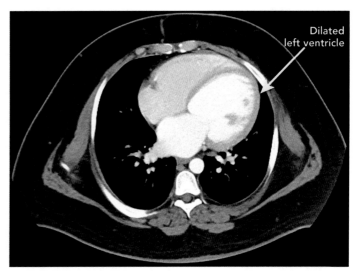

FIGURE 4. CT with intravenous contrast, axial image. Although the heart was not an intended imaging target, it appears in the uppermost CT slice of the series. The left ventricle appears markedly enlarged, an indication of the patient's dilated cardiomyopathy.

CASE RESOLUTION

The patient was treated with intravenous heparin and admitted. He underwent echocardiography, which revealed a left ventricular thrombus, likely the consequence of his low ejection fraction. At discharge, he was prescribed apixaban.

REFERENCES

1. Domanovits H, Paulis M, Nikfardjam M, et al. Acute renal infarction. Clinical characteristics of 17 patients. *Medicine (Baltimore)*. 1999 Nov;78(6):386 394.
2. American College of Radiology ACR Appropriateness Criteria® acute onset flank pain — suspicion of stone disease (urolithiasis). American College of Radiology. Revised 2023. https://acsearch.acr.org/docs/69362/Narrative/
3. Yuh BI, Cohan RH. Different phases of renal enhancement: role in detecting and characterizing renal masses during helical CT. *AJR Am J Roentgenol*. 1999 Sep;173(3):747-755.
4. Kawashima A, Sandler CM, Ernst RD, Tamm EP, Goldman SM, Fishman EK. CT evaluation of renovascular disease. *Radiographics*. 2000 Sep-Oct;20(5):1321-1340.
5. ACR-SABI-SAR-SPR practice parameter for the performance of computed tomography (CT) of the abdomen and computed tomography (CT) of the pelvis. American College of Radiology. Revised 2021. https://www.acr.org/-/media/ACR/Files/Practice-Parameters/CT-Abd-Pel.pdf
6. Dym RJ, Duncan DR, Spektor M, Cohen HW, Scheinfeld MH. Renal stones on portal venous phase contrast-enhanced CT: does intravenous contrast interfere with detection? *Abdom Imaging*. 2014 Jun;39(3):526-532.

Feature Editor: Joshua S. Broder, MD, FACEP. See also *Diagnostic Imaging for the Emergency Physician* (Winner of the 2011 Prose Award in Clinical Medicine, the American Publishers Award for Professional and Scholarly Excellence) and *Critical Images in Emergency Medicine* by Dr. Broder.

Managing Opioid Use Disorder

By Aaron D'Amore, MD; and
Andrew J. Eyre MD, MS-HPEd
Harvard Affiliated Emergency Medicine
Residency, Boston, Massachusetts

Objective

On completion of this article, you should be able to:

- Explain how patients with untreated OUD can be identified and treated in the emergency department.

Hawk K, Hoppe J, Ketcham E, et al. Consensus recommendations on the treatment of opioid use disorder in the emergency department. *Ann Emerg Med.* 2021 Sep;78(3):434-442.

KEY POINTS

- OAT initiation in the emergency department is proven to reduce mortality from opioid overdose.

- Effectively treating OUD in the emergency department aligns with emergency medicine's goal of intervening for high-mortality diseases.

- Emergency departments are often the only access patients with OUD have to health care. Thus, emergency physicians must identify patients with untreated OUD and provide them treatment.

People in the United States are more likely to die from unintentional opioid overdoses than from motor vehicle collisions. There is strong evidence to support that opioid agonist therapy (OAT) significantly reduces mortality from opioid use disorder (OUD). Patients with OUD often access health care only through the emergency department. Even though patients who present for a nonfatal opioid overdose are 100 times more likely to have a fatal overdose in the following year, only one-third receive OAT for this subsequent overdose. Hawk et al present consensus guidelines for the treatment of OUD in the emergency department based on a review of the pertinent literature and recommendations from an expert panel.

Three main pharmacologic agents are used to treat OUD: naltrexone, methadone, and buprenorphine. Naltrexone is a long-acting, competitive μ-opioid receptor antagonist used for both OUD and alcohol use disorder. Naltrexone precipitates opioid withdrawal; patients must abstain from opioids 7 to 10 days prior to using it, which significantly limits its use in emergency departments. Methadone is a synthetic μ-opioid receptor full agonist that can treat both OUD and chronic pain. Although it can potentially cause fatal respiratory depression if doses are rapidly escalated, methadone's benefit is that it does not precipitate opioid withdrawal. Buprenorphine, a synthetic μ-opioid receptor partial agonist, has a ceiling effect on respiratory depression but can precipitate withdrawal if initiated prior to abstinence- or naloxone-related withdrawal.

The guidelines recommend that emergency physicians treat opioid withdrawal, offer buprenorphine initiation, and provide a means for access to ongoing medication. Strong evidence indicates that patients with OUD treated with OAT outside of emergency departments have significant reductions in morbidity and mortality. The evidence also indicates that emergency departments are effective settings to engage patients in formal addiction treatment. A randomized controlled trial demonstrated that 78% of patients with OUD who were initiated on buprenorphine in the emergency department and referred for ongoing buprenorphine treatment participated in formal addiction treatment at 30 days and reduced their opioid use from 5.4 to 0.9 days per week.

Experts also recommend normalizing buprenorphine initiation in the emergency department for patients with untreated OUD and using nonstigmatizing language when discussing patients' drug use and treatment to maintain their trust. This language should be patient centered, professional, and objective, avoiding words such as *abuse*, *addict*, and *being clean*. Recommended person-first language to use would be phrases such as *person who injects drugs* or *patient with an opioid use disorder*. After buprenorphine initiation, patients should be sent home with a prescription for buprenorphine to bridge them to care with a trusted outpatient opioid treatment physician or program, ideally within 1 week.

Evidence-based, institution-specific protocols should be used to identify and treat patients with OUD to ensure buy-in and consistency. Most emergency department protocols include a validated assessment for OUD, an assessment of opioid withdrawal, and a determination of pregnancy status. Many protocols suggest that buprenorphine should be initiated with at least 8 mg for patients with clinical signs of opioid withdrawal and can be increased to 24 mg or more throughout the course of the visit. Emergency departments should engage their community stakeholders in developing treatment protocols to ensure that patients initiated on buprenorphine have direct, reliable, and specific referrals to outpatient programs for continuity. When no such connections exist, emergency physicians can identify programs in their area by using the Substance Abuse and Mental Health Services Administration (SAMHSA) website. Hospitals can also provide health advocates and navigators in the emergency department who help motivate patients and assist them with getting to their appointments to ensure better outcomes.

Collaboration with hospital leadership and strong advocacy are critical for adopting OUD protocols in a hospital system. Integrating clinical decision support into the electronic health record has been shown to be highly effective in streamlining emergency department OUD treatment and referrals for continued treatment. A pilot study showed that these decision-making tools more than doubled prescription rates for buprenorphine and the number of physicians who adopted the prescribing practice.

Critical Decisions in Emergency Medicine's LLSA literature reviews feature articles from ABEM's 2024 Lifelong Learning and Self-Assessment Reading List. Available online at acep.org/moc/llsa and on the ABEM website.

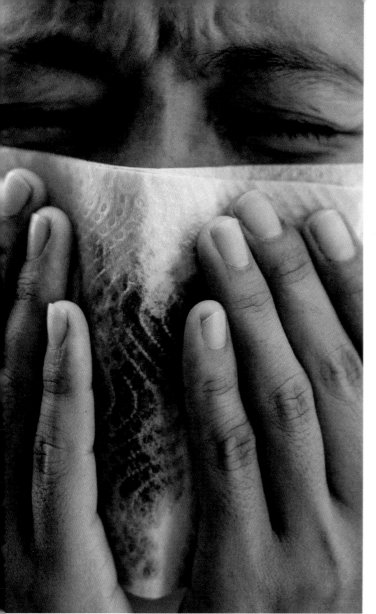

Red Alert

Hemoptysis Evaluation and Management

LESSON 24

By Alan John, MD; Jonathan Reeder, MD; and Kyle Thomas, MD
Dr. John and Dr. Reeder are assistant professors and Dr. Thomas is a resident in the Department of Emergency Medicine at the University of Texas Southwestern Medical Center.

Reviewed by Walter L. Green, MD, FACEP

Objectives

On completion of this lesson, you should be able to:

1. Distinguish between minor and massive hemoptysis.

2. Differentiate hemoptysis from its imitators.

3. Recognize history and examination findings that suggest a more severe disease course.

4. Identify and treat the spectrum of hemoptysis presentations.

From the EM Model

1.0 Signs, Symptoms, and Presentations
    1.3 General
        1.3.23 Hemoptysis

■ CRITICAL DECISIONS ■

- What is hemoptysis, and how is it classified?

- Which conditions commonly mimic hemoptysis?

- What are the important elements of history and physical examination findings in hemoptysis?

- What are the options for evaluation and management of hemoptysis?

- What disposition is appropriate in cases of hemoptysis?

Hemoptysis is a common complaint that exists on a spectrum of disease — ranging from benign and self-limited to critical and life-threatening. The challenge for emergency physicians is to accurately classify the severity of the disease causing the hemoptysis and apply the appropriate critical interventions to patients who present with life-threatening hemorrhage.

CASE PRESENTATIONS

■ CASE ONE

A 75-year-old woman arrives via EMS for coughing up blood. She appears cachectic and chronically ill, with increased respiratory effort and wet blood in her oropharynx. Her mentation is good, but she appears to be very anxious. EMS reports that she had two to three episodes of frank hemoptysis during transport. Her vital signs on arrival include BP 121/77, P 98, and T 36.9°C (98.4°F); SpO$_2$ is 84% on room air. Wearing a nonrebreather mask set to 15 L/min, the patient has an SpO$_2$ of 94%. EMS reports a medical history notable for hypertension, diabetes, and unspecified lung cancer. The patient struggles to provide her history because difficulty breathing and frequent coughing are interfering with her ability to speak. Shortly after arrival, she has a prolonged coughing fit and begins continuously expectorating a large volume of blood.

■ CASE TWO

A 52-year-old man presents with shortness of breath for the past week. He is a truck driver and just finished a long trip across the country. He complains of a cough and hemoptysis over the last 2 days. He is tachycardic, hypertensive, and hypoxic; his SpO$_2$ is 88% on room air. His physical examination reveals clear lungs, and CT angiography is positive for a pulmonary embolism.

■ CASE THREE

An 18-year-old man with a recent history of upper respiratory infection with excessive coughing presents for a new-onset, bloody cough. When the patient is asked to quantify how much blood, he responds with "a lot." On further questioning, the patient states that he has likely coughed a few teaspoons of blood since onset. The patient's history includes attention deficit hyperactivity disorder, no recent travel, and no family history of blood clots. His vital signs are stable. The patient is without hemoptysis in the emergency department, but he has photographs on his phone that show blood on tissue paper. A chest x-ray shows no acute cardiopulmonary pathology. Laboratory results show leukocytosis (13 × 10^9/L) and a hemoglobin level of 12.5 g/dL.

Introduction

Hemoptysis can have several causes, thus requiring differentiation; it can also carry high risks. Emergency physicians must be able to recognize and treat true hemoptysis because timely intervention can decrease the likelihood of death in high-mortality cases.

CRITCAL DECISION

What is hemoptysis, and how is it classified?

Hemoptysis is defined as the expectoration of blood from the respiratory tract below the vocal cords.[1] Hemoptysis can be separated into two main categories: minor and massive, which are differentiated by the volume of blood loss. Massive hemoptysis accounts for only 1% to 5% of total cases of hemoptysis, but it carries an exceedingly high mortality rate.[2] These patients do not die from acute blood loss but rather from asphyxiation. In a typical adult, respiratory failure and a high risk of death can result from just 150 mL of blood in the conducting airways.[2,3]

Pathophysiology

Most cases of hemoptysis result from vascular disruption within the trachea, bronchi, bronchioles, or lung parenchyma.[2] The bronchial arteries account for only 1% of total blood supply to the lungs (the remaining supply is from the pulmonary arteries), yet they are believed to cause up to 90% of hemoptysis cases. Minor hemoptysis is usually due to injury to tracheobronchial capillaries, whereas massive hemoptysis typically originates in the bronchial or pulmonary arteries. Causes of injury include inflammation, local infection, infarction, trauma, malignant invasion, and fistulization.[1-3] Each of these etiologies carries its own unique pathophysiology.

Acute and chronic inflammatory states can cause hemoptysis. In acute inflammatory states such as bronchitis, the frequent trauma from coughing can lead to bleeding in otherwise healthy lungs.[2] In chronic inflammatory states such as chronic obstructive pulmonary disease (COPD), proliferation of bronchial arteries creates fragile vessels that are at high risk of bleeding.[1] Bronchiectasis is a common disease marked by chronic inflammation, which leads to hypertrophy and tortuosity of bronchial arteries that can cause large volumes of blood to be lost into the small airways.[4] Lupus, yet another cause of chronic inflammation, can cause hemoptysis by the recruitment of macrophages and neutrophils, eventually degrading the alveolar-capillary membrane and leading to massive hemoptysis.[5]

The cavitary lesions of tuberculosis (TB) or aspergillosis are another common cause of hemoptysis. These lesions can both erode bronchial vessels and promote proliferation of fragile, friable vessels that are prone to near-spontaneous hemorrhage. TB continues to be the leading cause of massive hemoptysis worldwide and is most common in low- and middle-income countries. Pulmonary infarction causes direct hemorrhage due to tissue necrosis. It also causes decreased flow through primary arteries, leading to an increase in pressure through surrounding bronchial arteries to compensate. This pressure can cause hemorrhage within the alveoli. Deceleration injuries, penetrating trauma, and iatrogenic injuries from procedures such as lung biopsies, right heart catheterizations, and bronchoscopy can all lead to pulmonary hemorrhage.[1]

Classification

Although the definition of massive hemoptysis varies, it is generally accepted as a loss of 100 to 600 mL of blood from the airway per 24 hours.[1,2,4] Some authors suggest an additional requirement of unsteady vital signs. The new criteria may include an oxygen requirement, pressors for blood pressure stability, or airway obstruction.[4] Minor hemoptysis is defined as a self-limited, small volume of blood loss in healthy lungs of patients with stable vital signs, adequate oxygenation and ventilation, and no risk factors for continued bleeding.[2]

Although the mechanisms of bleeding are similar, the sources are commonly different in minor and massive hemoptysis. Minor hemoptysis originates from tracheobronchial capillaries and is believed to be caused by vigorous coughing or minor bronchial infections. By contrast, massive hemoptysis derives from the bronchial or pulmonary arteries directly.[1] Massive hemoptysis is predominantly from the bronchial arteries secondary to the pathologies noted above, most commonly from TB, bronchiectasis, necrotizing pneumonia, and bronchogenic carcinomas.[4] The differentiation between minor and massive hemoptysis can be challenging in real time. It is imperative to obtain a detailed history from the patient or family and perform a careful physical examination to determine the severity of hemoptysis. Typically, hemoptysis should be presumed to be massive unless ruled out because these patients can deteriorate rapidly.

CRITICAL DECISION

Which conditions commonly mimic hemoptysis?

Physicians must remember that not all blood that exits the oropharynx comes from the lungs. Sources of expectorated blood must be differentiated because their management varies. Common mimics of hemoptysis are:

- **GI bleeding:** Upper GI bleeding that leads to hematemesis is commonly confused with massive hemoptysis. Both involve large volumes of blood from the mouth and represent severely unstable disease processes. The color of the blood can suggest its source. The acidic milieu of the upper GI tract tends to darken and fragment blood cells, leading to the classic *coffee-ground* emesis, whereas hemorrhage from a pulmonary source is typically bright red with a nonacidic pH level.[2]
- **Epistaxis:** Large-volume epistaxis often leads to a cough reflex, causing expectorated blood. History and physical examination findings are key to establishing the diagnosis. Patients generally report nasal trauma or a history of frequent nosebleeds.
- **Oral or hypopharyngeal bleeding:** Like epistaxis, large-volume bleeding from the pharynx can trigger a cough reflex. The posterior oropharynx should be examined to evaluate for oropharyngeal sources of bleeding that may descend to the bronchial tree.

If the origin of bleeding is unclear with traditional physical examination, a flexible fiberoptic endoscope can be useful to view the nasopharynx and oropharynx.[6] History and physical examination are often sufficient to make the distinction, however.

CRITICAL DECISION

What are the important elements of history and physical examination findings in hemoptysis?

History

In history gathering, emergency physicians must:

- Distinguish hemoptysis from its mimics;
- Quantify the hemorrhage; and
- Obtain a medical history that can point to an etiology of the bleeding.

To distinguish hemoptysis from its mimics, establishing the setting of the bleeding can be useful:

- Has the patient had recent nosebleeds or nasal trauma?
- Is the expectorated blood truly coughed up, or does it appear to be vomited?
- How early into the coughing episodes was blood noted?
- Is the blood dark like coffee grounds, or is it bright red?

Any amount of expectorated blood is distressing to most patients; as such, patients' attempts to quantify the hemorrhage are notoriously unreliable. However, most patients can differentiate between blood-tinged sputum and frank hemorrhage or clots, and an exact measurement of the volume of hemorrhage is unnecessary. With the widespread use of cell phones, patients increasingly use their phones to photograph medical issues; therefore, physicians should ask the patient or family if they have any photographs of the sputum or blood.

A focused medical history must be obtained. Since massive hemoptysis is unlikely to occur spontaneously, medical comorbidities provide useful information to distinguish causes of hemoptysis that are at risk of massive hemorrhage from those likely to be less severe. Inquire about:

- Inflammatory disorders that are known to attack lung parenchyma, such as eosinophilic granulomatosis with polyangiitis, Goodpasture syndrome, and lupus;
- Lung infections, especially TB and fungal infections such as aspergillosis;
- Chronic pneumonia;
- Risk factors for pulmonary embolism, such as a smoking history, recent surgery, estrogen replacement therapy, and recent long drives or flights;
- Coagulopathy, such as hemophilia, von Willebrand disease, thrombocytopenia, and anticoagulant medications (warfarin, apixaban, heparin, rivaroxaban, dabigatran, and clopidogrel);
- Signs of malignancy, which can cause hypercoagulability or increased bleeding (both risk factors for hemoptysis), such as unintentional weight loss, melena, hematochezia, a smoking history, and active chemotherapy; and
- Recent pulmonary instrumentation, which increases the risk of bleeding from the vasculature with local trauma.

✔ Pearls

- Quantify hemoptysis to guide the treatment algorithm.
- It is critical to rapidly differentiate massive from minor hemoptysis because massive hemoptysis has a high mortality rate.
- Most cases of hemoptysis are self-limiting. Treatment of the underlying cause often resolves the issue.
- Use a large-bore endotracheal tube if intubation is necessary in cases of massive hemoptysis.

Examination

The physical examination should first attempt to distinguish hemoptysis from its mimics. Identifying the source will help with treatment and resolution of a patient's bleeding. An examination of the nose can reveal active bleeding or sequelae of recent epistaxis. The posterior oropharynx must be examined to evaluate for an oropharyngeal source of bleeding. The initial physical examination can start with an otoscope and tongue depressor to assess for oro– or nasopharyngeal etiologies of bleeding. In patients with difficult anatomy, a fiberoptic laryngoscope can be helpful to visualize the nasopharynx and oropharynx. Keep in mind that extrapulmonary sources of bleeding can still lead to airway compromise. Establishing a protected airway must be the main priority if there is a concern.

The lung examination is essential in evaluating hemoptysis. Focal lung rales can suggest pneumonia. Wheezing can point to long-standing COPD. A patient with both of these findings is at greater risk of hemoptysis. Auscultation alone may be insufficient to rule in or rule out hemoptysis, but it can make a stronger case for lateralization of the bleeding if intervention is needed to protect the airway. Lateralizing the bleed can allow for quicker identification of the source via bronchoscopy or placement of a Fogarty catheter for source control.[2,7] Lateralization can also enable the physician to protect the healthy lung to prevent asphyxiation and death by involvement of both lungs.[3,4] Simple intubation may be inadequate for airway protection because the source of massive hemoptysis is generally distal to the endotracheal cuff. Lateralizing the source allows for more specific airway interventions to contain or resolve the bleed, preventing the bleeding region from overcoming the rest of the lungs and interfering with gas exchange.[7]

Other physical examination findings that suggest an etiology of hemoptysis include evidence of lower-extremity deep vein thrombosis (DVT) and evidence of possible coagulopathy. Unilateral edema and pain point to lower-extremity DVT. Notably, DVT findings may suggest that pulmonary embolism is the likely source (via DVT traveling to the pulmonary vasculature to cause an infarction and, ultimately, hemoptysis). However, negative findings do not rule out emboli as the cause. Evidence of possible coagulopathy includes scattered, unexpected ecchymosis; gingival bleeding; hematemesis; hematochezia; melena; and persistent bleeding with minor cuts or intravenous access. Recognizing patients with possible bleeding disorders or bleeding secondary to anticoagulants allows physicians to intervene or directly reverse the cause with appropriate medications.

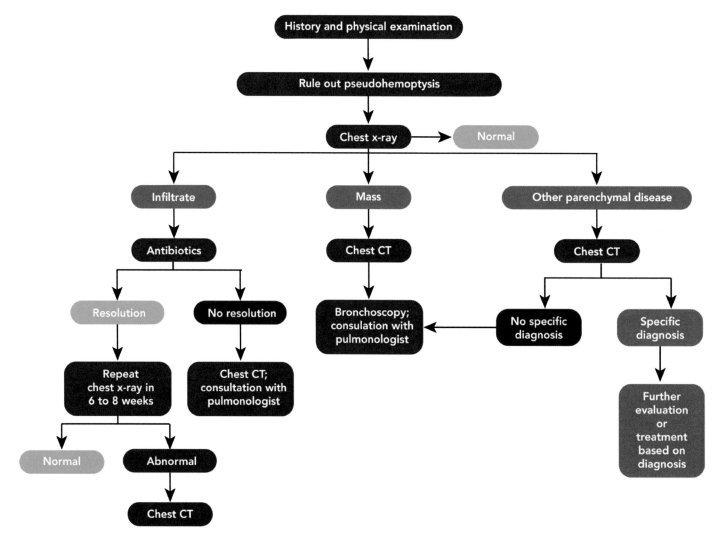

FIGURE 1. Evaluation of nonmassive hemoptysis. *Credit:* ACEP.

CRITICAL DECISION

What are the options for evaluation and management of hemoptysis?

Evaluation

In any case of hemoptysis, the immediate priority is to assess airway, breathing, and circulation. Hypoxic patients should receive supplemental oxygen. Airway protection should be considered in cases of massive hemoptysis. Although laboratory findings cannot confirm or rule out hemoptysis, they can aid in initial resuscitation to stabilize patients and reverse the potential underlying pathology that led to hemoptysis. Laboratory tests for initial diagnostics include:

- **CBC:** A drop in hemoglobin levels can suggest active bleeding. Leukocytosis can reveal pneumonia that causes a risk of hemoptysis.

- **Comprehensive metabolic panel:** Assess renal function to evaluate for a possible need for contrast or medications and to evaluate for uremia that causes platelet dysfunction and increases the risk of bleeding (BUN >35 mg/dL).[8]

- **Coagulation studies:** Assess PT, PTT, and INR for signs of bleeding disorders or supratherapeutic anticoagulation.

- **ABG:** Hypercapnia or hypoxia can show poor oxygenation, suggesting future or active respiratory failure that requires immediate intervention.

- **Lactate level:** An elevated lactate level may show hypoperfusion from poor gas exchange due to airway compromise, hypovolemia (from acute blood loss), or shock (obstructive or septic).

- **D-dimer level:** If considering pulmonary embolism, a D-dimer test is warranted.

- **Type and crossmatch tests:** These tests should be included if blood products will be required for stabilization and resuscitation.

The cause and location of hemoptysis are generally diagnosed with imaging (*Figure 1*). Imaging options include chest x-ray, CT scan of the chest, and bronchoscopy.[2] X-ray is typically recommended for first-line imaging. However, plain x-ray findings are normal in 20% to 30% of patients with massive hemoptysis. Additionally, it can be difficult to locate the source of bleeding if a large amount of blood has spilled into the nonbleeding lung.[2] Depending on findings, further imaging studies and interventions may be necessary to reach the most accurate diagnosis and determine the best treatment (*Figure 2*). In most emergency departments, a CT scan should be obtained if there is serious concern for hemoptysis after an x-ray.[9,10] A CT scan of the chest can be obtained without or with contrast. However, CT angiography is preferred because it can help identify the vessels that are causing the patient's massive hemoptysis and can guide consultants for future procedures required to stop the bleeding.[2]

Sometimes, imaging is impossible because of the patient's acuity. If x-ray studies are nondiagnostic or the patient is too unstable to travel to the CT scanner, bronchoscopy can be performed at the bedside. Bronchoscopy can provide diagnostic and therapeutic benefits. If available, consultation with

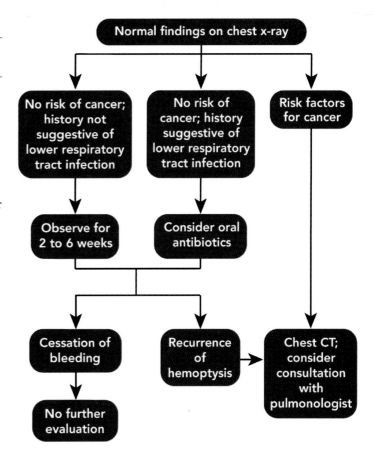

FIGURE 2. Management of nonmassive hemoptysis in patients with normal x-ray findings. *Credit:* ACEP.

pulmonology or interventional radiology can help with definitive treatment for massive hemoptysis.

Management

Management of hemoptysis differs by severity. For minor hemoptysis, the hallmark is to treat the underlying cause. Treatment is with antibiotics for pneumonia, steroids and antitussives for bronchitis, or inhaled bronchodilators for asthma. Minor hemoptysis is often self-limiting and tends to resolve on its own. By contrast, massive hemoptysis requires intervention; with conservative management, it has a mortality rate as high as 75%.[3,4] Admission is required for patients with proven massive hemoptysis and for those with minor hemoptysis at high risk of conversion to massive hemoptysis. Consider admission for patients with tachypnea (>30 breaths/min), hypoxia (SpO$_2$ <88% on room air or requiring >8 L/min of oxygen), hemodynamic instability (tachycardia, hypotension, or a hemoglobin level <8 mg/dL or dropping more than 2 g/dL from baseline), respiratory comorbidities such as COPD or cystic fibrosis, or current anticoagulant use.[4]

Massive hemoptysis has several considerations prior to disposition. Al-Adhoubi and Bystrom recommend nebulized tranexamic acid during initial resuscitation to encourage source control.[5] In critically ill patients, focus on airway protection quickly. Not all patients with suspected massive hemoptysis require endotracheal intubation. If patients are awake and alert with a strong cough, first attempt supplemental oxygen. These patients are generally able to maintain a patent airway.[2] However, these patients can deteriorate quickly, so physicians must continuously reassess their stability. When intubating, use an 8.5-mm or larger endotracheal tube, if possible. Larger tubes allow for passage of a flexible bronchoscope for balloon tamponade, passage of a Fogarty catheter, or laser therapy (*Figure 3*).[2,7] Consider mainstem intubation, either to block the bleeding lung or to protect the healthy lung. If possible, left-sided bronchus intubation is recommended because the left bronchus is longer than the right.[7,11]

For ventilation, it may be possible to contain the bleeding and protect the unaffected lung by placing the patient in a decubitus position with the bleeding lung down.[4] In many pulmonary pathologies, placing the healthy lung in a dependent position improves ventilation-perfusion matching. However, in cases of hemoptysis, this position can allow bleeding from the affected lung to spread to the unaffected lung. If both lungs are bleeding, the patient should be placed in the Trendelenburg position. If there is coagulopathy, transfuse blood products like packed RBCs, vitamin K, and fresh frozen plasma, or prothrombin complex concentrates for warfarin reversal. Give platelets if there is thrombocytopenia to less than 50×10^9/L.[2] Administer desmopressin for uremic platelet dysfunction (BUN >35 mg/dL). Provide specific anticoagulant reversal if the patient is on oral anticoagulants (idarucizumab for dabigatran; andexanet alfa for apixaban or rivaroxaban).[8]

Bronchoscopy must be used urgently if the patient is considered unstable. Instability is marked by an increasing need for supplemental oxygen, an inability to protect the airway, a change in mental status, or hemodynamic instability. Bronchoscopy can be used to improve gas exchange by inserting a balloon-tipped catheter into the affected bronchus to allow oxygen into the healthy lung. It can also be used to ensure successful intubation, if required.[12] More specifically, bronchoscopy can be used on unstable patients when intubation and lung isolation are necessary, when a bronchial blocker is urgently needed, or for clot extraction. Local tamponade is also possible using bronchoscopy, as well as electrocautery, argon plasma coagulation, or Nd:YAG laser. Some studies describe success with ice-cold saline, endobronchial epinephrine, or norepinephrine. However, success and safety vary.[9] If these methods do not control bleeding, consult interventional radiology for bronchial artery embolization (BAE), which is the standard therapy of choice.[1-3,7,13] Bronchoscopy prior to BAE is believed to be unnecessary because of BAE's ability to provide more long-term resolution of bleeding.[11]

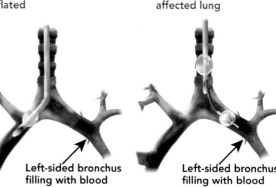

Right main bronchus endotracheal tube intubation with cuff inflated

Fogarty catheter passed by endotracheal tube to tamponade the affected lung

Left-sided bronchus filling with blood

Left-sided bronchus filling with blood

FIGURE 3. Intubation without and with Fogarty catheter. *Credit:* ACEP.

These nonsurgical interventions are becoming the gold standard for treating hemoptysis, either through bronchoscopy or BAE. Complete cessation is achieved in 70% to 99% of cases. However, recurrence rates remain high, most commonly due to nonbronchial systemic collaterals, bronchopulmonary shunting, aspergillomas, reactivation TB, or multidrug-resistant TB.[7,14,15] Historically, surgical interventions such as thoracotomies were the best intervention to decrease mortality, which declined to 20% in the 1970s. Today, surgery is only recommended in specific circumstances: iatrogenic pulmonary artery rupture; complex arteriovenous malformations; refractory hemoptysis due to aspergilloma, lung abscess, or chest trauma; or when primary interventions have failed. BAE and local methods of bronchoscopic control remain the preferred first-line therapies in most cases.[7]

CRITICAL DECISION

What disposition is appropriate in cases of hemoptysis?

Patients with minor hemoptysis can be discharged with close primary care follow-up. Provide these patients with strict return precautions. Patients with massive hemoptysis require admission to the ICU and consultation with pulmonology and other indicated specialists. Ensure airway protection early, reverse anticoagulation, and replace blood products as needed to stabilize the patient before admission or transfer to the appropriate facility. The length of hospital stay can vary depending on the intervention used to resolve hemoptysis. Lee et al. report that with BAE as the primary intervention, the length of stay is 14.9 ± 15.8 days (range: 1-71 days); for those who receive surgical treatment, the length is 20.9 ± 16.3 days (range: 7-81 days).[16]

Summary

Hemoptysis represents a spectrum of disease and is categorized by its volume. Brisk bleeding into the bronchial tree (100-600 mL per 24 hours) carries a staggeringly high mortality rate. By contrast, most minor cases of hemoptysis related to acute respiratory infection are self-resolving and can be managed on an outpatient basis. Because of this dichotomy

━━━━━━━━━━━━━━━━ ✖ **Pitfalls** ━

- Failing to consider the full spectrum of underlying causes for hemoptysis.

- Being unprepared to resuscitate patients with massive hemoptysis, who can deteriorate quickly.

- Delaying specialist consultation.

- Missing more sinister underlying pathologies that present with hemoptysis.

CASE RESOLUTIONS

CASE ONE
Shortly after the patient arrived, the decision was made to intubate her because of hypoxia and concern for massive hemoptysis, likely secondary to lung malignancy. Despite an airway contaminated with bright red blood, she was successfully intubated with an 8.0-mm endotracheal tube. Pulmonology and interventional radiology were consulted immediately after her arrival. Because of the large volume of blood, pulmonology was unable to locate the source of the bleeding during bronchoscopy other than that it was coming from the left lung. The bronchoscope end was placed into the right mainstem bronchus, and the endotracheal tube was advanced over the bronchoscope to facilitate a right mainstem intubation. The patient was placed in a left lateral decubitus position. CT angiography showed active extravasation from a left-sided bronchial artery, and interventional radiology successfully embolized the culprit vessel. The patient had a prolonged stay in the ICU. She was discharged 22 days after admission.

CASE TWO
The patient was given enoxaparin sodium and admitted to the ICU for close hemodynamic monitoring. His hemoptysis and shortness of breath improved, and he was discharged home on an oral anticoagulant.

CASE THREE
The patient remained stable throughout the visit, without vital sign abnormalities or new oxygen requirements. He was not found to be anemic on CBC. The bleeding was controlled prior to his arrival, and suspicion of massive hemoptysis was low. Given the patient's healthy background and lack of risk factors for DVT and pulmonary embolism, the patient was thought to have a mild hemoptysis episode from recent bronchitis. He was prescribed antitussives and was given strict return precautions, with primary care follow-up recommended.

of disease severity, the central focus of emergency physicians must be to recognize the severity of hemoptysis and quickly escalate care for patients with massive hemoptysis or at risk of developing it. Certain risk factors and red flags raise suspicion for large-volume hemorrhage. The diagnostic and management options for massive hemoptysis start with early airway protection, proper resuscitation, advanced imaging techniques to identify bleeding sources, and early involvement of pulmonary and interventional radiology consultants for definitive hemorrhage control.

REFERENCES

1. Sims TC. Hemoptysis. In: Tintinalli JE, Ma OJ, Yealy DM, et al, eds. *Tintinalli's Emergency Medicine: A Comprehensive Study Guide.* 9th ed. McGraw-Hill Education; 2020:432-436.

2. Brown CA III. Hemoptysis In: Walls RM, Hockberger RS, Gausche-Hill M, et al, eds. *Rosen's Emergency Medicine: Concepts and Clinical Practice.* Vol 1. 10th ed. Elsevier; 2023:189-193.

3. Prey B, Francis A, Williams J, Krishnadasan B. Evaluation and treatment of massive hemoptysis. *Surg Clin North Am.* 2022 Jun;102(3):465-481.

4. Earwood JS, Thompson TD. Hemoptysis: evaluation and management. *Am Fam Physician.* 2015;91(4):243-249.

5. Al-Adhoubi NK, Bystrom J. Systemic lupus erythematosus and diffuse alveolar hemorrhage, etiology and novel treatment strategies. *Lupus.* 2020 Apr;29(4):355-363.

6. Larici AR, Franchi P, Occhipinti M, et al. Diagnosis and management of hemoptysis. *Diagn Interv Radiol.* 2014 Jul-Aug;20(4):299-309.

7. Kalva SP. Bronchial artery embolization. *Tech Vasc Interv Radiol.* 2009 Jun;12(2):130-138.

8. Atchinson PRA, Hatton CJ, Roginski MA, Backer ED, Long B, Lentz SA. The emergency department evaluation and management of massive hemoptysis. *Am J Emerg Med.* 2021 Dec;50:148-155.

9. Mori H, Ohno Y, Tsuge Y, et al. Use of multidetector row CT to evaluate the need for bronchial arterial embolization in hemoptysis patients. *Respiration.* 2010;80(1):24-31.

10. Jeudy J, Khan AR, Mohammed TL, et al; Expert Panel on Thoracic Imaging. ACR Appropriateness Criteria hemoptysis. *J Thorac Imaging.* 2010 Aug;25(3):W67-W69.

11. Jean-Baptiste E. Clinical assessment and management of massive hemoptysis. *Crit Care Med.* 2001 May;29(5):1098.

12. Fartoukh M, Khoshnood B, Parrot A, et al. Early prediction of in-hospital mortality of patients with hemoptysis: an approach to defining severe hemoptysis. *Respiration.* 2012;83(2):106-114.

13. Tom LM, Palevsky HI, Holsclaw DS, et al. Recurrent bleeding, survival, and longitudinal pulmonary function following bronchial artery embolization for hemoptysis in a US adult population. *J Vasc Interv Radiol.* 2015 Dec;26(12):1806-1813.e1.

14. Lu GD, Yan HT, Zhang JX, Liu S, Shi HB, Zu QQ. Bronchial artery embolization for the management of frequent hemoptysis caused by bronchiectasis. *BMC Pulm Med.* 2022 Nov 1;22(1):394.

15. Panda A, Bhalla AS, Goyal A. Bronchial artery embolization in hemoptysis: a systematic review. *Diagn Interv Radiol.* 2017 Jul-Aug;23(4):307-317.

16. Lee BR, Yu JY, Ban HJ, et al. Analysis of patients with hemoptysis in a tertiary referral hospital. *Tuberc Respir Dis (Seoul).* 2012 Aug;73(2):107-114.

MDCALC REFERENCES

Wells' Criteria for Pulmonary Embolism. https://www.mdcalc.com/calc/115/wells-criteria-pulmonary-embolism

Revised Geneva Score for Pulmonary Embolism. https://www.mdcalc.com/calc/1750/geneva-score-revised-pulmonary-embolism

CME Questions

Reviewed by **Danya Khoujah, MBBS, MEHP, FACEP**; and **Walter L. Green, MD, FACEP**

Qualified, paid subscribers to *Critical Decisions in Emergency Medicine* may receive CME certificates for up to 5 ACEP Category I credits, 5 *AMA PRA Category 1 Credits™*, and 5 AOA Category 2-B credits for completing this activity in its entirety. Submit your answers online at acep.org/cdem; a score of 75% or better is required. You may receive credit for completing the CME activity any time within 3 years of its publication date. Answers to this month's questions will be published in next month's issue.

1 In outlining a continuing certification program for its member boards to tailor and implement, the American Board of Medical Specialties was responding not only to the rapid advancements in medicine but also to patient safety concerns raised by which organization in 1999?

A. American College of Emergency Physicians
B. American Medical Association
C. Institute of Medicine
D. The Joint Commission

2 What is the best way for emergency physicians to locate a clear, up-to-date description of both their completed and pending American Board of Emergency Medicine continuing certification requirements?

A. Ask a colleague who has recently completed requirements
B. Call member services at the American College of Emergency Physicians
C. Look on their American Board of Emergency Medicine profile at abem.org
D. Refer to the American Board of Emergency Medicine annual report

3 MyEMCert modules are the new way to maintain American Board of Emergency Medicine certification. Which statement is correct about how physicians should plan to take a MyEMCert module?

A. Modules can be taken together with a group of other emergency physicians like the Lifelong Learning and Self-Assessments
B. Modules can be taken an unlimited number of times during any calendar year
C. Modules must be completed in 4 hours without pausing
D. Physicians can access resources, such as key advances, synopses, and module study points while taking the examination in an open-book format

4 The Resuscitation module is available to American Board of Emergency Medicine–certified physicians at no cost. What is true about this module?

A. The module can be taken again immediately if failed the first time
B. The module counts toward the American Board of Emergency Medicine continuing certification requirements
C. The module has an optional continuing medical education opportunity that could potentially count toward state and local requirements
D. The module is a closed-book examination, and resources are not allowed during the test

5 The American Board of Emergency Medicine recently implemented an annual fee for physicians who are on a 5-year certification cycle. What is true about the annual fee?

A. Certification can be maintained even if the fee is not paid
B. The annual fee is in addition to fees for continuing certification activities
C. The annual fee is rare among the American Board of Medical Specialties member boards
D. The annual fee must be paid to access continuing certification activities

6 The Improvement in Medical Practice component of certification emphasizes practice-based learning activities related to patient care and professionalism. What best represents the American Board of Emergency Medicine's current requirements for these activities?

A. 5 continuous years of data are required
B. Improvement projects are verified by the American Board of Emergency Medicine every year
C. Quality improvement projects that emergency medicine groups are already doing can fulfill this requirement
D. Patient satisfaction survey data must be uploaded to the American Board of Emergency Medicine's website

7 In 2021, a physician took the ConCert Exam early, in her 8th year of certification. Which statement about the situation is true?

A. If she fails the examination, she will lose her American Board of Emergency Medicine certification
B. She can take the examination early and will be certified for 10 years beyond her current certification date if she passes
C. She will recertify and receive 10 years of certification if all other requirements are met
D. She will recertify for 5 years from the expiration date of her most recent certification, not from when she took the ConCert Exam early

8 What is true about the American Board of Emergency Medicine's Lifelong Learning and Self-Assessment readings and test?

A. A group or journal club format for article review is prohibited
B. A passing score of the open-book examination is 75% or higher
C. Subspecialty activities do not count toward meeting primary continuing certification
D. They will be discontinued in 2026

9 How many MyEMCert modules must be taken every 5 years to meet continuing certification requirements?

A. 4
B. 5
C. 6
D. 8

10 What percentage of physicians who took the Lifelong Learning and Self-Assessment test and MyEMCert modules selected the optional CME activity in 2022?

A. 30%
B. 50%
C. 80%
D. 100%

11. An 85-year-old woman presents with injury to her right ribs from a ground-level fall. She reports chest pain, shortness of breath, and hemoptysis of around 600 mL in the last 6 hours. She is on warfarin for atrial fibrillation. A chest x-ray shows multiple rib fractures from ribs 3 through 8 with pulmonary contusions. Her INR is 8. What is the best disposition?
   A. Admission to the floor for pain control
   B. Admission to the ICU for pain control, close hemodynamic monitoring, and anticoagulant reversal with vitamin K
   C. Discharge with pain control and instructions to hold her warfarin for 2 days
   D. Discharge with return precautions

12. A 21-year-old man presents with 2 days of fever, chills, cough, and blood-streaked sputum. He has sick contacts with similar symptoms. He has no medical history. His vital signs are within normal limits, and his examination findings are unremarkable. Laboratory findings, including a D-dimer level, are within normal limits. Chest x-ray results are negative. What is the best treatment plan?
   A. Admit for monitoring, intravenous antibiotics, and echocardiography
   B. Discharge with supportive care and close primary care follow-up
   C. Initiate oral antibiotics
   D. Obtain a CT angiogram of the chest

13. A 45-year-old woman presents with hemoptysis. She is toxic appearing and in respiratory distress. Her vital signs are significant for tachycardia, tachypnea, and hypoxia. She has bright red blood in her sputum and is having active, large-volume hemoptysis of 500 mL. What is the best next step?
   A. Antitussives
   B. CT of the chest
   C. Endotracheal intubation
   D. Intravenous antibiotics

14. A 36-year-old woman presents with 2 weeks of right-sided chest pain and shortness of breath. She reports associated cough and hemoptysis. She is on oral contraceptives and reports unilateral leg swelling 1 month ago that has since improved. On examination, she is afebrile, hypoxic with an SpO_2 of 88% on room air, tachycardic (110 bpm), and tachypneic (35 breaths/min). A chest x-ray is normal. What is the most appropriate next step?
   A. Discharge with close primary care follow-up
   B. Intravenous antibiotics
   C. Intubation
   D. Oxygen supplementation and a CT angiogram of the chest

15. A 65-year-old woman presents with large amounts of blood with coughing (>600 mL in 24 hr). The patient has a history of chronic obstructive pulmonary disease and currently smokes one pack of cigarettes per day. She complains of burning chest pain and denies abdominal pain, NSAID use, or a history of alcohol abuse. The patient is found to be tachycardic, hypotensive, and actively coughing up bright red blood. What is the likely source of her blood loss?
   A. Bronchial arteries
   B. Esophageal varices
   C. Gastroduodenal artery
   D. Tracheobronchial capillaries

16. How is massive hemoptysis differentiated from mild hemoptysis?
   A. Massive hemoptysis is defined by blood loss of 100 to 600 mL within a 24-hour period
   B. Massive hemoptysis is defined by greater than 25 mL of blood loss in a 24-hour period
   C. Massive hemoptysis is defined by new anemia that necessitates blood transfusion
   D. Massive hemoptysis is defined by vital sign abnormalities

17. A 35-year-old woman on estrogen replacement therapy presents for hemoptysis that began this morning after getting home late from a road trip the night before. The patient has no medical history but states she may have had an upper respiratory infection last week that has since fully resolved. The results of a CBC and comprehensive metabolic panel are within normal limits. Her D-dimer level is elevated, and a chest x-ray shows no acute pathology. What is the likely etiology of her hemoptysis?
   A. Acute emboli with secondary alveolar hemorrhage
   B. Chronic inflammatory changes
   C. Epistaxis
   D. Persistent coughing from a recent upper respiratory infection

18. A 65-year-old man presents with massive hemoptysis. He is actively coughing up large quantities of blood and is hypoxic with an SpO_2 of 82% on room air. The patient has been resuscitated but appears to still be actively coughing up blood. He is beginning to desaturate again despite receiving oxygen at a rate of 15 L/min on a nonrebreather mask. The bleeding source is determined to be from the lungs, distal to the left primary bronchus. What is an appropriate definitive airway?
   A. Continuous positive airway pressure
   B. Endotracheal intubation
   C. Intubation to the left mainstem bronchus
   D. Intubation to the right mainstem bronchus

19. A 68-year-old man presents with hemoptysis. Which element of the patient's history would be most concerning for a large-volume hemorrhagic source?
   A. History of recent unintentional weight loss
   B. Persistent cough that lasts 10 days
   C. Personal history of chronic obstructive pulmonary disease
   D. Recent fever with rhinorrhea

20. Which statement about hemoptysis is true?
   A. Massive hemoptysis carries a mortality rate of about 75%
   B. Most hemoptysis originates from the pulmonary arterial system
   C. Once hemoptysis is diagnosed, the patient should be intubated for airway protection
   D. Patients with hemoptysis should be placed in a decubitus position with the unaffected lung toward the ground

ANSWER KEY FOR NOVEMBER 2023, VOLUME 37, NUMBER 11

1	2	3	4	5	6	7	8	9	10	11	12	13	14	15	16	17	18	19	20
C	A	B	C	B	C	D	D	C	C	B	D	B	A	A	C	A	A	D	D

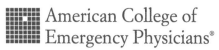
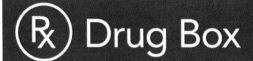

2023 GOLD Report for COPD

By Frank Lovecchio, DO, MPH, FACEP
Valleywise Health Medical Center and ASU, Phoenix, Arizona

Objective
On completion of this column, you should be able to:

- Explain GOLD's latest recommendations for patients with COPD.

The Global Initiative for Chronic Obstructive Lung Disease (GOLD) 2023 report emphasizes that patients with chronic obstructive pulmonary disease (COPD) are at an increased risk of other medical conditions, including heart failure, ischemic heart disease, myocardial infarction, pneumonia, and gastroesophageal reflux disease. The GOLD guidelines recommend spirometry; classifying patients with COPD into groups by their symptom and exacerbation history to guide treatment; and increasing therapy in a stepwise approach. The three classification groups are A, B, and E. Patients in group A are less symptomatic and at a low risk of exacerbations. Patients in groups B and E are more symptomatic and at a high risk of exacerbations. Updated pharmacotherapy recommendations state that patients in groups B and E should be started on a combination of long-acting β-2 agonists (LABAs) and long-acting muscarinic antagonist (LAMAs) instead of either alone. The use of LABA and inhaled corticosteroids (ICS) (when ICS are indicated) has been phased out because triple therapy with LABA, LAMA, and ICS has been shown to be superior in reducing all-cause mortality and exacerbations in patients with moderate to severe COPD and a history of exacerbations.

Removing LABA and ICS from COPD recommendations is consistent with the current evidence that ICS are most effective when eosinophilic inflammation is present. Triple therapy is recommended if patients have a blood eosinophil count of 300 cells/µL or greater, concomitant asthma, or two or more COPD exacerbations in a year. If patients fall into group B with blood eosinophil counts between 100 and 300 cells/µL, consider their individual risks and benefits from ICS treatment and decide if this treatment is appropriate based on shared decision-making. ICS are not recommended for patients who have had multiple pneumonia events, blood eosinophil counts less than 100 cells/µL, or histories of mycobacterial infections.

GOLD newly defines COPD as a heterogeneous lung condition characterized by chronic respiratory symptoms due to abnormalities of the airways or alveoli that cause persistent, often progressive airflow obstruction. GOLD redefines a COPD exacerbation as an event characterized by dyspnea or cough and sputum that worsens over 14 or more days and is caused by airway infection, pollution, or other insults to the airways. Tachypnea or tachycardia may accompany an exacerbation. The latest GOLD report also outlines a new classification for exacerbation severity and recommends nonpharmacologic therapies of smoking cessation and flu and pneumococcal vaccinations for patients in group A.

For patients in group A, a long-acting rather than a short-acting bronchodilator alone is recommended (grade 2B). For patients with COPD in groups B and E, initial treatment with dual long-acting bronchodilator therapy is recommended instead of a single long-acting bronchodilator alone (grade 2C).

REFERENCE
Agustí A, Celli BR, Criner GJ, et al. Global Initiative for Chronic Obstructive Lung Disease 2023 report: GOLD executive summary. *Am J Respir Crit Care Med.* 2023 Apr 1;207(7):819-837.

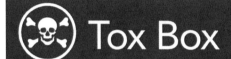

Vitamin A Toxicity

By Christian A. Tomaszewski, MD, MS, MBA, FACEP
University of California San Diego Health

Objective
On completion of this lesson, you should be able to:

- Discuss hypervitaminosis A and its treatment options.

Introduction
Acute hypervitaminosis A is well-known to occur after ingestion of polar bear liver, a vitamin A–rich food. Other sources of hypervitaminosis A include supplements, analogues (acitretin), and prescription drugs (isotretinoin). Although acute ingestions are rarely a problem, excessive amounts taken acutely or chronically can lead to toxicity, including conditions like pseudotumor cerebri (ie, intracranial hypertension).

Mechanism of Action
- Inhibits keratinization of epithelial tissue

Kinetics
- 80% oral bioavailability with toxic effects in hours to days
- Metabolized in the liver and excreted in feces and urine

Toxic Dose
- >300,000 IU in children
- >1 million IU in adults

Clinical Manifestations
- **GI:** nausea and vomiting
- **CNS:** pseudotumor cerebri, headache, blurred vision, and papilledema
- **Metabolic:** hypercalcemia (with chronic ingestion)
- **Hepatic:** hepatotoxicity
- **Dermal (delayed):** desquamation and alopecia

Diagnostics
- Electrolyte levels, calcium levels for chronic ingestions
- Lumbar puncture if altered mental status

Treatment
- Can give oral activated charcoal if <1 hr post ingestion
- Supportive care
- Treat intracranial hypertension (acetazolamide, furosemide, or lumbar puncture)
- Treat any hypercalcemia (fluids and appropriate therapeutics)

Disposition
- Refer acute overdoses >300,000 IU for evaluation
- Observe if symptomatic

Made in United States
Orlando, FL
23 December 2024

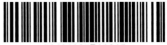

56491265R00215